Atlas of ANESTHESIA

Volume II

Scientific Principles of Anesthesia

Atlas of ANESTHESIA

Series Editor
Ronald D. Miller, MD
Professor and Chairman of Anesthesia
Professor of Cellular and Molecular Pharmacology
University of California, San Francisco, School of Medicine
San Francisco, California

Volume II

Scientific Principles of Anesthesia

Volume Editor
Debra A. Schwinn, MD
Associate Professor of Anesthesiology, Pharmacology, and Surgery
Department of Anesthesiology
Director, Molecular Pharmacology Laboratory
Duke University Medical Center
Durham, North Carolina

With 28 contributors

CHURCHILL LIVINGSTONE

Developed by Current Medicine, Inc., Philadelphia

Current Medicine, Inc.
400 Market Street
Suite 700
Philadelphia, PA 19106

Managing Editor:	Lori J. Bainbridge
Developmental Editor:	Marian A. Bellus
Editorial Assistant:	Deborah Singer
Art Director:	Paul Fennessy
Design and Layout:	Christine M. Keller
Illustration Director:	Ann Saydlowski
Illustrators:	Liz Carrozza, Wieslawa Langenfeld, Beth Starkey, Larry Ward, Lisa Weischedel, Debra Wertz
Production:	Lori Holland, Sally Nicholson
Indexing:	Alexandra Nickerson

Scientific principles of anesthesia / volume editor, Debra Schwinn
p. cm. -- (Atlas of anesthesia : v. 2)
Includes bibliographical references and index.
ISBN 0-443-07901-3
1. Anesthesiology--Atlases. I. Schwinn, Debra. II. Series.
[DNLM: 1. Anesthesia--methods--atlases. WO 517 P927 1997 v.2]
RD81.S376 1997
617.9'6--DC21
DNLM/DLC
for Library of Congress 97-11333
CIP

ISBN 0-443-07901-3

Although every effort has been made to ensure that drug doses and other information are presented accurately in this publication, the ultimate responsibility rests with the prescribing physician. Neither the publishers nor the author can be held responsible for errors or for any consequences arising from the use of the information contained therein. Any product mentioned in this publication should be used in accordance with the prescribing information prepared by the manufacturers. No claims or endorsements are made for any drug or compound at present under clinical investigation.

Printed in Singapore by Imago Productions (FE) Ltd.
10 9 8 7 6 5 4 3 2 1

SERIES PREFACE

This multi-volume series *Atlas of Anesthesia* organizes the largest and most comprehensive collection of teaching visuals in the field of anesthesiology. The publisher, volume editors, and I have invited the most prominent members of the anesthesiology community to provide the most up-to-date information in a format that offers not only the finest images available but also unique schematic presentations of how and why we feel pain. Combined with the slide atlas and CD-ROM, *Atlas of Anesthesia* provides teaching materials of the finest quality in easily accessible formats and allows anesthesiology to become a visual specialty in a way that has never been attempted previously. The topics of the volumes include Critical Care, Scientific Principles, Preoperative Preparation and Intraoperative Monitoring, Principles of Anesthetic Techniques and Anesthetic Emergencies, Subspecialty Care, Pain Management, Cardiothoracic Anesthesia, and Pediatric Anesthesia.

The specialty of anesthesia originally was restricted to operating room anesthesia with some involvement in preoperative evaluation. Furthermore, in the past, patients with severe medical conditions were considered too high risk to be anesthetized (*eg*, those who had suffered a myocardial infarction within the previous 3 to 6 months or those with severe obstructive pulmonary disease). In the last 25 years, it has become possible for patients with extensive medical disease (*eg*, acute myocardial infarction, failure of one or more organs, immunosuppression) to be successfully anesthetized for major invasive surgery.

With far more challenging situations, the specialty has responded by the development of new drugs, monitoring techniques, and subspecialties. The new drugs act on receptors that were not even known a few years ago, necessitating extensive knowledge of receptors (*eg*, opioid) of various functions and selection of drugs for specific effects. Improvements in monitoring include the development of the pulmonary catheter, transesophageal echocardiography, evoked potentials, pulse oximetry, and multiple gas analysis. New techniques such as hemodilution, infusion and warming devices, and fiberoptic endotracheal intubation have also been introduced. Cardiac, neurologic, pediatric, transplant, ambulatory, and obstetric subspecialties have expanded to encompass the entire perioperative period, including extensive preoperative evaluation and therapy, critical care medicine, and pain management, in both acute and chronic settings.

In response to the impressive expansion of the specialty, many educational devices (including books and journals) have been developed. The educational transmission of the combined cognitive and technical aspects of anesthesia can be markedly facilitated by illustrations including images, graphs, decision-making trees, and algorithms.

In bringing this series to publication, credit is due to the volume editors and to the many contributors who have shared their expertise and their time. Credit is also due to Abe Krieger, President of Current Medicine, who conceived the atlas, to Marian Bellus, Senior Developmental Editor, and to Jackie Dunn, who coordinated work on this project in my office.

Ronald D. Miller, MD

PREFACE

Anesthesiology encompasses many clinical disciplines, varying physiologic settings, and sophisticated pharmacological principles. Hence, designing a volume focusing on scientific principles underlying anesthesiology is a daunting task. In a volume covering such a large body of literature, by nature the editor is somewhat capricious in choosing specific scientific areas to present. I have decided to focus on the basic science behind various clinically relevant areas of anesthesiology. Individual authors represent a cross-section of scientific and clinical experts, each writing his or her chapter with a keen eye toward ensuring that the underlying principles are made as clear as possible. Therefore, each chapter in this volume provides a "state of the art" review of clinical physiology and scientific principles. Frequently the busy clinician learns just enough underlying pharmacology and physiology to safely treat complicated patients. This volume therefore gives a unique opportunity for clinicians to enhance their understanding of basic science concepts underlying anesthesiology. Figures and tables are designed to provide a concise description of complex phenomena, giving the reader the flexibility to focus on a specific topic to gain new insights and a more complete understanding of particular aspects of anesthesiology.

The volume begins with an overview of general pharmacologic and physiologic concepts, starting with the cell and moving to whole organ systems such as intact animals/patients. Included in this section are topics such as physics principles underlying patient monitoring, pharmacokinetic/pharmacodynamic principles, as well as overviews of cardiovascular, respiratory, and cerebral physiology. The next section focuses on specific topics within anesthesiology, such an neuromuscular transmission, coagulation, injury/inflammation, pain, and the new frontier of molecular biology. Finally, the last section deals with anesthetic agents themselves including inhaled, intravenous, and local anesthetics. The science underlying anesthesiology becomes increasingly important as we understand more about mechanisms underlying human disease in general. It is my hope that by delving into the science underpinning the daily practice of anesthesiology, each reader can gain useful insights to take back to their clinical practice.

Debra A. Schwinn, MD

CONTRIBUTORS

Dan E. Berkowitz, MBBCh
Assistant Professor
Department of Anesthesiology and Critical Care Medicine
The Johns Hopkins Medical Institutions
Baltimore, Maryland

Gregory H. Botz, MD
Associate Professor
Department of Anesthesiology and Surgery
Duke University School of Medicine;
Staff Anesthesiologist and Intensivist
Durham Veterans Affairs Medical Center
Durham, North Carolina

Johnny E. Brian, Jr., MD
Assistant Professor
Department of Anesthesia
University of Iowa;
Assistant Professor
University of Iowa Hospitals and Clinics
Iowa City, Iowa

John Butterworth, MD
Professor
Department of Anesthesiology
Bowman Gray School of Medicine;
Anesthesiologist
North Carolina Baptist Hospital
Winston-Salem, North Carolina

Marcel E. Durieux, MD
Assistant Professor
Departments of Anesthesiology, Pharmacology and Neurological Surgery
University of Virginia School of Medicine
Charlottesville, Virginia

Stanley Feldman, MBBS, FRCA
Professor Emeritus
Magill Department of Anesthetics
Charing Cross and Westminster Medical Schools;
Honorary Consultant
Chelsea and Westminster Hospital
London, United Kingdom

Leonard Firestone, MD
Safar Professor and Chairman
Department of Anesthesiology and Critical Care Medicine
University of Pittsburgh School of Medicine;
Pittsburgh, Pennsylvania

Philip S. Gibbs, MD
Professor of Anesthesia
Department of Anesthesia
Indiana University School of Medicine;
Medical Director of Surgical Intensive Care Unit
Indiana University Hospitals
Indianapolis, Indiana

Peter S.A. Glass, MB, ChB, FFA (SA)
Associate Professor
Director of Clinical Research
Department of Anesthesiology
Duke University School of Medicine
Durham, North Carolina

Michael A. Gropper, MD, PhD
Assistant Professor
Department of Anesthesia
University of California, San Francisco, School of Medicine
San Francisco, California

Ferenc Gyulai, MD
Assistant Professor
Department of Anesthesiology and Critical Care Medicine
University of Pittsburgh Medical Center
Pittsburgh, Pennsylvania

Peter C. Houck, M.D., Ph.D.
Clinical Assistant Professor
Department of Anesthesia
Indiana University School of Medicine
Indianapolis, Indiana

Scott T. Howell, MD
Assistant Professor
Department of Anesthesiology
Duke University School of Medicine
Durham, North Carolina

Jonathan B. Mark, MD
Associate Professor
Department of Anesthesiology
Duke University School of Medicine;
Chief, Anesthesiology Service
Veterans Affairs Medical Center
Durham, North Carolina

Richard E. Moon, MD
Associate Professor
Departments of Anesthesiology and Pulmonary Medicine
Duke University School of Medicine;
Anesthesiologist, Pulmonologist
Duke University Medical Center;
Durham, North Carolina

Joseph Quinlan, MD
Associate Professor
Department of Anesthesiology and Critical Care Medicine
University of Pittsburgh School of Medicine;
Director of Cardiac Anesthesia
University of Pittsburgh Medical Center
Pittsburgh, Pennsylvania

Ira Rampil, MD
Associate Professor
Department of Anesthesia
University of California, San Fransisco, School of Medicine;
Attending Physician, Medical Director
Neurophysiologic Monitoring Services
University of California Medical Center
San Francisco, California

Allison Kinder Ross, MD
Assistant Professor
Department of Anesthesiology
Duke University School of Medicine;
Chief, General Pediatric Anesthesia
Duke University Medical Center
Durham, North Carolina

Teiji Sawa, MD, PhD
Assistant Research Anesthesiologist
Department of Anesthesia
University of California, San Francisco, School of Medicine
San Francisco, California

Steven L. Shafer, MD
Associate Professor
Department of Anesthesia
Stanford University School of Medicine
Stanford, California;
Staff Physician
Palo Alto VA Health Care System
Palo Alto, California

Thomas F. Slaughter, MD
Assistant Professor
Department of Anesthesiology
Duke University School of Medicine;
Attending Physician
Durham Veterans Affairs Medical Center
Durham, North Carolina

Linda S. Sorkin, PhD
Associate Professor
Department of Anesthesiology
University of California, San Diego
La Jolla, California

Wolf H. Stapelfeldt, MD
Assistant Professor
Department of Anesthesiology and Critical Care Medicine
University of Pittsburgh;
Staff Anesthesiologist and Director of Research
Veterans Affairs Medical Center
Pittsburgh, Pennsylvania

Robert K. Stoelting, MD
Professor and Chair
Department of Anesthesia
Indiana University School of Medicine
Indianapolis, Indiana

Bryant W. Stolp, MD, PhD
Assistant Professor
Department of Anesthesiology
Associate Professor
Department of Cell Biology
Duke University School of Medicine;
Anesthesiologist
Duke University Medical Center
Duke University Hyperbaric Medicine Center
Durham, North Carolina

David S. Warner, MD
Professor
Department of Anesthesiology
Duke University School of Medicine
Durham, North Carolina

Jeanine P. Wiener-Kronish, MD
Professor
Director, Preoperative Care
Departments of Anesthesia and Medicine
University of California, San Francisco, School of Medicine
San Francisco, California

Tony L. Yaksh, PhD
Professor of Anesthesiology
Adjunct Professor of Pharmacology
Vice Chairman for Research, Anesthesiology
University of California, San Diego
La Jolla, California

CONTENTS

Chapter 6

The Lung During Anesthesia and in Adverse Environments

Richard E. Moon and Bryant W. Stolp

Chapter 7

Cerebral Anatomy and Physiology

Johnny E. Brian, Jr, and David S. Warner

Chapter 8

Neuromuscular Transmission

Stanley Feldman

Chapter 9

Hemostasis and Thrombosis

Thomas F. Slaughter

Chapter 10

Injury and Inflammation

Teiji Sawa, Jeanine P. Wiener-Kronish, and Michael A. Gropper

Chapter 11

Mechanisms of Pain Transmission

Tony L. Yaksh and Linda S. Sorkin

1

Cellular Signal Transduction

Dan E. Berkowitz

Receptors and their signal transduction mechanisms provide the link between pharmacologic agents (either endogenous hormones or exogenous drugs) and their ultimate physiologic actions. The exact mechanisms by which receptors and their signal transduction mechanisms alter cellular, organ, and organism function are complex and depend on the receptor system involved. Understanding these cellular signaling mechanisms and their regulation allows us to more easily understand rational drug therapy aimed at modulating receptors. Recently, molecular biologic approaches have defined the putative structure, signal transduction mechanisms, and regulation of many receptors and channels. These advances have further enabled researchers to gain insights into the molecular basis of ligand specificity that ultimately will enable development of receptor-specific drugs to exploit desired clinical effects while avoiding adverse side effects.

Most receptor systems of interest to the anesthesiologist are located in cell membranes and can be defined as excitable transmembrane proteins [1]. The mechanisms by which they transduce their signals are distinct and can be broadly classified into 6 different groups, as described in the paragraphs that follow. G protein–coupled receptors bind their ligands on the extracellular surface of the cell and couple to intracellular effector systems (channels or enzymes) via intermediary guanine nucleotide proteins (G proteins) [2–4]. G protein–coupled receptors represent the largest family of membrane-associated receptors with many diverse functions and many different signal transduction mechanisms. Examples of these receptor classes include the adrenergic, muscarinic, cholinergic, opioid, serotonin, histamine, cannabinoid, cholecystokinin, endothelin, and substance P receptors, to name but a few. They mediate their functions by coupling to G proteins. G proteins are a highly conserved family of membrane-associated proteins (with three distinct subunits), which require GTP for their function [5,6]. Although diverse in their binding of ligands and physiologic functions, these integral cell membranes proteins have several striking common structural features. These receptors consist of a single polypeptide with seven stretches of 20 to 25 hydrophobic amino acids that represent potential membrane-spanning portions, three intracellular loops, and an extracellular amino and intracellular carboxyl terminus. Using various molecular biologic techniques it has been demonstrated that various portions of the receptor are important for different receptor functions. Transmembrane regions form a pocket for ligand binding. Cytoplasmic domains contain regions capable of interacting with G proteins, and various regulatory enzymes appear to be important in the transduction of receptor occupancy signals and coupling as well as in receptor regulation.

Ligand-gated ion channels contain ion channels as part of their overall receptor structure and are specialized for gating ion movement and generating electrical signals in response to specific chemical neurotransmitters [7–10]. In addition to G protein–coupled receptors, ligand-gated ion channels mediate responses to drugs frequently used by anesthesiologists. Members of this superfamily of receptors contain ion channels as part of their overall structure. *Gating* refers to the process whereby opening and closing of the channel is controlled. These channels thus gate ion movements and generate electrical signals in response to specific chemical neurotransmitters such as acetylcholine, glutamate, glycine, or γ aminobutyric acid (GABA). Ligand-gated ion channels are structurally more complex than G protein–coupled receptors because they are composed of several subunits (each containing transmembrane domains) surrounding and forming an ion channel. These channels may also contain more than one receptor site, making it under modulatory control of a complex of several receptors and ligands. One of the primary examples of a ligand-gated ion channel is the nicotinic cholinergic receptor, the receptor complex responsible for neurotransmission at the motor end plate. Other more centrally located ligand-gated ion channels of clinical importance include the amino acid receptors. Amino acid receptors are ubiquitous transducers of inhibitory synaptic neurotransmission (exemplified by the $GABA_A$ receptors, which bind GABA, benzodiazepines, barbiturates, and ethanol) and of excitatory synaptic transmission (exemplified by the *N*-methyl-D-aspartate or NMDA receptor, which binds NMDA, phencyclidine—for which ketamine is an analogue—glycine, and various ions).

Voltage-gated ion channels are the elementary excitable elements in cell membranes of nerve, muscle, and other tissue that are responsible for transduction of electrical signals. These channels or pores open and close primarily in response to changes in membrane electrical potentials [11–13]. In contrast to ligand-gated ion channels, which open and close channels in response to binding of ligands, voltage-gated ion channels conduct current in response to changes in membrane potentials. Voltage-gated ion channels are characterized by their selectivity for ions, as well as the kinetics of movement of ions through the particular channels (opening and closing characteristics). They are critical in signal tranduction in all excitable tissue (neural tissue, heart, and muscle).

Growth factor receptors constitute a superfamily of receptors that are distinct from the G protein–coupled receptors in that they have the target effector enzyme (tyrosine kinase) as an integral part of the receptor complex. Growth factor receptors such as epidermal growth factor and platelet-derived growth factor have profound effects on the growth and differentiation of cells. In the short term, they lead to protein phosphorylation of tyrosine residues by the tyrosine kinase–containing domain of the receptor. These lead to short-term effects on the function of channels as well as secretory activities of cells by increasing phosphoinositol turnover. They also lead to long-term effects by altering gene expression resulting in differentiation or growth of cells.

Transmembrane guanylate cyclase type receptors are also distinct from G protein–coupled receptors and are characterized by the ability to catalyze GTP to synthesize the ubiquitous second-messenger molecule cGMP [14,15]. The prototypic receptor in this group is the atrial naturetic peptide receptor. These receptors have one transmembrane segment linking a large glycosylated extracellular ligand-binding domain with an intracellular domain that contains the guanylyl cyclase activity domain.

The nitric oxide (NO) system represents a recently described novel gaseous signal transduction mechanism. NO is a potent labile diffusible gas that mediates many functions in many organs, including endothelial-dependent vasodilation, neurotransmission, and cytotoxicity, to name but a few [16,17]. Of clinical importance to the anesthesiologist is that NO is the mediator of the commonly used drugs sodium nitroprusside and nitroglycerin. Inhaled NO is the most effective therapy for the treatment of pulmonary hypertension.

The molecular pharmacology of receptor channels and their signal transduction mechanisms is complex and is one of the hottest topics in neurobiology today. It is beyond the scope of this chapter to review all receptors, channels, and transduction mechanisms in detail; however, the chapter stresses principles and clinically relevant signal transduction pathways. The references cite detailed reviews on each superfamily of receptors, which will in turn provide information on receptor subtypes and their functions.

G PROTEIN–COUPLED RECEPTORS

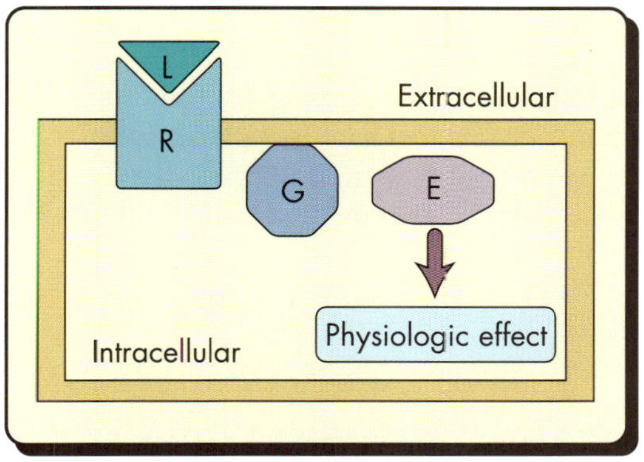

Figure 1-1. G protein–coupled receptors. The receptor (R) is a transmembrane protein that binds ligand (L). The ligand may be a peptide, an endogenous nonpeptide neurotransmitter or hormone, or an exogenous drug. The membrane receptor interacts with a G protein (G) that transduces the signal from the receptor to the effector (E). Energy derived from the hydrolysis of GTP enables the G protein to interact with the effector molecule, resulting in a change in the intracellular chemistry, thereby eliciting a physiologic effect.

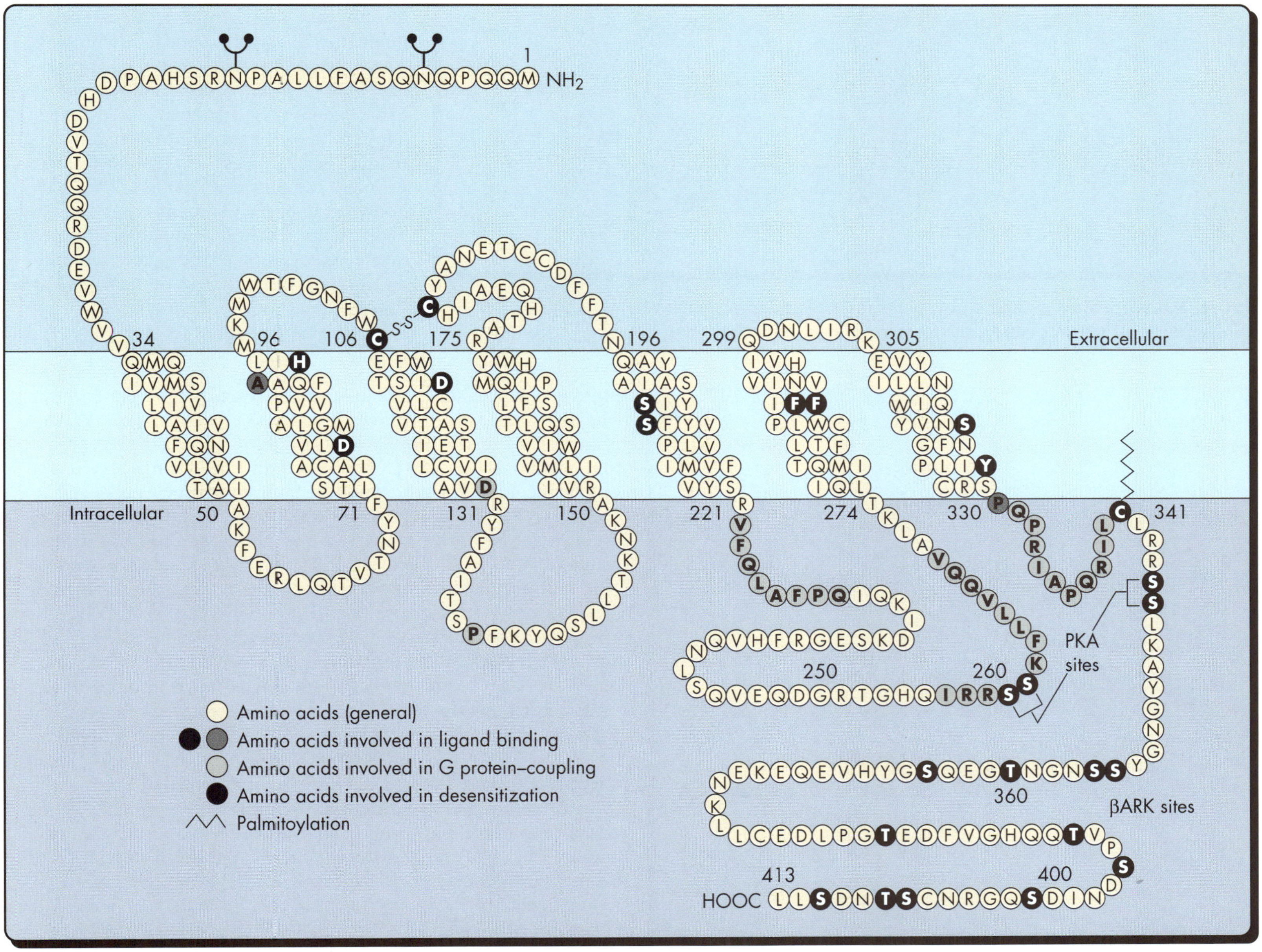

Figure 1-2. Regions of β2-adrenoceptor important in ligand binding, G protein coupling, and regulation. The β2-receptor has been the most well defined in terms of its molecular-structure function relationship. Thus, it represents the paradigm for understanding regions of importance in ligand binding, signal transduction, and regulation in G protein–coupled receptors. Using molecular biologic techniques such as the creation of chimeric receptors (receptors created by combining different regions of two distinct receptor genes) or mutagenesis (engineering of distinct mutations in the receptor to examine specific functional changes), regions important in different receptor functions have been defined. βARK—β-adrenoceptor kinase; PKA—protein kinase A. (From Berkowitz and Schwinn [18]; with permission.)

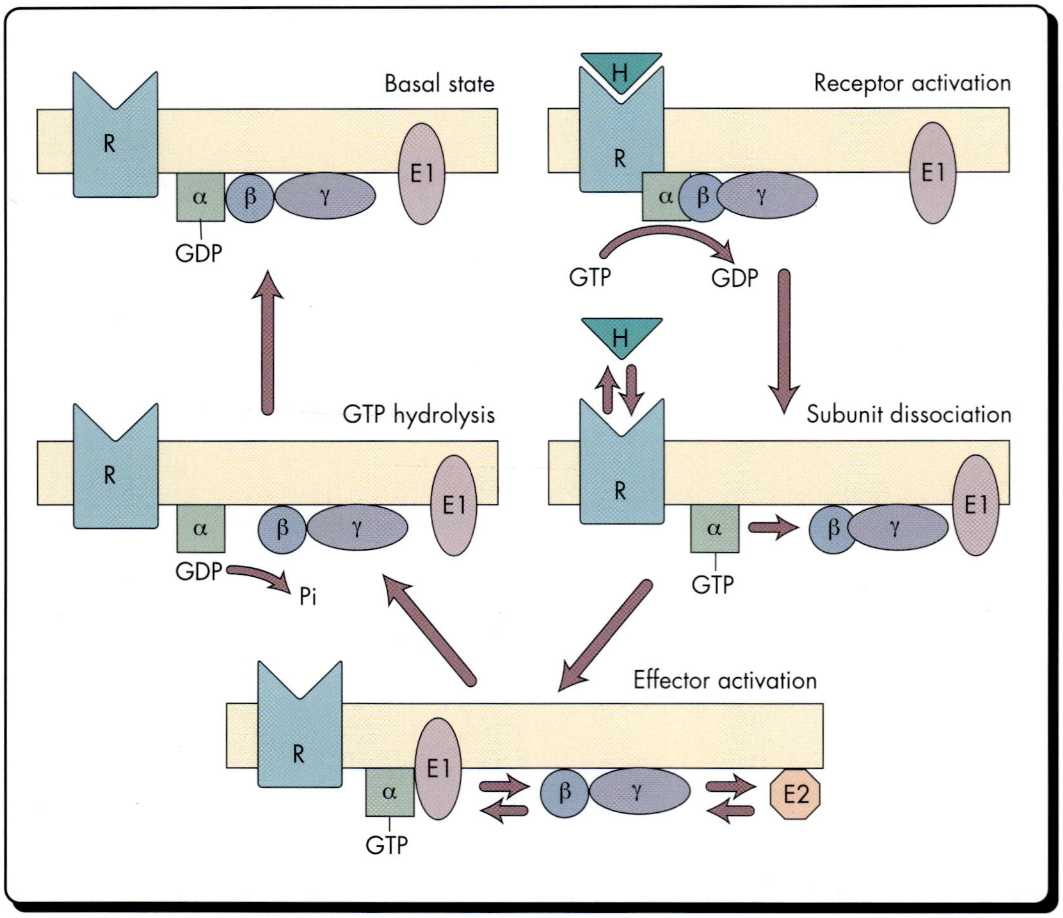

Figure 1-3. G-protein cycling and G protein–mediated transmembrane signaling. In the basal state, G proteins exist as heterotrimers with guanosine diphosphate (GDP) bound tightly to the α subunit. The receptor (R) is unoccupied and the effector (E) is inactive. After binding of the hormone or ligand (H), the receptor undergoes a conformational change and interacts with the G protein. This results in the dissociation of GDP from the guanine nucleotide binding site. Binding of guanosine triphosphate (GTP) to the G protein α subunit has two consequences. First, the G protein dissociates from the H-R complex, reducing the affinity of the hormone for the receptor. Second, a reduced affinity of the G protein α subunit for the βγ subunits occurs, resulting in βγ subunit dissociation from the alpha subunit. The α-GTP–bound subunits bind the effector (E1), which in turn induces a change in intracellular chemistry. The βγ subunit may interact directly with a different effector (E2) or may modulate the activity of the α-E1 complex. The α subunit possesses intrinsic GTPase activity. The alpha subunit catalyzes the hydrolysis of GTP, resulting in GDP being left bound to alpha subunit nucleotide binding sites, a process that results in deactivation of the activated complex. The GDP-bound form of the G protein α subunit has a high affinity for the βγ subunits, with subsequent reassociation of these three subunits and a return of the system to the basal state. Pi—phosphate. (*From* Berkowitz and Schwinn [18]; with permission.)

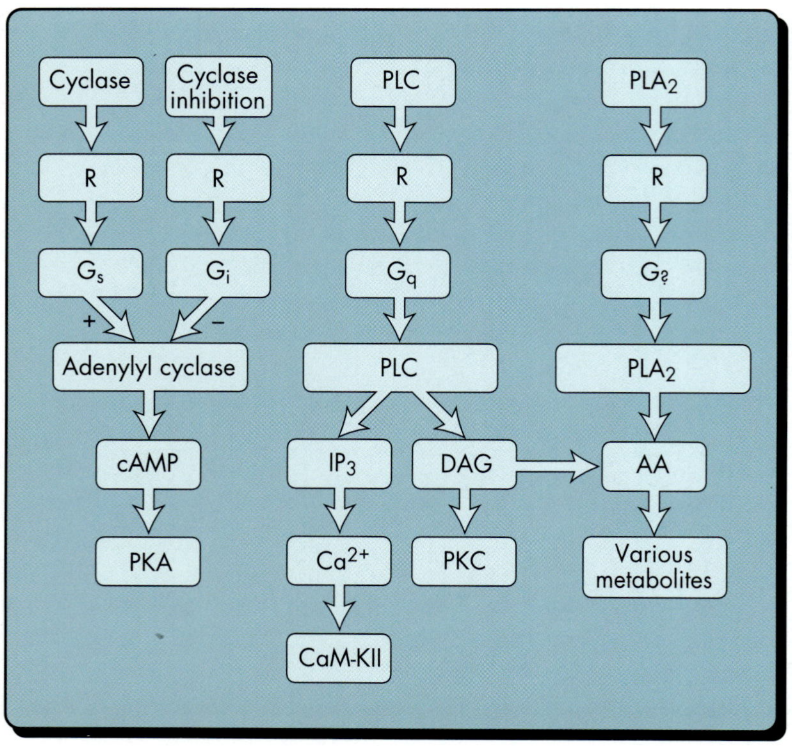

Figure 1-4. Classic G protein–coupled pathways present in the cell. The first is the cAMP pathway discovered by Sutherland [19]. Its G protein is called Gs (stimulatory G protein). The classic receptor (R) that couples to Gs is the β_2-adrenoceptor. This distinguishes it from Gi (the second pathway), which mediates inhibition of adenylyl cyclase. The classic receptor that couples to Gi is the α_2-adrenoceptor. The third pathway couples to phospholipase C (PLC) through a group of G proteins called Gq. PLC hydrolyzes a membrane phospholipid (phosphoinositol [PIP_2]) to form two intracellular messengers: inositol-1,4,5-triphosphate (IP_3) and diacyglycerol (DAG). Both are active second messengers. DAG activates protein kinase C (PKC) and IP_3 releases Ca^{2+} from intracellular stores in the endoplasmic reticulum. Ca^{2+} has many second-messenger functions. The classic receptor that couples to Gq is the α_1-adrenoceptor. The final pathway uses another phospholipase (PLA_2) to liberate a highly unsaturated fatty acid, arachidonic acid (AA), that is quickly metabolized to at least 20 short-lived but potent intermediates (prostaglandins and leukotrienes). A unique feature of many of the AA metabolites is that, being lipid soluble, they can leave the cell and act on neighboring cells in the tissues. CaM-KII—type II Ca-calmodulin-dependent protein kinase; cAMP—cyclic adenosine monophosphate; PKA—protein kinase A; R—receptor.(*From* Hille [11]; with permission.)

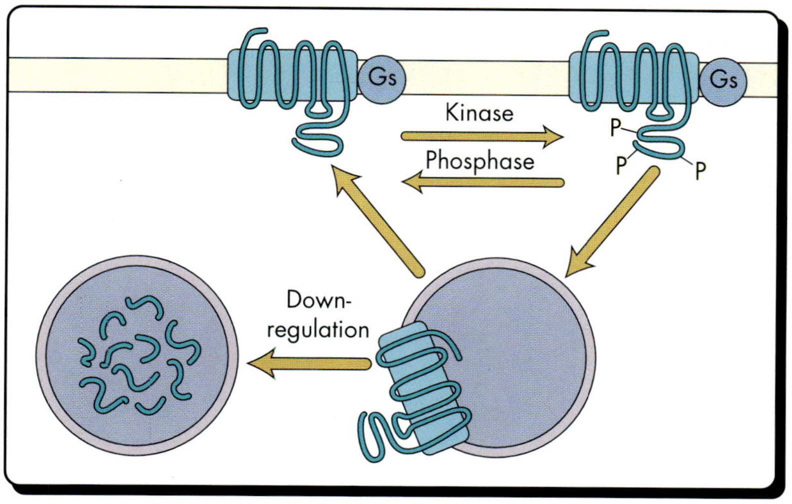

Figure 1-5. Mechanisms of regulation of G protein–coupled receptors. The physiologic response to a particular hormone may decrease over time. This process, initially referred to as tachyphylaxis, is now known to be the result of dynamic regulation of the receptor giving rise to the observed pharmacologic dampening phenomenon. The most extensively investigated mechanism of regulation is that of desensitization, which is the reduction in a physiologic response to a stimulus that remains constant over time. Desensitization is the result of three interrelated processes that have been well worked out in the β_2-adrenoceptor system [20,21].

Receptor uncoupling refers to a rapid process (seconds to minutes) that results in the inability of the receptor to bind G protein, resulting in uncoupling of the receptor from the G protein. Uncoupling results when intracellular portions of the receptors (and possibly the G protein) are phosphorylated by specific enzymes, changing the affinity of the receptor for its corresponding G protein.

Receptor sequestration is a process that occurs more slowly (minutes to hours) and results in the movement of receptors from the cell surface to intracellular compartments that are not accessible to ligands. However, with termination of agonist stimulation, sequestered receptors are available for recycling to the cell surface.

Downregulation is a more prolonged process (hours to days) that results in a decrease in the amount of transcribed mRNA, necessary for translation into new receptor protein. This regulation thus occurs at a nuclear rather than a cytoplasmic level and involves the interaction of the products of signal transduction (*eg*, cAMP) with DNA binding proteins that affect the transcription of DNA (and thus ultimately affect the amount of membrane protein expressed). Gs—stimulatory G protein. (*From* Berkowitz and Schwinn [18]; with permission.)

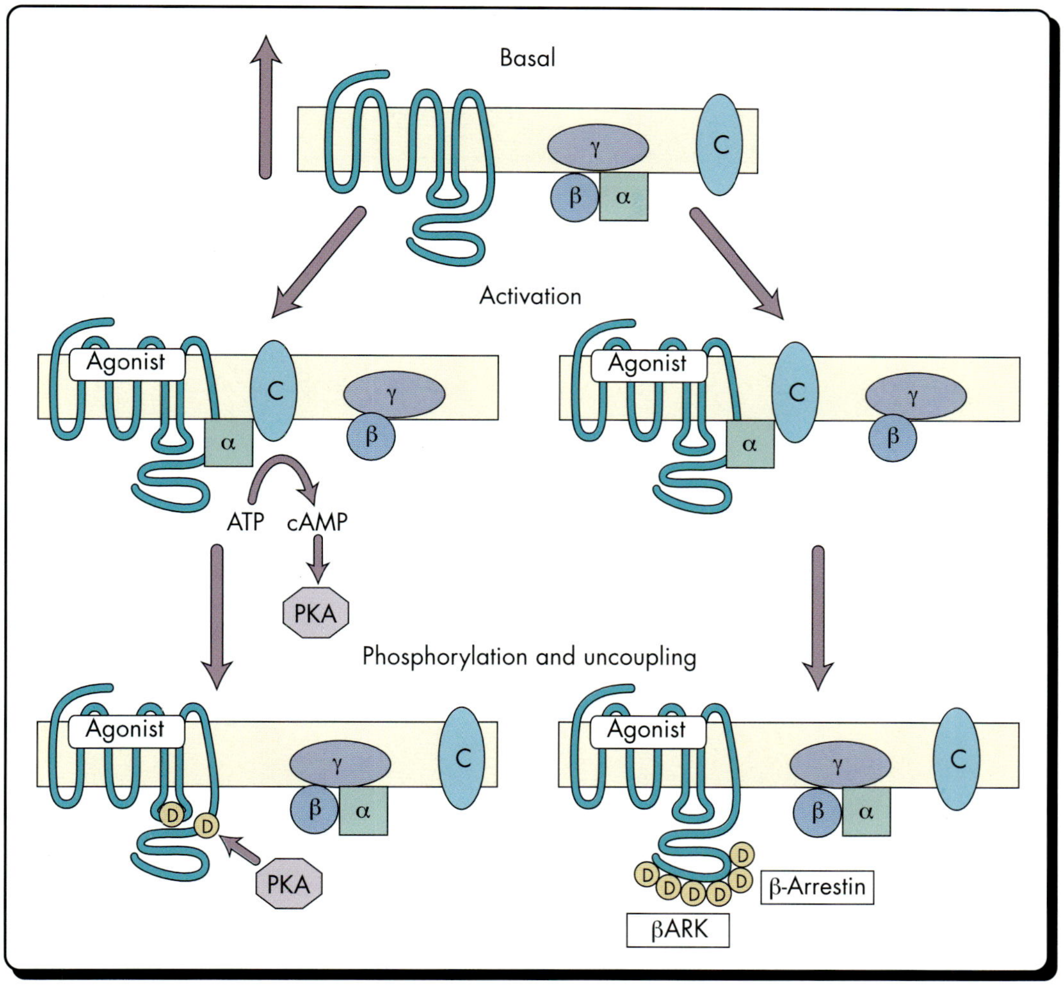

Figure 1-6. Mechanisms of uncoupling of β-adrenoceptors (β-AR) as a paradigm for other receptor systems. The most rapid form of desensitization, receptor uncoupling, is associated with phosphorylation of the carboxyl terminus of the β-AR. Phosphorylation is dependent on enzymes called protein kinases that catalyze the transfer of phosphate groups from ATP to a distinct amino acid in a specific receptor sequence. Two distinct protein kinases, protein kinase A (PKA, also known as cAMP-dependent kinase) and β-AR kinase (β-ARK, a member of a group of G protein–coupled receptor kinases [22]), are known to be involved in the regulation of the β-ARs. Agonist binding to the beta-AR results in the activation of adenylate cyclase. This in turn results in the activation of cAMP. cAMP-dependent kinase or PKA is regulated by the upstream second messenger. PKA phosphorylates the sites in the third intracellular loop of the carboxyl terminus, resulting in uncoupling. Thus, the cAMP-dependent protein kinase (a target protein for cAMP) regulates β-AR, the downstream second messenger of which is cAMP. This process is known as heterologous desensitization because cAMP may be generated by other receptor systems. β-ARK has a high affinity for the agonist-occupied form of the receptor and phosphorylates sites on the carboxyl terminus. β-Arrestin binds to the phosphorylated form of the receptor, disrupting G protein coupling. Because β-ARK phosphorylates the agonist-occupied form of the receptor, its major function is homologous desensitization. C—adenylyl cyclase. (*Adapted from* Berkowitz and Schwinn [18].)

ELECTROPHYSIOLOGIC CHARACTERISTICS OF LIGAND- AND VOLTAGE-GATED ION CHANNELS

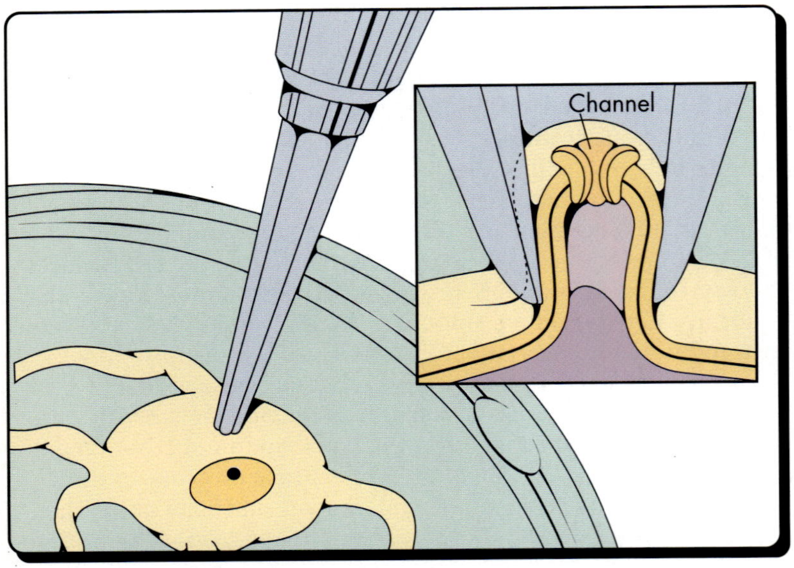

Figure 1-7. Patch clamp technique. The transmission of signals within and between cells is mediated by ion channels, pore-forming proteins embedded in the plasma membrane of all cells. When activated these channels produce the flickers of electrical activity that stimulate neurons and muscle cells. In sensory organs, the channels translate physical or chemical stimuli into electrical signals for the nervous system. Nonneural cells also use ion channels for signaling processes. The initial concept invoked by Hodgkins and Huxley [23] (that electrical signals in neurons are mediated by proteins in lipid membranes) has exploded with the development of the patch clamp technique by Neher and Sackmann [24] (for which they received the Nobel Prize). By pressing a patch pipette against the surface of a cell and applying gentle suction, a high-resistance seal can be made around the patch. An experimenter can then apply various stimuli from within the pipette and measure the behavior of the isolated channels by measuring the flow of minute currents (amplitude and number) through the channel. Using these techniques researchers have been able to determine the electrophysiologic characteristics of channels whose opening and closing are controlled by changes in the binding of ligands (ligand-gated ion channels) and changes in membrane potentials (voltage-gated ion channels). (*From* Neher and Sakmann [24]; with permission.)

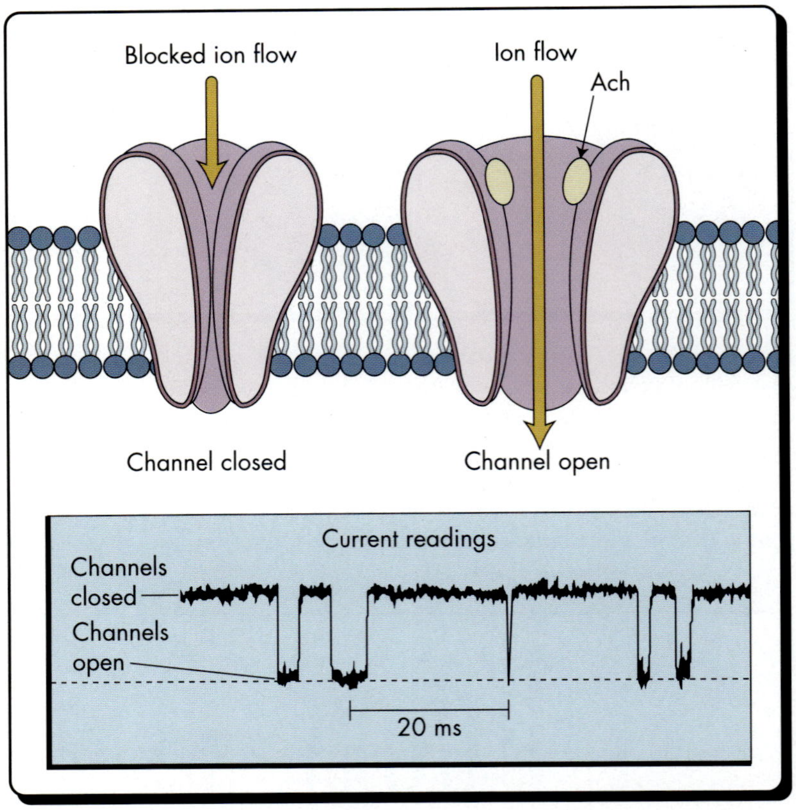

Figure 1-8. Receptor channels found at the neuromuscular junction. When the ligand (in this case acetylcholine) is absent, no current passes through the channel. When acetylcholine binds to the channel, a small current measured in picoamperes flows. The measured durations of the current and the intervals between them are dependent on the interactions of acetylcholine molecules with the receptor and are governed by probability. (*From* Neher and Sakmann [24].)

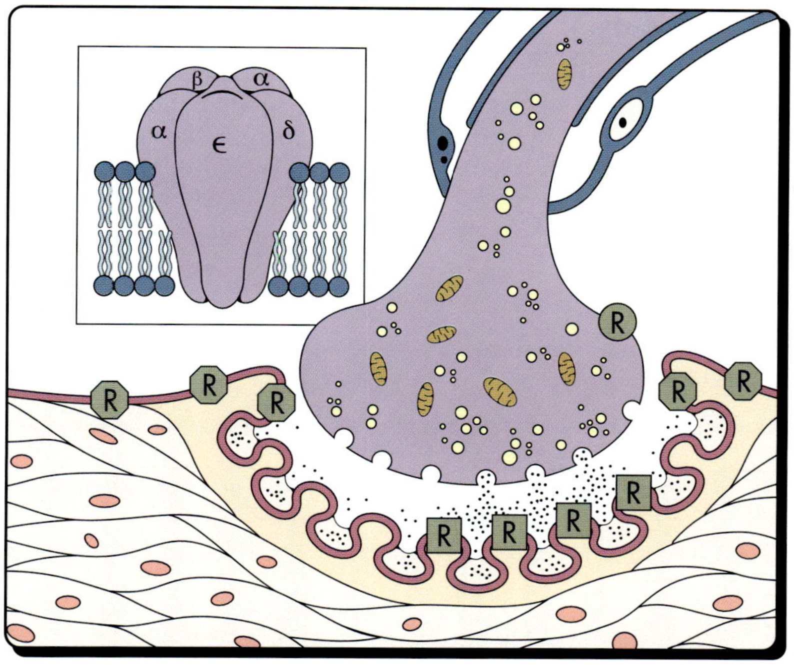

Figure 1-9. The nicotinic acetylcholine receptor-channel complex within the muscle membrane. Nicotinic acetylcholine is known to exist in a pentameric complex consisting of subunits designated as α, β, γ, and δ, with a stoichiometry of two α and one each of the other subunits [25]. These five subunits are arranged in a petal-like fashion around a central cavity that represents the ion channel. Only the α subunits appear to possess the recognition sites for acetylcholine and other agonists and antagonists. The binding site for both α subunits must be occupied by an agonist for receptor (R) activation and subsequent channel opening. (*From* Standaert [26]; with permission.)

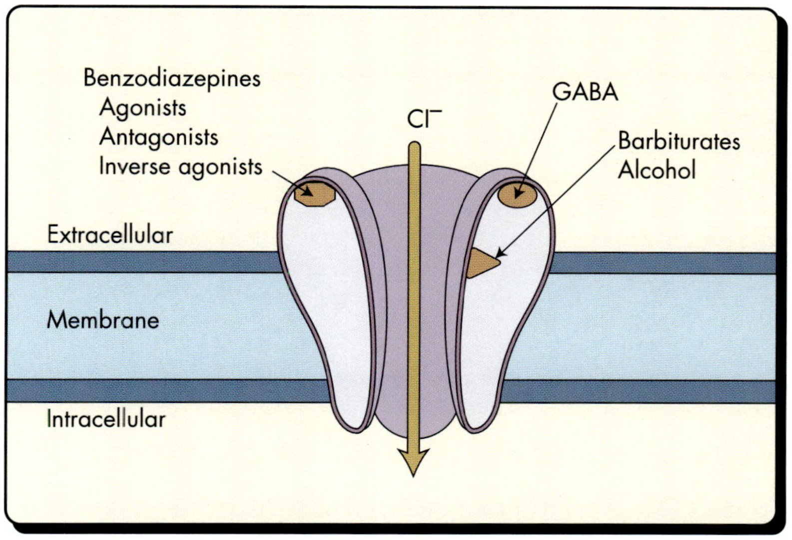

Figure 1-10. The GABA/benzodiazepine receptor. The GABA receptor is a prototypic ligand-gated receptor that inhibits synaptic transmission. The $GABA_A$ receptor is a complex macromolecule containing binding sites for several drugs as well as a chloride channel within the complex [27,28]. Within this complex are discrete benzodiazepine, GABA, and barbiturate receptors as well as sites of action for alcohol. GABA itself causes a rapid increase in neuronal permeability to chloride ions. Barbiturates facilitate GABA neurotransmission by increasing the mean open time of the chloride channel. The benzodiazepine receptor is an allosteric modulatory site within the GABA receptor–chloride channel complex [29]. They facilitate GABAergic neurotransmission by increasing the frequency of chloride channel openings. The benzodiazepine receptor is unique among receptors in that it recognizes three classes of ligand, two of them producing opposite modulatory effects on GABA receptor function, and the third acting as an antagonist of the other two. Agonists and partial agonists of the benzodiazepine receptor belong to various classes and have various applications as anesthetics, anxiolytics, and anticonvulsants (diazepam, midazolam, and lorazepam). Benzodiazepine receptor antagonists bind reversibly to benzodiazepine receptor but have no intrinsic activity (flumazenil). This drug enhances the versatility of benzodiazepine receptor agonists in therapy by simplifying treatment of agonist overdose. Inverse benzodiazepine receptor agonists reduce the efficiency of GABAergic transmission resulting in central nervous system stimulation. Although not clinically useful, these drugs provide interesting probes for analyzing the basis of anxiety-related emotional disorders. (*From* Berkowitz and Schwinn [30]; with permission.)

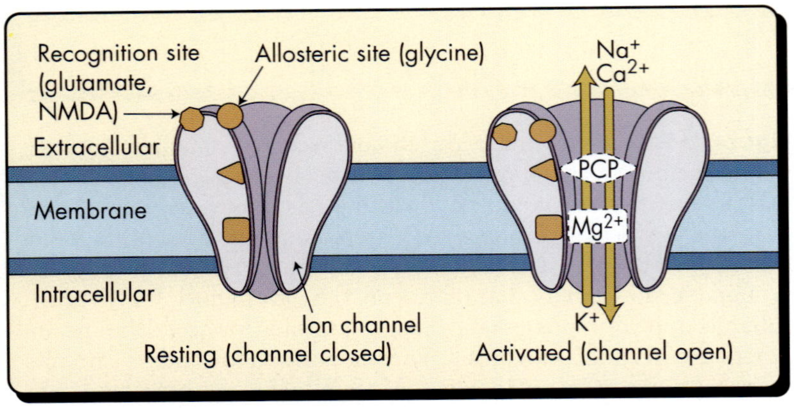

Figure 1-11. The NMDA receptor complex. The NMDA receptor is a prototypic amino acid receptor responsible for mediating excitatory synaptic transmission in the brain. Not only are this group of ligand-gated ion channels important targets for anesthetics (ketamine) but they also remain important target for agents that show promise as neuroprotectants [31]. Like the GABA receptor complex, the NMDA receptor is a macromolecule with multiple binding and modulatory sites including NMDA, glycine, a phencyclidine (PCP) ion binding site for Mg^{2+}, and a cation channel permeable to K^+ and Ca^{2+}. The ion channel is thus positively modulated by NMDA/glycine and negatively modulated by PCP and Mg^{2+} [32]. (*From* Berkowitz and Schwinn [30]; with permission.)

VOLTAGE-GATED ION CHANNELS

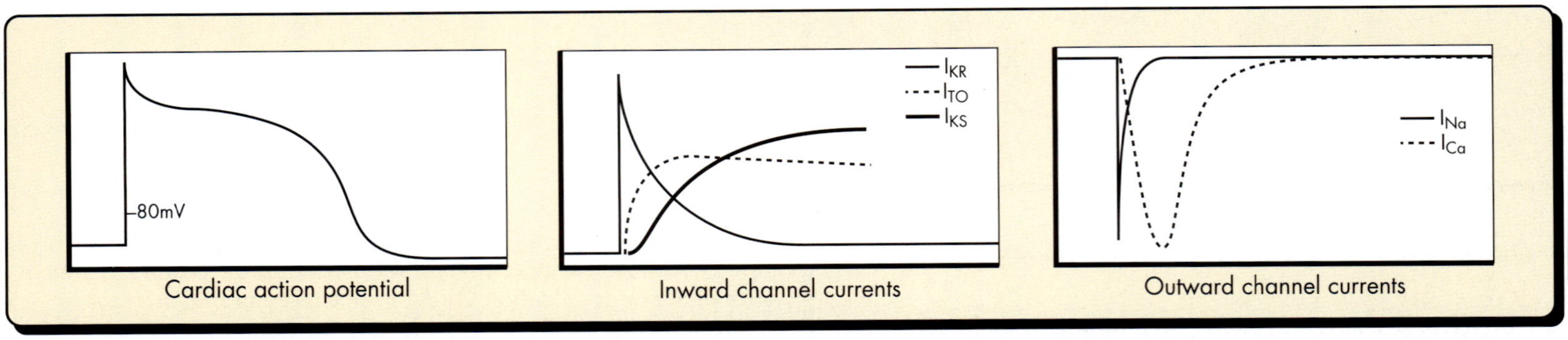

Figure 1-12. Various ionic currents flow through voltage-gated ion channels during a cardiac action potential. Inward currents (downward) include the Na current (I_{Na}), with very rapid kinetics, which is the principal determinant of the action potential upstroke and the rate of conduction through cardiac tissue. The inward calcium current (I_{Ca}) follows the Na current and supports the action potential plateau. Outward potassium currents tend to shorten or terminate the action potential and include the transient outward current (I_{TO}), which activates early and may be downregulated during heart failure, and the rapid (I_{KR}) and slow (I_{KS}) delayed rectifier potassium currents. I_{KR} is a target for class III antiarrhythmic compounds, and mutations in the gene for this channel are responsible for a type of congenital long-QT syndrome. I_{KR}, the inward rectifier potassium current, is active primarily during diastole and maintains the resting membrane potential.

GROWTH FACTOR RECEPTORS

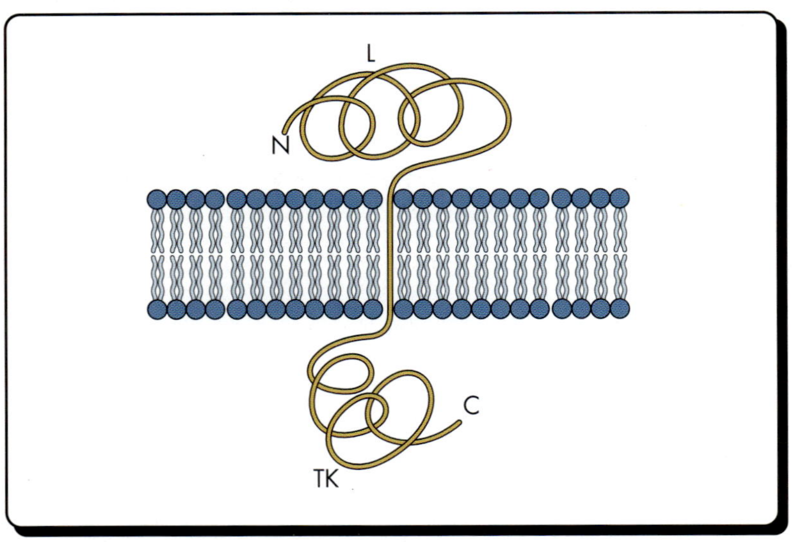

Figure 1-13. A growth factor receptor. Growth factor receptors have one transmembrane domain linking a large glycosylated extracellular ligand-binding domain (L) with a large intracellular domain that usually includes a protein kinase domain (TK). Ligand binding initiates dimerization of the receptor, a process that results in stimulation of TK activity [33]. C—carboxy terminus; N—amino terminus.

TRANSMEMBRANE GUANYLATE CYCLASE RECEPTORS

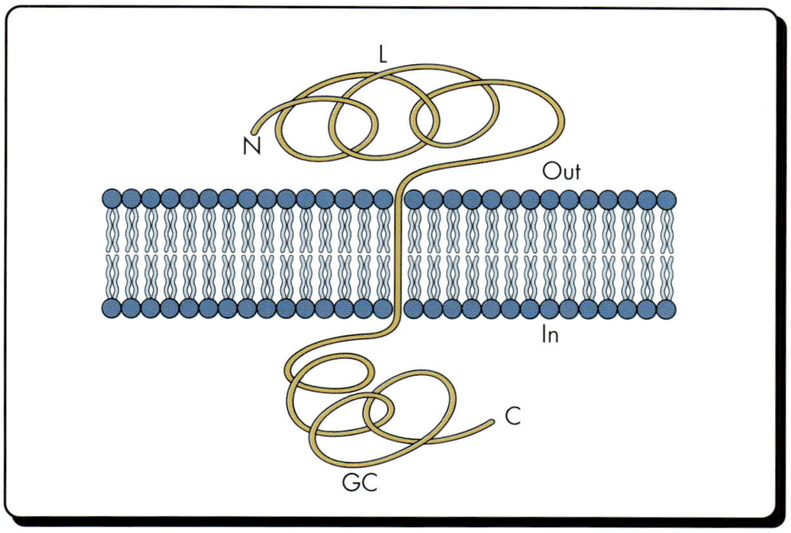

Figure 1-14. Receptor guanylyl cyclase (GC). The GC receptors have a structure that is very similar to that of the growth factor receptors. They have a single transmembrane domain with an NH_2^- and $COOH^-$ terminus. The extracellular domain is important in ligand binding (ligands include atrial natriuretic peptide, or ANP) and the intracellular portion of the receptor contains the GC domain, which will catalyze the conversion of GTP to cGMP. Like cAMP, cGMP can activate protein kinases. Thus when ANP acts on the kidney collecting duct cells, protein phosphorylation results in closure of an apical cation channel and resorption of Na^+ ions is blocked, with resultant diuresis [34]. C—carboxy terminis; L—ligand-binding domain; N—amino terminus.

NITRIC OXIDE

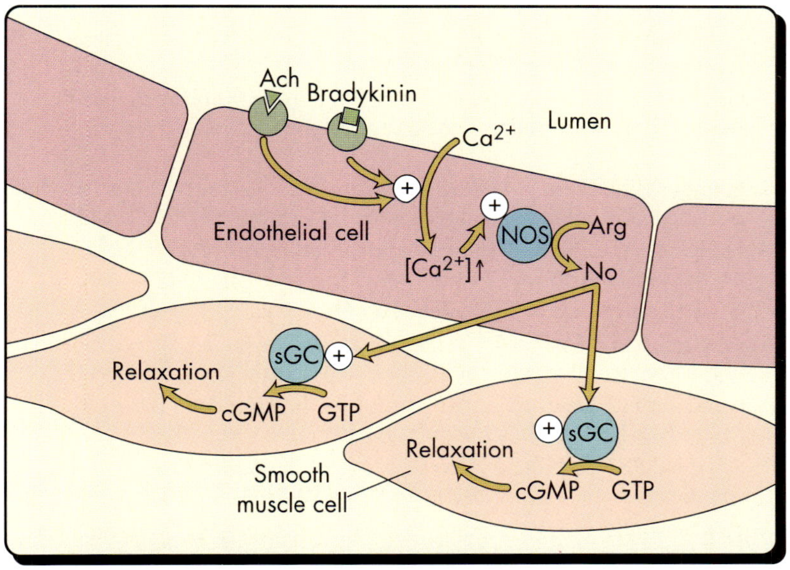

Figure 1-15. Nitric oxide synthase (NOS) and its signal transduction in endothelial/smooth muscle cells. NO is one of the most ubiquitous and widespread biologic mediators in mammalian cells. It produces many diverse physiologic functions, including vascular smooth muscle relaxation, neurotransmission, inhibition of platelet aggregation, and leukocyte cytotoxicity, to mention but a few. In high concentrations, NO produces pathophysiologic actions leading ultimately to cell destruction. These diverse actions are attributed to the unique chemistry of the molecule, which is a small, lipophilic, reactive nitrogen radical that binds with high affinity to hemoproteins. NO is synthesized in mammalian cells from L-arginine by the monooxygenase flavoprotein NOS, which catalyzes the conversion of L-arginine to NO and citrulline. The constitutive isoform of NOS in vascular endothelial cells is activated by Ca^{2+}-calmodulin interactions. Endothelium-dependent vasodilators such as acetylcholine, histamine, and bradykinin interact with selective receptors on the endothelial cell surface to promote calcium influx and NOS activation. NOS activation is also promoted by shear forces on the vascular wall. The physiologic actions of NO are mediated by cGMP. NO binds to the heme prosthetic group of cytosolic guanylyl cyclase, thereby activating the enzyme. cGMP results in the sequestration of intracellular Ca^{2+} with a resultant decrease in smooth muscle tone. The major importance of this signal transduction mechanism is that the organic and inorganic nitrates (nitroglycerin and sodium nitroprusside) are NO donors and cause vascular smooth muscle relaxation through this signal transduction mechanism. Also, inhaled NO in concentrations up to 80 ppm is fast becoming the treatment of choice for acute pulmonary hypertension. Inhaled NO is almost completely devoid of systemic effects because it is rapidly quenched in the lung by hemoglobin, which is converted to met-hemoglobin. Ach—acetylcholine; Arg—arginine; NOS—nitric oxide synthase; sGC—soluble guanylyl cyclase. (*From* Knowles and Moncada [17]; with permission.)

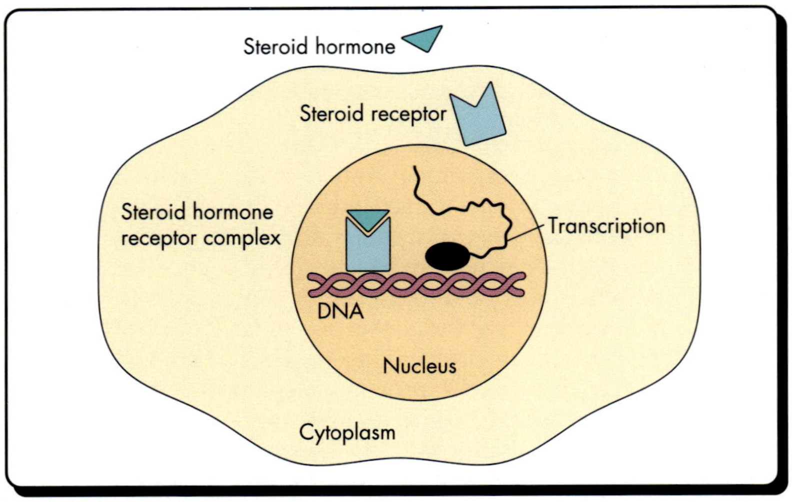

Figure 1-16. Nuclear hormone receptor signal transduction. The steroid or nuclear hormone receptors are a group of intracellular receptors that bind steroid hormones, thyroid hormone, retinoic acid, and other lipid-soluble vitamins. They share the same modular structure and are composed of a ligand-binding domain and a DNA-binding domain. Intracellular receptor binds the hydrophobic ligand, a steroid, thyroid hormone, or vitamin that diffuses into the cell. The nuclear hormone receptor binds to specific nucleotide sequences in the target gene. These targets are called response elements. Activation of the receptor by the ligand results in enhancement or repression of transcription of this target gene [35]. A clinically important example of this is the mechanism of action of steroids as anti-inflammatory agents. Steroids result in the repression of proinflammatory cytokine expression, thus attenuating the inflammatory response.

REFERENCES

1. Hollenberg MD: Structure activity relationships for transmembrane signalling: The receptors' turn. *FASEB J* 1991, 5:178–186.
2. Gudermann T, Nurnberg B, Schultz G: Receptors and G proteins as primary components of transmembrane signal tranduction: Part 1: G-protein-coupled receptors: structure and function. *J Mol Med* 1995, 73:51–63.
3. Schwinn DA, Caron MG, Lefkowitz RJ: The beta-adrenergic receptor as a model for molecular structure-function relationships in G-protein-coupled receptors. In *Scientific Basis of Cardiovascular Disease*, Edited by Fozzard HA. New York: Raven Press; 1992:1657–1684.
4. Strader CD, Fong TM, Graziano MP, *et al.*: The family of G-protein-coupled receptors. *FASEB J* 1995, 9:745–754.
5. Gilman AG: G proteins: Tranducers of receptor-generated signals. *Annu Rev Biochem* 1987, 56:615–649.
6. Helper JR, Gilman AG: G proteins. *Trends Biochem Sci* 1992, 17:383.
7. Dani JA, Mayer ML: Structure and function of glutamate and nicotinic acetylcholine receptors. *Curr Opin Neurobiol* 1995, 5:310–317.
8. Hille B: Ligand-gated channels of fast chemical synapses. In *Ionic Channels of Excitable Membranes*. Sunderland, MA: Sinauer; 1991:140–169.
9. Ortells MO, Lunt GG: Evolutionary history of the ligand-gated ion-channel superfamily of receptors. *Trends Neurosci* 1995, 18:121–127.
10. Unwin N: Neurotransmitter action: Opening of ligand-gated ion channels. *Cell* 1993, 72(suppl):31–41.
11. Hille B: *Ionic Channels of Excitable Membranes*. Sunderland, MA: Sinauer; 1991:1–20; 170–201.
12. Catterall WA: Structure and function of voltage gated ion channels. *Annu Rev Biochem* 1995, 64:493–531.
13. Keynes RD: The kinetics of voltage-gated ion channels. *Q Rev Biophys* 1994, 27:339–434.
14. Ullrich A, Schlessinger J: Signal transduction by receptors with tyrosine kinase activity. *Cell* 1990, 61:203–212.
15. Schultz S, Chinkers M, Garbers DL: The guanylate cyclase/receptor family of proteins. *FASEB J* 1989, 3:2026–2035.
16. Nathan C, Xie Q: Regulation of biosythesis of nitric oxide. *J Biol Chem* 1994, 269:13725–13728.
17. Knowles RG, Moncada S: Nitric oxide as a signal in blood vessels. *Trends Biochem Sci* 1992, 17:399–402.
18. Berkowitz DE, Schwinn DA: Basic pharmacology of α- and β-adrenoceptors. In *The Pharmacologic Basis of of Anesthesiology*. Edited by Bowdle TA, Horita A, and Kharasch ED. New York: Churchill Livingstone; 1994:581–605.
19. Sutherland EW: Studies on the mechanisms of hormone action. *Science* 177: 401–408.
20. Freedman NJ, Kefkowitz RJ: Desenitization of G protein coupled receptors. *Recent Prog Horm Res* 1996, 51:319–351.
21. Hausdorff WP, Caron MG, Lefkowitz RJ: Turning off the signal: Desensitization of β-adrenergic receptor function. *FASEB J* 1990, 4:2881–2889.
22. Premont RT, Inglese J, Lefkowitz RJ: Protein kinases that phosphorylate activated G protein-coupled receptors. *FASEB J* 1995, 9:175–182.
23. Hodgkins AL, Huxley AF: Action potentials recorded from inside a nerve fiber. *Nature* 1939, 144: 710–711.
24. Neher E, Sakmann B: The patch clamp technique. *Sci Am* 1992, 28 –35.
25. McCarthy MP, Earnest JP, Young EF, *et al.*: The molecular neurobiology of the acetylcholine receptor. *Annu Rev Neurosci* 1986, 9:383–413.
26. Standaert FG: Neuromuscular physiology. In *Anesthesia* Edited by Miller RD. New York: Churchill Livingstone; 1990:659–684.
27. Schofield PR: The $GABA_A$ receptor: Molecular biology reveals a complex picture. *Trends Pharmcol Sci* 1989, 10:476–478.
28. Stephenson PA: Understanding the $GABA_A$ receptor: A chemically gated ion channel. *Biochem J* 1988, 249:21–32.
29. Haefely W: The $GABA_A$-benzodiazepine interaction fifteen years later. *Neurochem Res* 1990, 15:169–174.
30. Berkowitz DE, Schwinn DA: New advances in receptor pharmacology. *Curr Opin Anesthesiol* 1991, 4:486–496.
31. Muir KW, Lees KR: Cliical experience with excitatory amino acid antagonist drugs. *Stroke* 1995, 26:503–513.
32. Mori H, Mishina M: Structure and function of NMDA receptor channel. *Neuropharmacology* 1995, 34:1219–1237.
33. Eppenberger U, Mueller H: Growth factor receptors and their ligands. *J Neurooncol* 1994, 22:249–254.
34. Nakao K, Itoh H, Suga S, *et al.*: The natriuretic peptide family. *Curr Opin Nephrol Hypertens* 1993, 2:45–50.
35. Lopes da Silva S, Burbach JPH: The nuclear hormone-receptor family in the brain: classics and orphans. *Trends Neurosci* 1995, 18:542–548.

2

Physics Principles Important in Anesthesiology

Ira Rampil

Physical laws and the mathematical equations that describe them form the nucleus by which we understand the physical world. Many phenomena associated with the practice of anesthesia are direct expressions of classical physics, including the behavior of compressed gases, the processes of vaporization, heat transfer or fluid flow, and resonance phenomena. Most patient monitoring techniques rely on physical principles, and the common artifacts and distortions can often be eliminated or compensated for with a grasp of the underlying physics.

With the passing of the Copper Kettle vaporizer into obsolescence, clinicians are now rarely called upon to perform physics-related calculations in the operating room. Nonetheless, a qualitative understanding of the basic principles illustrated in this chapter can provide practitioners with facility in understanding the tools of their trade and a patient's response to physical phenomena, and with a framework for formulating appropriate therapeutic interventions.

The illustrations that follow introduce a small subset of the physical principles that play a role in anesthesia. Many are accompanied with demonstrations of clinical relevance.

FIRST PRINCIPLES

UNITS OF MEASURE

Quantity	Unit of Measure	Abbreviation
Time	second	s
Length	meter	m
Mass	kilogram	kg
Temperature	degree Kelvin	°K
Current	ampere	A
Atomic quantity	mole	mol
Luminosity	candela	cd

Figure 2-1. Units, standards, dimensions. Our understanding of the physical laws that govern our reality is based on empirical observation, *ie*, measurements. The units, scales, and benchmark standards for these measurements are codified by international agreement expressed in the Systéme Internationale (SI) d'Unités. Modern physics relies on fundamental constants of matter to define all but one of the benchmark values. For example, a second (sec) is defined as the time required for exactly 9,192,631,770 gyroscopic precessions of the outer electron of an undisturbed cesium atom, and the meter (m) is defined as the distance traveled in vacuum by a photon in 1/299,792,458 of a second. At present, the benchmark kilogram (kg) is a bar of platinum kept in Sevres, France.

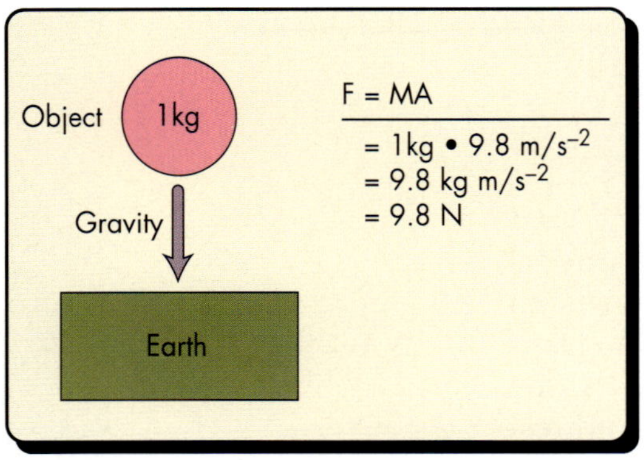

Figure 2-2. Force. Force (F) is an influence on matter that tends to create movement. In fact, force was defined by Sir Issac Newton in terms of its ability to accelerate a mass (M). Because movement has direction, so too must force: force is a vector. On the surface of a planet, such as Earth, force must also be exerted on an object to render it stationary by counteracting the constant force of gravity. The International System of Units (SI) unit of force is the newton (N), defined as an influence with sufficient magnitude to accelerate a 1.0 kg mass at a rate of 1 m per sec per sec. Since a 1.0 L bag of saline has a mass of approximately 1 kg, and at sea level the gravitational acceleration is approximately 9.8 m/s/s, a force of 9.8 N is required to hold the bag.

PRESSURE

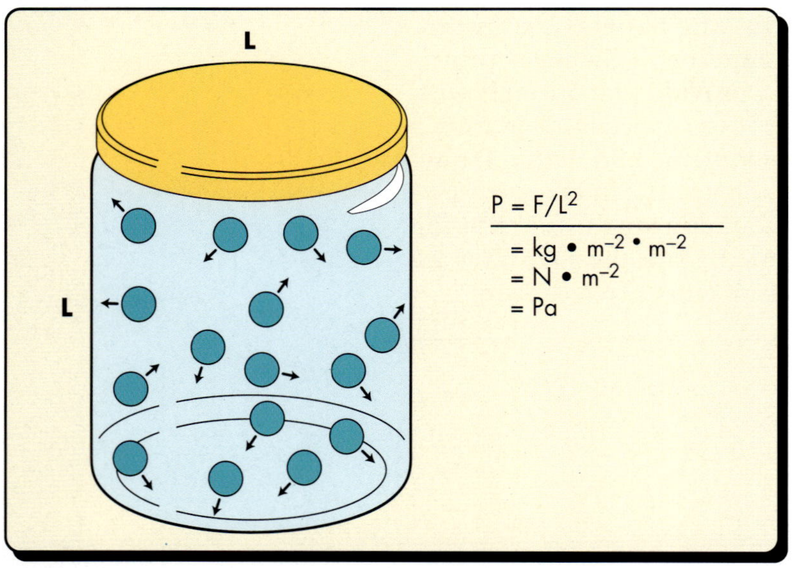

Figure 2-3. Definition of pressure. Gravity causes a solid object lying on the ground to exert a force (weight) on the ground. In a similar fashion the thermal energy in a gas or liquid leads to motion of the constituent molecules. The constant barrage of these molecules against a container wall exerts a force we know as pressure. Pressure (P) is measured as the force (F) per surface area (L^2)of the container, *ie*, as N per m^2, or pascals (Pa).

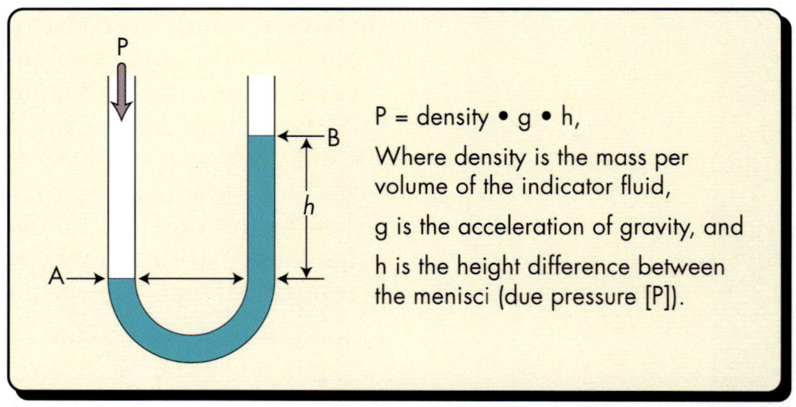

Figure 2-4. Manometry. A difference in gas pressure (P) in the two arms of the manometer tube performs work by moving the indicator fluid out of the higher pressure arm until it reaches that point where the gravitational force (g) on the excess fluid in the low pressure arm balances the difference in pressure. If the diameters of the two arms are matched, then the difference in pressure is a simple function of the difference in height (h) of the two menisci.

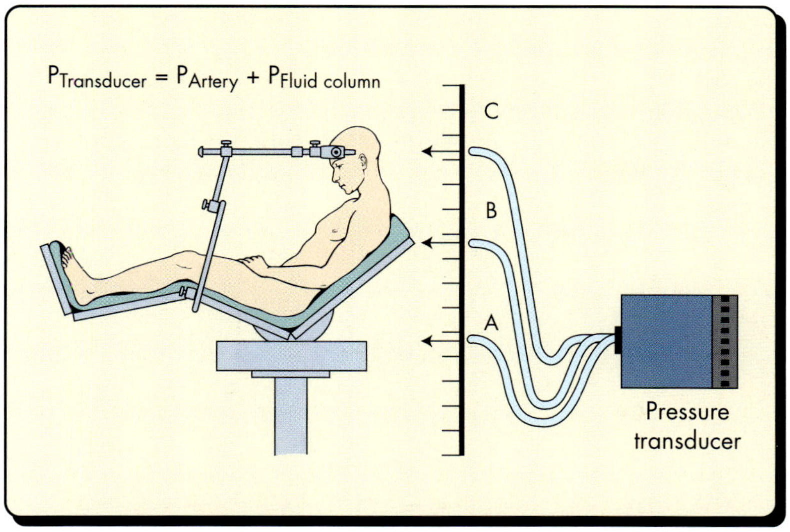

Figure 2-5. Zero level pressure. The principle of the manometer applies in the operating room, where one must decide on an appropriate zero or reference level for arterial pressure monitoring. If the transducer is placed at the level of the table (A) and electrically zeroed to that height, the measured pressure (P) is higher than at the aortic root (B) and even higher compared with the pressure within the Circle of Willis (C) because of the manometer effect, *ie*, the added weight of the saline within the tubing rising from A to B or C.

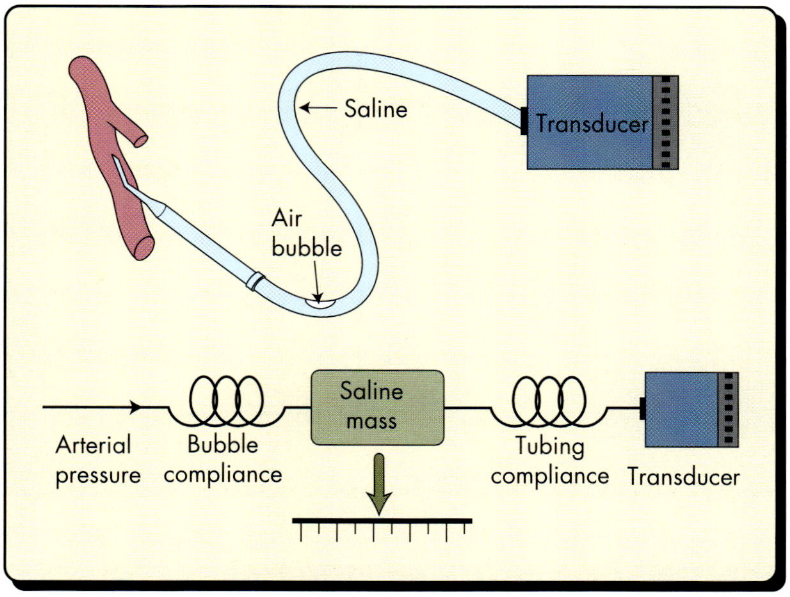

Figure 2-6. Blood pressure measurement. Arterial blood pressure waveforms are usually distored by the catheter/tubing/transducer system. The dynamics and artifacts of such pulsatile pressure recordings can be understood by considering the simple model in the illustration. An ideal pressure measurement would be derived from an intraluminal transducer, but these are not very practical. Therefore, the pressure variations are carried in a saline-filled plastic tube to a relatively large external transducer. In the process of transferring the pressure wave to the transducer, one must consider the mass (and hence inertia) of the saline and the compliance of the tubing and retained air bubbles. Like a mass suspended on springs, any movement can lead to a series of oscillations (commonly misinterpreted as "whip" or "fling").

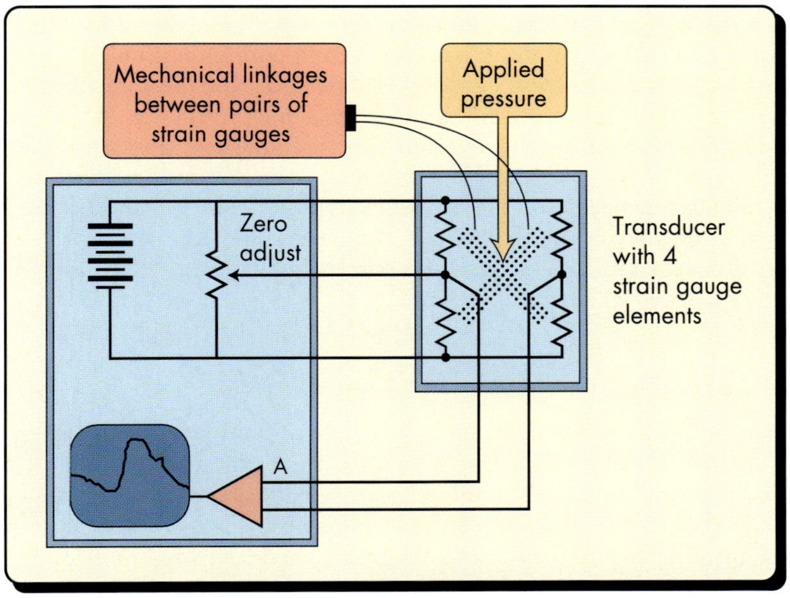

Figure 2-7. Direct measurement. Disposable pressure tranducers in wide clinical use are based on a "bridge circuit" arrangement of four strain gauges. Strain gauges alter their electrical resistance in proportion to applied mechanical force. The bridge arrangement, by placing in series strain gauges in both tension and compression, maximizes the detectable signal. The pressure force is applied to mechanical linkages that simultaneously compress and stretch strain gauges on both sides of the bridge. During a zero-adjust, an adjustable resistor is set to a point where the "zero" pressure load produces no output voltage from the bridge circuit. A—amplifier.

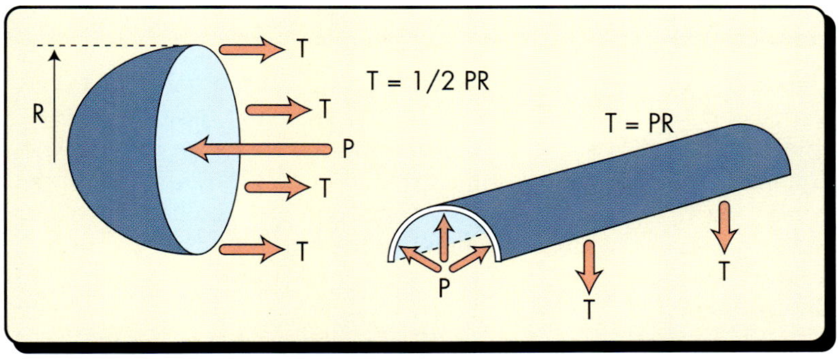

Figure 2-8. Surface tension. Surface tension (T) is the result of forces of mutual attraction between the molecules of the fluid. In the interior of a liquid, a molecule's neighbors exert mutual attraction. At the surface, there are few neighboring molecules in the gas phase, leading to a net attractive force back into the liquid. Likewise, in a bubble, the attractive force is everywhere tangential to the surface, trying to attract the bubble surface into a smaller radius. This wall tension increases the internal pressure of the bubble. Laplace's Law states that the pressure (P; force applied to separate the bubble's hemispheres) within the bubble must equal the wall tension (force attempting to hold the sphere together). For a spherical shape, the wall tension is equal to the internal pressure times half the radius (R); for a cylindrical shape, the wall tension is the pressure times the radius.

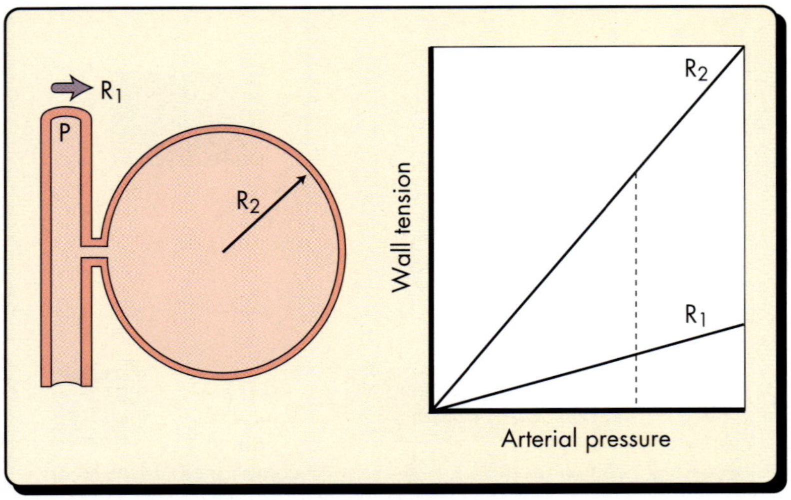

Figure 2-9. Aneurysmal rupture. When wall tension exceeds the mechanical strength of wall, the wall will tear apart. Vascular aneurysms are at particular risk of wall rupture because they have larger radii (R) and thinner walls compared to the surrounding vasculature. Therefore, at a given arterial pressure (P), an aneurysm has a higher wall tension and that tension acts on thinner, weaker tissue.

FLUID FLOW

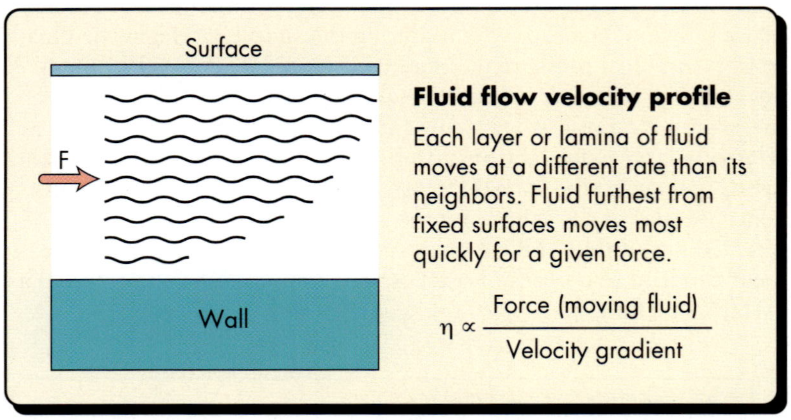

Figure 2-10. Viscosity. The same forces (F) of mutual attraction responsible for surface tension in liquids also resist movement of adjacent molecules and are therefore responsible for an internal friction or viscosity. Viscosity is measured in unit of Poise and given the symbol eta (η) equals shearing force per unit area divided by velocity change per unit thickness. Certain problems in fluid flow require reckoning with the weight of the fluid, *eg*, when flow accelerates or changes direction. The usual approach to these problems is to divide the viscosity by the density (weight per unit volume) of the fluid. This ratio is known as the *kinematic viscosity* or υ.

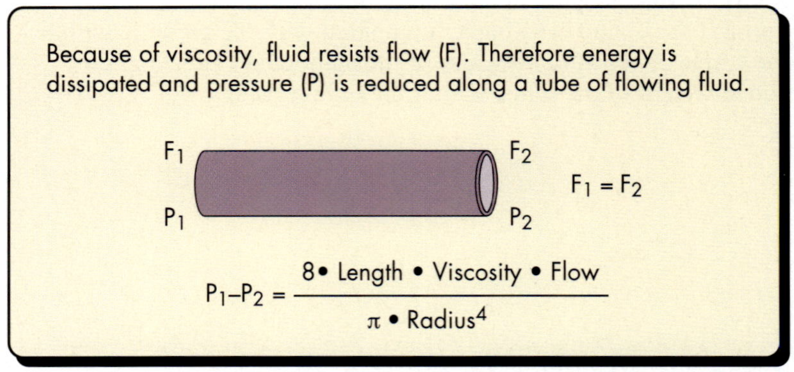

Figure 2-11. The Hagen-Poiseuille equation. The Hagen-Poiseuille equation illustrated in this figure relates to smooth (nonturbulent) flow and is analogous to Ohm's Law for electricity, *ie*, that pressure difference (voltage) is proportional flow (current) times resistance. In the case of fluid flow in a pipe, the resistance term is exquisitely sensitive to the radius of the pipe. When rapid infusion is required, it may be useful to recall the dependence on radius. For example, an 8-in, 16-gauge central venous pressure catheter (0.85 mm radius) has nine times the flow resistance of a 2-in, 14-gauge (1.05 mm radius) catheter.

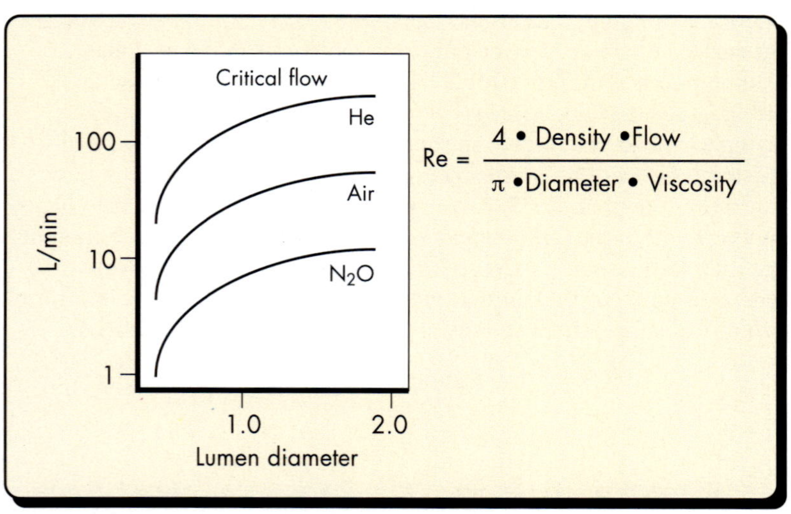

Figure 2-12. Reynold's number. Turbulent fluid flow results when the parallel, orderly structure of laminar flow chaotically breaks down in random eddies, impinging on neighboring eddies and the walls of the pipe. Turbulence causes inefficiency, wasting kinetic energy. Turbulence is promoted by increased density and increased flow rate or by decreased viscosity or a more restricted channel of flow. The onset of turbulence can be predicted by the Reynold's number (Re): Assuming the system under consideration is flow in a smooth pipe, when Re > 2000, flow becomes turbulent instead of laminar, and the pressure force to create a certain flow increases. Alternatively, for a given fluid and geometry, flow becomes turbulent at a critical flow velocity. He—helium; N_2O—nitrous oxide.

Work = Force (exerted against an object) x Distance (moved by that object)

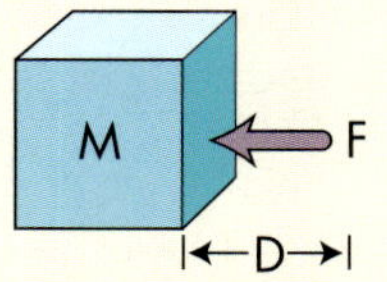

Energy = Capacity to perform work. Energy can exist in many forms, *eg*:
- Mechanical:
  - Potential (due to position) or Kinetic (due to motion)
- Thermal
- Chemical bond
- Electrical

Power = Work/Time (rate of doing work)

Figure 2-13. Measurment of work and energy. D—distance; F—force; M—mass.

The mechanical work of the heart (moving blood) can be calculated as F • D, or more conveniently as

Work = Pressure • Flow • Time

However, mechanical work is a small fraction of the heart's work load:

Basal metabolism	= 20%
Activation	= 25%
Tension development	= 50%
Mechanical work	= 5%

Figure 2-14. Myocardial work. The issue of work performed in physiologic systems is often more complex than might be assumed from first principles. For example, the work performed by the heart in moving blood through the circulatory system is easily calculated. However, that calculation results in only 1/20 the energy expended by the myocardium when measured by other means. D—distance; F—force. (*Data from* Ream and Fogdall [1].)

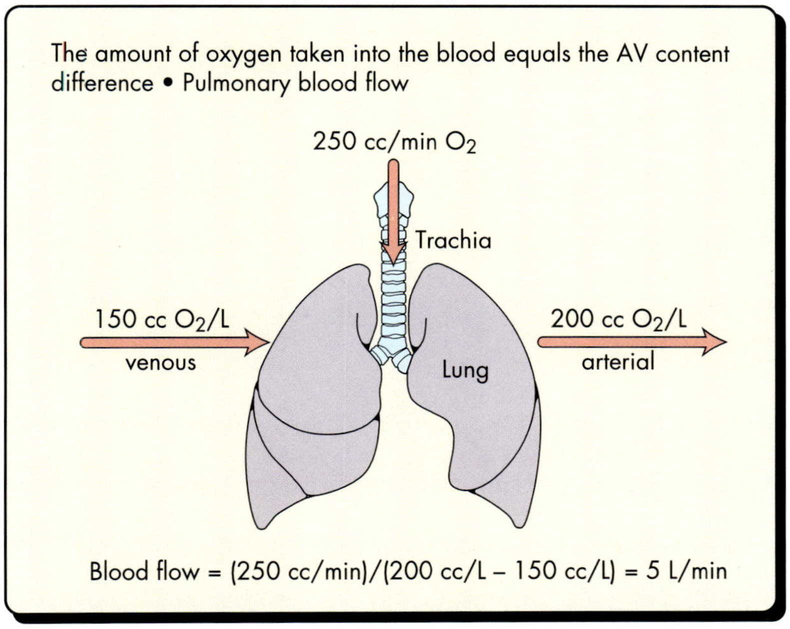

Figure 2-15. Fick principle. It is inconvenient or dangerous to directly measure blood flow *in vivo*. One can, however, apply physical principles to make indirect or noninvasive estimates of blood flow. An early example is the Fick method of calculating cardiac output, which is shown in this figure. The method relies on the principle of conservation of mass: One assumes that the quantity of an indicator substance in blood can be completely accounted for by a simple mass balance equation and that blood flow into an organ is the same as the blood flow out. If the content per unit of blood of an indicator substance such as oxygen (O_2) can be measured on both the inflow and outflow sides of the lungs, and the whole body oxygen consumption can also be determined, then one can write an equation stating that the rate of oxygen flowing out of the lungs (*via* blood in the pulmonary veins) equals oxygen flowing in through the pulmonary arteries plus that flowing in through the trachea. Rearranging this equation yields the equations shown here.

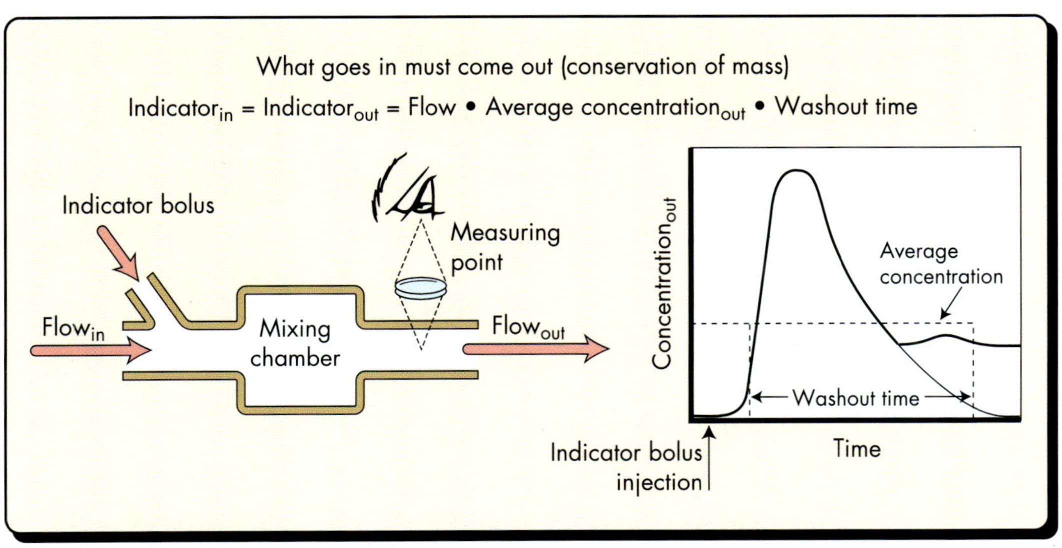

Figure 2-16. Indicator dilution. The Stewart-Hamilton theory for estimating cardiac output by indicator dilution is another application of conservation of mass. The underlying principle is that an unknown volume of liquid can be measured by mixing in a known quantity of indicator and measuring the resulting concentration. Here, an indicator (*ie*, indocyanine green dye or cold saline) is bolused into the inflow of a mixing chamber (like a capillary bed of an organ), where it is transported into the mixing chamber, diluted, and eluted, producing the washout curve in the figure. Two other methods of measuring blood flow are based on Doppler shifts and electromagnetic induction. These techniques are covered later in the chapter.

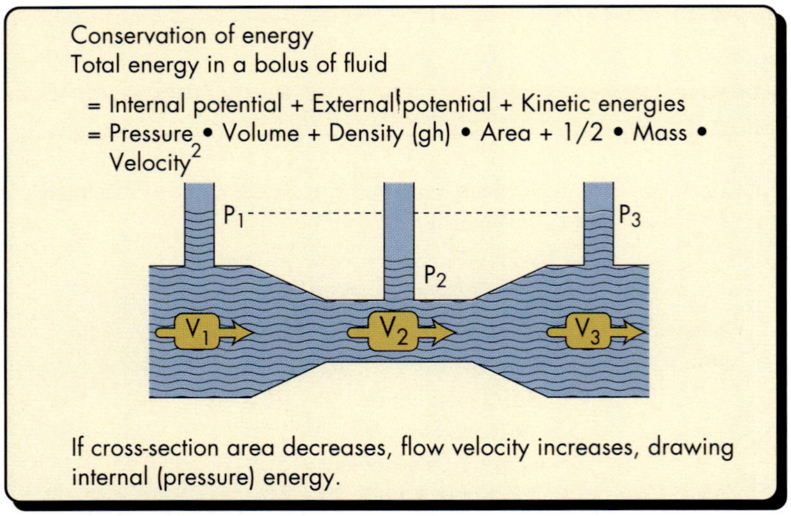

Figure 2-17. Venturi equation. Assuming no energy is lost to such factors as turbulence or wall friction, the product of the flow velocity (V) times cross-sectional area is constant. Therefore, when the diameter of a fluid-carrying tube decreases, the velocity of the fluid must increase. Because increasing speed requires energy and none is added from outside, some of the internal potential (pressure [P]) energy of the fluid is converted to the required kinetic energy. The reduction in pressure at the constriction can be used to measure fluid flow velocity or used to entrain other liquids or gases into the fluid stream.

GAS LAWS

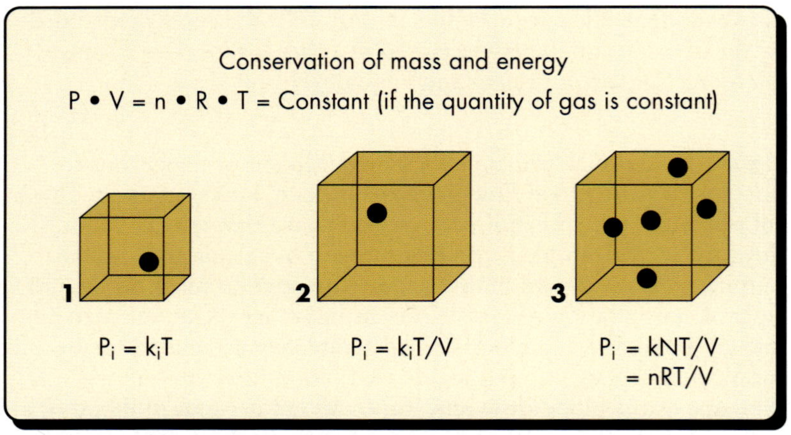

Figure 2-18. Ideal gas laws. The ideal gas laws combine conservation of mass and energy. The dependencies on volume (V), temperature (T), and number of molecules can be understood by examining the illustration.

In *box 1*, a single molecule occupies a unit volume of space. The pressure (P) it generates is due to the collisional energy it imparts to the wall. The molecule's movement is due to thermal energy: the higher the temperature, the faster the molecule bounces around in its space. The k factor is dependent on the molecule's mass and other properties.

In *box 2*, the same molecule is now in a larger volume (V) of space. Because the distances are larger, the number of collisions with the wall are less frequent. The exerted pressure is inversely proportional to the volume.

In *box 3*, more (N) molecules of the same species are added. The frequency of collisions with the wall increases with the number of molecules. If moles (n) is used instead of N, the k is replaced by a new factor R.

When a gas consists of a mixture of molecules, then each species contributes to the total vessel pressure in proportion to the number of molecules present of each species:

$$PV = (N_1 + N_2 + N_3 ... + N_i)\, kT$$

or

$$\frac{P_1}{N_1} = \frac{P_2}{N_2} = \frac{P}{N_1 + N_2}$$

Figure 2-19. Partial pressure. The equations in this illustration are a statement of Dalton's Law, which simply says that in a mixture of gases, each molecular species exerts the same pressure it would if it were alone in a container. kT—proportionality constant times degrees Kelvin; N—number of molecules of a particular species; PV—vessel pressure.

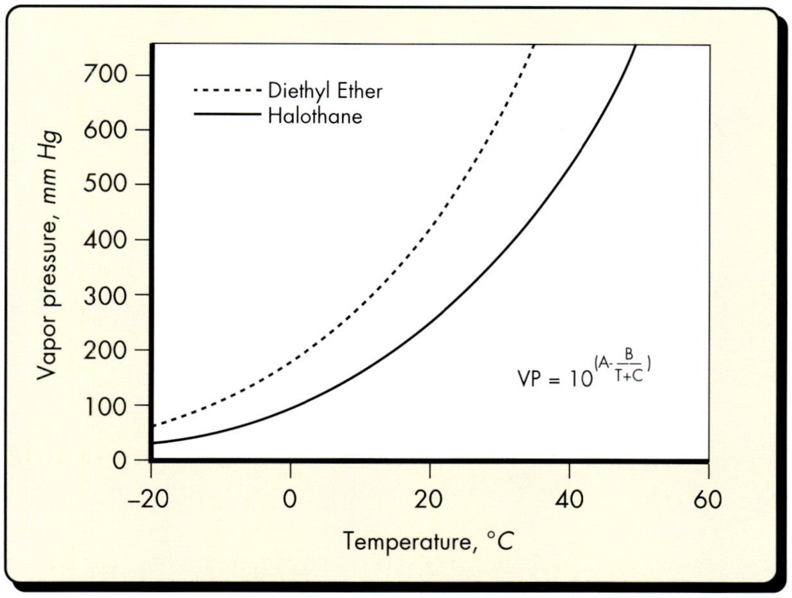

Figure 2-20. Vapor pressure (VP). Molecules of a liquid may escape a liquid by virtue of their thermal (kinetic) energy. For a given liquid, the number of molecules that can escape into vapor phase (creating a vapor pressure) is dependent on the temperature (T) and some empirically derived constants (A,B,C) as described by Antoine's equation. The graph illustrates typical vapor pressure curves. At a given temperature, the more volatile diethyl ether exerts a higher vapor pressure than halothane. The boiling point is that temperature at which the vapor pressure equals ambient atmospheric pressure (about 760 mm Hg).

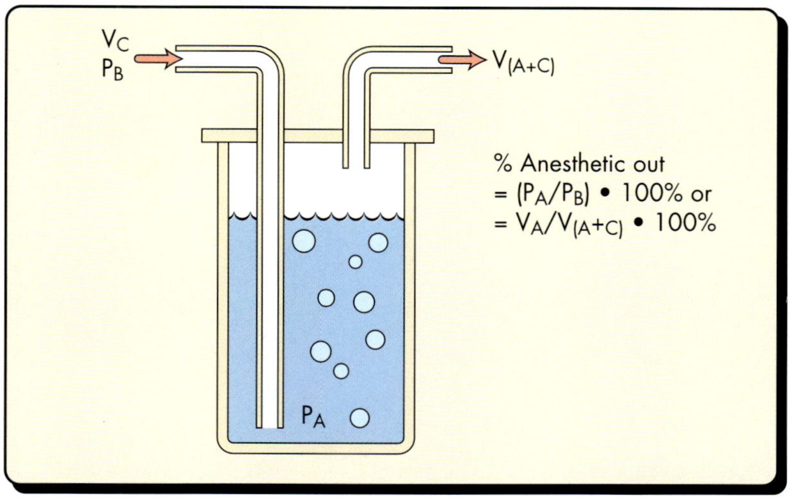

Figure 2-21. Vaporizers. Anesthetic vaporizers provide a controlled, efficient means of converting liquid anesthetic into the gas phase. In its simplest form, the copper kettle, a carrier stream of oxygen (V_C) at standard barometric pressure (P_B) enters the vaporizer and is bubbled through the anesthetic. Anesthetic molecules vaporize into the bubbles until each bubble contains a partial pressure of anesthetic equal to the vapor pressure (P_A). The addition of anesthetic to the oxygen increases the volume of the bubbles ($V_C + V_A$). Note that the Copper Kettle vaporizer is manufactured from a massive piece of copper, which serves as a heat sink. The heat sink is useful in moderating the temperature decrease that would be expected in the process of vaporization. The output of a kettle-type vaporizer must be further diluted before administration because the vapor pressure of commonly used agents is far above a lethal concentration.

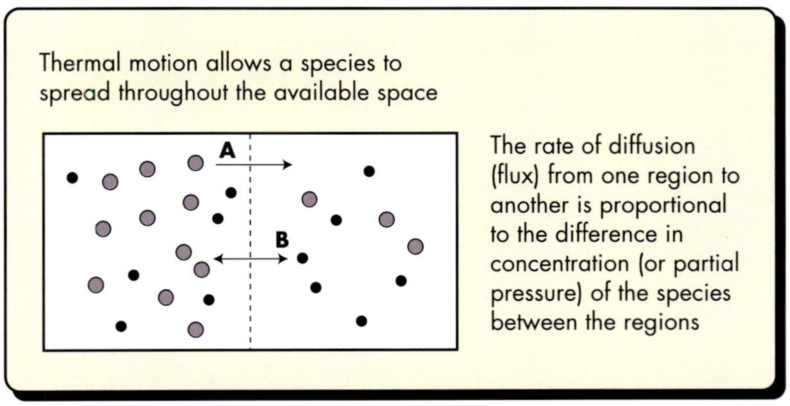

Figure 2-22. Diffusion. In this illustration, the B species (*black circles*) is roughly evenly distributed, leading to no net flux, whereas the A species (*purple circles*) is far more numerous on the left side, leading to a partial pressure gradient and a net flux to the right. If several ionically charged species are mixed, and a barrier between compartments is not equally permeable to all species, stable concentration gradients develop, as the forces that act to balance concentration must now also balance separated electrical charges.

WAVES

A disturbance that propagates through a medium:

Wave velocity = wave frequency • wavelength

Sample wave propagation velocities

Name	Disturbance	Media	Velocity
Sound	Pressure	Air	330 m/sec
Sound	Pressure	Tissue	1550 m/sec
Sound	Pressure	Bone	4000 m/sec
Light	Electromagnetic	Vacuum	299,792,458 m/sec

Figure 2-23. Wave propagation velocity of various media. Note that electromagnetic waves like light, radio, and x-rays also have a particle-like nature (photons) and do not require a physical medium for propagation as do sound waves.

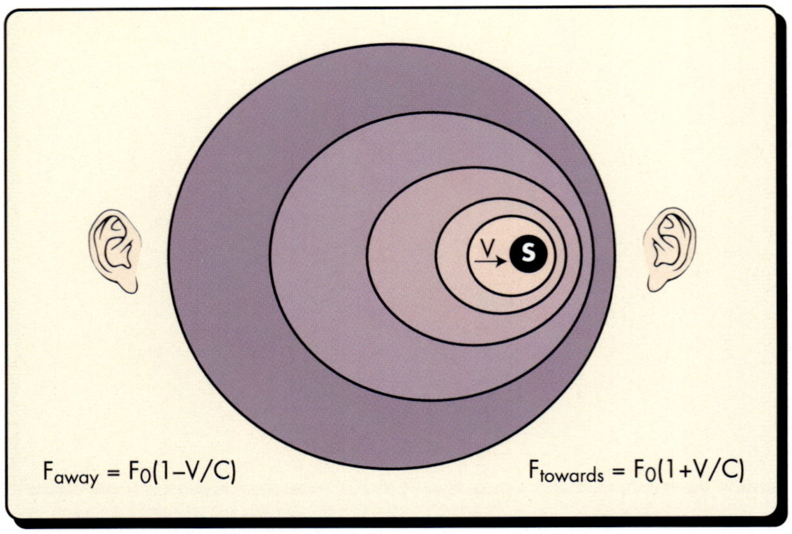

Figure 2-24. Doppler shift. When a source (S) of waves (of frequency F_0) moves relative to observers, the observers sense a frequency shifted from its original value. Since the pitch or frequency of sound is our perception of the rate at which our ear detects passing wavefronts, a motion towards the source (or the source towards our ear) will allow the detection of more wavefronts per unit of time—an increase in pitch. Knowing the original frequency, the new shifted frequency, and the speed of wave propagation (C) allows the observer to calculate the speed of the moving source (V). This technique is widely used in ultrasonography and police radar guns.

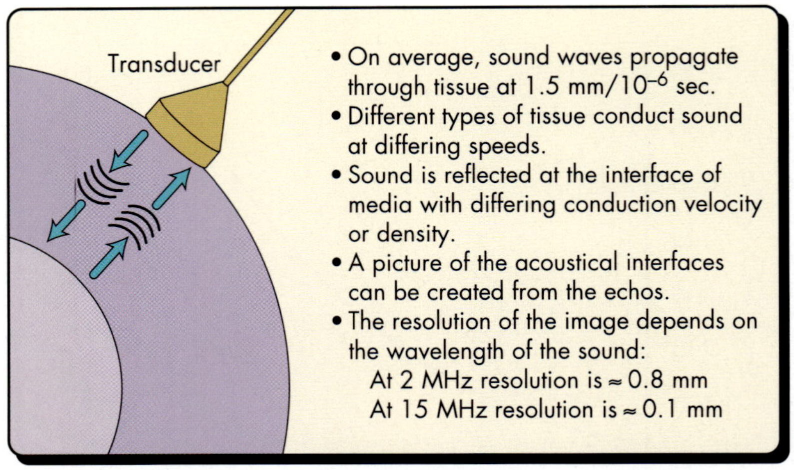

Figure 2-25. Ultrasound. Ultrasonic waves are generated by electrically pulsing a piezoelectric crystal at the desired frequency. Since these crystals change shape with applied voltage, they generate the required sound waves. This transduction also works in reverse, that is, when mechanically deformed by sound waves reflected by the target, the crystals generate electricity.

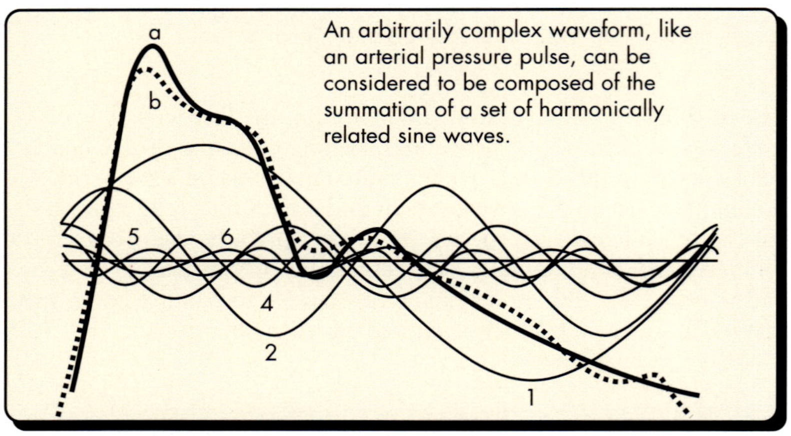

Figure 2-26. Fourier's theorem. Fourier's theorem states that any arbitrary, complex but repetitive waveform (like an arterial pressure wave or an electrocardiogram) can be considered to be composed of a series of simple sine waves. The slowest sine wave is called the fundamental and is the frequency of the repetition rate of the complex wave. The other sine waves are all harmonics (integer multiples of the fundamental frequency) but may vary in amplitude or phase as required to summate to the original waveform. An original arterial waveform "a" is decomposed into six sine waves. Adding the six sine waves together yields "b," a close representation of "a." One may add higher harmonic sine waves (*ie*, waves 1 through 6) until the desired level of accuracy in reproduction is attained.

ELECTRICITY

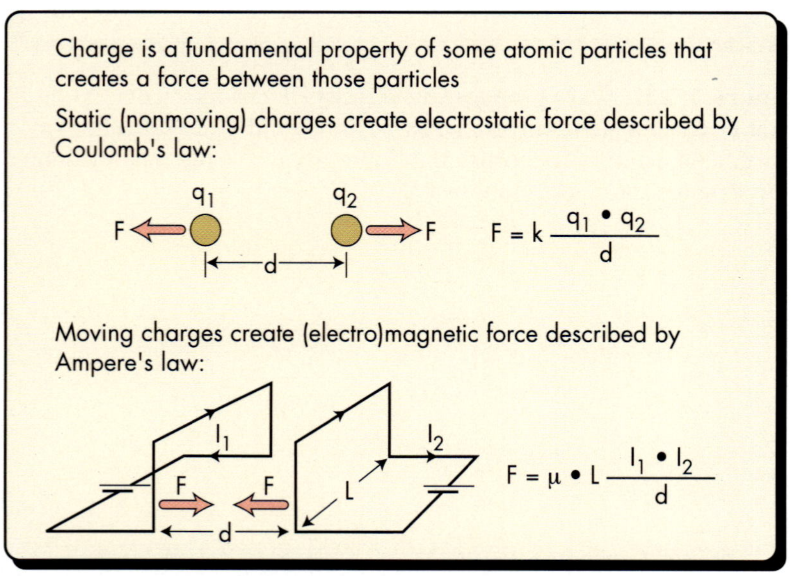

Figure 2-27. Electric charge. Electric charge is a fundamental property of electrons and protons. Each complete atom has an equal number of positive and negative particles, leading to a net charge of zero. If an atom loses or acquires electrons, it becomes an ion with a net nonzero charge. The unit of charge is the Coulomb, which is equal to the charge carried by 6.25 x 10^{18} electrons or protons. Like charges repel each other, and unlike charges attract. The force is proportional to the product of the net charges (q_i) and inversely proportional to the square of the distance (d) between them.

A moving charge is known as a current (I), which is measured in amperes (coulombs/second). Currents create another force, electromagnetism, which forms the basis for electromagnets and motors. In a model of parallel wires, this force is proportional to the product of current flow and the length of the parallel run (L) and inversely proportional to the distance (d) between them. Finally k and μ are proportionality constants relating charge to force.

The volt is a measure of potential energy created by separating charge:

$$1 \text{ volt (V)} + \frac{1 \text{ joule (S)}}{1 \text{ coulomb (C)}}$$

where 1 C = the charge carried by $6.25 \bullet 10^{18}$ electrons

Wires provide some resistance to current flow, defined as:

Resistance = voltage/current (Ohm's Law)

Figure 2-28. Current flow. Separating unlike charges requires work, which is stored in the system as potential energy. The volt is the unit of this potential energy. Voltage (potential energy) is always measured between two points, usually a point of interest and a reference site that is considered to have zero potential, the earth, otherwise known as "ground."

When the potential energy of charge separation is consumed by current flow in a wire (reuniting charge), some of the energy is lost to heat due to inefficiencies in moving the charge through the material of the wire. Materials like metals that allow passage of current with high efficiency are called conductors; materials that have very low efficiency are insulators. The efficiency of conduction is measured in terms of "resistance," measured in ohms. As summarized by Ohm's Law, for a given voltage across a wire, the higher the resistance of the wire, the smaller the current flow.

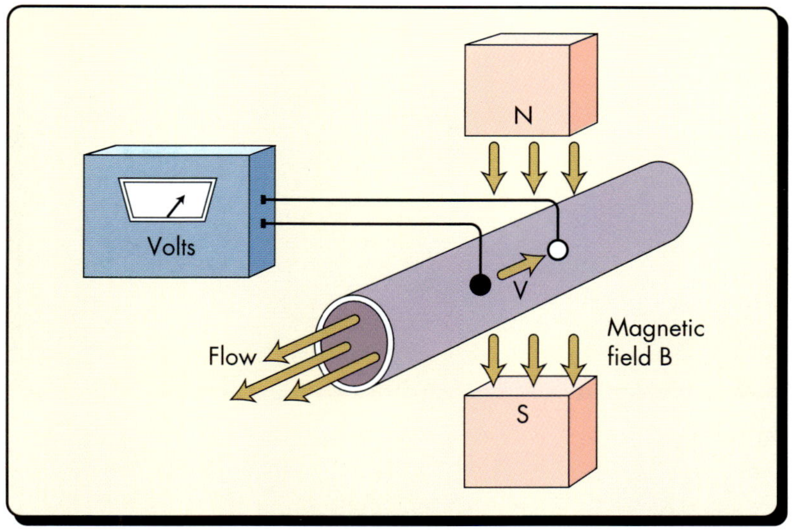

Figure 2-29. Electromagnetic flowmeter. The electromagnetic flowmeter is an application of Faraday's Law, which states that voltage is generated within a conductor that moves across a magnetic field. The voltage is proportional to the rate at which the moving conductor cuts magnetic field lines, *ie*, the speed of the fluid and the intensity of the magnetic field. N—north pole of magnet; S—south pole of magnet; V—voltage.

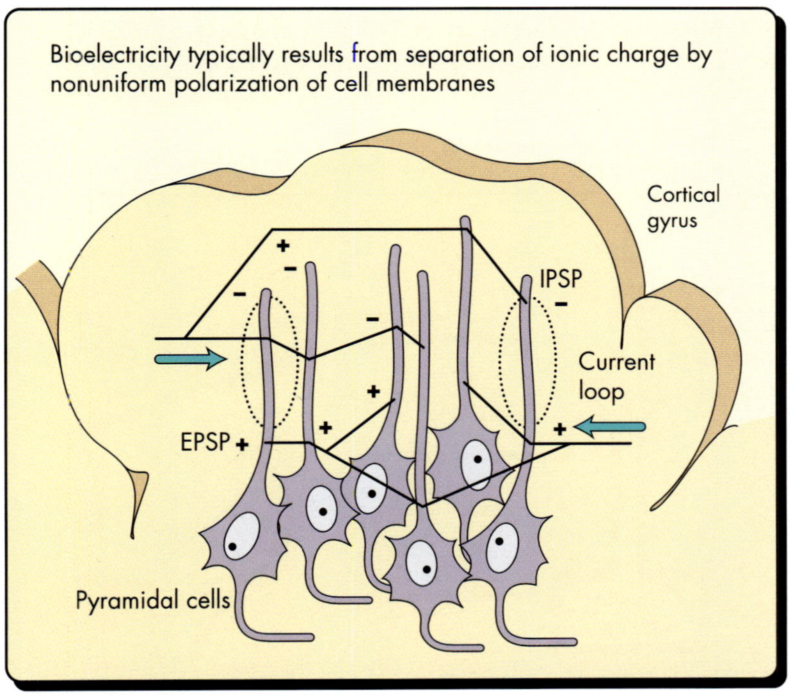

Figure 2-30. Bioelectricity. The brain and the heart generate relatively large electrical signals. These signals are due to the synchronous depolarization and hyperpolarization of thousands to millions of cells. If the geometry is favorable, the minute current loops surrounding each electrically active cell summate to produce relatively large ionic currents that can be detected on the skin. EPSP—excitatory post-synaptic potential; IPSP—inhibitory post-synaptic potential.

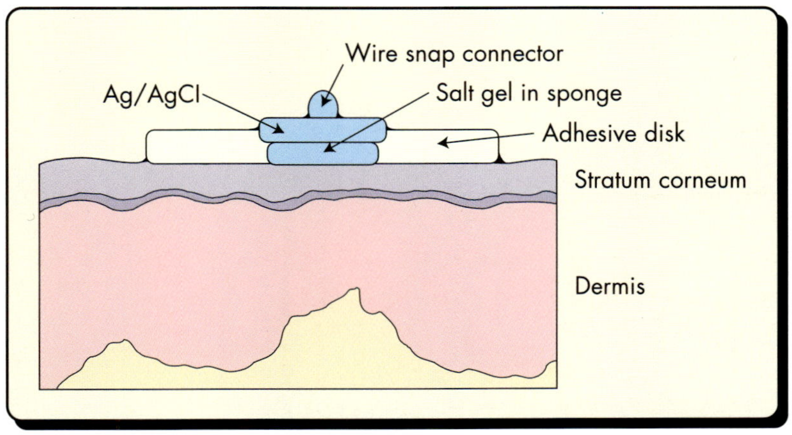

Figure 2-31. Bioelectric electrodes. In tissue, electric currents are carried by the flow of chemical ions, both positively or negatively charged, whereas in metal wires, current is carried by the flow of electrons. Skin electrodes are transducers, converting between these different types of current. Many types of metal have been discovered to be suboptimal for this purpose because they form a kind of unstable battery at the interface of the metal and body fluid. The ubiquitous electrode combination of silver (Ag) with a silver chloride (AgCl) coating minimizes this electrode potential and thus provides the least distortion of bioelectric signals. The noise immunity of skin electrodes can be improved further by scratching through the stratum corneum, which lowers the resistance of the contact [2].

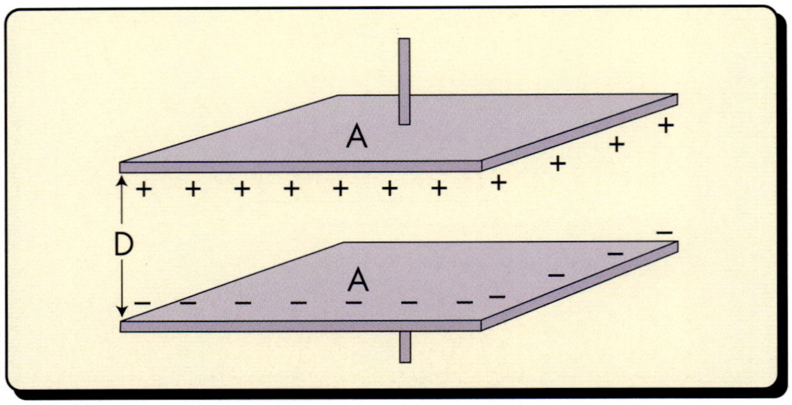

Figure 2-32. Capacitance. In mechanical systems, energy may be stored in springs. Capacitors serve the same purpose in electrical systems. The separation of equal quantities of unlike charges on metal plates separated by an insulator creates a potential (voltage). The voltage is equal to a ratio of the quantity of charge (in coulombs) divided by a geometric factor called capacitance. Capacitance has the units of farads and is proportional to the area (A) of the plates and inversely proportional to the distance (D) separating them and to a property of the interposed insulator known as the dielectric constant.

Electrical energy can also be stored in a magnetic field created by current flowing through a wire. This type of energy storage can be enhanced by winding wire into a coil, which increases magnetic field strength.

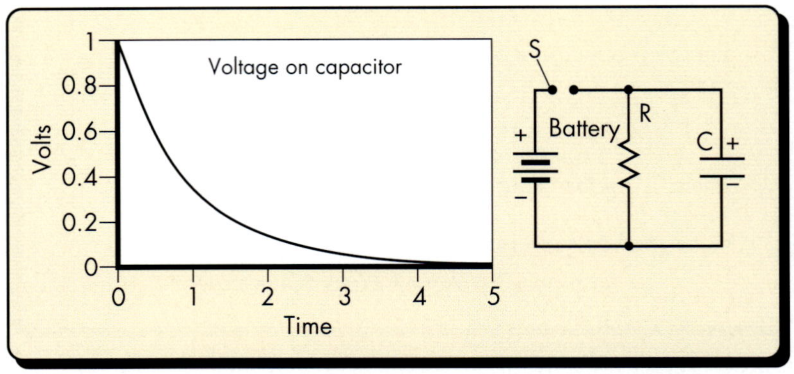

Figure 2-33. Time constants. Capacitors tend to retard changes in applied voltage. In the illustration, when the switch (S) is closed, the battery applies a voltage of, say, 1 V across both the resistor (R) and the capacitor (C). When the switch opens, there is no longer an extrinsic energy source to maintain the voltage. If there were no resistor in the circuit, the capacitor might remain charged forever since there would be no way for the charges separated by the battery to reunite. With the resistor present, electrons can run through this circuit element and eventually completely discharge the capacitor.

The rate at which the capacitor voltage changes can be simply determined by differentiating the equation describing the voltage as the ratio of charge over the capacitance. Therefore, the rate of voltage change equals the current flowing into or out of the capacitor over the capacitance. Replacing the capacitor current with its Ohm's law equivalent (voltage/resistance) yields $dV/dt = I_C/C = -V/RC$.

The solution to this differential equation is: $V(t) = V_0\theta^{(-t/RC)}$, and RC is known as the time constant. The time constant is the time, in seconds, required for the voltage to decrease to $1/\theta$ or 0.367 of its initial value. After 5 time constants, the voltage is less than 1% of the initial voltage.

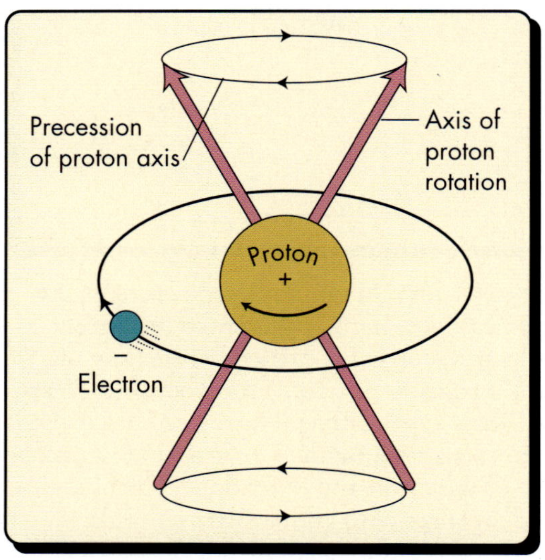

Figure 2-34. Magnetism. Magnets are recognized as objects that exert a force at a distance on ferrous metals and some other materials. Magnetic force has polarity, *ie*, poles commonly referred to as north and south, that appears to exist at diametric ends of the object and that attracts opposite poles and repulses like poles. Atomic nuclei and electrons spin and precess (the axis of spin itself rotates around another axis) like toy tops. They therefore comprise moving charges and generate, on a microscopic scale, the same kind of magnetic force as charges moving in a wire. Each nucleus forms a tiny bar magnet, and in most materials, the axes of the poles are oriented randomly. Some materials like iron allow their constituent nuclei to be coerced into a uniform orientation, creating an object with grossly discernible magnetic properties. The effect of a magnetic field is the same whether the field was created electrically, by the rotation of the Earth's metallic core, or by bar magnet.

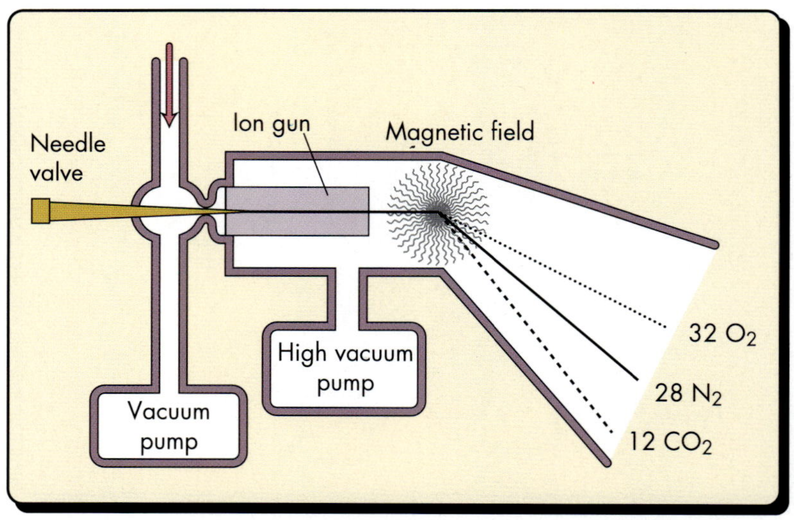

Figure 2-35. Mass spectrometry. A static magnetic field exerts a force on moving charged particles, forming the basis for mass spectrometry. In this device, a rarified stream of gaseous atoms and molecules is pulled into a vacuum chamber, one or more electrons are removed, and each resulting ion is accelerated to high velocity by strong electric fields (an ion gun). These freshly formed ions then pass through a magnetic field that is oriented perpendicular to their path, causing them to deflect from a straight line. Lightweight ions are deflected more than heavier species. The magnetic field thus spreads out a mixed stream of ions, like a glass prism separates the individual wavelengths of light. An ion detector at the end of the vacuum chamber measures the number of ions (sorted by weight) that impact on a moment-to-moment basis. CO_2—carbon dioxide; N_2—nitrogen; O_2—oxygen.

RADIATION AND SAFETY

- Photons are particles with enough energy to knock electrons from stable atomic orbits.
- Radioactivity is measured in curies (Li) (3.7 • 10^{10} disintegrations/sec
- Exposure (density of irradiations) is measured as the ionization of air in the path of a radiation beam. A roentgen (R) = 2.58 • 10^{-4} coulombs (C)/kg of air.
- Absorbed dose is measured in rads: 1 rad = 0.01 J/kg.
- Biological effect in rem (roentgen-equivalent-man) is a function of the number of rads times a quality factor dependent on the type of radiation.
- Natural radiation dose in the United States is about 80 mrem, a chest x-ray about 25 mrem, and a CT scan about 1 rem.

Figure 2-36. Ionizing radiation. CT—computed tomography.

Distance
- Stay out of the direct beam axis; collimated x-rays decrease linearly with distance
- Backscattered radiation decreases with the square of the distance

Shielding
- 1 mm of lead will stop 99.8% of a 100 keV x-ray
- Standard lead aprons have 0.25 or 0.5 mm of lead

Figure 2-37. Minimizing physician exposure.

ELECTRICAL SAFETY

Current	Effect
10 μA	Maximal allowable leakage current through indwelling catheters or electrodes
50 μA	Ventricular fibrillation (current applied via intra-cardiac electrode)
500 μA	Threshold of perception at skin;
1 mA	Ventricular pacing pulse applied to myocardium
5 mA	Maximal "harmless" skin current
10 mA	Maximal "let go" current
100 mA	Pain, possible fibrillation
-2.5 A	Ventricular fibrillation
≥ 6 A	Sustained myocardial and muscular contraction, tissue burns

Figure 2-38. Electrical safety. Nonphysiologic current flow through biological tissue is poorly tolerated, particularly if the current passes through organs that rely on electrical signalling, such as the heart and brain. Electrical safety is therefore centered on eliminating inadvertent currents and minimizing current flow around sensitive organs when electrical devices must be used in and near the body. The table identifies the thresholds of current flow associated with various levels of phsyiologic effect for a 1-sec exposure to 60–Hz (power line frequency) alternating current. These thresholds are not absolute and vary depending on the condition of the skin, the type of contact electrode, and so on. High current density causes heating, even cooking tissue.

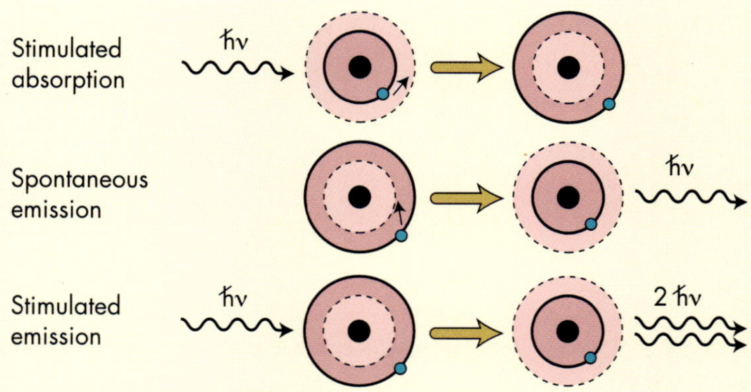

- Laser light is all one wavelength.
- All the photons travel in the same direction and all are in phase with each other.
- Thus there is no destructive interface or beam spread and the light can be precisely focused to create very high-power densities.

Figure 2-39. Stimulated emission and laser light. Photons may interact with orbital electrons in three ways: (1) stimulated absorption—a photon striking an electron may transfer its energy to the electron, pushing the electron into a higher energy orbit; (2) spontaneous emission—an electron in an orbit higher than the minimal energy state may spontaneously lose energy in the form of an emitted photon; (3) stimulated emission—an incoming photon may interact with an electron that is already in a high-energy orbit, with the result that two perfectly coherent, collimated photons leave the electron. ħ—Planck's constant; ν—wavelength of photon.

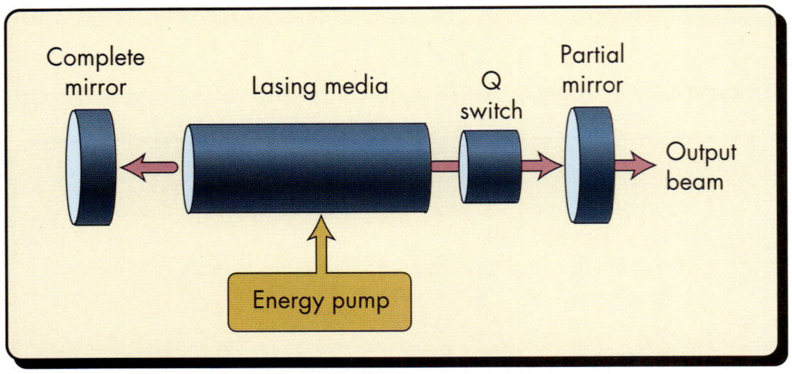

Figure 2-40. Generic laser hardware. A laser system consists of several components, irrespective of whether the laser is based on solid-, liquid-, or gas-based media. The central component is the lasing media itself. This may be a solid crystal of yttrium-aluminum-garnet with a small concentration (doping) of neodymium, or a tube containing carbon dioxide. The energy pump provides the means of pushing orbital electrons to a higher energy state. A pair of axial mirrors allow repeated passes of collimated photons through the media, allowing maximal amplification by stimulated emission. The mirror on the right is not 100% reflective, allowing the beam to eventually escape. The optional Q-switch increases the efficiency of pulsed lasers by allowing a small delay to increase pumping [3].

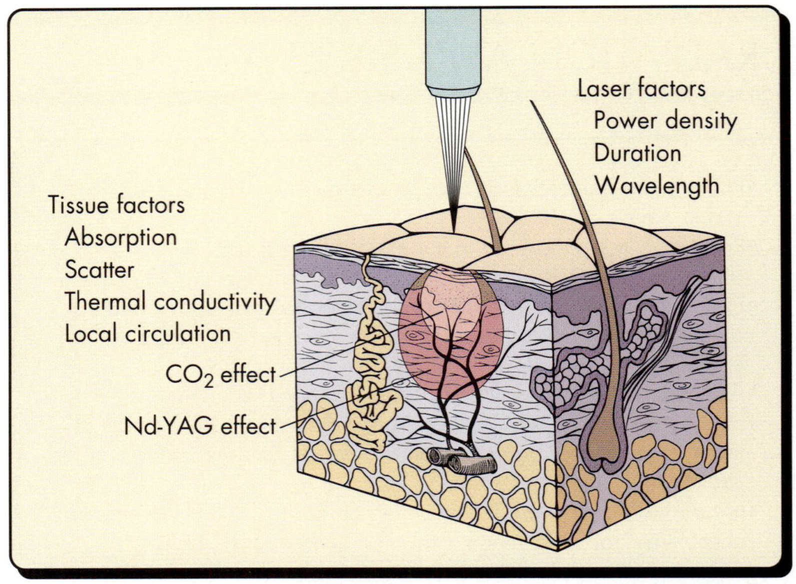

Figure 2-41. Laser light interactions with tissue. The therapeutic or surgical effects of laser light are due to the transfer of energy from the laser to the tissue. Long wave infrared from a carbon dioxide (CO_2) laser is strongly absorbed by water molecules, explosively converting superficial tissue to steam. Shorter wavelength infrared from a neodymium-yttrium-aluminum-garnet (Nd-YAG) laser is less completely absorbed by water, allowing coagulation of tissue to the depth of several millimeters. Alternatively, this near-infrared can be used to heat a sapphire probe which, in turn, is used as a direct contact scapel. Argon laser light is strongly absorbed by hemoglobin, making it useful in coagulating vascular lesions. New (excimer) ultraviolet lasers are intensely absorbed by tissue and can be used to shave the cornea by a few cell layers at a time.

REFERENCES

1. Ream AK, Fogdall RP: Acute Cardiovascular Management. Philadelphia: JB Lippincott; 1982:11.
2. Geddes LA, Baker LE: Principles of Applied Biomedical Instrumentation, edn. 3. New York: Wiley; 1989:315–452.
3. Rampil IJ: Anesthesia for Laser Surgery. In Anesthesia, edn. 4. Edited by Miller RD. New York: Churchill-Livingstone; 1994:2197–2211.

3

Pharmacokinetics and Pharmacodynamics for the Anesthesiologist

Scott T. Howell and Steven L. Shafer

An overview of the mathematical models that help define the clinical pharmacology of drugs used by anesthesia providers is presented in this chapter. The purpose of focusing on pharmacokinetic (PK) and pharmacodynamic (PD) models is to provide the reader with pictures that illustrate general pharmacologic principles. The types of drugs used by anesthesiologists are emphasized, *ie*, drugs given intravenously to achieve a rapid but short-lived duration of action. The derivation of mathematical models and the finer points of PK/PD modeling are discussed in less detail, since these topics are beyond the scope of this chapter and can be obtained from other texts. This chapter is organized by first explaining the role of mathematical modeling in general. These concepts are followed by actual PK/PD models presented as equations, computer simulations, and theory (pictoral form). More sophisticated models that take into account population variability and drug interactions follow. This information should provide a solid foundation to begin studying clinical anesthetic drug action. Whenever possible, clinically relevant examples will be used to "drive home" the importance of these concepts.

Before we begin our discussion, it should be noted that large numbers of anesthesiologists practice successfully without knowing *anything* about pharmacologic models. This raises a simple question: who *requires* a PK/PD model? There is a simple answer: *no one does!* We can titrate our anesthetic drugs based on clinical training and experience without complex models. However, by turning to models we can perhaps glean insight into choices of drug and doses that may provide for more rapid induction, reduced side effects, or more rapid emergence. In fact, the offset of drug effect is of great clinical importance. To achieve a timely offset of drug effect, the clinician constantly attempts to decrease the patient's blood concentrations as much as possible and yet still provide for unconsciousness and hemodynamic stability. The structure of the basic PK and PD models is explored, and their mathematical descriptions briefly considered, to try to convey the elegant simplicity of PK/PD models. Part of the elegance of these models is reflected in the small number of parameters that provide for surprisingly accurate predictions of the relationship between drug dose and drug effect.

THE ROLE OF PHARMACOKINETIC AND PHARMACODYNAMIC MATHEMATICAL MODELS

RELATIONSHIPS AMONG PHARMACOKINETIC PARAMETERS FOR A THREE-COMPARTMENT MODEL

Model Type		
Exponential Form (coefficients/exponents)	**Central Volume/Microrate Constants**	**Volumes/Clearances**
$A = (k_{21}-\lambda_1) \times (k_{31}-\lambda_1)/(\lambda_1-\lambda_2)/(\lambda_1-\lambda_3)/V_1$	$V_c(V_1)$	V_1
$B = (k_{21}-\lambda_2) \times (k_{31}-\lambda_2)/(\lambda_2-\lambda_1)/(\lambda_2-\lambda_3)/V_1$	$k_{10} = Cl_1/V_1$	$V_2 = V_1 \times k_{12}/k_{21}$
$C = (k_{21}-\lambda_3) \times (k_{31}-\lambda_3)/\lambda_3-\lambda_2)/(\lambda_3-\lambda_1)/V_1$	$k_{12} = Cl_2/V_1$	$V_3 = V_1 \times k_{13}/k_{31}$
$\alpha = \lambda_1$	$k_{13} = Cl_3/V_1$	$Cl_1 = V_1 \times k_{10}$
$\beta = \lambda_2$	$k_{21} = Cl_2/V_2$	$Cl_2 = V_1 \times k_{12} = V_2 \times k_{21}$
$\gamma = \lambda_3$	$k_{31} = Cl_3/V_3$	$Cl_3 = V_1 \times k_{13} = V_3 \times k_{31}$

Where λ_1, λ_2, λ_3 are complex functions of solutions to a cubic equation involving the microrate constants

Figure 3-1. The multicompartment model. Literature reports almost always employ the same general model for pharmacokinetic analysis, namely the "multicompartment model" (sometimes called the mammillary model). This model performs the most basic function required of PK models: the prediction of plasma (or blood) concentration over time when given a dosing scheme for a particular drug. The reason for popularity of the model is simple: it very often describes the clinical data! In addition to fitting the data, the model translates easily between various forms: the exponential form and compartmental models ("bucket and pipe" model). Furthermore, many of the details have been worked out for the use of these models in computer controlled infusion pumps and in "off the shelf" curve-fitting programs for PK/PD analysis. The mathematical form of the three-term (compartment) exponential equation (also called the drug disposition function, because it describes the "disposition" of drug over time) is $C_p(t) = \text{dose x } (Ae^{-\alpha t} + Be^{-\beta t} + Ce^{-\gamma})$, where $C_p(t)$ is the blood (plasma) concentration at time t, dose is the dosing input and A, α, B, β, C, and γ are constants whose values determine the shape of the disposition curve. For a two-compartment model, there would only be an A and B term (*ie* C = 0); for a one-compartment model, there would only be the A term. This equation incorporates many assumptions when used to describe PK data, among them: 1) all constants are just that—they don't change over time or over the range of drug concentrations, and 2) that the model is linear with respect to dose (simply put, if you give twice the dose over the same time, you will get twice the plasma concentrations). For clinical doses of most drugs, these assumptions are generally valid.

As already mentioned, the terms of the equation can be mathematically transformed to describe the components of the compartmental model that suggests some idea of the underlying clearances and physiology of volumes of distribution. The mathematical relationships between the coefficients/exponents, rate constants, and volume/clearances for a three-compartment model are given in the table shown here. Figure 3-8 illustrates the curve resulting from a bolus dose input into this equation.

As shown in Figure 3-7, drug is placed into the central compartment, and most PK models predict central compartment concentration (C_p). However, it is possible to examine drug concentrations in the other (peripheral) compartments (Fig. 3-9) and, by doing so, we can gain some insight into how C_p declines when drug input is stopped (Figure 3-10).

***Errata**: To properly comprehend the content of Chapter 3: Pharmacokinetics and Pharmacodynamics for the Anesthesiologist, the figures should be read in the following order:* 3.1, 3.8, 3.7, 3.9, 3.10, 3.4–3.6, 3.2, 3.11–3.13, 3.3, *and* 3.14–3.25.

$$C_e(t) = \text{Dose} \times k_{e0} \times \left[\frac{A}{\alpha(k_{e0}-\alpha)} e^{-\alpha t} + \frac{B}{\beta(k_{e0}-\beta)} e^{-\beta t} + \frac{C}{\gamma(k_{e0}-\gamma)} e^{-\gamma t} + De^{-k_{e0} t} \right]$$

Figure 3-2. Coefficient/exponent equation corresponding to the three-compartment kinetic model. Up to this point, only the blood (or plasma) concentrations over time have been discussed. However, we don't (usually) give drug to achieve a certain blood level, rather we are interested in achieving a particular effect. Therefore, what we really want is a description of kinetics where "the action is." This is accomplished mathematically by adding an "effect site" to the compartmental model (Figure 3-11). The coefficient/exponent equation that corresponds to the 3 compartment kinetic model with an effect compartment is shown in this figure. The equation includes the rate constant, k_{e0} which describes the rate at which drug moves from the central compartment into the effect site.

The terms are the same as discussed in Figure 3-1, except the $C_e(t)$ is the effect site concentration at time t, and D is a function of the coefficients (A, B, C), exponents (α, β, γ), and k_{e0} such that, at time 0, $C_e = 0$. (The curve resulting from a bolus dose input into this equation is shown in Fig. 3-12).

The preceding discussion of plasma concentration (C_p) profiles over time can be translated to similar discussions for effect site concentrations (C_e) over time. In general, C_e mirrors C_p but with a slight delay. For example, the same phenomenon of prolonged C_p decline for longer infusion periods (see Fig. 3-4) is also seen for C_e, except that the time required for the C_e decline is slightly longer than for C_p (due to the k_{e0} "delay"; see Fig. 3-13).

1 $$\text{Effect} = E_0 + \frac{E_{max} * C_e^{\gamma}}{C^{\gamma}_{50} + C_e^{\gamma}}$$

2 $$\text{probability} = \frac{C^{\gamma}_e}{C^{\gamma}_{50} + C_e^{\gamma}}$$

3 $$\text{Occupancy} = \frac{[L]}{K_{\alpha} + [L]}$$

4 $$\text{Occupancy} = \frac{C_e}{K_d + C_e}$$

Figure 3-3. Sigmoid Emax model. Up to this point, we've discussed the plasma and effect site concentrations and their behavior over time. However, the effect site concentration is often related to the actual drug effect in some "nonlinear" way. Said differently, if we double the effect site concentration, we may or may not double the drug effect. The nonlinear relationship between effect site concentration and drug effect is often described by an S-shaped curve (see Fig. 3-14B) called the Sigmoid Emax model (also referred to as the Hill equation). The shape of the Sigmoid Emax model is sigmoidal (of course), and has a maximal effect plateau (the "effect max" or Emax). The relationship is shown mathematically in *1*, where *effect* is the drug effect, E_0 is the minimal effect ("no drug effect"), E_{max} is the maximal change from baseline effect, E_0+E_{max} is the maximal effect, C_e is the effect site concentration, C_{50} is the effect site concentration that achieves a 50% response (*ie* an effect precisely halfway between E_0 and E_{max}), and gamma (γ) is a "steepness factor" that determines the shape of the response curve. This equation can easily be modified to reflect drug effects that are inhibitory rather than "excitatory", that is, this form illustrates a "positive" effect with increasing drug concentration, but many anesthetic drugs inhibit an effect (*eg*, opioids depress minute ventilation) and would use the inhibitory form.

It is interesting that the same general mathematical form found in the Hill equation also appears in the logistic regression equation and in the receptor occupancy equation. Logistic regression is a way of relating concentration to the probability of an effect. The minimum alveolar concentration (MAC) of inhaled anesthetic agents, well known to anesthesiologists, is based on logistic regression techniques and represents the end tidal concentration (and presumed effect site [brain] concentration) required to prevent 50% of patients from moving in response to skin incision. Therefore, at 1 MAC there is a 50% probability that a certain effect (no movement in response to incision) will be achieved. A logistic regression of a hypothetical drug is shown in Figure 3-15. The form of the logistic regression equation is shown in 2, where *probability* is the probability that the response (effect) will occur (value ranges between 0 and 1), $C_e$is the effect site concentration, C_{50} is the effect site concentration that produces a 50% probability of response, and γ is the "steepness factor" that determines the shape of the response curve (analogous to gamma in *1*).

Likewise, the receptor occupancy equation (for a simplified receptor system characterized by ligand molecule/receptor binding in a 1:1 ratio and receptors having a single affinity state) has a form very similar to that found in 2, where occupancy is the percentage of receptors occupied relative to total number of receptors available (value ranges between 0 and 1), [L] is the ligand concentration, K_d is the ligand concentration when 50% of the available receptors are bound (at steady state), as determined by receptor affinity. There is no "steepness factor" (γ) for receptor occupancy, provided it follows standard reaction kinetics. If we assume that the concentration of the ligand *in vivo* is proportional to the measured drug concentration, and consider K_d as the drug concentration associated with 50% receptor binding, then we can rewrite the equation in *3* to that shown in *4*.

The similarity of the equations in *1*, *2*, and *4* is not accidental. It is reasonable that there be agreement among mathematical descriptions relating concentration to either the magnitude of effect, the probability of an effect, or the occupancy of receptors that bring about the effect. However, receptor pharmacology is complex. Notice that the equation in *4* relates concentration to "occupancy", while the equation in 2 relates concentration to "drug effect." Fractional occupancy does not equal fractional drug effect, and thus K_d does not equal C_{50}. For example, the presence of "spare" receptors can alter the traditional concentration-occupancy-effect relationships (see Fig. 3-16B).

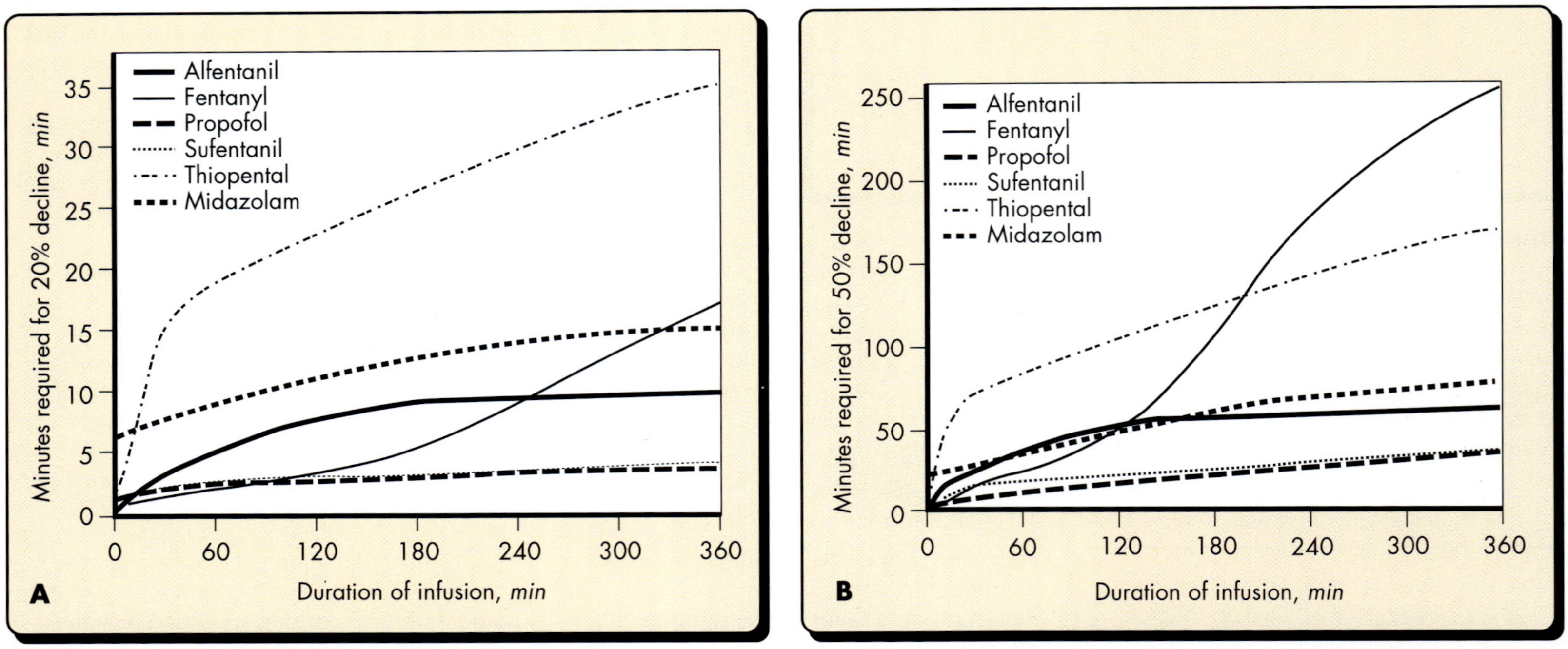

Figure 3-4. Time required for a 20% decline in plasma concentration of anesthetic. **A**, A graph illustrating the time required to get a 20% decrease in plasma concentrations (y axis) following a steady state intravenous infusion of varying duration (x axis) for selected drugs. Even for thiopental, whose elimination half-life is approximately 5.9 hours, a 20% decline takes only 35 minutes after a 6 hour (360 min.) infusion. For the other drugs shown, a 20% decrease in concentration occurs within 20 minutes, even after a 6 hour steady state infusion.

B, When a greater percent decrease is required, more time is needed. Shown here is the time required for a 50% decrease of the same drugs (sometimes referred to as the "context-sensitive half-time"; the context is infusion duration). As an example, fentanyl requires less than 9 minutes following a 4-hour infusion to achieve a 20% drop in plasma concentration, but for a 50% drop, 172 minutes are needed. This illustrates why careful drug titration is essential for timely recovery after lengthy procedures. *Panel B* also demonstrates that the published elimination half-life (sometimes called terminal half-life) poorly predicts how drug levels will decline following drug administration. Using the thiopental example, its elimination half-life of 5.9 hours grossly over-exaggerates the time to get a 50% decline, which is actually 166 minutes after a 6 hour infusion. (*Adapted from* Shaker and Varvel [1] and Hughes and coworkers [2].)

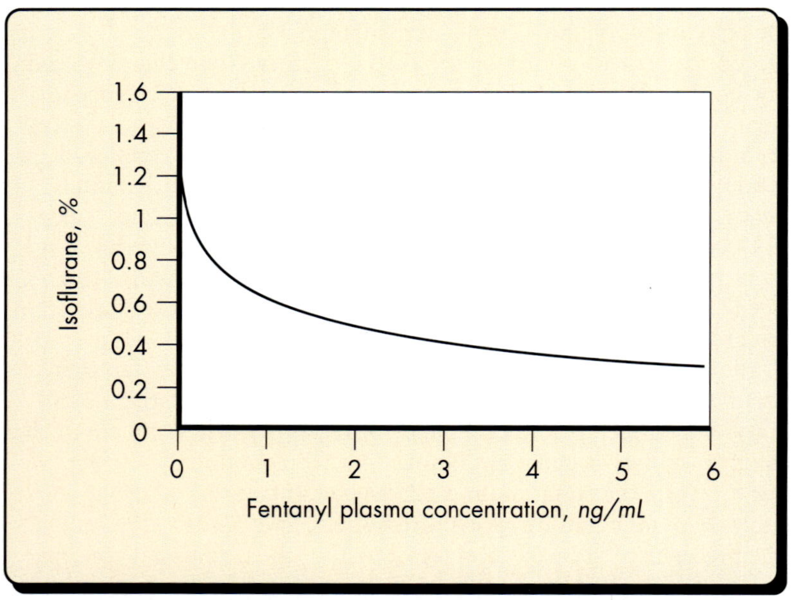

Figure 3-5. Mean alveolar concentration (MAC) reduction of isoflurane by fentanyl. Graph of end-tidal isoflurane concentration (in oxygen) versus mean fentanyl plasma concentration required for a 50% likelihood of no movement in response to skin incision (known to anesthesiologists as mean alveolar concentration [MAC]). The line shows that there is great benefit to achieving fentanyl concentrations of about 1.5 ng/ml, but that higher concentrations don't offer much in the way of MAC reduction. Even for very high fentanyl concentrations, some isoflurane is required to reliably suppress movement in response to incision. This supports the widely held belief that anesthesia is a combination of analgesic and hypnotic effects. Fentanyl is a poor hypnotic and thus requires a hypnotic contribution from isoflurane. The graph illustrates how useful clinical information provided by mathematical models can be. In this example, while the reader likely recognized that opioids reduce inhalational agent requirement, the lack of MAC reducing effect from very high fentanyl doses may offer new clinical insights. (*Adapted from* Westmoreland and coworkers [3].)

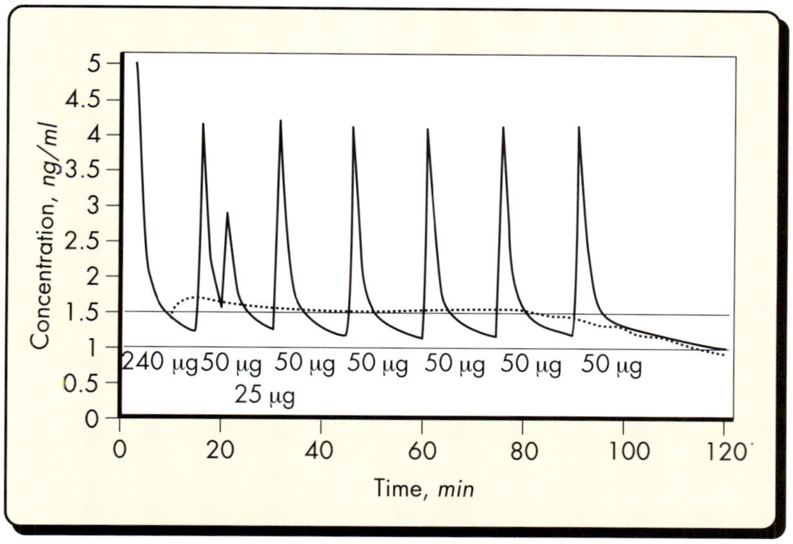

Figure 3-6. Comparison of simulated multiple bolus versus bolus/infusion dosing schemes for fentanyl. The bolus/infusion scheme is a "cookbook" approach based on PK models. The multiple bolus approach (*solid line*) simulates a theoretical 120-minute surgery where a 3 µg/kg bolus of fentanyl was given at induction and followed by 50 or 25 µg boluses as indicated. The bolus/infusion scheme (*dotted line*) also started with a 3 µg/kg induction bolus, which was followed by a 0.04 µg/kg/min infusion after 10 minutes. This was continued until 80 minutes when it was reduced to 0.03 µg/kg/min for ten minutes, when the surgeon announced he needed about 30 minutes to finish. The infusion was reduced to 0.02 µg/kg/min (90-min. mark) and then to 0.01 µg/kg/min at 100 minutes. Ten minutes prior to intended emergence, the infusion was stopped. The goal of the infusion "cookbook" was to achieve high plasma levels at intubation, then "drop and hold" at approximately 1.5 ng/ml for efficient MAC reduction (see Fig. 3-5). For emergence, the goal was to awaken the patient at 1 ng/ml to provide some analgesia at extubation. It is clear that the infusion approach provides a much more stable plasma level and avoids the high concentration peaks that accompany the boluses. By avoiding these periods of relative "overdosing," the patient actually receives less total drug (512 µg versus 565 µg). Note that even with careful titration, the bolus method has short concentration "dips" below the 1.5 ng/ml level. During the last 20 minutes of the case, the concentration profiles of the bolus and infusion approaches are nearly identical, suggesting that emergence times should be similar for both techniques.

If the infusion were carried out with a computer-controlled infusion pump (programmed with a pharmacokinetic model), the plasma targets of 1.5 and 1.0 ng/mL could be achieved precisely (in simulation). Furthermore, the use of a computer controlled infusion would permit the targeting of "effect site" concentration (that is, targeting a mathematical "site" where the drug is presumed to act), which some believe to be more useful than targeting plasma concentration. (*Adapted from* Scott and Stanski [4].)

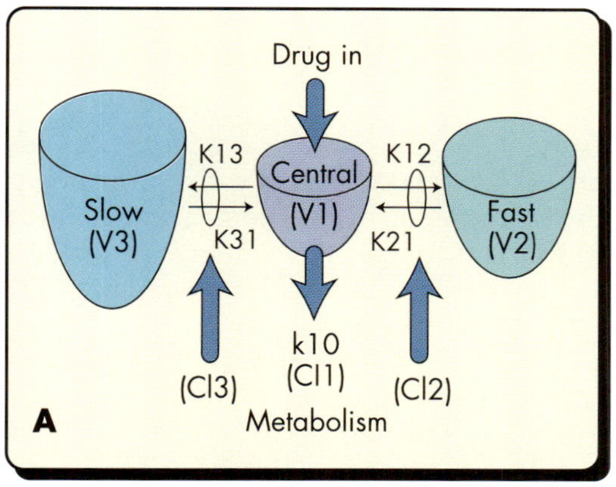

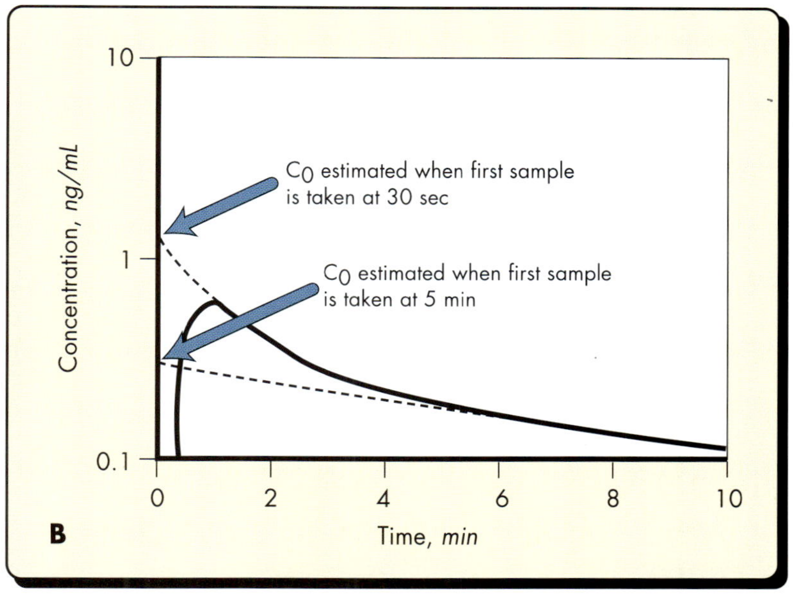

Figure 3-7. A three-compartment mammillary pharmacokinetic model. **A**, Following injection into the central compartment, drug moves between the different buckets (compartments) through pipes of various diameters. Drug is both infused into and sampled from the central compartment (V_c or V_1). The drug concentration in V_c immediately following an intravenous bolus dose represents the dilution observed by putting the dose (*eg*, 1 mg) into a volume (*eg*, 10 L) to get an initial concentration, C_0 (100 µg/L for 1 mg into 10 L). The V_c of 10 L might suggest that the drug "goes somewhere else" after given as a bolus, since, if it stayed in the exclusively in the blood, the expected volume of dilution would be 5 to 6 L (*ie*, total blood volume) in the average person. However, the V_c isn't a true volume, merely an "apparent volume" needed to get agreement between dose given and concentration measured immediately after dosing. V_c differs from actual blood volume because of several factors, the first being the assumption that the dose input is instantaneously mixed throughout the central compartment. This is not true for the first minute or two following a dose [5]. Other reasons why V_c is different from blood volume relate to assay technique, including whether protein bound or unbound drug is assayed, and when the first sample is drawn after dosing—the longer you wait, the lower the apparent C_0 (**B**), and thus the larger the apparent dilution volume. However, while all of these factors may lead to somewhat inaccurate estimates of the central volume, kinetic analyses usually ignore these phenomena and still produce reasonable predictions of the overall kinetic profile, provided the first minute or two is not of particular clinical interest.

Drug transfer among the compartments is described by rate constants (usually called microrate constants to avoid confusion with other rate constants) or by clearances, each of which is mathematically related to the other (see Fig. 3-1). In most literature, the kinetic parameters are reported either as coefficients/exponents, central volume/microrate constants, or as volumes/clearances. Regardless of which form is used there must always be two parameters specified for each compartment of the model, *ie*, a three-compartment model requires six parameters, a two-compartment model requires four and so on.

We shall discuss the behavior of drug concentrations in the each of the compartments later, but for now we caution that the volumes and clearances illustrated are not representative of any anatomic structures, just as V_c doesn't represent blood volume. Reports in the literature may refer to the slow peripheral compartment (V_3) as the "fat" compartment and the fast peripheral compartment (V_2) as the "vessel rich" compartment, but we stress that the size of the buckets, and the rate of drug transfer between them is purely a mathematical convenience that gives the disposition curve the proper shape to best describe the observed data. In other words, when a computer program is finding the best line to fit through the data, it does not consider any anatomic correlation whatsoever. That being said, there may be some correlation between central clearance (Cl_1) and actual total drug clearance from the body and the volume of distribution at "steady state" ($Vd_{ss} = V_1 + V_2 + V_3$) with the overall distribution of the drug in the body (as dictated by properties of the drug, such as lipid solubility).

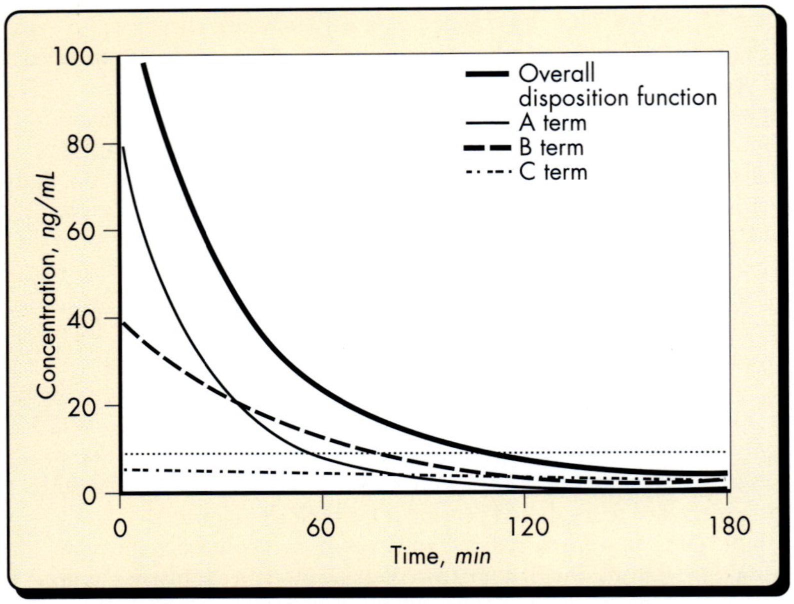

Figure 3-8. A generic three-compartment disposition function (see equation in Legend of Fig. 3-1) showing the contribution of the three components (A, B, and C terms) following a single bolus dose, given at time 0. As shown in Figure 3-1, the relationship between the A, B, and C terms and the volumes and rate constants shown in Figure 3-7 are fairly complex for three-compartment models. In the case of a one-compartment model, the A term (the only term) is 1 divided by the volume of the central (and only) compartment. As more compartments are added, the complexity of drug exchange prevents any single term of the equation in Figure 3-1 from completely describing drug behavior in the central volume.

As indicated in the equation of Figure 3-1, concentration of drug in the plasma (*thick solid line*) is equal to the sum of the three individual component lines. For early time points, *eg*, less than 60 minutes following the dose, the contribution of the C term to the overall disposition function is small compared with the A and B terms. This explains why the same drug may be reported in the literature as a two-compartment model in one paper and as a three-compartment model in another; if the first paper only sampled drug concentrations for 60 minutes, then the C term would not be needed to describe the measured data (thus requiring only two terms or a two-compartment model). In addition, the drug's assay sensitivity may influence the model structure. For example, if the lower detection limit of a drug assay was indicated by the *thin dotted line* (around 10 concentration units), then models using this assay would almost always be two-compartment models because there are few data above the limit of detection that would benefit from including the third exponential (the C term). This also explains why PK literature rarely uses more than three-compartments: the assay would need to be extremely sensitive and, for most drugs, the duration of a study designed to gather enough data to adequately describe the D term (not shown, but would lie between the C term line and the x-axis) would be impractical. In addition, clinical usefulness of the "trace" concentrations described by the fourth term would be dubious. Nearly all drugs in the anesthesia literature are reported as two- or three-compartment models.

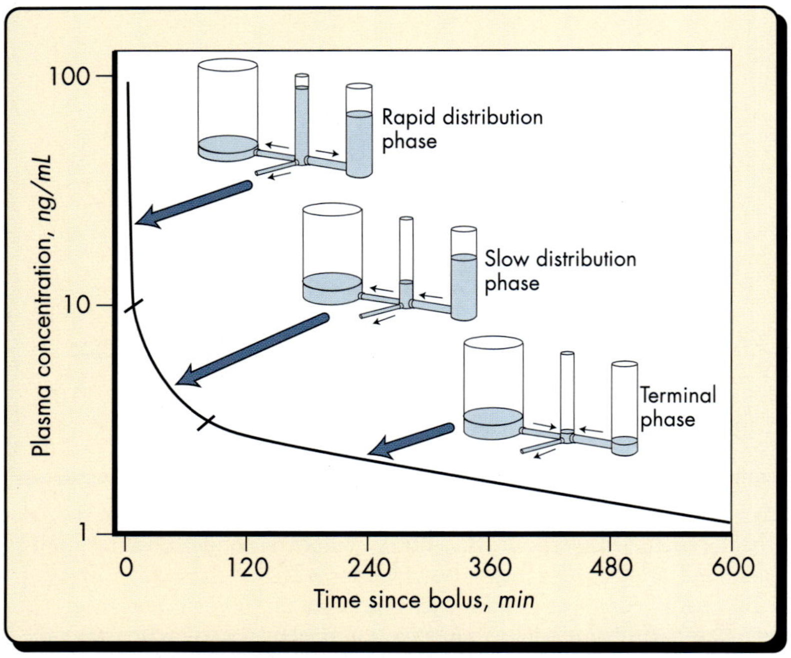

Figure 3-9. Illustration of the three phases of drug disposition in a three-compartment system with correlation to a hydraulic model. The fluid volume in each compartment illustrates the amount of drug in that compartment at any given time and the height is proportional to drug concentration in the compartment. The central compartment (V_1) is located in the middle of the diagram, the "fast" (V_2) and "slow" (V_3) peripheral compartments are to the right and left, respectively (as viewed)). Note that soon after bolus dosing, drug is contained almost exclusively in V_1 and V_2. As time passes, the relative contribution of V_3 increases to the point where it becomes a reservoir infusing drug into V_1 during the terminal phase. This "peripheral to central infusion" is an important consideration when understanding the longer decrement times required for infusions of increasing duration shown in Figure 3-4. This is discussed further in Figure 3-10. (Hydraulic model diagrams courtesy of Dr. Elizabeth Youngs, Palo Alto Veterans Administration Hospital, Palo Alto, CA).

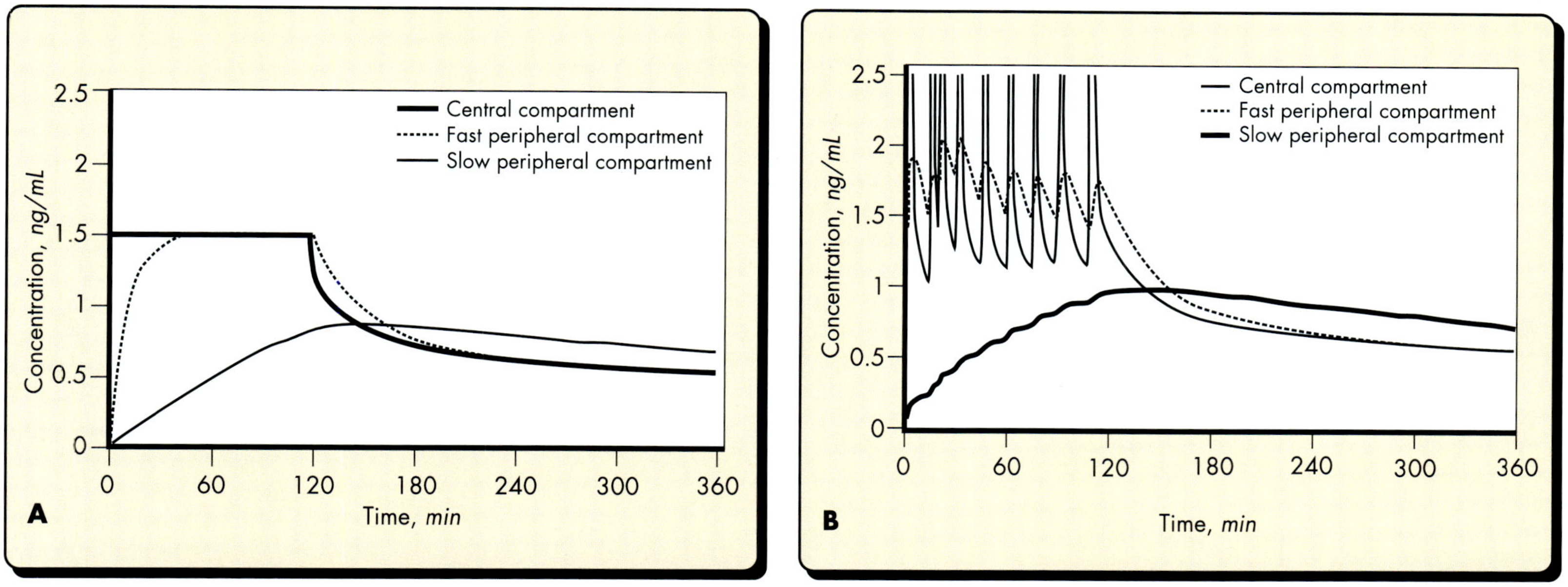

Figure 3-10. Drug concentrations in various compartments. **A**, A theoretical "instant" steady state infusion that achieves a plasma concentration of 1.5 ng/ml and maintains it for 120 minutes, at which point the infusion is terminated. The decline in plasma concentration after stopping the infusion is determined both by the clearance out of the central compartment (Cl_1) and the amount of drug returned to the central compartment from the peripheral compartments. During infusion, the fast peripheral compartment equilibrates (in this example) with plasma concentration at around 45 minutes, while the slow compartment doesn't achieve equilibrium, reaching 54% of plasma concentration at 120 minutes. When the infusion is stopped, plasma concentration drops below the concentrations in the two peripheral compartments, setting up concentration gradients that return drug to the central compartment. The fast peripheral compartment returns all of its "surplus" drug by about 220 minutes (100 minutes after infusion end), while the slow peripheral compartment maintains a concentration gradient for a great deal longer. As one "fills up" the slow peripheral compartment with greater amounts of drug (as would occur during a longer infusion), there is more drug stored that will eventually return to the central compartment, thus prolonging the decline of plasma concentration when the infusion is stopped. This is the basis for the longer "context-sensitive half-times" in Figure 3-4. **B**, Bolus dosing. The same general phenomena can occur for multiple bolus dosing. Because of higher concentration peaks after bolus dosing, more drug is "driven" into the peripheral compartments, thus "filling" them more than a comparable steady state infusion. In this example, both dosing schemes maintained a median plasma concentration of 1.5 ng/ml for 120 minutes. The greater amount of drug returning from the "fuller" peripheral compartments prolongs the plasma concentration decline; for a 50% decline (from the concentration at 120 minutes), the bolus approach required 85 minutes, while the infusion scheme required only 48 minutes.

EFFECT SITE

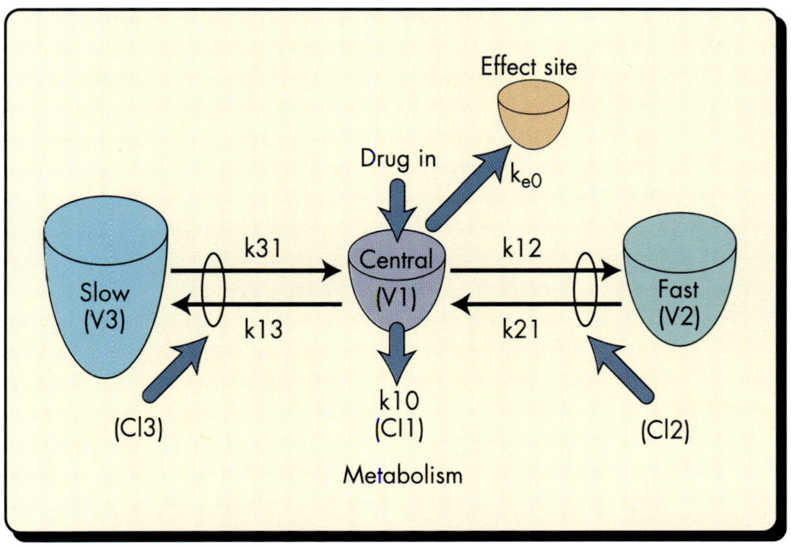

Figure 3-11. Pharmacokinetic model from Figure 3-2 incorporating the effect site (sometimes called "effect compartment" or "biophase"). The assumptions of the effect compartment include (1) it is too small to affect drug concentrations in the central compartment (we arbitrarily assign a volume of V_c/10,000) and (2) that effect itself is an instantaneous manifestation of the drug concentration in the effect site. The term "k_{e0}" is the equilibration rate constant between the plasma and the site of drug effect. The half time of equilibration is $0.693/k_{e0}$. If the plasma concentration is held constant, then in one plasma-effect site equilibration half time ($0.693/k_{e0}$) the concentration in the effect site will be half the plasma concentration, in two plasma-effect site equilibration half-times the concentration in the effect site will be three fourths of the concentration in the plasma, and so on.

Even though the actual amount of drug in the effect compartment is small, the concentration of drug in the effect site (called C_{effect} or C_e) is extremely important; in essence, we attribute *all* of the observed drug effect to whatever C_e is obtained following drug dosing. As in Figure 3-7, there is no defined anatomic correlation to the effect compartment. The effect site, if it exists at all, is the immediate milieu of the receptor. Thus, were one to measure drug concentration in CSF or ground brain, it is unlikely that the concentration measured would ever correspond to the effect site concentration. Additionally, the effect site concentration is normalized to the plasma concentration at steady state. The "true" concentration in the effect site will be offset by the relative solubilities of the drug in plasma and at the site of drug effect. However, the effect site remains an effective mathematical device that permits us to calculate the time course of drug effect: a prediction of great clinical relevance. That being said, we expect that there *are* some true effect sites in the body; in the case of opioids, for example, we attribute drug effect to the binding of various opiate receptors.

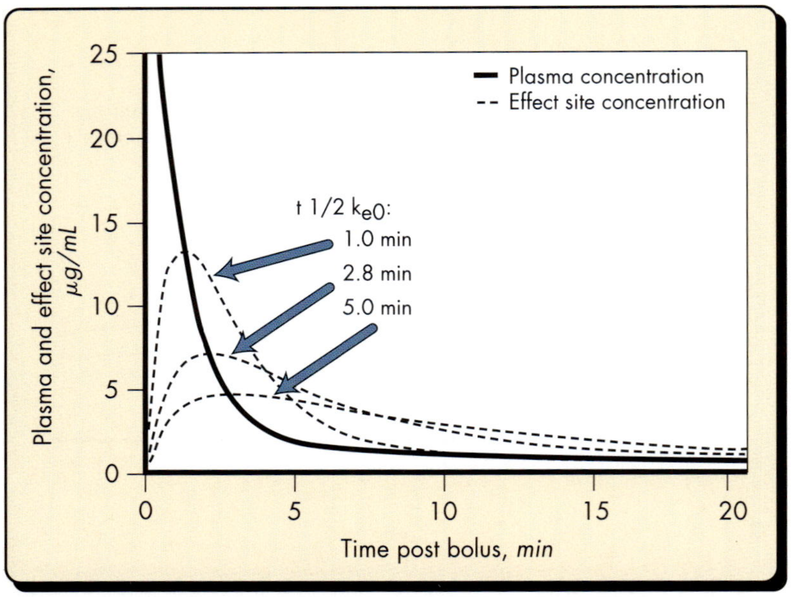

Figure 3-12. Plasma and effect site concentrations resulting from a bolus dose input, according to the equation in Figure 3-2. The effect site concentration ($C_e(t)$) is represented by the dashed lines. For comparison, the solid line shows the concurrent plasma concentration ($C_p(t)$)7 from the equation in Figure 3-1). As shown, there is a delay between the peak plasma concentration and the peak C_e because of the time required for drug to move from the central compartment into the effect compartment (See Fig. 3-11). This delay is dependent on the k_{e0}; a larger k_{e0} implies faster drug movement into the effect site and therefore higher (and faster) peak C_e for the same plasma concentrations. The graph indicates the "speed" of effect site equilibration by illustrating different $t_{1/2}k_{e0}$ (the k_{e0} "half-life" presented in Figure 3-11 as equal to $0.693/k_{e0}$). If a steady plasma level were "instantly" established, the effect site would require 4.5 $t_{1/2}k_{e0}$s to get to 95% of the plasma concentration. For a steady state plasma infusion, the C_e profile would appear similar to that of the fast compartment concentration profile as shown in Figure 3-10A.

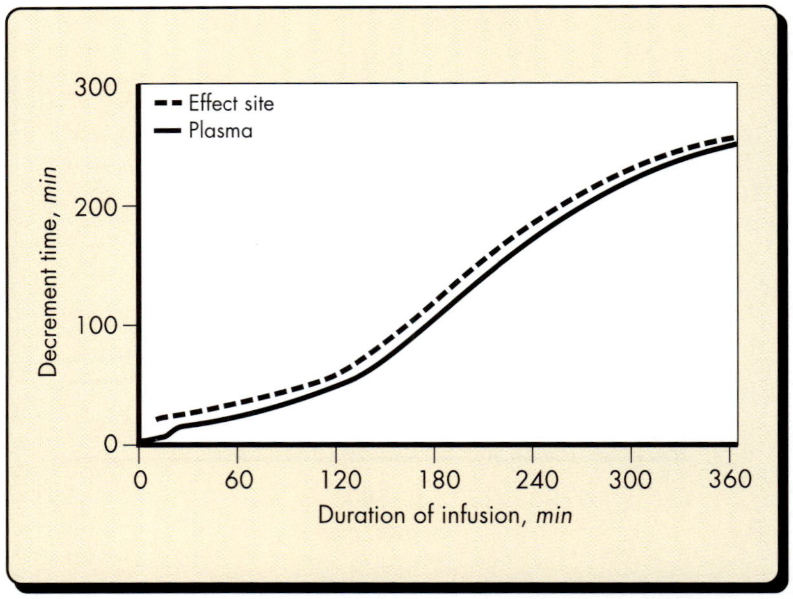

Figure 3-13. Plasma and effect site decrement times. The time required for a 50% decline in plasma and effect site concentrations for fentanyl following a steady state plasma infusion. To extend the terminology presented in Figure 3-4, we'll call the time required for effect site concentration decline the "effect site decrement time" (ESDT) and note that the ESDT parallels that for plasma, with an "offset" due to the time required to move drug out of the effect compartment (determined by the k_{e0}). The effect site decrement time has also been called the "relevant effect-site decrement time" when linked to a specific clinical effect [6].

SIGMOID EMAX MODEL

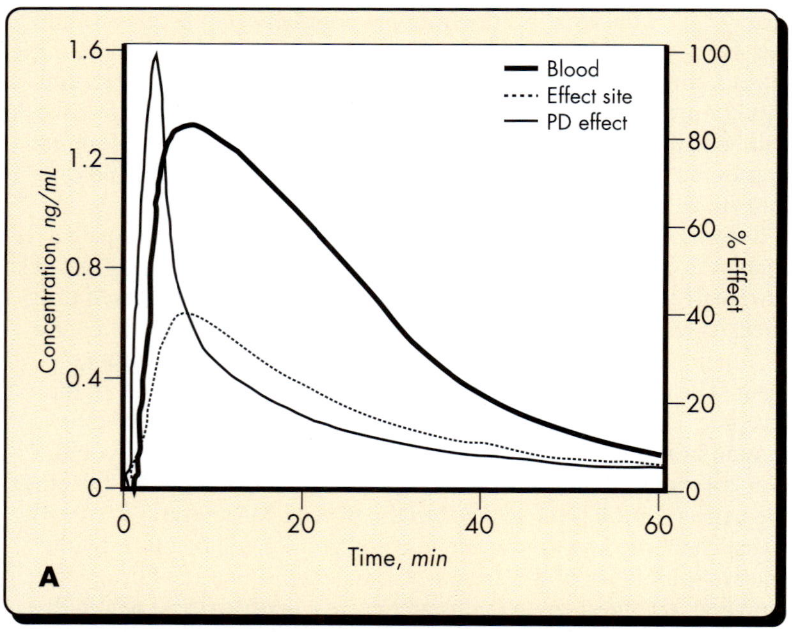

Figure 3-14. Effect site concentration. **A**, Concurrent plots of blood concentration, effect site concentration (left-hand y axis), and pharmacodynamic (PD) effect following a bolus dose (right-hand y axis). As shown in Figure 3-12, the effect site concentration peak is delayed compared with the blood peak. Since effect site concentration determines the magnitude of PD effect, the effect peak is delayed by the same amount as peak C_e.

(Continued on next page)

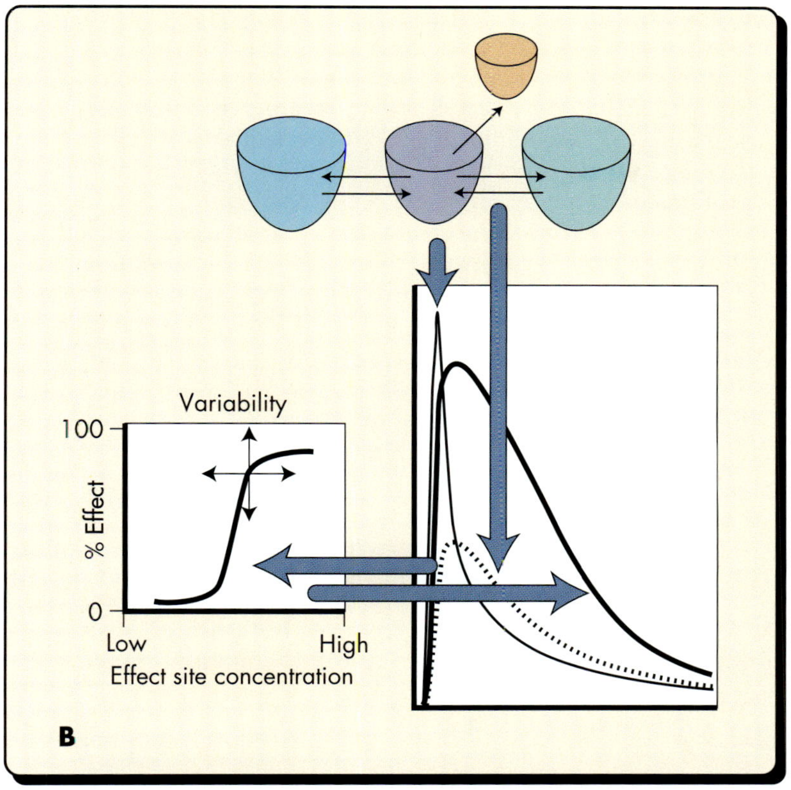

Figure 3-14. (*Continued*) B, Relationship between the compartmental model, effect site concentration, and PD effect. The concentration/effect profiles are the same as shown in *panel A*. The relationship between effect site concentration and PD effect is determined by the Sigmoid Emax model (Hill equation) as shown in the *lower left corner*. In any given population of patients, there is a variability between the amount of drug given and the magnitude/duration of the PD response, indicated by the *crossed arrows* on the sigmoidal curve. Variability is usually attributed to two areas: pharmacokinetic variability and pharmacodynamic variability. The kinetic variability results from the same dose producing different effect site concentrations in different people (*horizontal arrow*). This is compounded by dynamic variability, *ie*, a given effect site concentration produces a variable magnitude PD effect for different people (*vertical arrow*). Inability to accurately record drug doses and measure drug concentrations, as well as imprecise measures of drug effect, also contribute to variability.

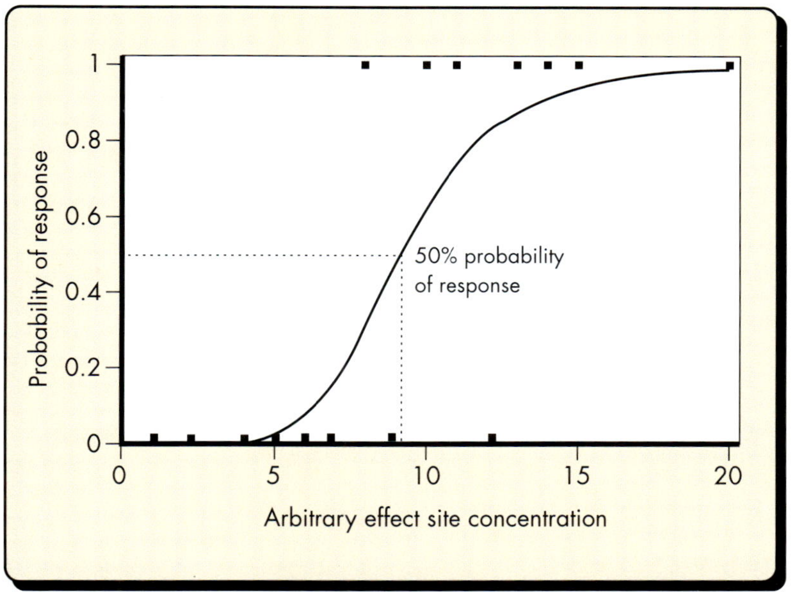

Figure 3-15. A hypothetical logistic regression fit from the equation in Figure 3-3B. The squares represent the presence or absence of a response at a given effect site concentration for various individuals. As shown, there is some overlap in effect site concentrations that produce positive/negative responses in different subjects. In this example, the C_e that produces a 50% probability of a response (C_{50}) is approximately 9.2 concentration units. The "steepness factor" (γ) in this example is 5.6. In general, the steeper the curve (*ie*, larger γ), the more predictable the response is, since the transition from low to high response probability occurs over a narrow range of effect site concentrations. Note the similarity of this curve with those shown in Figure 3-16.

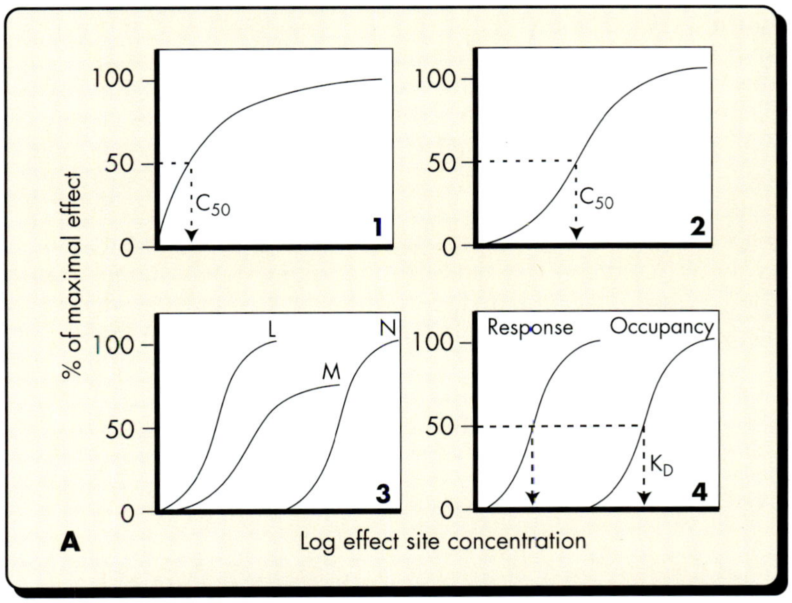

Figure 3-16. Effect site concentration, PD effect, and receptor interactions. A, Relationship among effect site concentration, magnitude of PD effect, and receptor occupancy. *Graph 1*, plot of the equation in Figure 3-3A, where agonist concentration (on the x axis) is taken to be equal to C_e. For this curve shape, γ approx 1. *Graph 2*, same as A except that the x axis is now on a log scale. Note that the curve reveals a sigmoidal shape using this scale. If γ were > 2 in graph 1, the shape of the curve (on a linear scale) would appear similar to graph 2; the larger the γ value the more "vertical" (steeper) the center portion of the curve. *Graph 3*, the effect of varying potency and efficacy for different drugs. Drug L is more potent than drugs M or N (has a lower C_{50}, *ie*, achieves 50% effect at a lower concentration); drugs L and N have more efficacy (have a higher E_{max}) than drug M, which would occur if M were a partial agonist. *Graph 4*, receptor occupancy doesn't always parallel the PD response due to signal amplification and second messenger activation. Therefore dose-response curves often fall to the left of receptor-occupancy curves.

(*Continued on next page*)

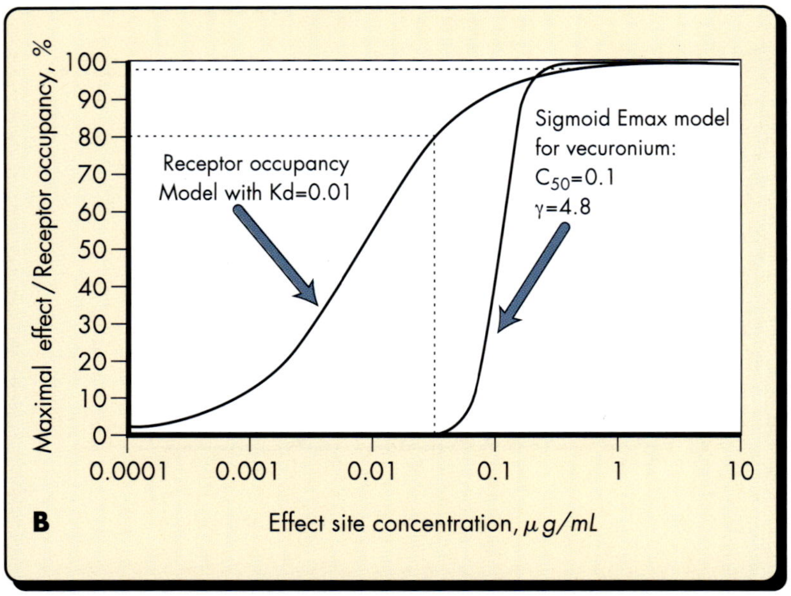

Figure 3-16. (*Continued*) This is not true when there are spare receptors, as in B, which shows the effect of spare receptors as found for neuromuscular blockade by vecuronium. The motor endplate of skeletal muscle has more acetylcholine receptors than needed to cause muscle contraction for the amount of neurotransmitter released into the synaptic space. The result is that while more than 75% of post-synaptic receptors are occupied by drug, paralysis is not present (0% effect). Neuromuscular blockade (the PD effect) requires that a greater percentage of receptors be blocked, thus the 0% to 100% PD effect (no blockade to paralysis) occurs over the range of receptor occupancy from about 80% to 100%. Unlike in *Graph 4*, the dose-response curve falls to the *right* of the receptor-occupancy curve. (Part A *adapted from* Ross [7]; part B *adapted from* Rupp and coworkers [8].)

THERAPEUTIC WINDOW

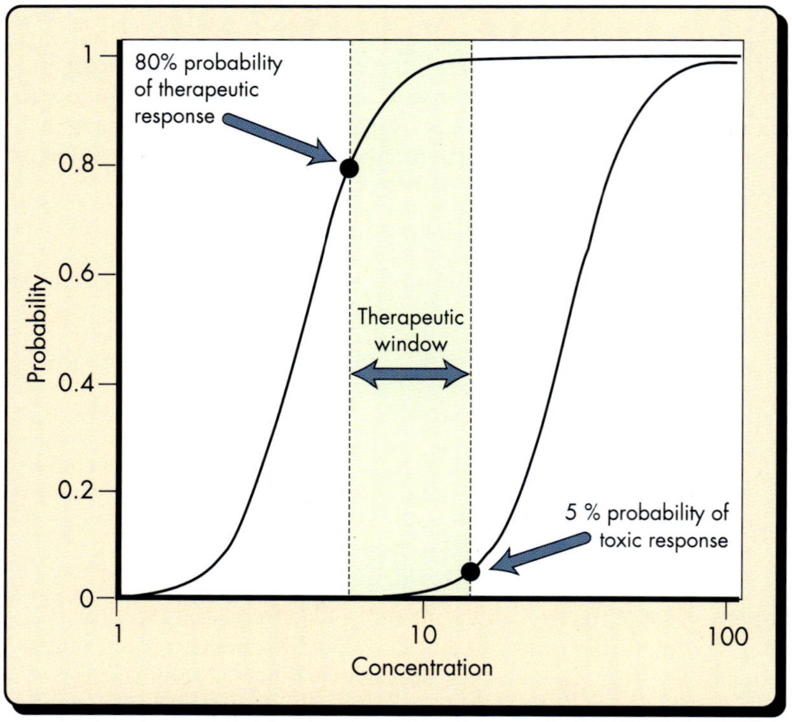

Figure 3-17. The probability of desirable and undesirable effects for a hypothetical drug. The *left curve* shows the probability of a desired (therapeutic) response, while the *right curve* shows the probability of an undesired response (toxicity). The distance between the curves, the therapeutic window, is determined by the properties of the drug and the type of effects being represented. For example, fentanyl doesn't exhibit significant hepatotoxicity or nephrotoxicity even in large doses, so the distance between the analgesia effect curve and the hepato/nephrotoxicity curve would be large. However, if respiratory depression and analgesia were plotted together, the therapeutic window would appear fairly narrow. Ultimately, clinicians (or lawyers) decide what the therapeutic window for a given drug is, depending on what is considered efficacious or toxic for a given patient.

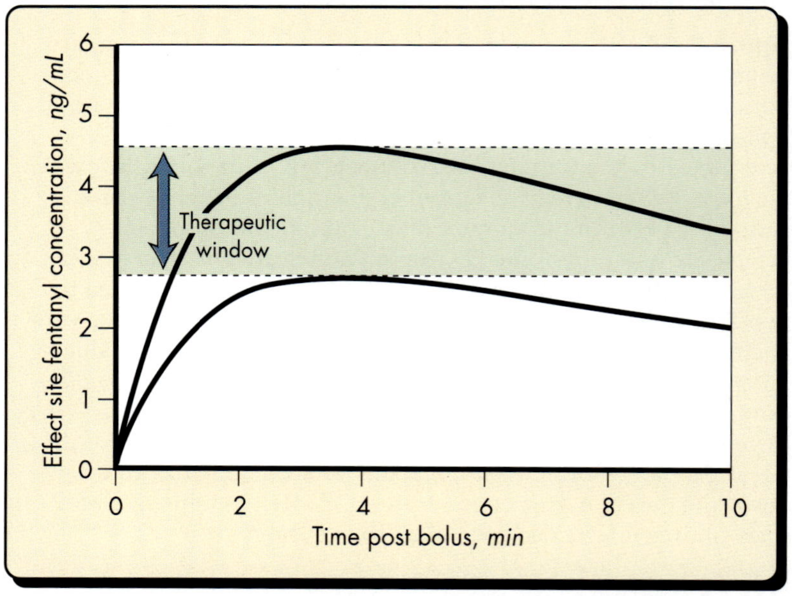

Figure 3-18. The effect site concentration curves resulting from a 3 μg/kg and a 5 μg/kg bolus of fentanyl. The therapeutic window shown is the Ce range recommended for anesthetic induction, when combined with an intravenous hypnotic. As illustrated, the smaller dose produces "therapeutic" effect site concentrations, but at a later time, and only transiently, when compared to the larger dose. One can achieve effective concentrations rapidly and for a longer duration by giving large doses. If a drug has a wide therapeutic window, this may be an acceptable technique. If the resulting concentration "overshoot" is associated with toxicity, such as muscle rigidity or delayed emergence, then the "overshoot" approach has obvious problems.

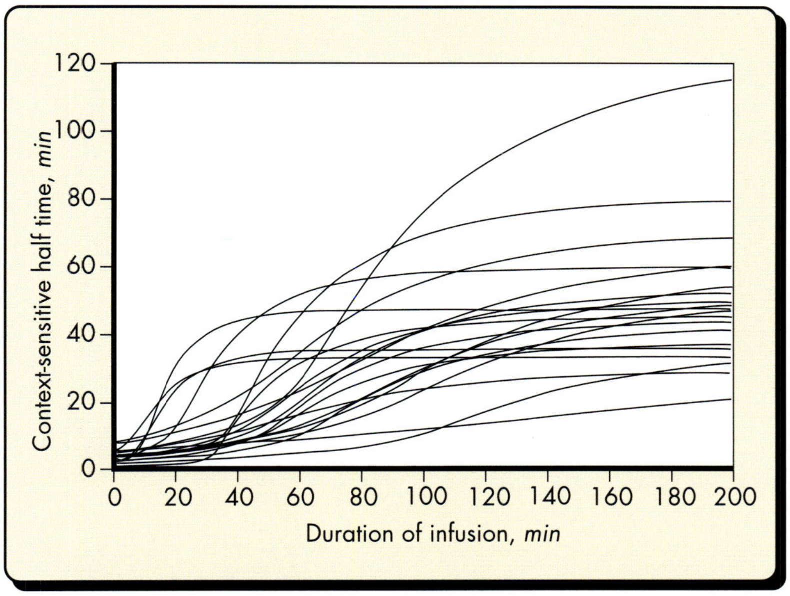

Figure 3-19. Estimates of context-sensitive half-times for fentanyl in individual pediatric patients. Note that the variability (in this instance, *kinetic* variability), covers a wide range of values and that a given individual may be at the lower end of the range at one point and at the high end at other points. As shown in Figure 3-13, the effect site concentration (C_e) mirrors the plasma concentration and subsequently would result in a variety of effect site decrement times similar to those shown for plasma. The variability of drug effect (dynamic variability) would likely be even greater than kinetic variability. A goal of PK/PD population modeling is to define the various patient characteristics that cause such variability in an effort to improve the accuracy of model predictions across a population.

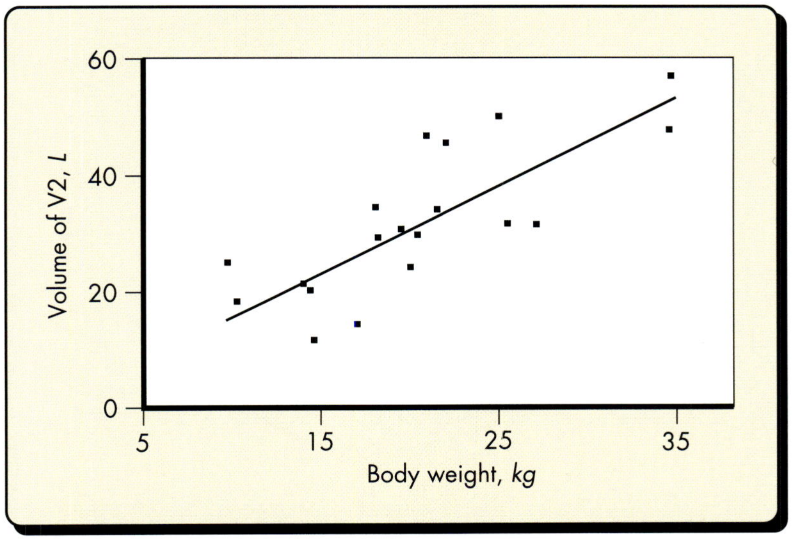

Figure 3-20. Individual volumes of V2 versus body weight. The estimates of the peripheral compartment volume (V_2) for fentanyl in the individual pediatric patients shown in Figure 3-19. Note the correlation between body weight and the volume of V_2. By taking this kinetic parameter-weight relationship into account, the PK model can improve its prediction accuracy. In effect, the variability seen in Figure 3-19 is partially explained by the inter-patient differences in V_2. Therefore, the observed variability in Figure 3-19 is not entirely random "noise" but is related to some measurable patient characteristic. Taken to theoretical extreme, if all significant characteristics (usually called covariates) could be accounted for, then all inter-subject variability could be explained. In the real world, we can never completely account for all factors that introduce noise into the measurements, but a PK/PD model that incorporates most significant covariates can improve prediction accuracy from an overall error of around 40% to a *prediction error* around 20% or less for many kinetic/dynamic analyses. Prediction error in this case is the amount that the model prediction "misses" the measured value; for example, if the PK model predicted a plasma concentration for a given person of 4 ng/ml at a specific time and the actual concentration was 2 ng/ml, then there would be a 50% prediction error at this time point. For a population model, the errors for all individuals at all time points constitute the overall percentage prediction error. For simplicity, the median (or mean) of these percentage prediction errors are reported.

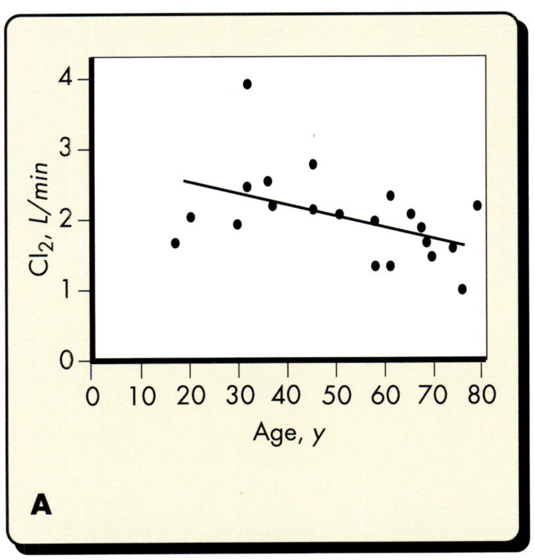

Figure 3-21. The clinical observation that older patients require less thiopental for induction has been examined by many investigators. It seemed reasonable that older patients would be more sensitive to the effects of barbiturates; that is, they would have a pharmacodynamic basis for their decreased dosage requirement (more effect for a given C_e). However, patient age did not change EEG patterns resulting from a given concentration of barbiturate [9].

(Continued on next page)

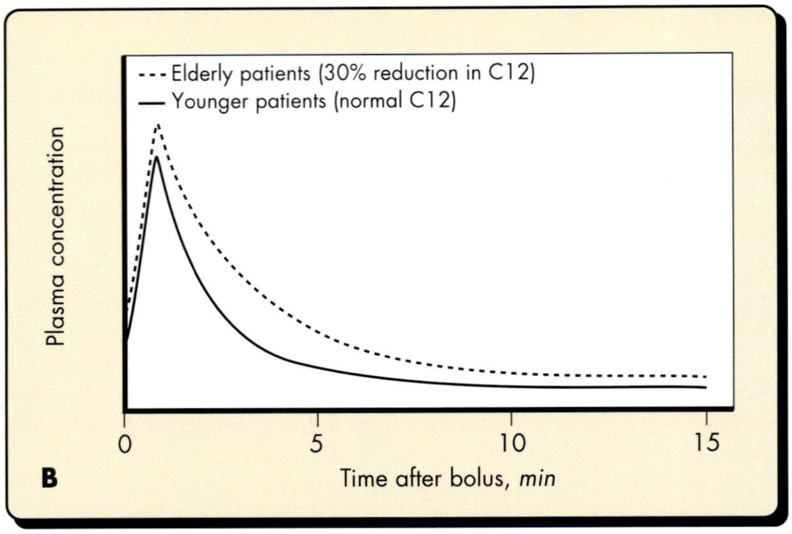

Figure 3-21. (*Continued*) It was subsequently shown that clearance into the second peripheral compartment (Cl_2) was reduced by approximately 30% in older patients [10] and that this reduction produces higher plasma (central compartment) concentrations (*ie*, less of the drug bolus moves from the central compartment into the second compartment in the early time period, **B**). Therefore, it is higher plasma (and higher effect site) drug levels that reduce thiopental requirements and not increased brain sensitivity with advancing age.

DRUG INTERACTIONS

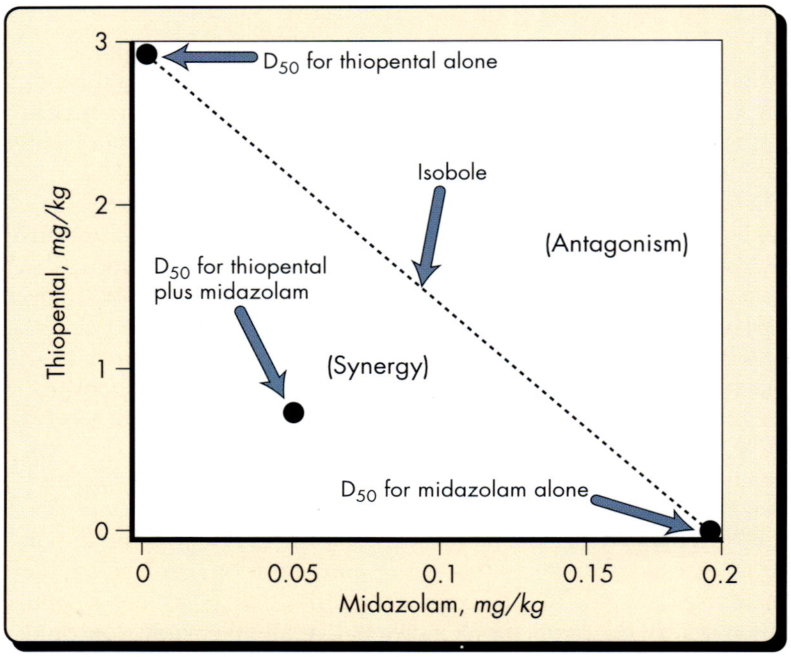

Figure 3-22. Interaction of thiopental and midazolam for induction of unconsciousness. The graph illustrated is called an isobologram and relates the effect of the two drugs as single agents and as combinations. The dose that induces unconsciousness in 50% of patients (D_{50}) by either drug alone is indicated by the x and y intercepts. If the drugs had a purely additive effect in producing unconsciousness, then various drug combinations would line up on the isobole. Combinations that fall to the left of the isobole are synergistic; those that fall to the right are relatively antagonistic. In this case, midazolam and thiopental are clearly synergistic. The isobologram illustrates a single probability of effect (here, it shows the doses to produce unconsciousness in 50% of patients); however, it is possible to derive a continuous "response surface" that shows a range of probabilities of effect, as shown in Figure 3-23.

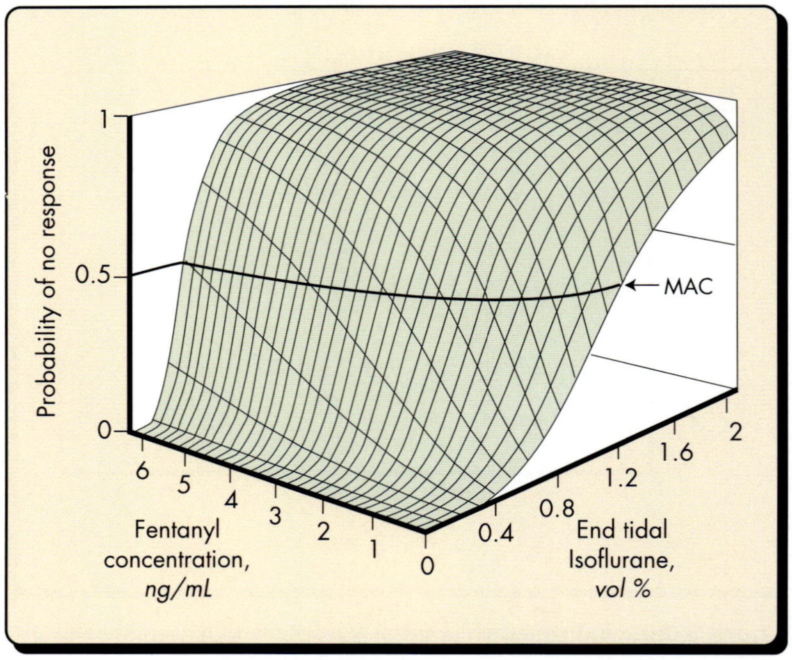

Figure 3-23. The response surface of various combinations of fentanyl and isoflurane in producing lack of movement to skin incision. This surface is an extension of the graph shown in Figure 3-5, which only shows the 50% probability of no response line (the traditional definition of MAC). However, if we were interested in the combination that produces a 90% chance that there would be no movement, we cannot get this information from Figure 3-5. It is available from the plot shown, as are other probabilities.

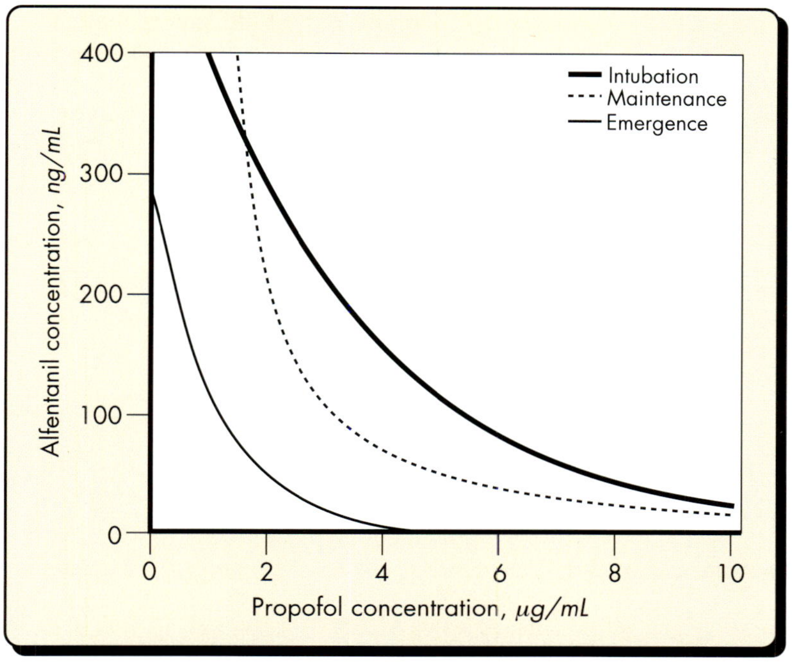

Figure 3-24. Concentration interactions between alfantamil and propofol for various anesthetic conditions. In addition to plotting a single effect isobologram as done in Figure 3-22, we can also plot a range of effects for a given combination of drugs. This graph illustrates the concentration interactions between alfentanil and propofol for various anesthetic scenarios (intubation, maintenance, and emergence). By choosing a given amount of narcotic or hypnotic (*ie*, "heavy" narcotic or mostly propofol techniques), the appropriate amount of adjunct drug can be given to achieve the desired effect. This type of graph allows the clinician to make educated guesses for a given anesthetic technique. (*Adapted from* Vuyk and coworkers [11].)

DOSING NOMOGRAMS

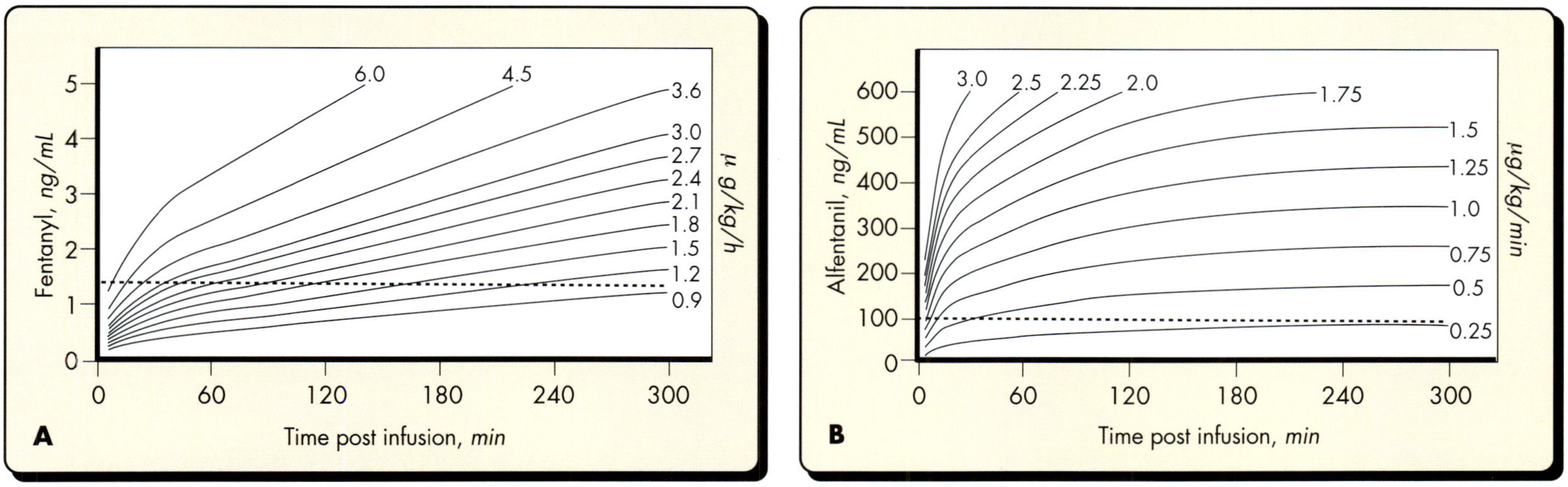

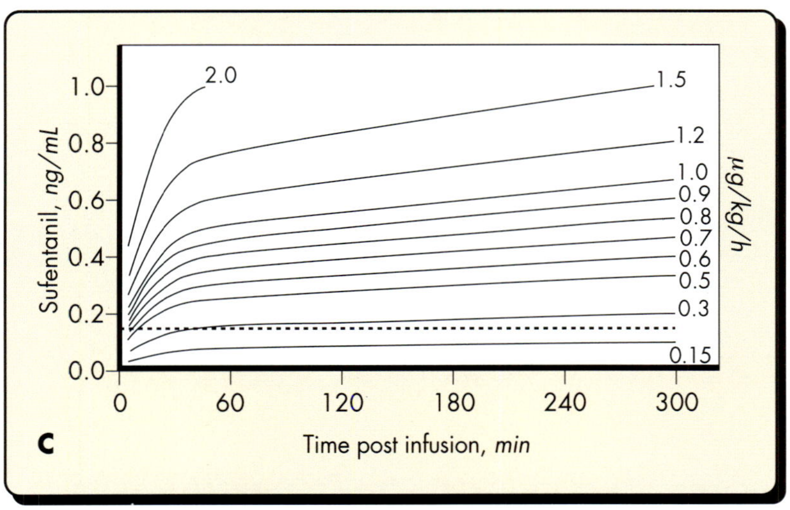

Figure 3-25. A potential application of PK models: dosing nomograms to maintain a stable plasma concentration of several anesthetic drugs. To use the graphs in this figure, pick a desired target concentration (left-hand y axis) and draw a horizontal line from that point. At each point in time, the necessary infusion rate is given by the nearest diagonal line, which corresponds to the infusion rate listed for that line on the right-hand y axis. The bold horizontal lines give the suggested initial target for use of the drug as an adjunct to general anesthesia using propofol/N_2O or a potent inhalational agent/N_2O (opioids) as the primary general anesthetic. For example, to obtain a plasma fentanyl concentration of 1.4 ng/mL, an initial infusion of 6.0 μg/kg/h is required, reduced to 4.5 μg/kg/h by 15 minutes, and further reduced to 3.0 μg/kg/h by 30 minutes. The infusion rate would be continually tapered during the surgery so that the following "milestones" are achieved at given time points: 2.4 μg/kg/h at 60 minutes, 1.8 μg/kg/h at 120 minutes, and so forth.

(*Continued on next page*)

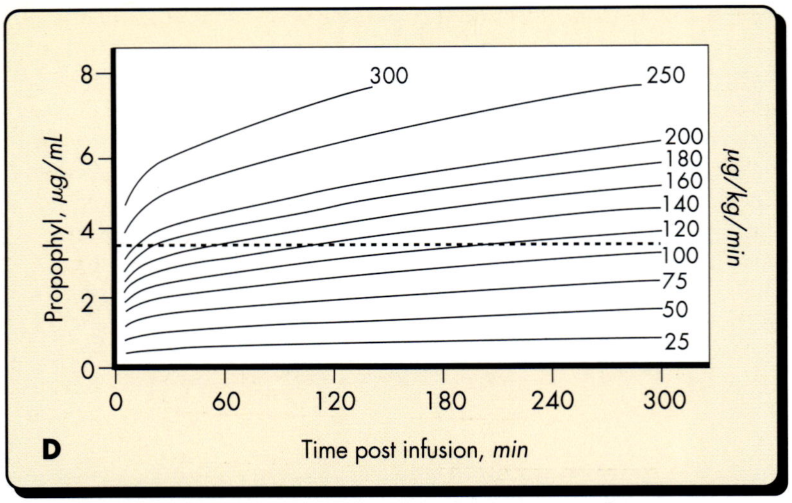

Figure 3-25. (*Continued*) Computer-driven infusion pumps "automatically" taper the infusion rate in an analogous manner to avoid drug accumulation. An alternative to a pure infusion approach is a bolus/infusion approach as presented in Figure 3-6. (*Adapted from* Vuyk and coworkers [11].)

REFERENCES

1. Shafer SL, Varvel JR: Pharmacokinetics, pharmacodynamics, and rational opioid selection. *Anesthesiology* 1991, 74:53–63.
2. Hughes MA, Glass PSA, Jacobs JR: Context-sensitive half time in multicompartment pharmacokinetic models for intravenous anesthetic drugs. *Anesthesiology* 1992, 76:334–41.
3. Westmoreland CL, Sebel PS, Gropper A: Fentanyl or alfentanil decreases the MAC of isoflurane in surgical patients. *Anesth Analg* 1994, 78:23–8.
4. Scott JC, Stanski DR: Decreased fentanyl and alfentanil dose requirements with age. A simultaneous pharmacokinetic and pharmacodynamic evaluation. *J Pharmacol Exp Ther* 1987, 240:159–66.
5. Henthorn TK, Avram MJ, Krejcie TC, *et al.*: Minimal compartmental model of circulatory mixing of indocyanine green. *Am J Physiol* 1992, 262:H903–10.
6. Schnider TW, Shafer SL: Evolving clinically useful predictors of recovery from intravenous anesthetics. *Anesthesiology* 1995, 83:902–5.
7. Ross EM: Chapter 2. In *Goodman & Gilman's The Pharmacological Basis of Therapeutics,* edn. 9. Edited by Hardman JG. New York: McGraw-Hill, 1996:38.
8. Rupp SM, Castagnoli KP, Fisher DM, Miller RD: Pancuronium and vecuronium pharmacokinetics and pharmacodynamics in younger and elderly adults. *Anesthesiology* 1987, 67:45–49.
9. Homer TD, Stanski DR: The effect of increasing age on thiopental disposition and anesthetic requirement. *Anesthesiology* 1985, 62:714–24.
10. Avram MJ, Krejcie TC, Henthorn TK: The relationship of age to the pharmacokinetics of early drug disposition: the concurrent disposition of thiopental and indocyanine green. *Anesthesiology* 1990, 72:403–11.
11. Vuyk J, Lim T, Engbers FHM, *et al.*: The pharmacodynamic interaction of propofol and alfentanil during lower abdominal surgery in women. *Anesthesiology* 1995, 83:8–22.

4

The Autonomic Nervous System

Wolf H. Stapelfeldt

A basic understanding of the structure and function of the autonomic nervous system (ANS) is of fundamental importance for the practice of anesthesia. The ultimate purpose of the ANS is the maintenance of system homeostasis, a task specifically shared by the anesthesiologist during the critical perioperative period. To the degree that autonomic responses such as cardiovascular reflex responses to ischemia or hypovolemia are maintained, the anesthesiologist must be prepared to anticipate, recognize, and treat their underlying causes; to the degree that they are diminished such as baroreceptor reflexes, he or she must be prepared to intervene and prevent undesirable hemodynamic changes through pharmacologic manipulation of the ANS.

The key observation by Loewi, in the 1920's, presented convincing evidence for the prevalence of *chemical* neurotransmission through the release of neurotransmitters. This discovery provided the scientific basis for the development and clinical use of neurotransmitter agonists or antagonists capable of altering ANS responses. More recent findings have indicated that neurotransmission in the ANS is not limited to actions of acetylcholine or catecholamines but may involve actions of more than 20 transmitters, including neuropeptides that typically coexist with classic transmitters in the same neurons. Although their occurrence is not limited to the ANS, it is in the ANS that we have recently begun to understand their *functional roles* and the underlying molecular structure and regulation of membrane receptor types and effector mechanisms used by these transmitters.

An outline of the system levels of ANS control mechanisms (network, cellular, and molecular) is followed by a review of the functional organization of the ANS, emphasizing the importance of afferent components such as chemosensory, low-pressure mechanosensory, and high-pressure mechanosensory (baroreceptor) fiber systems in cardiovascular control. The *baroreceptor reflex* and its alteration during anesthesia are reviewed in more detail. The overview of the organization of the ANS is concluded by a brief discussion of the *functional* subdivisions of sympathetic nervous system efferent neuronal populations and their *chemical coding* according to specific patterns of cotransmitters.

Next, the principles of autonomic ganglionic transmission of preganglionic impulses are discussed. It has become clear that the functional role of sympathetic ganglia is not merely that of simple relays but rather that of fairly sophisticated integrators processing multiple converging synaptic inputs of central and *peripheral afferent* origins, *functionally coded* via the differential release of acetylcholine and nonadrenergic-noncholinergic cotransmitters.

Synthesis, storage, release, postsynaptic action, and metabolism of acetylcholine are the subject of a specific review of cholinergic neurotransmission. This discussion concentrates on presynaptic mechanisms controlling the release of acetylcholine and on postsynaptic signal transduction molecular mechanisms invoked by the interaction of acetylcholine with nicotinic receptors and the various muscarinic (m1-m5)-receptor subtypes.

The remainder of the chapter is concerned with sympathetic neuroeffector transmission, including the mechanisms of synthesis, storage, release, presynaptic and postsynaptic actions, desensitization, downregulation, and termination of actions of norepinephrine, adenosine triphosphate, and neuropeptide Y (NPY), the principal transmitters at neurovascular junctions. Characteristic signal transduction molecular mechanisms invoked by the main types of adrenoceptors (α1, α2, β) are examined. The chapter is concluded by a review of evidence for a genuine transmitter role of NPY in humans and a schematic demonstration of multiple local neural-endothelial interactions which exert fine modulatory control of sympathetic neuroeffector transmission and resulting vascular smooth muscle tone at neurovascular junctions.

FUNCTIONAL ORGANIZATION OF THE AUTONOMIC NERVOUS SYSTEM

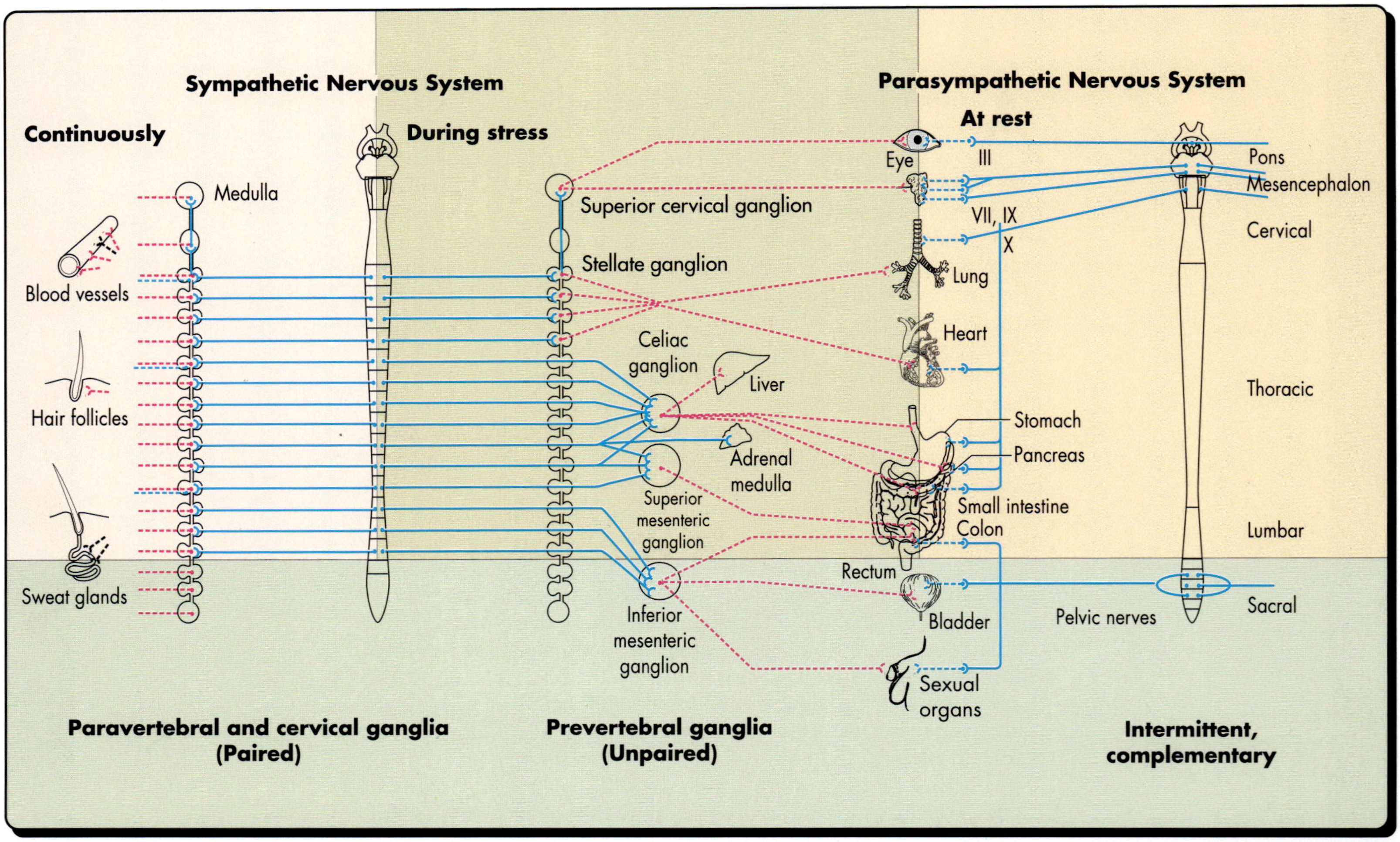

Figure 4-1. Structure of the autonomic nervous system (ANS). The ANS is historically divided in two major efferent components, the sympathetic (cervicothoracic, SNS) and parasympathetic (craniosacral, PNS) nervous systems. The main commonality between these systems is that in either case, end organ innervation is provided by nerve fibers originating from autonomic ganglia located outside the central nervous system (CNS), driven by preganglionic cholinergic input from the CNS (*solid blue lines*). Main differences consist of the types of principal transmitter used by postganglionic fibers (PNS: acetylcholine [*dotted blue*]; SNS: norepinephrine [*dotted red*]), the location of the ganglia (PNS: near or within the end organs; SNS: near the spinal cord, either paravertebral [22 pairs] or prevertebral [unpaired]), the degree of divergence and convergence of preganglionic input to postganglionic neurons (PNS: very little; SNS: considerable), and their respective functional roles. Most internal organs receive input from both PNS and SNS (shown in *middle*). Important exceptions include blood vessels and skin (pilomotor and sudomotor) functions, which are exclusively controlled by noradrenergic and cholinergic postganglionic fibers of SNS origin only (shown at *left*), and the adrenal gland, which functions as the equivalent of a sympathetic ganglion, causing systemic catecholamine release (80% epinephrine, 20% norepinephrine) in response to preganglionic cholinergic stimulation. In the case of most internal organs, SNS and PNS exert opposite effects. PNS effects normally prevail at rest, whereas SNS effects predominate during stress or exercise (flight or fight response). In genitourinary organs, SNS and PNS functions are complementary; for example, PNS mediates erection, SNS mediates ejaculation. (*Adapted from* Bannister and Mathias [1]; with permission.)

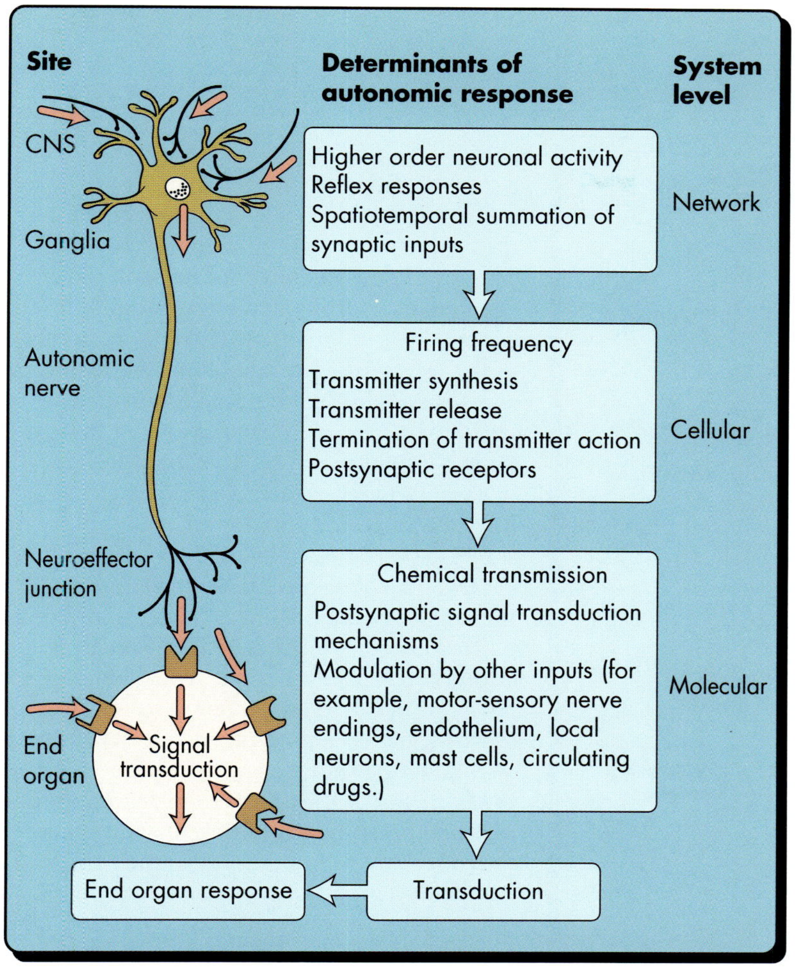

Figure 4-2. Determinants of end organ control by the autonomic nervous system (ANS). Control mechanisms operate concurrently at different system levels. At a neural network level, processing and integration of patterns of neuronal activity (including reflex responses) determine the **firing frequency** of autonomic efferent nerve fibers. Cellular mechanisms operative at the level of nerve terminals determine the types, amounts, and fates of chemical **transmitters released** at autonomic synapses and neuroeffector junctions. At a molecular level, membrane receptor and postsynaptic **signal transduction** mechanisms determine the types and magnitude of cellular effector responses. At each of these system levels, various interactions occur between distinct functional divisions of the ANS (sympathetic, parasympathetic, afferent, enteric, and local neuronal systems) involving classic (cholinergic and adrenergic) transmitters as well as a variety of nonclassic neurotransmitter systems [2]. CNS—central nervous system.

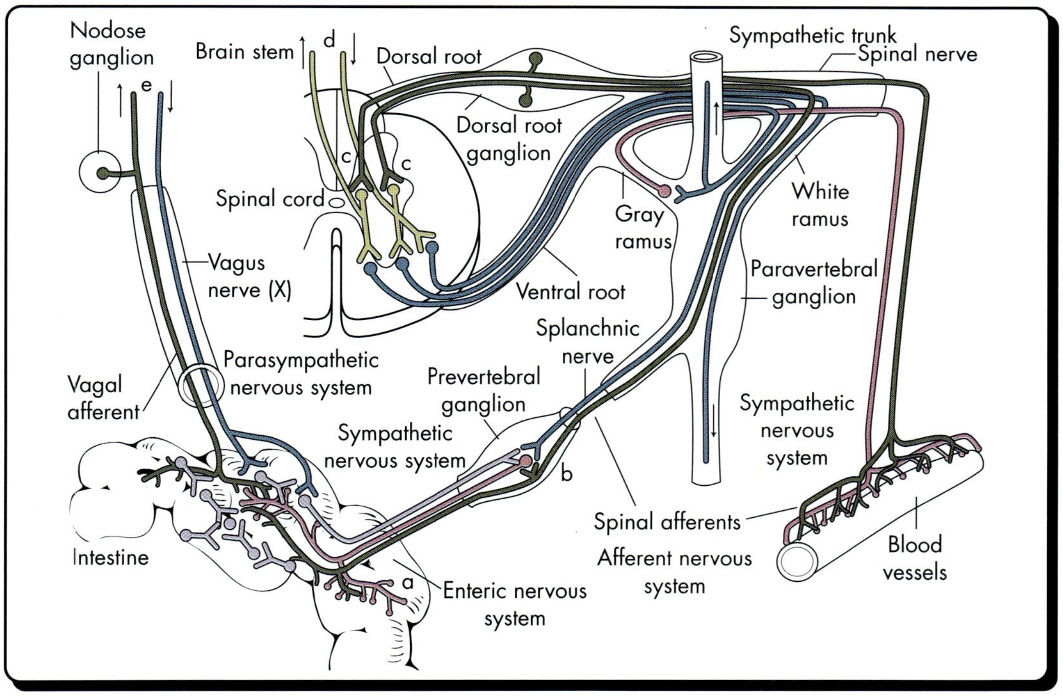

Figure 4-3. Functional components of the autonomic nervous system (ANS). Complementing the roles of parasympathetic (PNS) and sympathetic (SNS) nervous systems as the principal efferent fiber systems, two additional neuronal systems have been recognized as important functional components of the ANS: the afferent and the enteric nervous systems. Primary afferent unmyelinated C and sparsely myelinated Aδ fibers (shown in *green*) represent a substantial portion of autonomic nerves (such as 80% of fibers contained in the vagus nerve). They are the peripheral (sensory) projection of pseudounipolar neurons arising from either nodose ganglia (vagal and glossopharyngeal afferents) or dorsal root ganglia (sympathetic afferents). Their central projections terminate in sensory nuclei of the central nervous system (CNS), either the nucleus tractus solitarius (NTS) of the brain stem or the dorsal horn of the spinal cord. Functioning as chemosensors or mechanosensors (or as both), these afferents play important roles through synaptic actions at three different sites: perivascular arborizations within end organs from which transmitters are released in response to local reflex activation (termed *axon reflexes*) [3] (*a*); collateral synaptic terminals in prevertebral ganglia, which participate in peripheral ganglionic reflexes [4] (*b*); central synaptic terminations in the dorsal horn and NTS, which are responsible for the activation of spinally mediated (*c*) and brain stem–mediated (*d* and *e*) ANS reflex responses. The efferent limb of centrally mediated sympathetic reflex responses consists of preganglionic cholinergic fibers (indicated in *blue*) exiting the spinal cord via the ventral spinal roots and forming synaptic connections with postganglionic noradrenergic neurons (indicated in *red*) in either paravertebral (cardiovascular reflexes) or prevertebral ganglia (gastrointestinal reflexes). The enteric nervous system (indicated in *purple*) forms a fourth—and with a total of approximately 100 million neurons in humans by far the largest quantitatively—component of the ANS. It is responsible for the intrinsic control of gastrointestinal secretion and motility patterns such as peristalsis. It is also the source of afferent (centripetal) neural projections to prevertebral sympathetic ganglia, which take part in extrinsic intestino-intestinal sympathetic reflexes and pathophysiologic ANS conditions such as ileus.

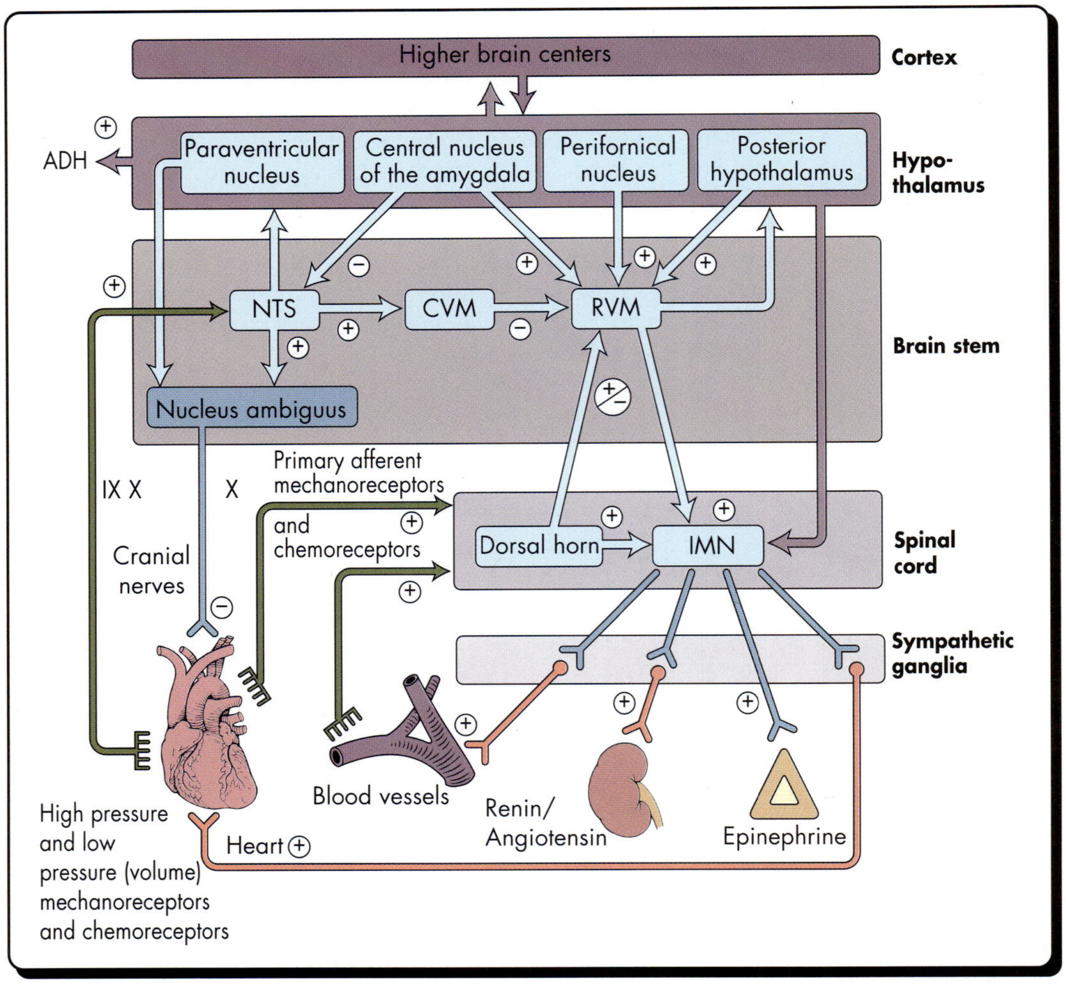

Figure 4-4. Schematic illustration of the autonomic nervous system (ANS) control of the cardiovascular system. The main integrative control of the cardiovascular system occurs in the brain stem. Brain stem nuclei maintain reciprocal connections with higher central nervous system (CNS) centers (hypothalamus, cerebral cortex) and lower CNS centers (spinal cord nuclei). The nucleus tractus solitarius (NTS) serves as the primary site for integration of sensory information received via arterial and cardiac high pressure mechanoreceptor (baroceptor), low pressure (volume) mechanoreceptor, and chemoreceptor afferent fibers contained in the glossopharyngeal and vagal nerves. NTS afferent input is processed in several ways, mainly via relays to hypothalamic nuclei and reflex pathways to the principal efferent (motor) brain stem nuclei of the cardiovascular system, the nucleus ambiguus (motor nucleus of the vagus), and the rostral ventrolateral medulla (RVM). The RVM consists of spontaneously active pacemaker neurons that exert excitatory control of sympathetic preganglionic nuclei in the intermediolateral column of the spinal cord (IML). Hypothalamic nuclei participate in cardiovascular regulation by controlling antidiuretic hormone (ADH) release (paraventricular and supraoptic nuclei) and by modulating the excitability of the NTS, nucleus ambiguus, RVM, and IML (paraventricular nucleus, central nucleus of the amygdala, perifornical nucleus, and posterior hypothalamus). The RVM receives additional ascending input from spinal mechanosensitive and chemosensitve fiber systems, which represent the sensory limb of sympathetic brain stem reflexes. The IML is the final site of integration of synaptic information controlling the efferent sympathetic nervous system. In addition to the principal descending inputs conveyed by hypothalamic and bulbospinal pathways (in particular from RVM and caudal raphe nuclei), it also receives direct intraspinal (reflex) collateral input derived from primary afferent synaptic terminals in the dorsal horn. These segmental connections play particularly important roles in patients with spinal cord transections, producing autonomic hyperreflexia. Subpopulations of IML neurons provide preganglionic input for postganglionic control of various cardiovascular neuroeffector mechanisms, that is, cardiac chronotropy and inotropy, vasomotor tone, release of renin/angiotensin, and release of epinephrine. CVM—caudal ventrolateral medulla.

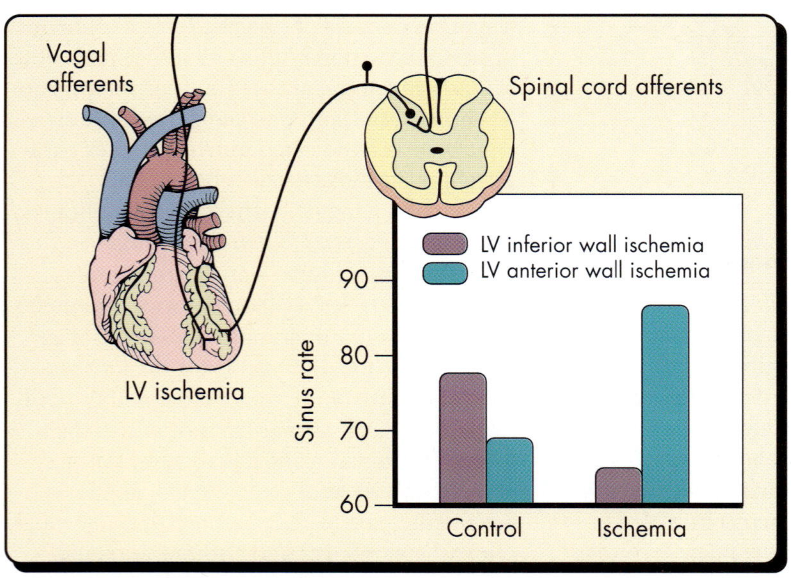

Figure 4-5. Example of the importance of chemosensory pathways in determining autonomic nervous system (ANS) hemodynamic responses. Inferior and anterior walls of the left ventricle (LV) are innervated along different sensory pathways. The inferior wall of the left ventricle is innervated by sensory arborizations of vagal afferents, whereas the anterior wall is innervated by sensory arborizations of spinal (sympathetic) afferents. In the presence of inferior ischemia, activation of vagal chemosensory afferents evokes reflex sinus bradycardia, whereas in the presence of anterior ischemia, activation of spinal (sympathetic) chemosensory afferents causes reflex sinus tachycardia. (*Adapted from* Shepherd [5]; with permission. Bar graphs based on data from Perez-Gomez and colleagues [6].)

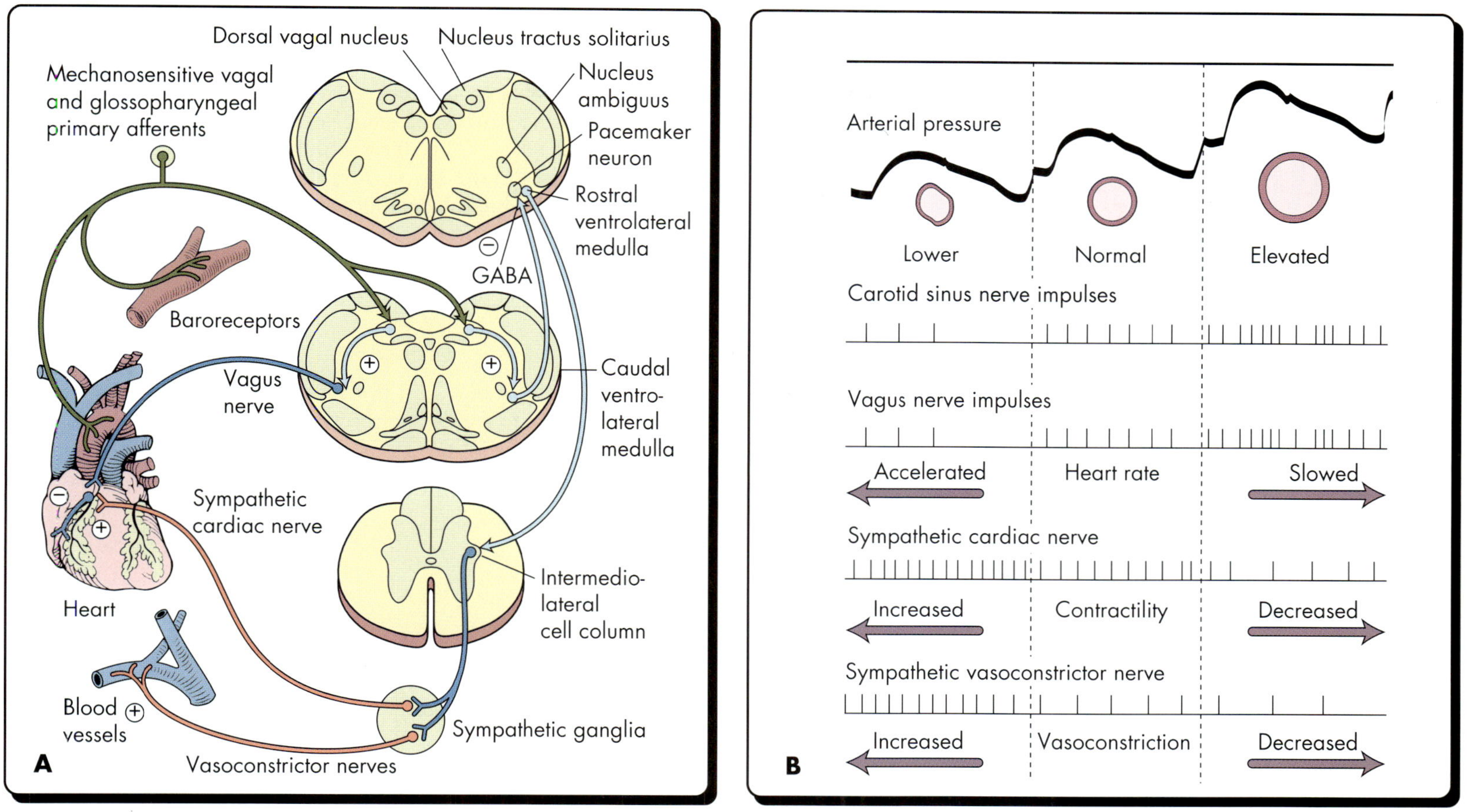

Figure 4-6. Baroreceptor reflex control. A, Baroreceptor reflex pathways. Primary afferent fibers arising from high-pressure mechanosensory endings in the heart, aorta, and carotid sinus project within the vagal and glossopharyngeal nerves to the nucleus tractus solitarius (NTS). Excitatory NTS outputs project to the vagal motor nucleus (nucleus ambiguus) and to the caudal ventrolateral medulla (CVM), activating an inhibitory (GABAergic) interneuron relay to the rostral ventrolateral medulla (RVM). Efferent limbs completing negative feedback loops consist of (inhibitory) vagal projections to the heart and sympathetic efferent projections from the RVM to the heart and vasculature via the interomedial column of the spinal cord (IML) and sympathetic ganglia. Heart rate reflex responses to changes in arterial pressure are determined by the balance between vagal and sympathetic efferent cardiac nerve activities. Reflex changes in systemic vascular resistance are determined by changes in vasoconstrictor nerve activities. GABA—γ-aminobutyric acid.

B, Beat-to-beat function of the baroreceptor reflex. Changes in arterial blood pressure result in parallel changes in the firing rate of carotid sinus nerve afferent impulses. These changes in the afferent nerve firing rate, in turn, cause parallel changes in vagal efferent and reciprocal changes in sympathetic efferent nerve firing rates. (*Adapted from* Spyer [7].)

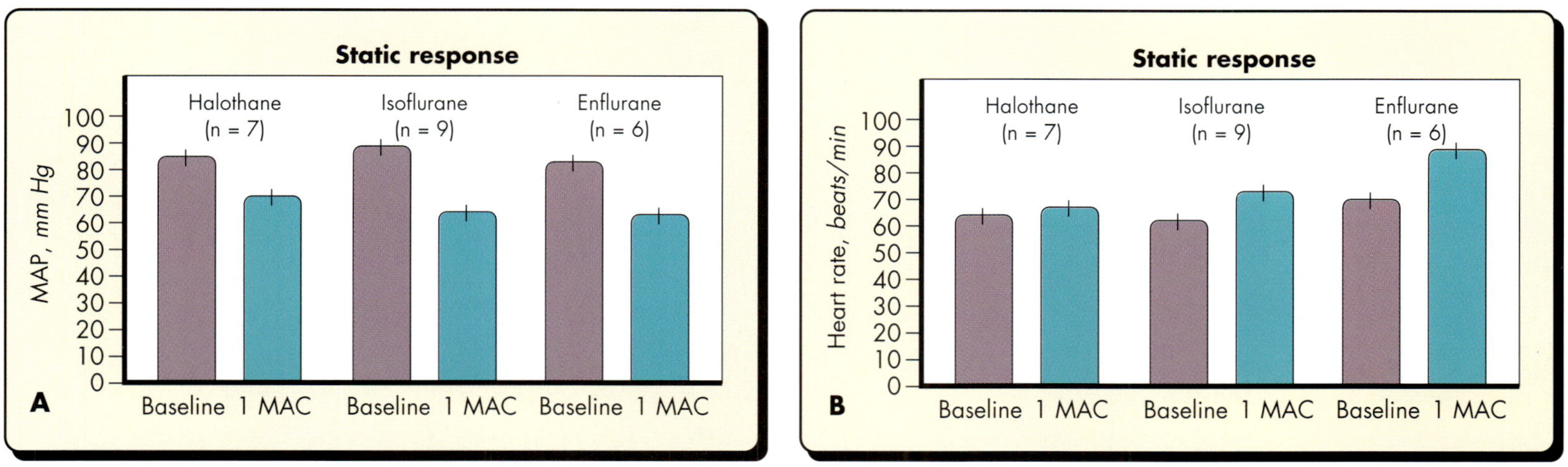

Figure 4-7. Anesthetic effects on baroreceptor reflex control of heart rate. When tested in a randomized, prospective comparison in age-matched healthy human volunteers, equipotent concentrations (1 MAC) of halothane, isoflurane, and enflurane cause a similar decrease in steady-state mean arterial blood pressure (MAP) from awake baseline (**A**). Despite the similar decrease in MAP, significant differences in steady-state heart rate result from the anesthetic action. Steady-state heart rate increases significantly in the presence of enflurane and isoflurane, but no significant change occurs in the presence of halothane (**B**).

(*Continued on next page*)

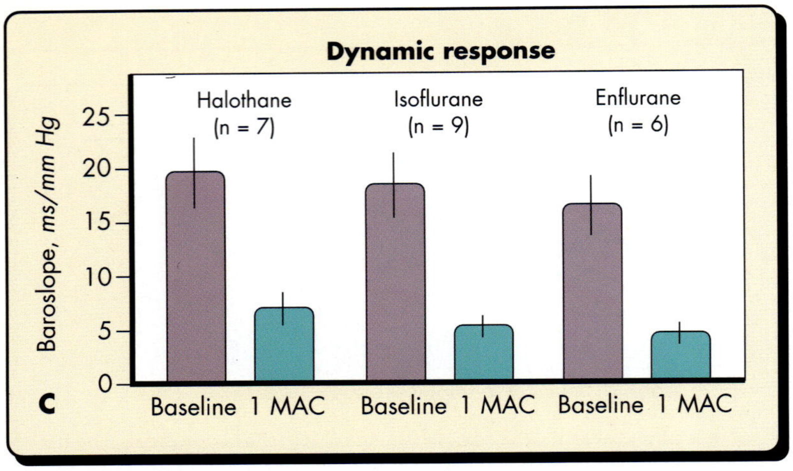

Figure 4-7. (*Continued*) In contrast, the dynamic heart rate response (reflex increase) to an acute (further) drop in MAP induced by a bolus of nitroprusside (100 µg) is equally blunted by all three anesthetics (C, baroslope expressed as change in R-R interval in ms per change in MAP in mm Hg). These data suggest that static and dynamic components of baroreceptor reflex control of heart rate are functionally distinct and that a static component of baroreceptor reflex control of heart rate is differentially affected by halothane (as compared with isoflurane and enflurane) whereas a dynamic component is similarly inhibited by equipotent concentrations of all three anesthetics. MAC—minimum alveolar concentration; error bars—standard error of the mean. (*Data from* Muzi and Ebert [8].)

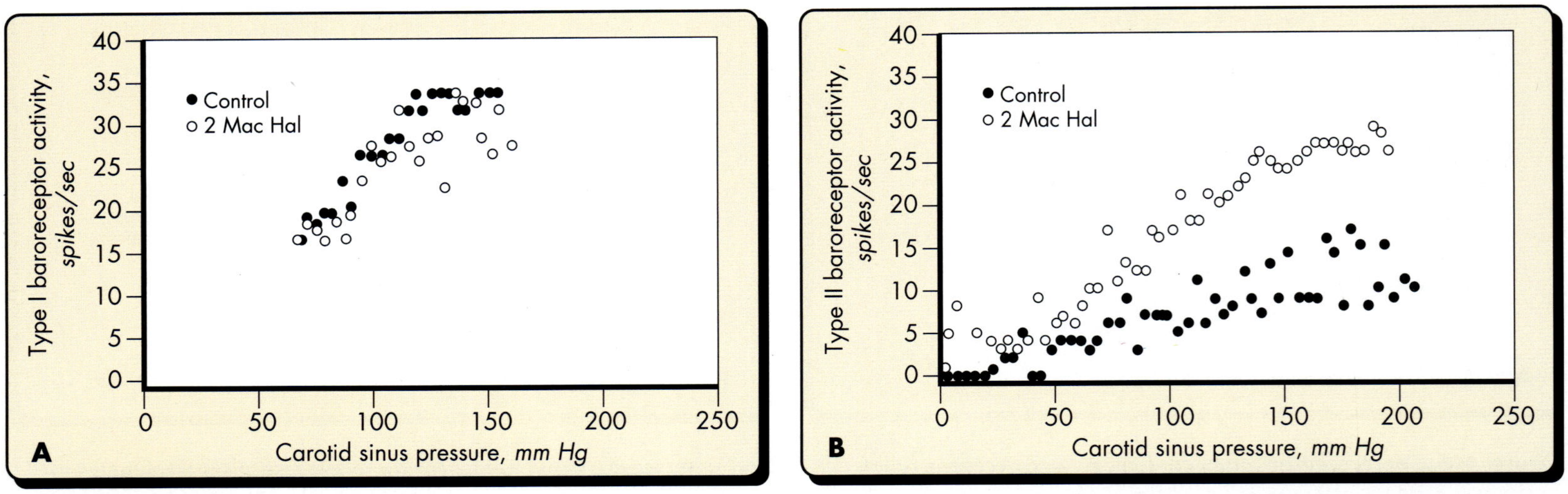

Figure 4-8. Effect of halothane on baroreceptor sensitivity. Two types of baroreceptor afferents have been functionally distinguished: **A**, larger A-fiber (type I) baroreceptor afferents that appear to preferentially mediate dynamic baroreflex regulation; and **B**, smaller A-fiber and C-fiber (type II) baroreceptor afferents that appear to be primarily involved in tonic baroreflex regulation of sustained changes in arterial pressure [9]. These two types of baroreceptor afferents are differentially affected by halothane. When tested in a vascularly isolated carotid sinus in dogs *in situ*, single unit recordings from the ipsilateral glossopharyngeal nerve identify members of each fiber type by their distinct response to a slow ramp increase in carotid sinus pressure as either type I baroreceptors (*panel A*) or type II baroreceptors (*panel B*) (control). When repeated in the presence of halothane (2 MAC) in the carotid sinus perfusate, the response of type I baroreceptor afferents is unchanged, whereas the response of the type II baroreceptor afferent is significantly *increased*. These data support the concept that anesthetic-induced changes in static baroreceptor control may in part be mediated by a halothane-evoked *increase in sensitivity* of type II baroreceptor afferents. MAC—minimum alveolar concentration. (*Adapted from* Seagard [9]; with permission.)

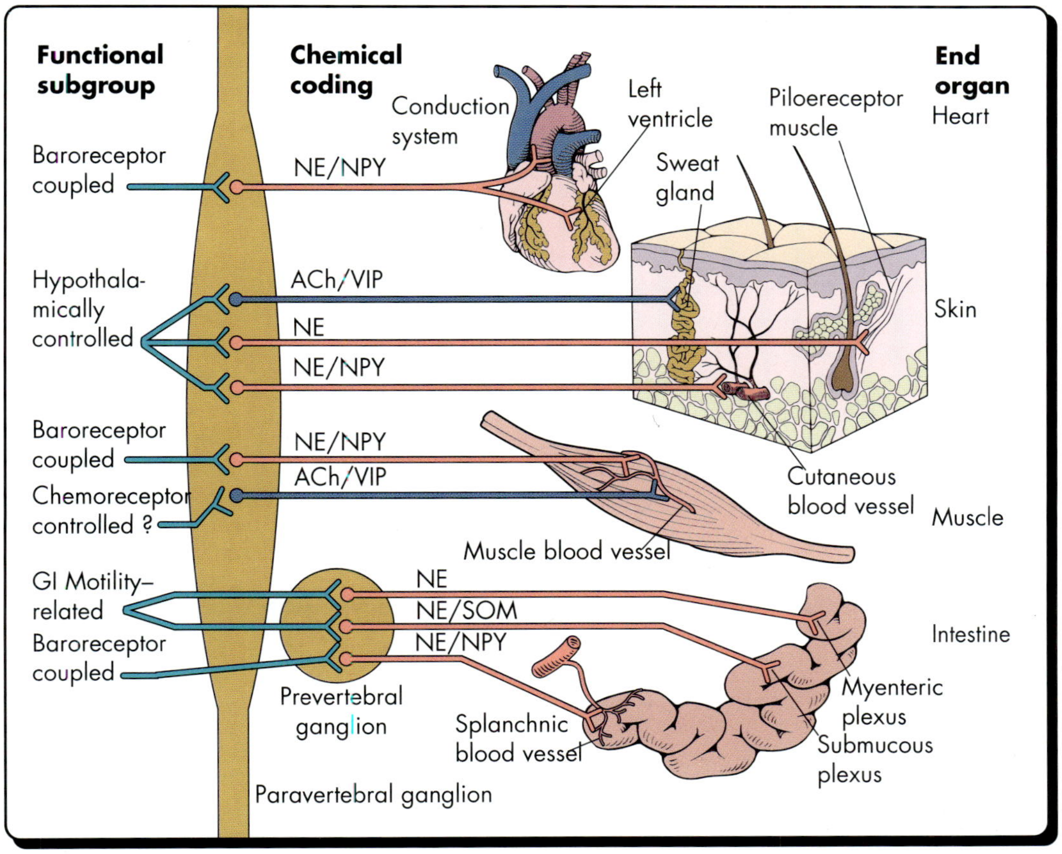

Figure 4-9. Chemical coding of functional subpopulations of postganglionic neurons within the sympathetic nervous system (SNS). This illustration schematically depicts subpopulations of neurons identified in immunohistochemical studies in human paravertebral sympathetic ganglia [10,11] and guinea pig prevertebral sympathetic ganglia [11]. In humans, approximately 75% of paravertebral ganglion cells are noradrenergic, and 25% are cholinergic. Approximately two thirds of noradrenergic ganglion cells project to the heart and vasculature (vasoconstrictor nerves). These neurons contain neuropeptide Y (NPY) as cotransmitter. Noradrenergic ganglion cells without apparent cotransmitter provide pilomotor innervation. Cholinergic neurons project to sweat glands (sudomotor) and skeletal muscle blood vessels (vasodilator nerves). These fibers contain vasoactive intestinal polypeptide (VIP) as a cotransmitter. Information about subpopulations of neurons in human prevertebral sympathetic ganglia is not available. Studies in guinea pigs have identified three subpopulations of noradrenergic ganglion cells: neurons without apparent cotransmitter projecting to the myenteric plexus of the enteric nervous system (ENS), neurons containing somatostatin (SOM) as cotransmitter projecting to the submucous plexus of the ENS, and neurons containing NPY as cotransmitter projecting to the splanchnic vasculature (vasoconstrictor nerves) [11]. Functional studies in various animal species including humans have established that only cardiac efferent, muscle vasoconstrictor, and splanchnic vasoconstrictor neuron populations receive baroreceptor-coupled preganglionic inputs, whereas cutaneous sympathetic fibers receive thermoregulatory hypothalamic inputs related to core temperature [12]. ACh—aceytlcholine; GI—gastrointestinal; NE—norepinephrine. (*Adapted from* Gibbins [10]; with permission.)

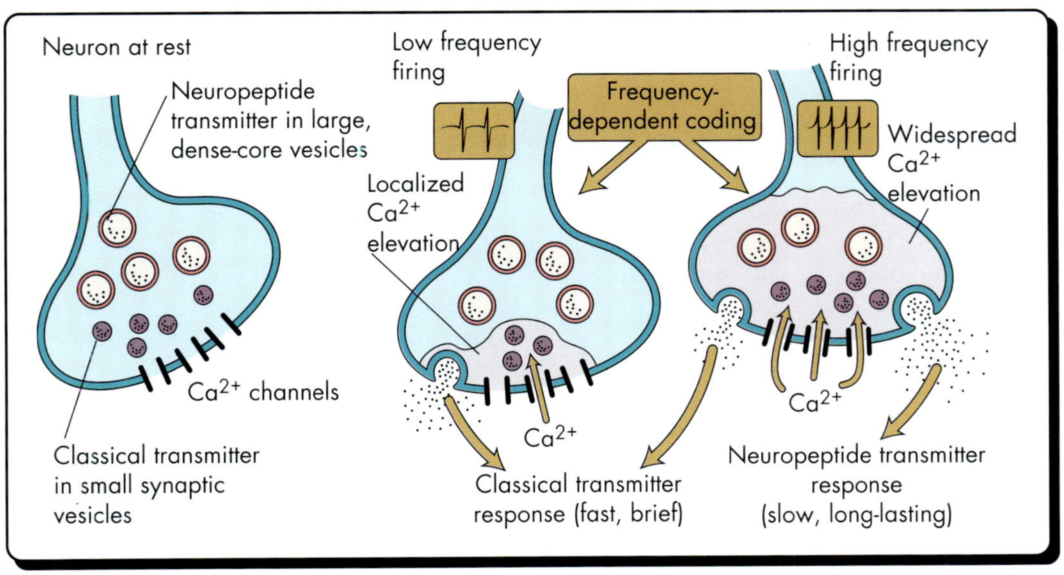

Figure 4-10. Role of neuropeptide cotransmitters in functional coding of postsynaptic responses. Neuropeptide cotransmitters are present not only in postganglionic autonomic nervous system (ANS) neurons but also in preganglionic neurons and in ANS pathways within the central nervous system. In general, classical transmitters such as acetylcholine are contained in small synaptic vesicles located near active zones high in Ca^{2+} channels and regulatory proteins controlling synaptic vesicle fusion with the neuronal membrane. In contrast, neuropeptide-containing larger (dense core) vesicles are located farther away from the neuronal membrane. As a consequence, low frequency neuronal firing, which typically causes only localized elevations in cytoplasmic Ca^{2+} (Ca_i^{2+}) near the cytoplasmic membrane, evokes predominant release of classic transmitters only, whereas high-frequency firing causes more widespread elevation in Ca_i^{2+} and, consequently, the additional release of neuropeptide cotransmitters as well. Classic transmitters such as acetylcholine typically evoke postsynaptic responses of rapid onset and short duration (fast synaptic responses), whereas neuropeptide transmitters characteristically produce postsynaptic responses of slower onset and longer duration (slow responses). Thus, within the ANS, the presynaptic firing frequency is encoded to some degree in the types and amounts of fast and slow transmitters released from nerve endings, which in turn, determine amplitude and duration of postsynaptic membrane responses.

AUTONOMIC GANGLIONIC TRANSMISSION

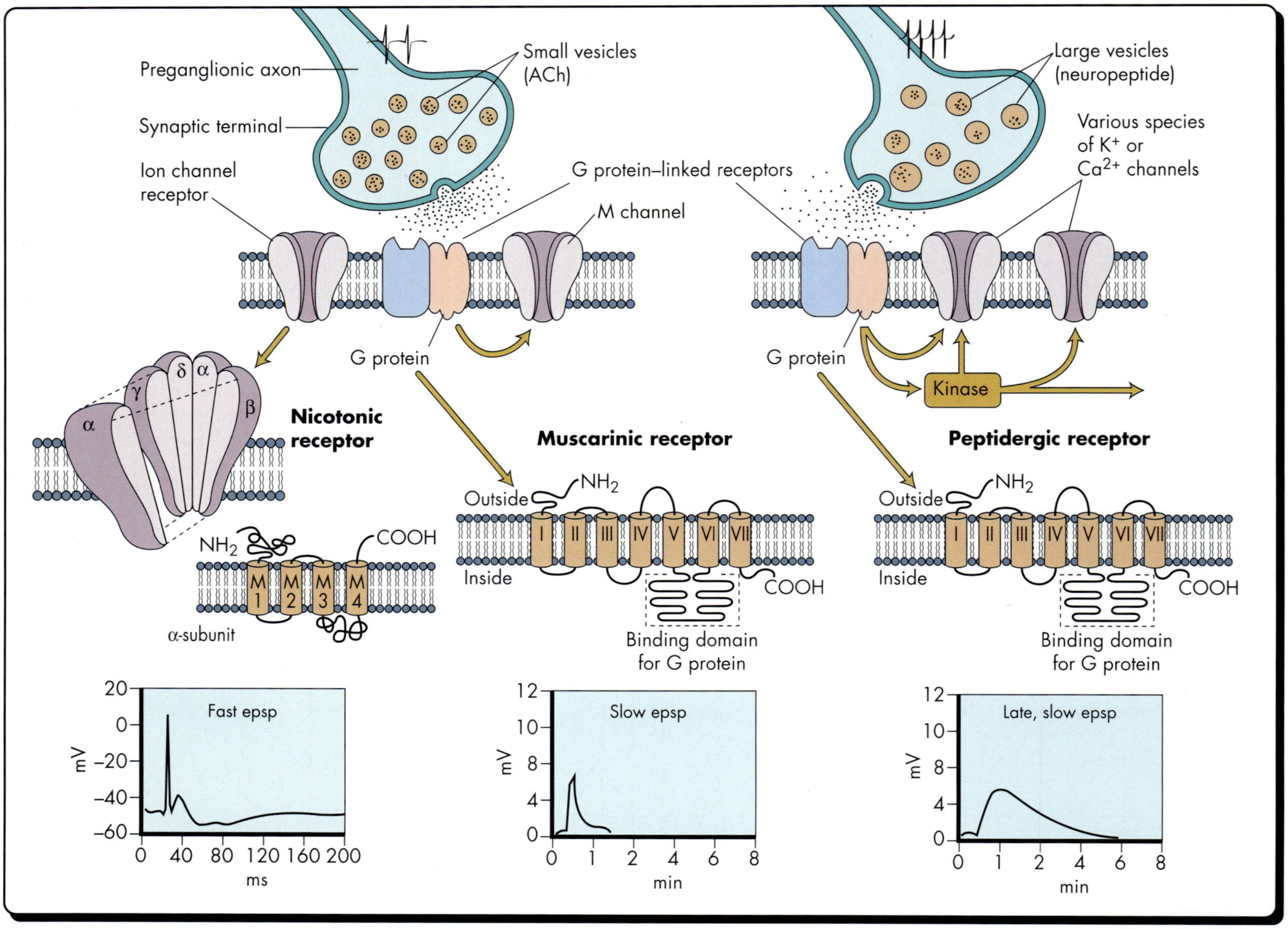

Figure 4-11. Determinants of autonomic ganglionic transmission. In sympathetic ganglia, low frequency preganglionic input causes predominantly release of acetylcholine (ACh). Acetylcholine acts on two types of postsynaptic cholinergic receptors, nicotinic and muscarinic (named after their particularly high affinity for nicotine and muscarine, respectively). Nicotinic receptors (n-ACH-R) are members of the family of ligand-gated ion channels consisting of pentameric subunits, each composed of a polypeptide chain with four hydrophobic transmembrane portions, as shown for an α-subunit. Acetylcholine occupation causes channel openings that produce fast excitatory postsynaptic depolarizing potentials (fast epsp) and action potentials (if of sufficient amplitude to reach the membrane firing threshold) (*lower left*). Muscarinic receptors (m-ACh-R) are members of the superfamily of G protein–linked transmembrane receptors consisting of seven hydrophobic transmembrane portions, an external agonist-binding site, and an internal G protein-binding site. In sympathetic ganglia, m-ACh-R–mediated G protein activation results in a decrease in conductance of an outwardly conducting (hyperpolarizing) ion channel species, the M channel (for muscarinically inhibited K^+ channel). M channel inhibition thus produces slow excitatory postsynaptic potentials (slow epsp) (*lower middle*). High-frequency preganglionic input evokes the additional release of neuropeptide transmitters contained in large dense core vesicles of subpopulations of preganglionic nerves such as luteinizing hormone-releasing hormone (LRH) in amphibian ganglia [13], or leu-enkephalin and neurotensin in mammalia ganglia [14,15]. Neuropeptides evoke via G protein–mediated signal transduction mechanisms postsynaptic changes in various (K^+ or Ca^{2+}) conductances to produce late slow excitatory postsynaptic potentials (noncholinergic late slow epsp) (*lower right*). The functional role of slow excitatory synaptic potentials is to increase postganglionic neuronal excitability and firing for extended periods of time [14,15]. EPSP—excitatory postsynaptic potential. (Recordings *adapted from* Jan and colleagues [13].)

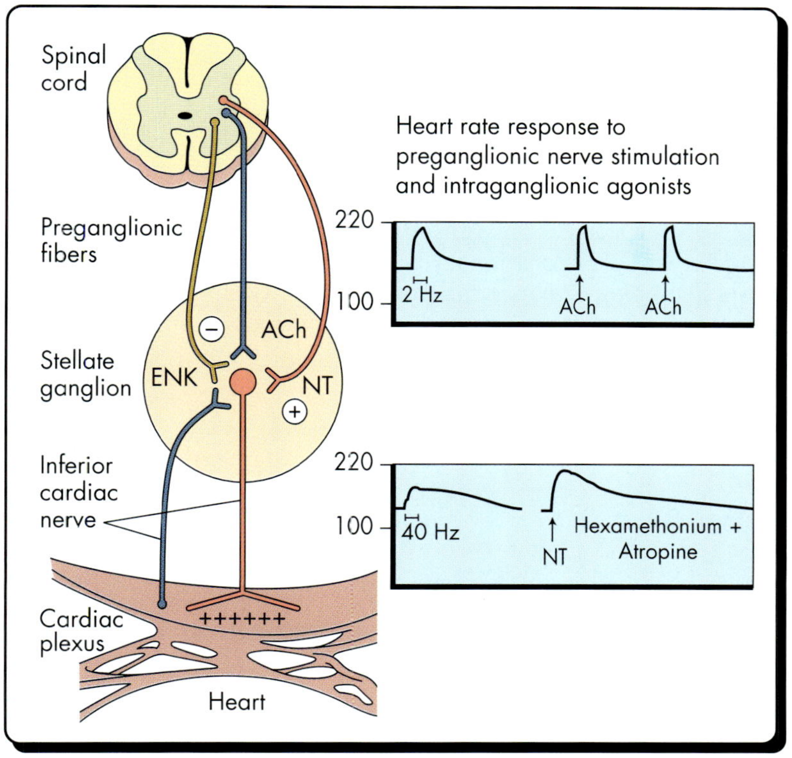

Figure 4-12. Role of cholinergic and noncholinergic synaptic inputs in paravertebral ganglionic control of heart rate (cat stellate ganglion). In addition to central preganglionic cholinergic inputs (shown in *blue*), ganglion cells receive preganglionic inputs from subpopulations of cholinergic neurons containing either leu-enkephalin (ENK) or neurotensin (NT) as a neuropeptide cotransmitter [14]. Ganglion cells also receive ongoing *afferent* synaptic input from fibers of peripheral origin, constituting a peripheral reflex arc [16]. Low-frequency preganglionic stimulation (2 Hz, 15 sec) of the *in situ* decentralized right stellate ganglion evokes a brief increase in heart rate that is mimicked by close *intraarterial* injection of acetylcholine (ACh) (*upper right*). Both of these actions are completely prevented by prior administration of the cholinergic antagonists hexamethonium (n-ACh receptor antagonist) and atropine (m-ACh receptor antagonist) (data not shown). Even in the presence of hexamethonium and atropine, high-frequency preganglionic stimulation (40 Hz, 15 sec) still evokes a prolonged increase in heart rate that is mimicked by close *intraarterial* injection of the noncholinergic neuropeptide transmitter neurotensin (*lower right*). All of these effects on heart rate are completely blocked by section of the (postganglionic) inferior cardiac nerve. (Tracings *adapted from* Bachoo and Polosa [14].)

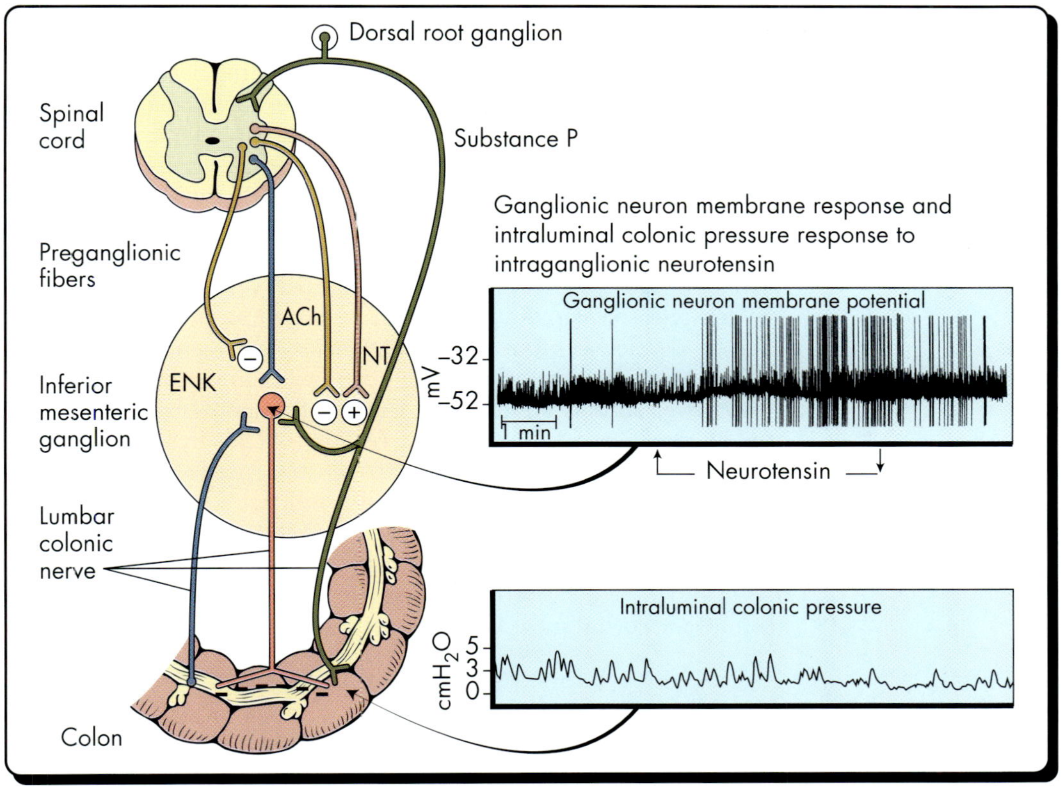

Figure 4-13. Multiplicity of cholinergic and noncholinergic synaptic inputs in sympathetic ganglionic control of colonic motor function (guinea pig inferior mesenteric ganglion). Prevertebral ganglion cells receive several synaptic inputs of central and peripheral origin [15]. Central preganglionic inputs consist of cholinergic fibers, subpopulations of which contain leu-enkephalin (ENK) or neurotensin (NT) as a cotransmitter. Afferent synaptic inputs consist of cholinergic fibers of peripheral origin containing neuropeptide cotransmitters such as vasoactive intestinal polypeptide (VIP) or cholecystokinin (CCK). In addition, ganglion cells receive sensory input from axon collateral terminals of primary afferent fibers containing the neuropeptide transmitters substance P and calcitonin gene-related peptide (CGRP). The output firing rate of ganglion cells is determined by spatiotemporal integration of all these various synaptic inputs. When tested with intracellular recording techniques in a decentralized ganglion-colon preparation *ex situ*, ganglion cells receive spontaneous, asynchronous afferent cholinergic synaptic input (subthreshold cholinergic fast excitatory postsynaptic potentials [epsps] resulting from ongoing colonic motor activity (*right panel*). High-frequency preganglionic nerve stimulation (15 Hz, not shown) or selective ganglionic administration of the noncholinergic transmitter neurotensin (*top right panel*) causes slow excitatory membrane responses (slow epsps) of ganglion cells that are associated with increased conversion of subthreshold fast epsps to action potentials. The resulting increase in the firing rate of sympathetic fibers causes a decrease in colonic motor activity (*bottom right panel*). Neurotensin causes such slow epsps by facilitating ongoing release of substance P from primary afferent axon collaterals (4). Leu-enkephalin presynaptically inhibits the release of acetylcholine (ACh) and substance P and thus depresses ganglionic firing. (Tracings *adapted from* Stapelfeldt and Szurszewski [15].)

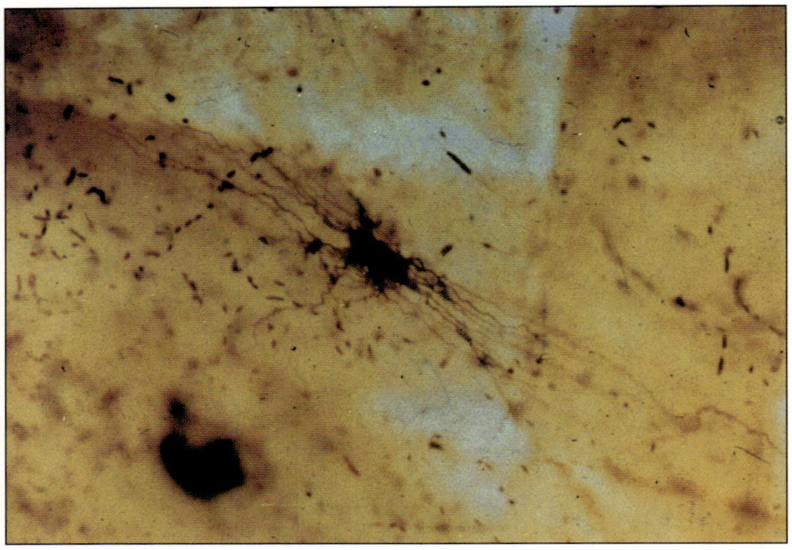

Figure 4-14. Morphology of a prevertebral sympathetic neuron in the inferior mesenteric ganglion of the guinea pig, stained after intracellular injection of horseradish peroxidase through a recording microelectrode [from Stapelfeldt, unpublished]. Multiplicity of synaptic inputs of central preganglionic and peripheral afferent origin is reflected in the complexity of dendritic arborizations projecting in both central and peripheral directions (the long process represents the axon of this ganglion cell, projecting peripherally to the upper left). The functional role of this complex dendritic structure is spatiotemporal integration of multiple synaptic inputs of central and peripheral origin rather than simple synaptic relay.

CHOLINERGIC NEUROTRANSMISSION

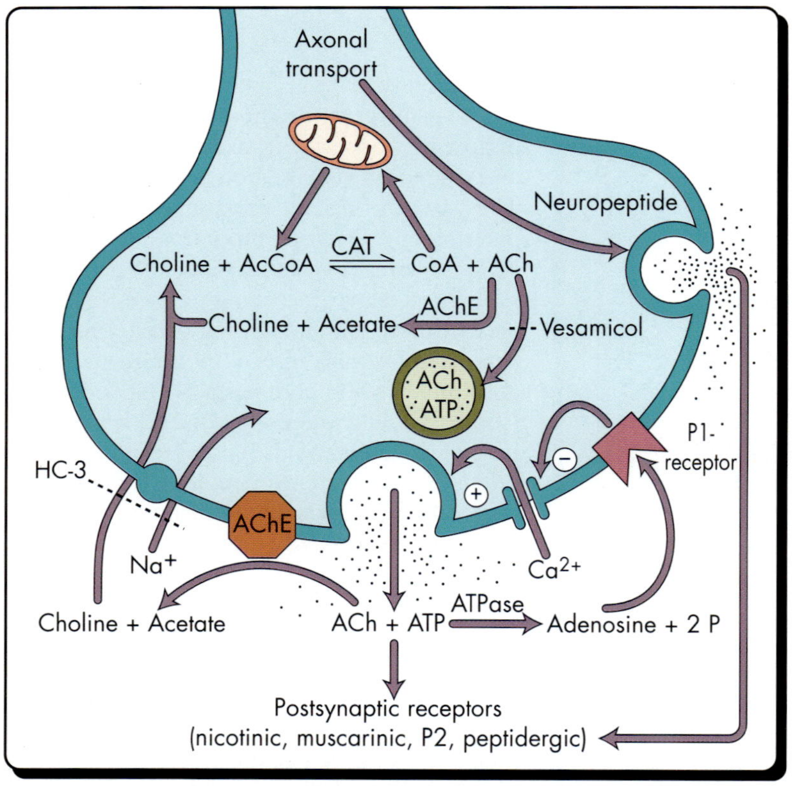

Figure 4-15. Mechanisms controlling transmitter synthesis and release at cholinergic nerve terminals. In contrast to neuropeptide cotransmitters and synthetic enzymes, which are exclusively produced in the cell soma and delivered to the nerve terminal via axonal transport, acetylcholine (ACh) is synthesized in the nerve terminal itself. The rate-limiting step for ACh synthesis is uptake of choline, which is acetylized by choline acetyltransferase (CAT), the characteristic biochemical marker of cholinergic neurons. ACh is taken up into synaptic storge vesicles and packaged together with adenosine triphosphate (ATP). Upon depolarization of the nerve terminal and an increase in cytoplasmic Ca^{2+} (Ca_i^{2+}) (predominantly through the opening of N-type Ca^{2+} channels near the active zones), ACh and ATP are released into the extracellular space through fusion of synaptic vesicles with the cytoplasmic membrane. Signal is transmitted by transmitter interaction with postjunctional receptors. ACh transmitter action is rapidly hydrolyzed within milliseconds by membrane-bound acetylcholine esterase (AChE). ATP is hydrolyzed by magnesium-dependent ATPase and 5′-nucleotidase to adenosine, which functions to feedback control transmitter release through inhibitory action on presynaptic P1-receptors. Neuropeptide transmitter action is terminated by extracellular peptidases and, predominantly, diffusion away from the nerve terminal. (*Adapted from* Nicholls and colleagues [17]; with permission.)

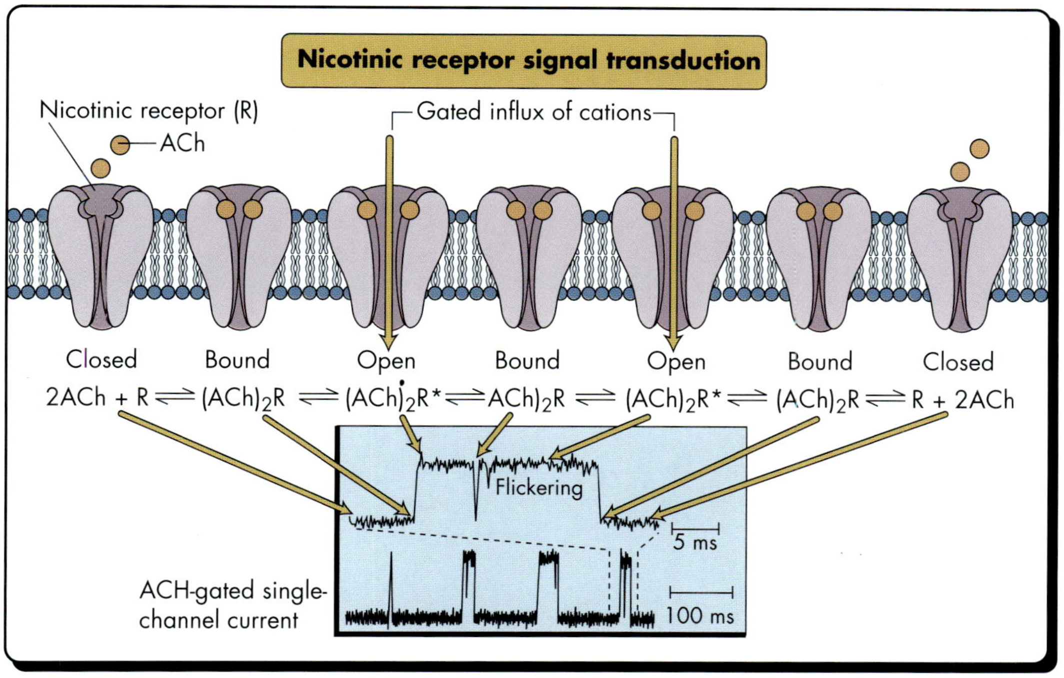

Figure 4-16. Signal transmission through nicotinic receptors. Nicotinic receptors are ligand-gated cationic ion channels consisting of five polypeptide subunits that vary in composition in different tissues (skeletal muscle, autonomic ganglia, different regions in the central nervous system), yet contain at least two identical alpha-subunits representing the binding sites for (each of) two aceytlcholine (ACh) molecules necessary to activate the channel. For the duration of its alpha-subunit occupation by ACh, the channel conformation changes to increase its permeability for cations such as Na^+, K^+, and Ca^{2+}, resulting in a net inward current (upward deflections in current traces). Specific agonist affinity and single channel ionic conductance are determined by the respective subunit composition. The amplitude of net inward current is determined by the single channel conductance and the driving forces (concentration gradients) for permeable ions. Open and closed conformational states of the agonist-occupied channel are in a dynamic equilibrium responsible for single channel "flickering" (shown in a faster time scale in the *insert*). Macroscopic summation of individual single channel currents contributed by all nicotinic receptors of neurons results in fast excitatory postsynaptic potentials (fast epsps). (*Adapted from* Nicholls and colleagues [17]; with permission.)

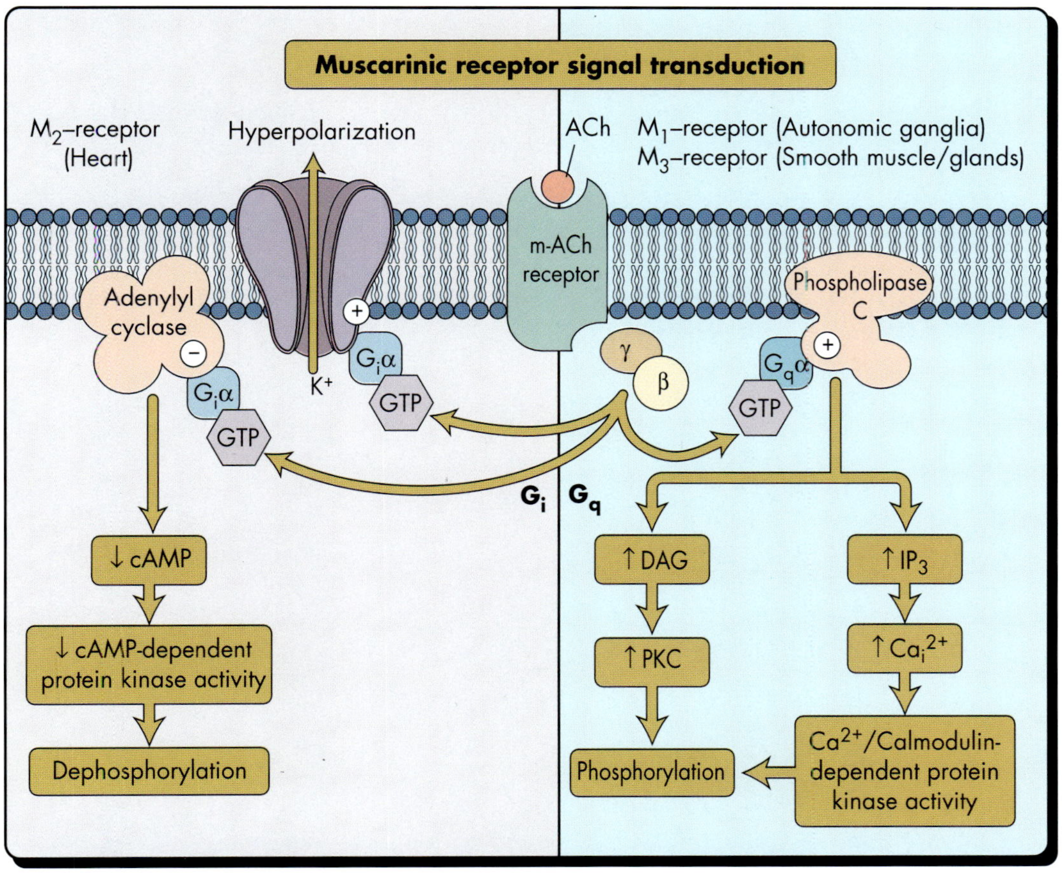

Figure 4-17. Signal transduction via muscarinic receptors. Muscarinic signal transduction is mediated by members of the G protein–linked membrane receptor superfamily. Extracellular occupation by acetylcholine (ACh) of the agonist-binding sites causes intracellular binding of guanosine triphosphate (GTP) to the α-subunit of receptor-bound heterotrimeric G proteins and their dissociation from the receptor into free activated α-subunits and βγ subunit complexes. Predominantly activated α-subunits are responsible for signal transduction by acting upon various effector systems. This action is terminated by intrinsic GTPase activity of α-subunits, resulting in spontaneous reassembly of inactivated guanosine diphosphate (GDP) α-subunits with βγ-subunit complexes into complete G proteins to be available again for binding to G protein–binding sites of transmembrane receptors. The particular family of G proteins bound and used by muscarinic receptors is determined by the receptor subtype. Three subtypes have been distinguished pharmacologically on the basis of different affinities for specific agonists/antagonists and differential localization in various target tissues (M_1, M_2, and M_3). Two more subunit types have been distinguished by gene expression (M_4, M_5). M_1, M_3, and M_5 receptors are coupled to members of the G_q family of G proteins. Their main functional role is to cause G_q-α–mediated activation of phospholipase C, resulting in liberation of inositol triphosphate (IP_3) and diacylglycerol (DAG). IP_3 produces an increase in cytoplasmic Ca^{2+} (Ca_i^{2+}) through release from intracellular stores and, secondarily, an increase in Ca_i^{2+}-dependent mechanisms such as activation of Ca_i^{2+}/calmodulin-dependent kinases, whereas DAG causes direct activation of protein kinase C. Both mechanisms thus produce secondary changes in effector cells through increases in protein phosphorylation and Ca_i^{2+}, resulting in increased secretion and smooth muscle contraction, respectively. M_2 and M_4 receptors have a particular affinity for members of the G_i family of G proteins. Their main functions are to cause G_i-α–mediated activation of K^+ channels (resulting in hyperpolarization) and to inhibit adenylyl cyclase activity. Decreases in cyclic adenosine monophosphate (cAMP) and cAMP-dependent protein kinase activity produce a state of decreased phosphorylation of effector systems such as voltage-sensitive Ca^{2+} channels, resulting in decreased channel opening probability (negative inotropy and diminished transmitter release, respectively, through resulting decreases in Ca_i^{2+}). PKC—protein kinase C.

CHOLINERGIC RECEPTORS

Receptor Class	Receptor Subtype	Agonists	Antagonists	Tissue	Responses	Molecular Mechanisms
Nicotinic	Muscle (N_M)	Phenyltrimethyl-ammonium	Tubocurarine α-Bungarotoxin	Neuromuscular junction	End-plate depolarization, skeletal muscle contraction	Opening of cation channel in N_M receptor
	Neuronal (N_N)	Dimethylphenyl-piperazinium	Trimethaphan	Autonomic ganglia	Depolarization and firing of postganglionic neuron	Opening of cation channel in N_N receptor
				Adrenal medulla	Secretion of catecholamines	
Muscarinic	M_1	Oxotremorine McN-A-343	Atropine Pirenzepine	Autonomic ganglia	Depolarization (late epsp)	Stimulation of PLC with formation of IP_3 and DAG; increased cytosolic Ca^{2+}
	M_2	—	Atropine	Heart		
			AF-DX 115	SA node	Slowed spontaneous depolarization: hyperpolarization	Activation of K^+ channels; inhibition of adenylyl cyclase
				Atrium	Shortened duration of action potential; decreased contractile force	
				AV node	Decreased conduction velocity	
				Ventricle	Slight decrease in contractile force	
	M_3	—	Atropine	Smooth muscle	Contraction	Stimulation of PLC with formation of IP_3 and DAG; increased cytosolic Ca^{2+}
			Hexahydro-siladifenidol	Secretory glands	Increased secretion	

Figure 4-18. Summary of the classes and subtypes of cholinergic receptors, specific agonists/antagonists, tissue localization, types of effector responses, and underlying molecular mechanisms of action. AV—atrioventricular; DAG—diacylglycerol; epsp—excitatory postsynaptic potentials; IP_3—inositol triphosphate; PLC—phospholipase C; SA—sinoatrial. (*Adapted from* Lefkowitz *and colleagues* [18]; with permission.)

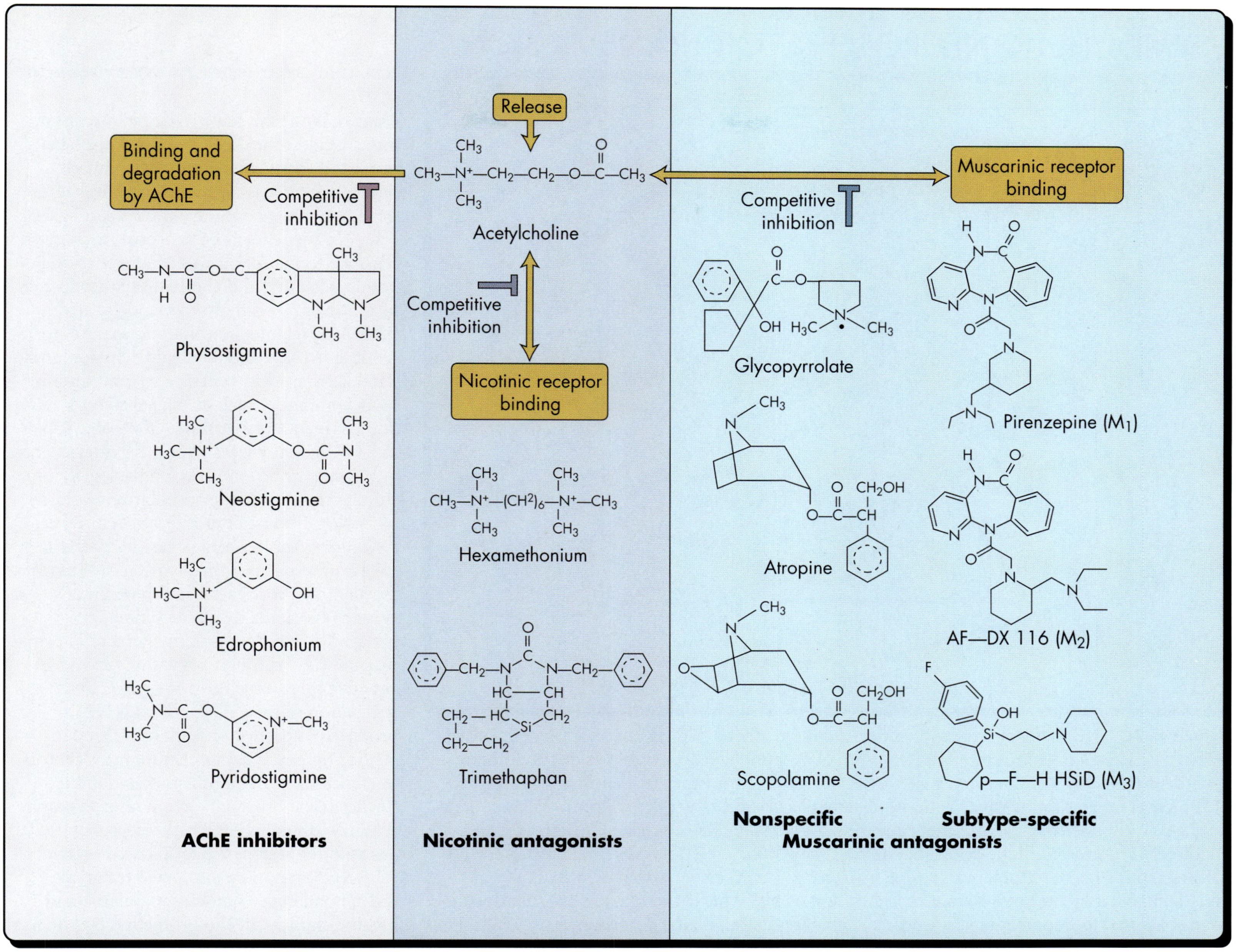

Figure 4-19. Pharmacology of cholinergic transmission. Various specific classes of acetylcholine (ACh) analogues are used clinically to alter cholinergic transmission through competitive inhibition. Competitive ACh esterase (AChE)-inhibitors are employed to increase the amount and duration of ACh available for binding to postsynaptic membrane receptors in skeletal muscle (during reversal of neuromuscular blockade), affecting cholinergic transmission in the autonomic nervous system (ANS) in an analogous manner. Competitive muscarinic receptor antagonists are used to inhibit excessive sialagogic or negative chronotropic effects mediated by muscarinic receptor occupation. The only antagonist with relative specificity for neuronal subtypes of nicotinic receptors (ganglionic blocker) in clinical use in the United States is trimethaphan. Competitive antagonists specific for skeletal muscle nicotinic receptors are clinically employed as nondepolarizing muscle relaxants. The majority of modern muscle relaxants are devoid of significant affinity for ANS cholinergic receptors.

SYMPATHETIC NEUROEFFECTOR TRANSMISSION

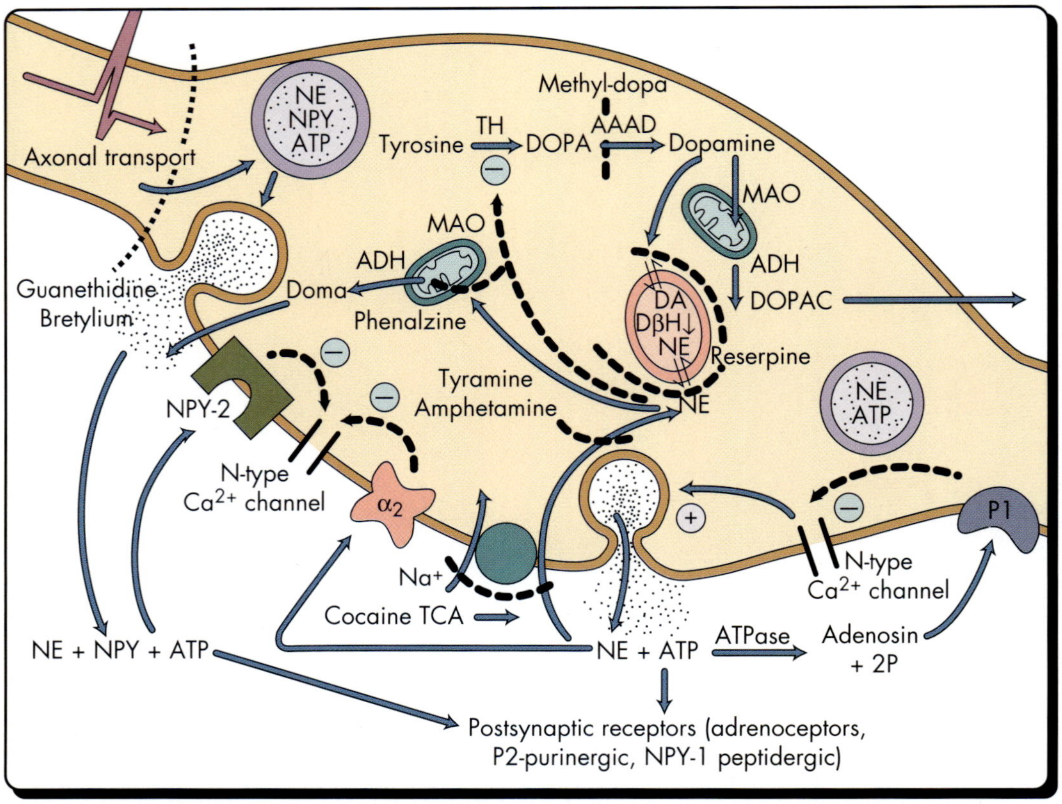

Figure 4-20. Mechanisms controlling transmitter synthesis and release at adrenergic nerve terminals. Transmitters are stored in two types of synaptic vesicles, small vesicles containing only the principal transmitter norepinephrine (NE) and cotransmitter adenosine triphosphate (ATP) (each synthesized within the nerve terminal itself) and larger dense-core vesicles containing the polypeptide cotransmitter neuropeptide Y (NPY) and chromogranin (both of which are exclusively synthesized in the cell soma) as well as NE and ATP. The rate-limiting step for NE synthesis in the nerve terminal is tyrosine hydroxylase (TH) enzyme activity, which is negatively controlled by the cytoplasmic concentration of NE. The TH enzymatic product dopa is decarboxylated to dopamine by (unspecific) aromatic L-amino acid decarboxylase (AAAD) in a step subject to therapeutic interference by provision of the "false" substrate α-methyl-dopa (resulting in the eventual formation of the "false transmitter" α-methyl-NE). Dopamine is to equal proportions either deaminated and excreted as DOPAC (3,4-dihydroxyphenylacetic acid) or taken up into dopamine-β-hydroxylase (DβH)—containing storage vesicles via a reserpine-sensitive active uptake process and hydroxylated to NE. The cytoplasmic concentration of NE is determined by a dynamic equilibrium established between diffusion (leakage) out of storage vesicles, reserpine-sensitive (active) reuptake into storage vesicles, cytoplasmic displacement and extrusion by indirect sympathomimetics such as tyramine and amphetamine, reuptake from the extracellular space via a Na^+-dependent cotransport mechanism sensitive to inhibition by cocaine or tricyclic antidepressants, and elimination after metabolization to 3,4-dihydroxymandelic acid (DOMA) by mitochondrial monoamine oxidase (MAO) and aldehyde dehydrogenase (ADH), a pathway sensitive to inhibition by MAO inhibitors such as phenelzine. In adrenal medullary neurons, 80% of cytoplasmic NE is methylized by *N*-methyl transferase into epinephrine before being packaged into storage vesicles. Nerve stimulation-evoked physiologic transmitter release occurs via fusion of synaptic storage vesicles with the cell membrane after the invasion of the nerve terminal by propagated action potentials (sensitive to blockade by guanethidine or bretylium) and the resulting increase in cytoplasmic Ca^{2+} through activation of voltage-sensitive (predominantly N-type) Ca^{2+} channels. Upon release, ATP, NE, and NPY produce neuroeffector responses through actions on postsynaptic membrane receptors. In addition, all three transmitters inhibit further release through action on presynaptic (P1, α2-adrenergic, NPY-2) receptors [19,20]. Transmitter actions are terminated by hydrolysis (ATP), reuptake into nerve terminals (NE), uptake into nonneuronal tissue and metabolism by catechol-O-methyl transferase (COMT) (NE), and diffusion away from the terminal and into the bloodstream (NE, NPY). ADH—aldehyde dehydrogenase; TCA—tricyclic antidepressants; TH—tyrosine hydroxylase; (*Adapted from* Nicholls *and colleagues* [17]; with permission.)

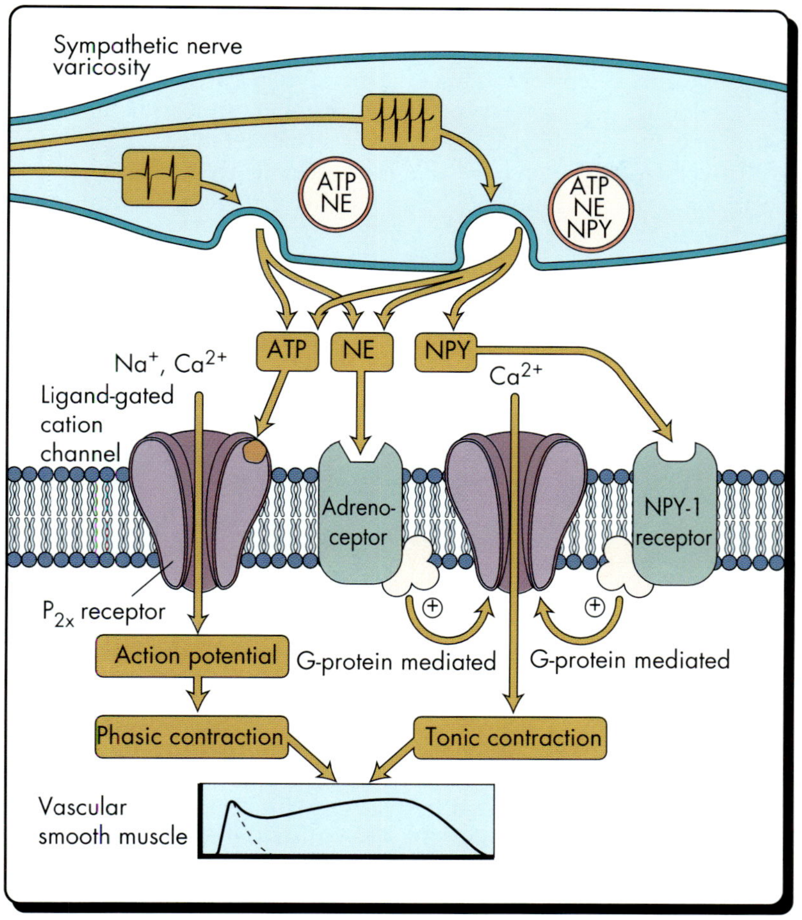

Figure 4-21. Sympathetic neuroeffector control of vascular smooth muscle. Firing of vasoconstrictor nerves is translated into junctional release of adenosine triphosphate (ATP), norepinephrine (NE), and neuropeptide Y (NPY). ATP binds to ligand-gated purinergic P_{2x}-receptors to evoke smooth muscle fast excitatory junction potentials (ejp) and action potentials resulting in phasic smooth muscle contractions, secondary to a transient influx of Ca^{2+}. Through activation of G-protein–linked receptors, NE and NPY prolong increases in Ca_i^{2+} via facilitated Ca^{2+} influx through voltage-gated Ca^{2+} channels and Ca^{2+} release from intracellular stores. Low-frequency prejunctional firing invokes primarily the release of ATP and NE. Higher frequency firing causes the additional release of NPY. NPY acts either indirectly to potentiate the postjunctional contractile response to NE or directly to evoke a particularly slow and long-lasting contractile response by itself, irrespective of NE. Such direct effects of NPY itself are found in forearm arteries, renal arteries, and mesenteric veins (but not arteries) [2]. (*Adapted from* Sneddon [21]; with permission.)

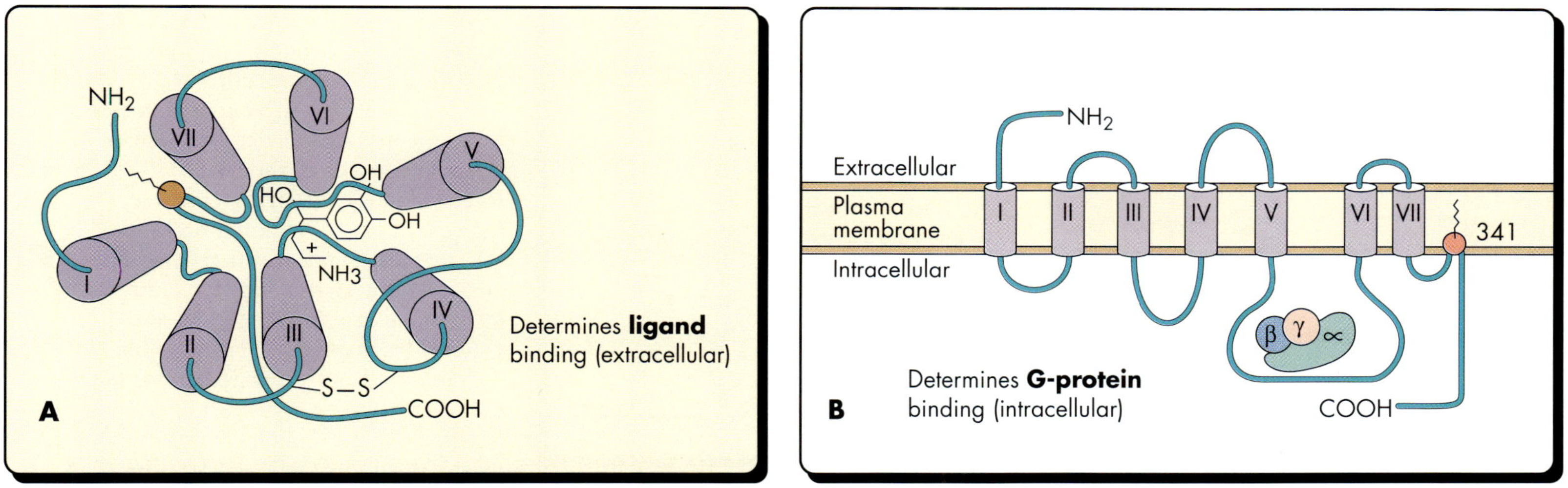

Figure 4-22. Adrenoceptor-mediated signal transduction mechanisms. Adrenoceptors are members of the superfamily of G protein–linked transmembrane receptors, similar to muscarinic ACh (m-ACh) receptors. Three different main families of adrenoceptors (α1, α2, and β) have been distinguished on the basis of particular affinities for specific extracellular agonists and antagonists, cytoplasmic affinities for distinct G protein families, and particular kinds of responses resulting from receptor activation (effector mechanisms) (**A**–**C**). Differences in extracellular agonist affinities are determined by selective differences in the transmembrane portions III, IV, and VII (indicated in *orange*) of the receptor molecules, whereas specific cytoplasmic affinities for different G proteins are determined by corresponding differences in their cytoplasmic loop between transmembrane portions V and VI (indicated in *blue*) [22]. α1-Adrenoceptors preferentially bind members of the G_q family of G proteins.

(*Continued on next page*)

Receptor type	Preferred G-protein	Effector mechanisms
α_1	G_q family members →	Phospholipase C (+) Phospolipase A_2 (+) Voltage-sensitive Ca^{2+} - channel activation (+)
α_2	G_i family members →	Adenylyl cyclase (–) K^+ - Channel activation (+) Voltage-sensitive Ca^{2+} - channel activation (–)
β	G_s family members →	Adenylyl cyclase (+) Voltage-sensitive Ca^{2+} - channel activation (+)

C

Figure 4-22. (*Continued*) Effector mechanisms include activation of phosphoplipases A_2 and C (in a manner similar to that described for the M_3, muscarinic receptor) and resulting increases in Ca^{2+}, mediating vasoconstriction. α2-Adrenoceptors preferentially bind members of the G_i family of G proteins. Effector mechanisms include inhibition of adenylyl cyclase activity, activation of K^+ channels mediating membrane hyperpolarization, and inhibition of voltage-sensitive Ca^{2+} channels mediating decreases in transmitter release (in a manner similar to that described for M_2 and M_4 muscarinic receptors). β-Adrenoceptors preferentially bind members of the G_s family of G proteins. Effector mechanisms include activation of adenylyl cyclase activity mediating vasodilatation and—indirectly, through increases in phosphorylation as well as directly through G protein linkage—activation of (L-type) voltage-sensitive Ca^{2+} channels mediating increased cardiac inotropy. Several genetic subtypes of each of these principal types of adrenoceptors have been identified and found to be differentially expressed in various tissues [23].

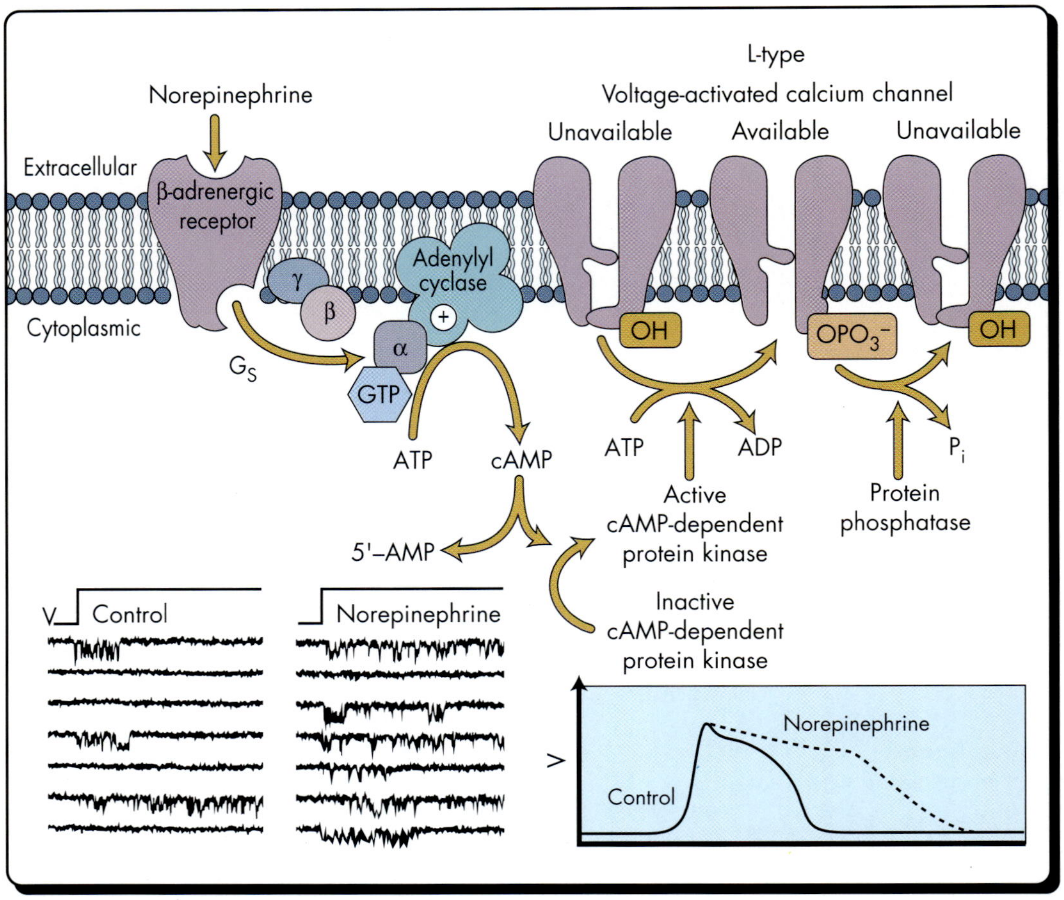

Figure 4-23. Mechanism of β-adrenoceptor-mediated control of myocardial inotropy. Upon agonist (norepinephrine, NE) binding to the extracellular agonist binding site of β-adrenoceptors, a conformational change causes intracellular binding of guanosine triphosphate (GTP) to the $G_s\alpha$ subunit of the associated heterotrimeric G_s protein and its dissociation from the receptor. GTP-activated $G_s\alpha$ binds to and increases the enzymatic activity of adenylyl cyclase, resulting in an increase in cytoplasmic cyclic adenosine monophosphate (cAMP) (second messenger). This increase in cAMP activates cAMP-dependent protein kinase (PKA). Activated PKA causes phosphorylation of serine and threonine moities of L-type Ca^{2+} channels. This phosphorylation alters their single channel voltage sensitivity in such a way that the same amount of membrane depolarization causes a larger increase in open-channel probability and thus increased Ca^{2+} inward current (*lower left*). Increased Ca^{2+} inward current, in turn, prolongs the myocardial action potential (*lower right*) and increases the resulting contractile force secondary to an increase in cytoplasmic Ca^{2+}. This functional organization of β-adrenergic signal transduction explains the clinically synergistic negative inotropic effects of β-adrenoceptor antagonists and Ca^{2+} channel blockers as well as the noncompetitive antagonism by glucagon or amrinone of the negative inotropic effect of β-adrenoceptor blockade through increases in the second messenger cAMP. ADP—adenosine diphosphate; ATP—adenosine triphosphate. (*Adapted from* Nicholls and colleagues [17]; with permission.)

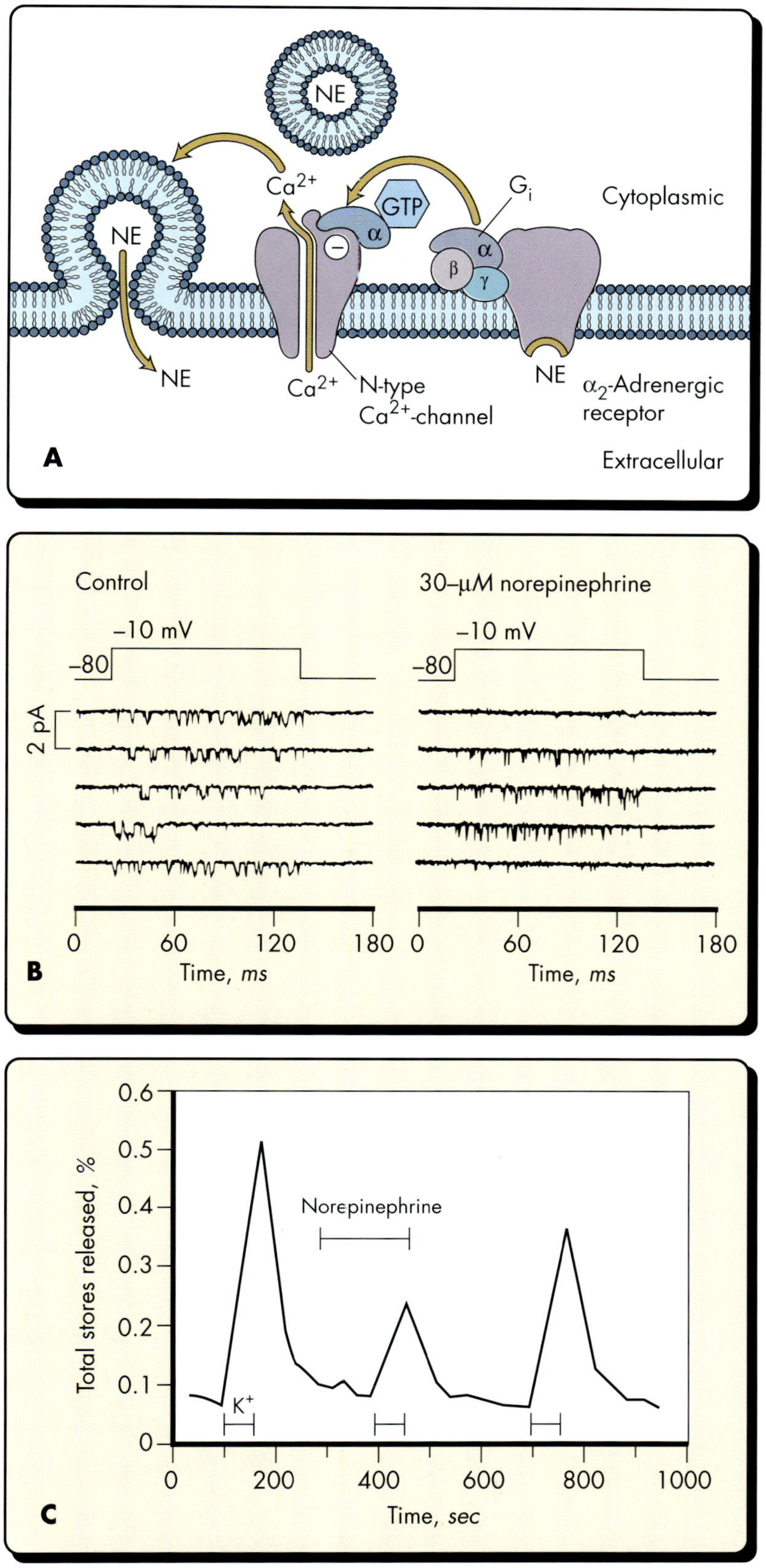

Figure 4-24. Mechanism of α2-adrenoceptor-mediated presynaptic inhibition of norepinephrine (NE) release. Upon binding of agonist NE to the extracellular agonist binding site of presynaptic α2-adrenoceptors (**A**), a conformational change causes intracellular binding of guanosine triphosphate (GTP) to the $G_i\alpha$ subunit of the associated heterotrimeric G_i protein and its dissociation from the receptor. GTP-activated $G_i\alpha$ binds to N-type Ca^{2+} channels and decreases their voltage sensitivity (**B**) in such a way that the same amount of membrane depolarization causes less of an increase in open-channel probability and thus decreased cytoplasmic Ca^{2+} inward current. The resulting decrease in Ca_i^{2+} transients in the presence of NE causes diminished K^+-depolarization–evoked presynaptic transmitter release (**C**). (*Adapted from* Nicholls and colleagues [17], based on data from Lipscombe and colleagues [19]; with permission.)

ADRENERGIC RECEPTORS

Receptor Type	Receptor Subtype	Agonists	Antagonists	Tissue	Responses	Molecular Mechanisms
				Adrenoceptors		
α_1	α_{1A} α_{1B} α_{1D}	Epi ≥ NE >> Iso Phenylephrine	Prazosin	Vascular smooth muscle	Contraction	Stimulation of PLC with formation of IP_3 and DAG; increased cytosolic Ca^{2+}
				Genitourinary smooth muscle	Contraction	Activation of Ca^{2+} channels
				Liver (α_{1A})	Glycogenolysis; gluconeo-genesis	(α_{1D})
				Intestinal smooth muscle	Hyperpolari-zation and relaxation	Activation of Ca^{2+}-dependent K^+ channels
				Heart (α_{1A})	Increased contractile force; arrhythmias	Inhibition of transient K^+ current
α_2	α_{2A} α_{2B} α_{2C} α_{2D}	Epi ≥ NE ≥ Iso Clonidine	Yohimbine	Pancreatic islets (β cells)	Decreased insulin secretion	Inhibition of adenylyl cyclase; activation of K^+ channels
				Platelets	Aggregation	
				Nerve terminals	Decreassed release of NE	Inhibition of neuronal Ca^{2+} channels
				Vascular smooth muscle	Contraction	Enhanced influx of Ca^{2+}; increased cytosolic Ca^{2+}
β	β_1	Iso > Epi = NE Dobutamine	Metoprolol CGP 20712A	Heart	Increased force and rate of contraction and AV nodal conduction velocity	Activation of adenylyl cyclase and Ca^{2+} channels
				Juxtaglomerular cells	Increased renin secretion	
	β_2	Iso > Epi >> NE Terbutaline	ICI 118551	Smooth muscle (vascular, bronchial, gastrointesti-nal, and genitourinary)	Relaxation	Activation of adenylyl cyclase
				Nerve terminals	Increased release of NE	
				Heart	Increased rate and force of contraction	
				Skeletal muscle	Glycogenolysis; uptake of K^+	
				Liver	Glycogenolysis; gluconeogenesis	
	β_1	Iso = NE > Epi BRL 37344	ICI 118551 CGP 20712A	Adipose tissue	Lipolysis	Activation of adenylyl cyclase
				Dopaminergic receptors		
D_{1A}, D_{1B}		Dopamine > NE Apomorphine	Droperidol Haloperidol	Smooth muscle (renal, mesenteric)	Relaxation	Activation of adenylyl cyclase
D_{2A}, D_{2B}, D_{2C}		Dopamine > NE Bromocriptine	Domperidone	Nerve terminals	Decreased release of NE	Inhibition of neuronal Ca^{2+} channels

Figure 4-25. Summary of the classes, types, and subtypes of adrenergic receptors, specific agonists/antagonists, tissue localization, types of effector responses, and underlying molecular mechanisms of action. AV—atrioventricular; DAG—diacylglycerol; Epi—epinephrine; IP_3—inositol triphosphate; Iso—isoproterenol; NE—norepinephrine; PLC—phospholipase C. (*Adapted from* Lefkowitz and colleagues [18]; with permission.)

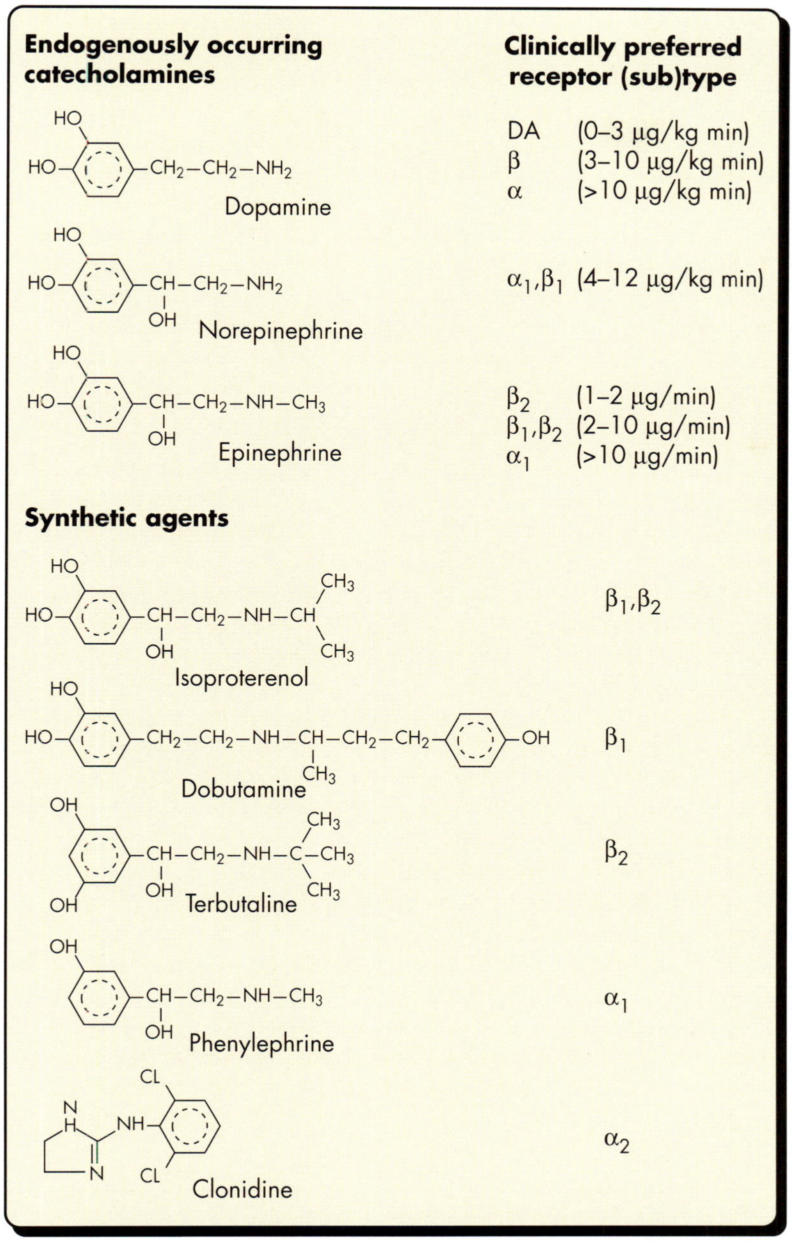

Figure 4-26. Clinically used adrenoceptor agonists. Adrenoceptor agonists in clinical use include endogenously occurring catecholamines such as dopamine, norepinephrine, and epinephrine and receptor type–specific synthetic derivatives. When exogenously applied by intravenous infusion, the clinically dominant target receptor types of endogenous catecholamines depend on the plasma concentration and thus the infusion rate. The relative clinical potencies for different receptor types are not fixed, however; they are subject to differential receptor desensitization or downregulation, which more commonly affects β-adrenoceptors than α-adrenoceptors and may occur even in response to the action of *endogenously released* catecholamines.

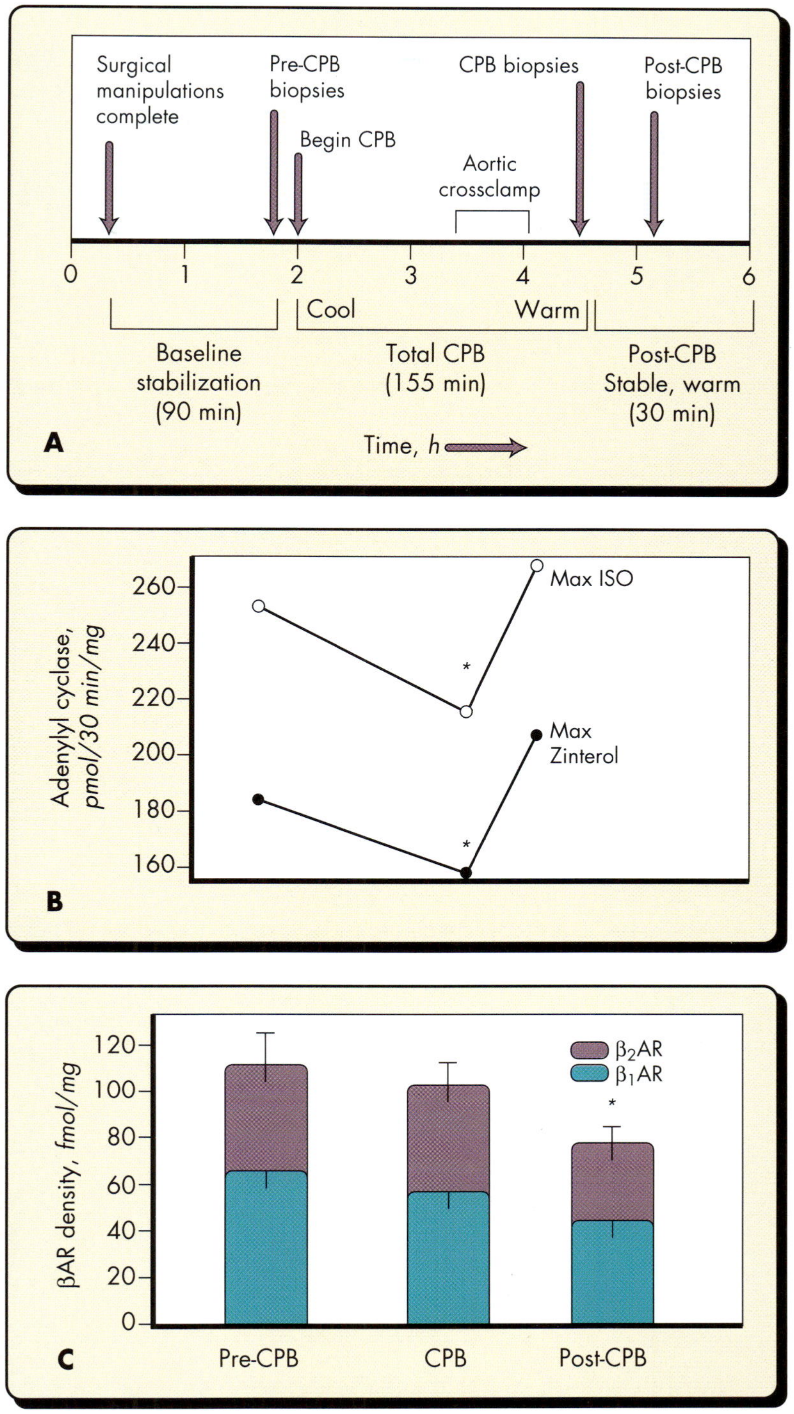

Figure 4-27. β-Adrenoceptor desensitization and downregulation after cardiopulmonary bypass. When myocardial biopsy samples are tested before and after hypothermic cardiopulmonary bypass (CPB) in dogs (**A**), significant changes are found with regard to β-adrenoceptor function. Compared with the prebypass maximal adenylyl cyclase activity stimulated with isoproterenol (ISO) (β1-and β2-adrenoceptor agonist) or zinterol (predominant β2-adrenoceptor agonist), there is an acute decrease in maximal adenylyl cyclase activity with either agonist immediately upon completion of CPB indicative for functional desensitization of β1-and β2-adrenoceptor agonist responses (**B**). This desensitization occurs in the absence of any simultaneous change in β1-or β2-adrenoceptor density (**C**). Thirty minutes postbypass, functional receptor desensitization is reversed (*panel B*); however, the total density of β-adrenoceptors is now significantly decreased, indicating receptor downregulation (*panel C*). Thus, receptor desensitization and downregulation both can occur independently of each other in response to endogenous catecholamine release during CPB. Either mechanism can significantly alter adrenergic responsiveness of cardiac myocytes in the postbypass period. (*Adapted from* Schwinn and colleagues [24]; with permission.)

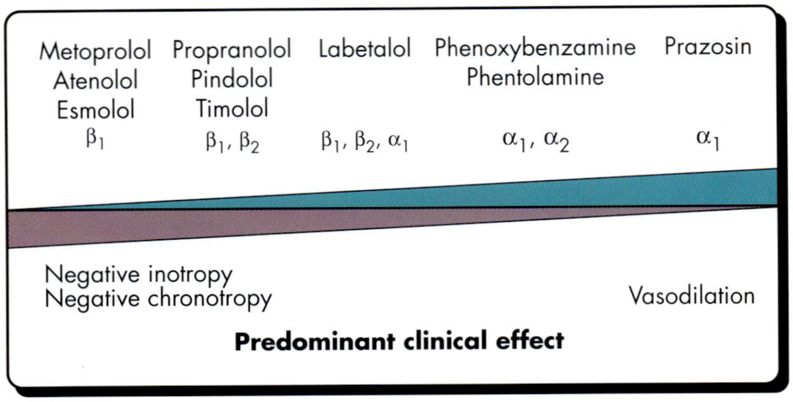

Figure 4-28. Clinically used adrenoceptor antagonists. Adrenoceptor antagonists with varying specificities for adrenoceptor (sub)types have been synthesized. The clinical responses vary accordingly. α-Adrenoceptor antagonists cause predominantly vasodilatation (and potentially a reflex increase in heart rate). β-Adrenoceptor antagonists cause predominantly a decrease in heart rate and inotropy (*ie*, a decrease in cardiac output) and bronchoconstriction. In response to physiologic sympathetic nervous system activity, end organ responses are altered by adrenoceptor antagonists to the degree that they are mediated by neurally released norepinephrine or circulating epinephrine, not however attributable to postjunctional effects of coreleased cotransmitters, in particular neuropeptide Y, which may contribute to vasoconstrictive responses during higher frequency sympathetic nerve activity.

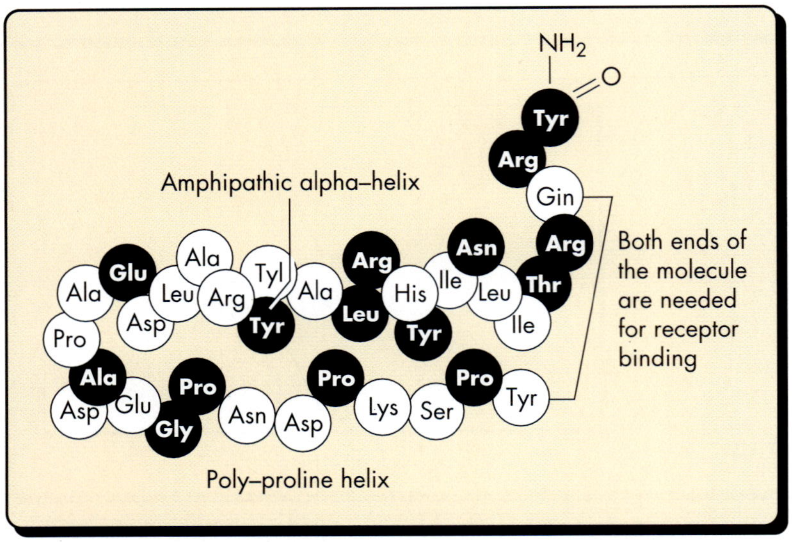

Figure 4-29. Structure of neuropeptide Y (NPY). Discovered in 1982 by Tatemoto *et al.* [25], NPY has been recognized as the single most abundant and widely distributed neuropeptide to date. It is a 36-amino acid polypeptide with completely conserved interspecies sequence homology among humans, rats, dogs, rabbits, and guinea pigs. In the peripheral autonomic nervous system, NPY is colocalized and coreleased with norepinephrine (NE) from postganglionic vasoconstrictor and cardiac efferent sympathetic nerve endings [8,10]. In addition, NPY is contained in various subpopulations of neurons within the central nervous system, and intrinsic neurons of the cardiac plexus. Based on a folded tertiary structure as suggested by radiograph reconstruction [26], NPY interacts via both C-and N-terminal ends with its G protein–linked transmembrane receptors. The two types of receptors identified to date are the postsynaptic NPY-1 receptor (which functions to either potentiate NE responses or cause postsynaptic vasoconstrictive responses by itself, even in the presence of adrenergic receptor blockade such as in human forearm arteries [27–29]) and the presynaptic NPY-2 receptor (which functions to inhibit presynaptic transmitter release through inhibition of N-type Ca^{2+} channels [20]). Favored post-versus presynaptic action may depend on the width of the junctional cleft [3]. Ala—alanine; Arg—arginine; Asn—asparagine; Asp—aspartic acid; Gln—glutamine; Glu—glutamic acid; Gly—glycine; His—histamine; Ile—isoleucine; Leu—leucine; Lys—lysine; Pro—proline; Ser—serine; Thr—threonine; Tyr—tyrosine. (*Adapted from* Schwartz and colleagues [26]; with permission.)

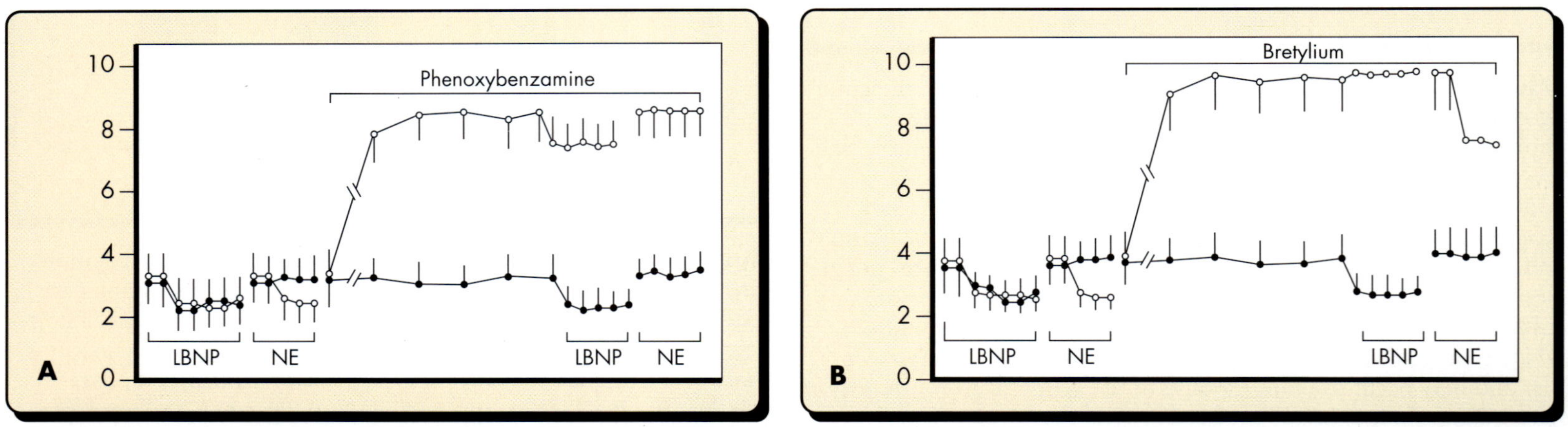

Figure 4-30. Evidence for a physiologic role of endogenously released neuropeptide Y (NPY) in human forearm vasoconstriction. Application of negative pressure to the lower body (LBNP, 10 mm Hg) in humans evokes a cardiac low-pressure mechanoreceptor-mediated bilateral sympathetic reflex increase in forearm vascular resistance (FVR) [30]. The postjunctional mediation of this reflex response is studied by unilateral pharmacologic intervention in one arm (*open circles*) compared with the contralateral control arm (*closed circles*), each studied by occlusion plethysmography. When tested on the study side, the reflex vasoconstriction is mimicked by intraarterial infusion of norepinephrine (NE). In the presence of the α-adrenoceptor antagonist phenoxybenzamine (PBZ) (and a resulting vasodilatation), the vasoconstrictive effect of NE is abolished, whereas the reflex increase in vascular resistance to LBNP is only partially diminished (**A**). In contrast, after infusion of bretylium, which blocks all transmitter release from sympathetic nerve endings, the ipsilateral reflex increase in vascular resistance to LBNP is completely abolished, whereas the vasculature still responds to exogenous NE (**B**) [29].

(*Continued on next page*)

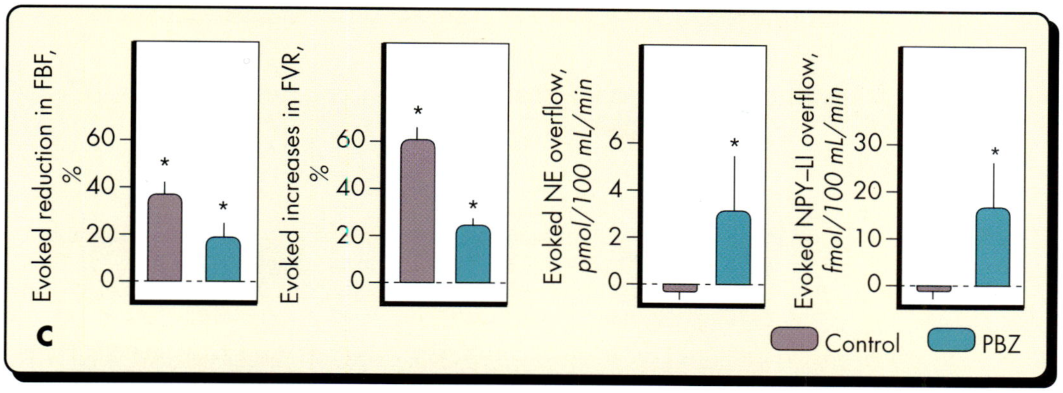

Figure 4-30. (*Continued*) The partially maintained reflex vasoconstrictive response to LBNP in the presence of PBZ is associated with increased overflow of NPY-like immunoreactive material (C) [28]. Finally, exogenous NPY has previously been shown to produce forearm vasoconstriction in the presence of doses of the α-adrenoceptor antagonist phentolamine, which block the response to exogenous NE (data not shown) [29]. Propranolol is present throughout. FBF—forearm blood flow. (Panels A and B *adapted from* Taddei and colleagues [27]; with permission; panel C *adapted from* Kahan and colleagues [28]; with permission.)

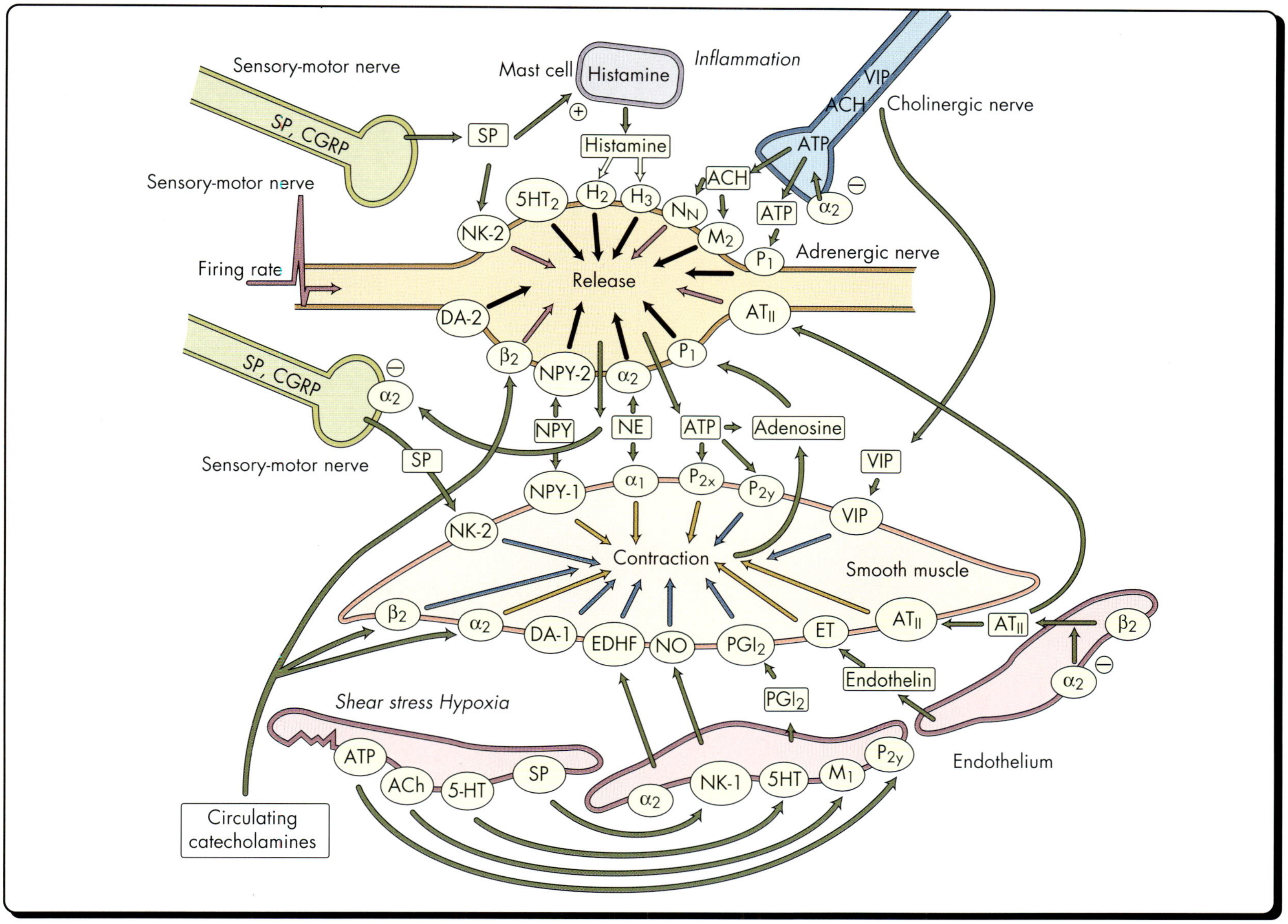

Figure 4-31. Neural-endothelial local interactions at adrenergic neuroeffector junctions. Vascular smooth muscle tone is determined not only by the firing rate of vasoconstrictor nerves but also by a large number of complex local interactions between adrenergic nerve endings, smooth muscle cells, vascular endothelium, circulating factors, cholinergic neurons, motor-sensory nerve endings, and other cells containing neuro- or vasoactive substances such as mast cells [3]. All of these regulatory mechanisms contribute to the local fine-tuning of vascular tone according to central *and* local needs under physiologic and, particularly, under pathophysiologic conditions such as shear stress, hypoxia, or inflammation. This is accomplished by interactive cross-modulation of transmitter release from these various regulatory elements and an integrative smooth muscle contractile response. Factors augmenting the release of adenosine triphosphate (ATP), norepinephrine (NE), and neuropeptide Y (NPY) from adrenergic nerve endings are indicated in *red*, and factors decreasing their release are indicated in *black*. Factors increasing smooth muscle tone are indicated in *orange*, and factors decreasing smooth muscle tone are indicated in *blue*. Contractile activity itself feeds back upon transmitter release through the extrusion of adenosine from active smooth muscle cells, which inhibits further transmitter release from adrenergic nerve endings. ACh—acetylcholine; AT_{II}—angiotensin II; CGRP—calcitonin gene-related peptide; DA-1—dopamine-1 receptor; EDHF—endothelium-dependent hyperpolarizing factors; $5HT_2$—5-hydroxy tryptamine-2 receptor; NK-1—neurokinin-1 receptor; NK-2—neurokinin-2 receptor; NO—nitric oxide; P_1—presynaptic purinergic receptor; $P_{2x, y}$—postsynaptic purinergic receptors; PGI_2—prostaglandin I_2; SP—substance P; VIP—vasoactive intestinal polypeptide.

REFERENCES

1. Bannister R, Mathias CJ: Introduction and classification of autonomic disorders. In *Autonomic Failure*. Edited by Bannister R, Mathias CJ. New York: Oxford University Press; 1992:1–12.
2. Milner P, Burnstock G: Neurotransmitters in the autonomic nervous system. In *Handbook of Autonomic Nervous System Dysfunction*. Edited by Korczyn AD. New York: Marcel Dekker; 1995:5–32.
3. Ralevic V, Burnstock G: *Neural-Endothelial Interactions in the Control of Local Vascular Tone*. Edited by Ralevic V, Burnstock G. Austin: RG Landes Company; 1993.
4. Stapelfeldt WH, Szurszewski JH: Neurotensin facilitates release of substance P in the guinea-pig inferior mesenteric ganglion. *J Physiol (Lond)* 1989, 411:325–345.
5. Shepherd JT: The heart as a sensory organ. *J Am Coll Cardiol* 1985, 5:83B–87B.
6. Perez-Gomez F, De Dios RM, Rey J, *et al.*: Prinzmetal's angina: reflex cardiovascular response during episode of pain. *Br Heart J* 1979, 42:81–87.
7. Spyer KM: CNS organization of reflex circulatory control. In *Central Regulation of Autonomic Functions*. Edited by Loewy AD, Spyer KM. New York: Oxford University Press; 1990:168–188.
8. Muzi M, Ebert TJ: Randomized, prospective comparison of halothane, isoflurane, and enflurane on baroreflex control of heart rate in humans. *Adv Pharmacol* 1994, 31:379–387.
9. Seagard JL: Differential control of blood pressure by two types of carotid baroreceptors. *Adv Pharmacol* 1994, 31:351–367.
10. Gibbins IL: Peripheral autonomic nervous system. In *The Human Nervous System*. Edited by Paxinos G. New York: Academic Press; 1990:93–123.
11. Elfvin LG, Lindh B, Hoekfelt T: The chemical neuroanatomy of sympathetic ganglia. *Annu Rev Neurosci* 1993, 16:471–507.
12. Jaenig W, McLachlan EM: Characteristics of function-specific pathways in the sympathetic nervous system. *Trends Neurol sci* 1992, 15:475–481.
13. Jan YN, Jan LY, Kuffler SW: A peptide as a possible transmitter in sympathetic ganglia of the frog. *Proceedings Natl Acad Sci U S A* 1979, 76:1501–1505.
14. Bachoo M, Polosa C: Cardioacceleration produced by close intra-arterial injection of neurotensin into the stellate ganglion of the cat. *Can J Physiol Pharmacol* 1988, 66:408–412.
15. Stapelfeldt WH, Szurszewski JH: Central neurotensin nerves modulate colo-colonic reflex activity in the guinea-pig inferior mesenteric ganglion. *J Physiol (Lond)* 1989, 411:347–365.
16. Bosnjak ZJ, Kampine JP: Intracellular recordings from the stellate ganglion of the cat. *J Physiol (Lond)* 1982, 324:273–283.
17. Nicholls JG, Martin AR, Wallace BG: *From Neuron to Brain*. Edited By Nicholls JG, Martin AR, Wallace BG. Sunderland MA: Sinauer Associates; 1992.
18. Lefkowitz RJ, Hoffman BB, Taylor P: Drugs acting at synaptic and neuroeffector junctional sites. In *The Pharmacological Basis of Therapeutics*. Edited by Gilman AG, Rall TW, Nies AS, *et al.* New York: Pergamon Press; 1990:84–121.
19. Lipscombe D, Kongsamut S, Tsien RW: α-Adrenergic inhibition of sympathetic neurotransmitter release mediated by modulation of N-type calcium-channel gating. *Nature* 1989, 340:639–642.
20. Toth PT, Bindokas VP, Bleakman D, *et al.*: Mechanism of presynaptic inhibition by neuropeptide Y at sympathetic nerve terminals. *Nature* 1993, 364:635–639.
21. Sneddon P: Co-transmission. In *Neurotransmitter Release and its Modulation*. Edited by Powis DA, Bunn SJ. Cambridge: Cambridge University Press; 1995:22–35.
22. Schwinn DA: Adrenoceptors as models for G-protein-coupled receptors: structure and regulation. *Br J Anaesth* 1993, 71:77–85.
23. Summers RJ, McMartin LR: Adrenoceptors and their second messenger systems. *Neurochem* 1993, 60:10–23.
24. Schwinn DA, Leone BJ, spahn DR, *et al.*: Desensitization of myocardial β-adrenergic receptors during cardiopulmonary bypass. *Circulation* 1991,84: 2559–2567.
25. Tatemoto K, Carlquist M, Mutt V: Neuropeptide Y—a novel brain peptide with structural similarities to peptide YY and pancreatic polypeptide. *Nature* 1982, 296:659–660.
26. Schwartz TW, Fuhlendorff J, Kjems LL, *et al.*: Signal epitopes in the three-dimensional structure of neuropeptide Y. *Ann N Y Acad Sci* 1990, 611:35–47.
27. Taddei S. Salvetti A, Pedrinelli R: Persistence of sympathetic-mediated forearm vasoconstriction after α-blockage in hypertensive patients. *Circulation* 1989, 80:485–490.
28. Kahan T, Taddei S. Pedrinelli R, *et al.*: Nonadrenergic sympathetic vascular control of the human forearm in hypersension: possible involvement of neuropeptide Y. *J Cardiovasc Pharmacol* 1992, 19:587–592.
29. Clark J, Benjamin N, Larkin S, *et al.*: Interaction of neuropeptide Y and the sympathetic nervous system in vascular control in man. *Circulation* 1991, 83:774:–777.
30. Mohanty PK, Thames MD, Arrowood JA, *et al.*: Impairment of cardiopulmonary baroreflexes after cardiac transplantation in humans. *Circulation* 1987, 74:914–922.

5

Cardiovascular Physiology and Pharmacology

Gregory H. Botz and Jonathan B. Mark

Cardiovascular disease remains the leading cause of death in the United States. Nearly one third of the 27 million patients undergoing surgery each year have coronary atherosclerosis or associated risk factors [1], and many hundreds of thousands more have valvular or congenital cardiac disease. These patients present a challenge to physicians responsible for their medical care in the perioperative period, who work to reduce the morbidity and mortality associated with surgery and the attendant costs that now exceed $20 billion per year.

A solid understanding of the scientific foundations of cardiovascular physiology and pharmacology is essential for the practice of clinical anesthesiology. This chapter attempts to summarize with figures and tables the principles that are most relevant for the anesthesiologist and perioperative physician.

Cardiac macro- and micro-anatomy are reviewed briefly, focusing on the critical cellular elements that are the functional units of physiologic actions and the targets of pharmacologic agents. Clinical anatomy of the cardiac chambers, valves, conduction system, and blood supply is presented.

Cardiac cellular physiology begins with a description of excitation-contraction coupling and neural control. The cardiac cycle and normal hemodynamic values are reviewed, followed by the physiologic insights provided by ventricular function curves and pressure-volume loops. These illustrative models help define the concepts of preload, afterload, and contractility, which are the factors that govern cardiac performance.

The final section on cardiovascular pharmacology combines the relevant receptor models with tabular summaries of the many drugs that act on these receptors. The focus here is on drugs given to alter the cardiovascular system acutely (vasopressors, inotropes, and vasodilators) and those given chronically to patients with a variety of cardiovascular disorders (adrenergic blockers, nitrates, diuretics, and calcium channel antagonists).

CARDIAC ANATOMY

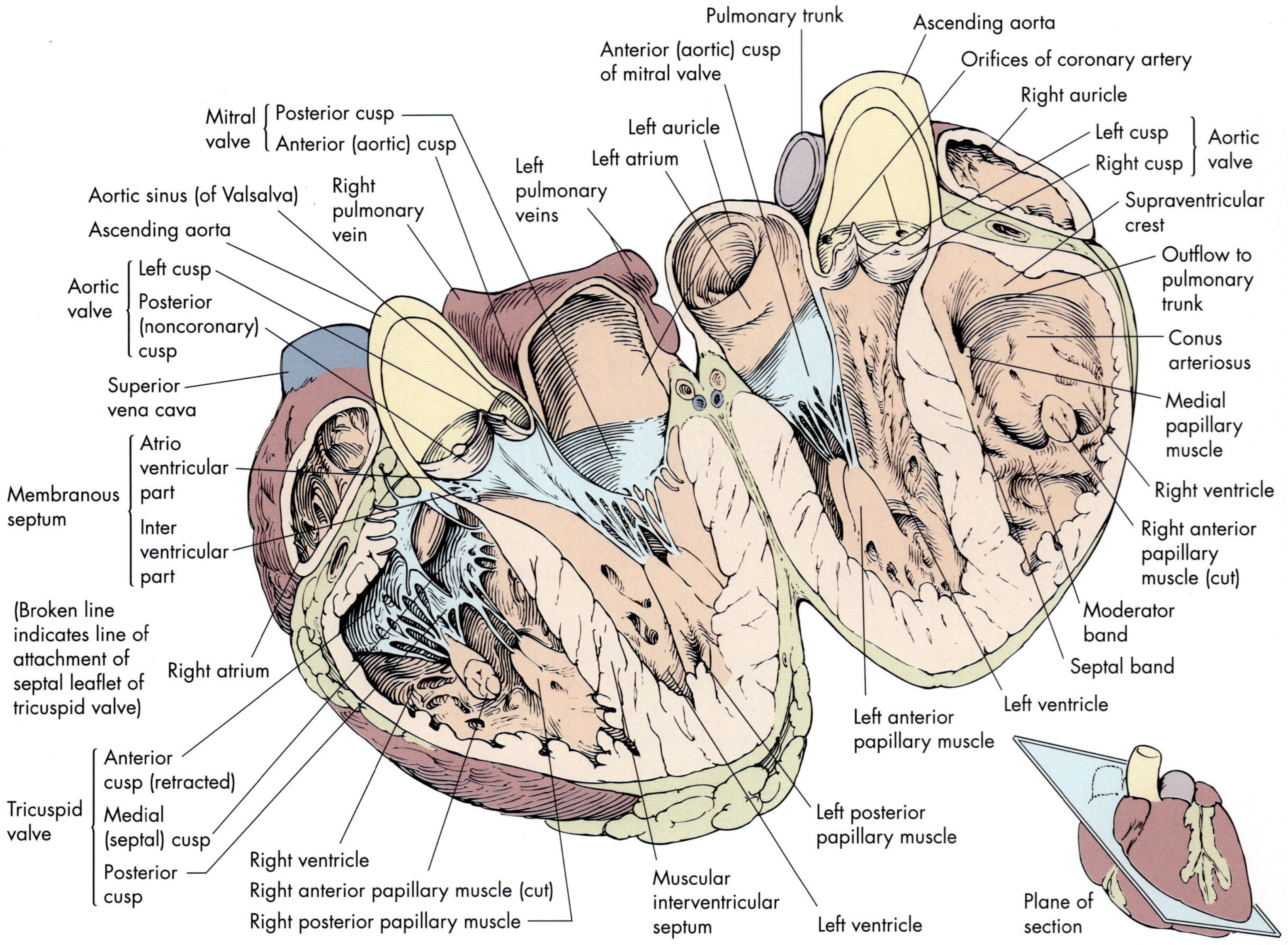

Figure 5-1. Detailed anatomy of the cardiac chambers and valves as seen on a long-axis cross-section (note the plane of the section). The four chambers of the heart include the right and left atria, separated by the interatrial septum, and the right and left ventricles, separated by the interventricular septum. The superior and inferior vena cavae deliver systemic venous return to the right atrium. Blood leaves the right atrium through the tricuspid valve and enters the right ventricle, a crescent-shaped, thin-walled chamber that lies anteriorly. Blood leaves the right ventricle through a distinct outflow tract that leads to the pulmonic valve and main pulmonary artery.

After traversing the lung, pulmonary venous blood enters the left atrium from the left and right pulmonary veins, then traverses the mitral valve into the muscular thick-walled left ventricle. The left ventricular outflow tract leads to the aortic valve and ascending aorta.

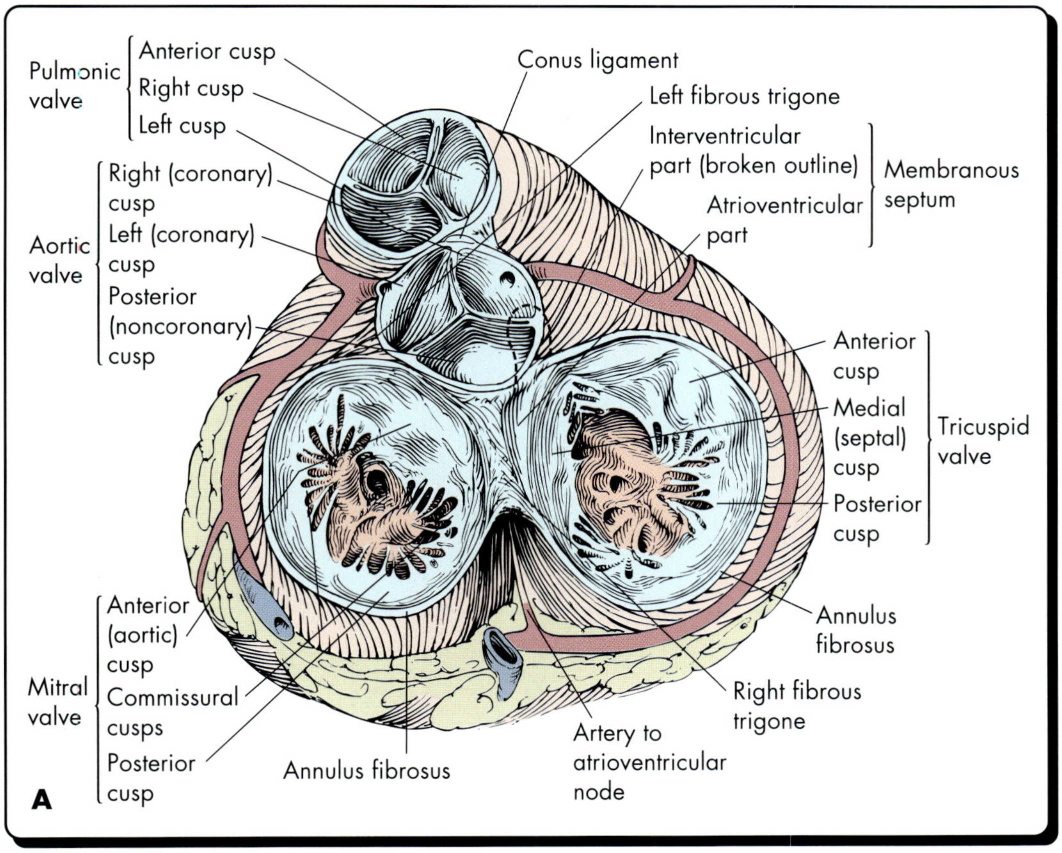

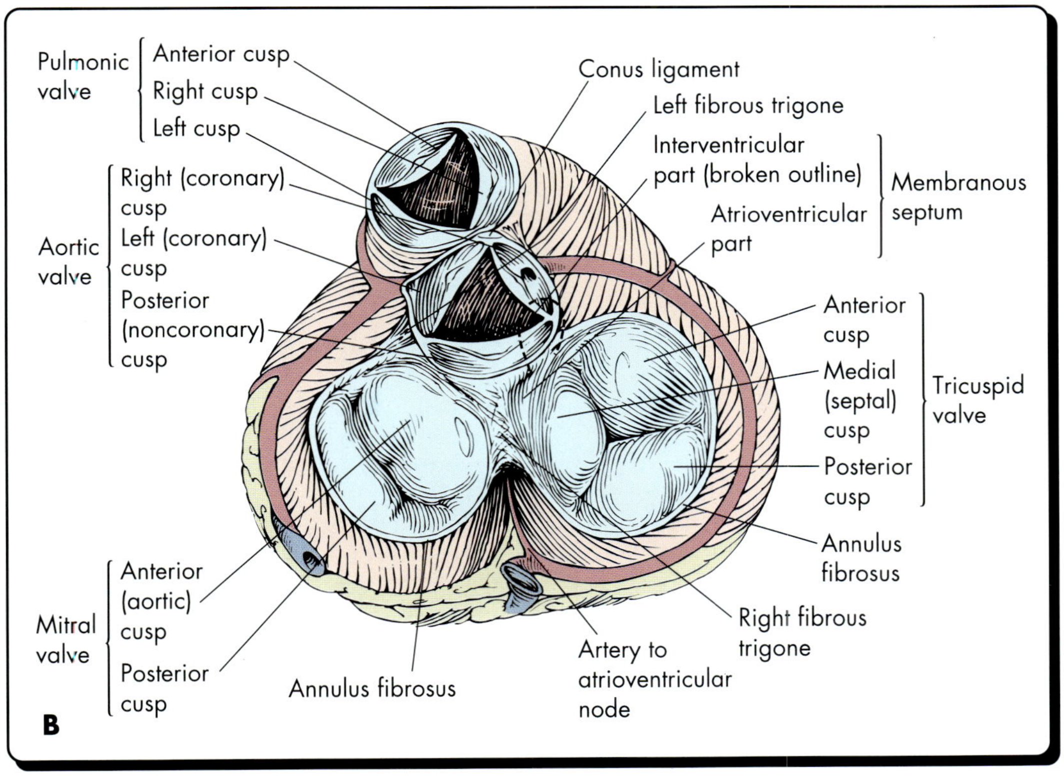

Figure 5-2. The important anatomic relationships of the four cardiac valves. **A**, The heart in diastole as viewed from the base with the atria removed. **B**, The heart in systole as viewed from the base with the atria removed. During diastole the two atrioventricular valves (mitral and tricuspid) are open and provide ventricular filling. During systole, these valves close, and the two semilunar valves (aortic and pulmonic) open to allow ventricular ejection of blood. The coaptation of the leaflets prevents backflow, thereby ensuring unidirectional flow. All four valves are supported by fibrous annular rings. In addition, papillary muscles and chordae tendineae tether the leaflets of the atrioventricular valves. The aortic and mitral valves are closely approximated within a single annular apparatus, whereas the tricuspid and pulmonic valves occupy distinct widely separated annulae.

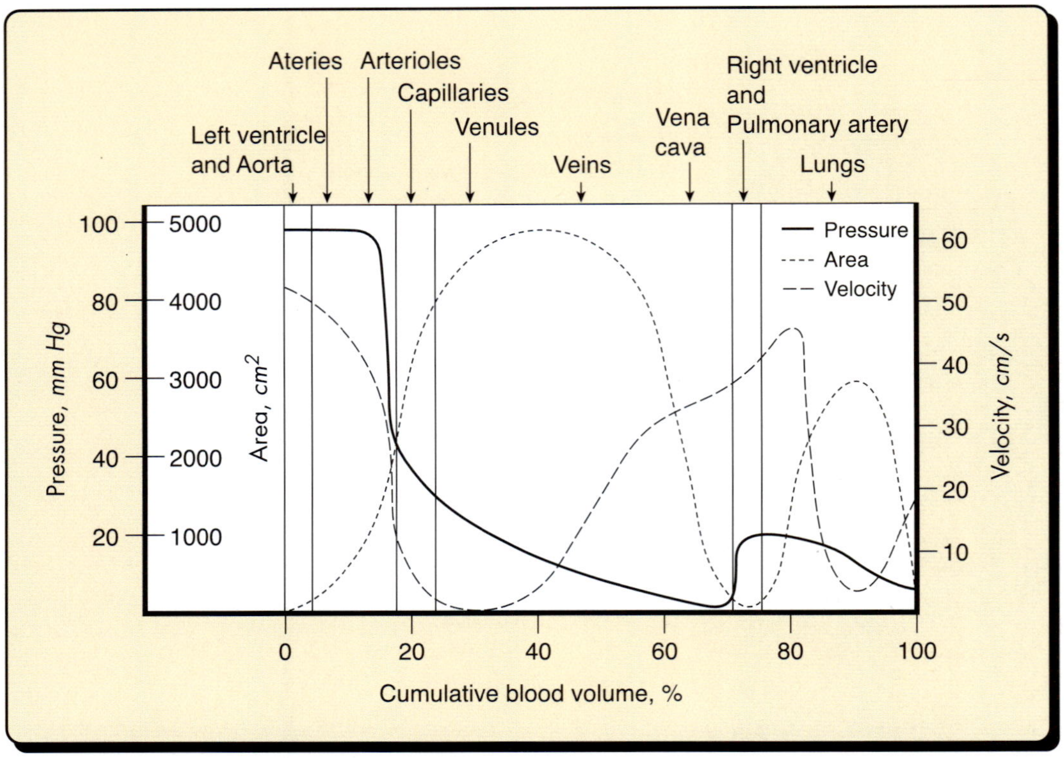

Figure 5-3. Relationship between velocity, area, volume, and pressure in various segments of the circulatory system. The same volume of blood must pass through each segment of the system per unit time, and therefore, the velocity and area are inversely related. The resistance of the large vessels is minimal, and therefore, pressure also is minimal until the small arterioles are reached. The important capacitance function of the systemic veins is demonstrated by the fact that approximately 45% to 50% of the total blood volume is contained within the venules and veins. (*From* Bullock and coworkers [2]; with permission.)

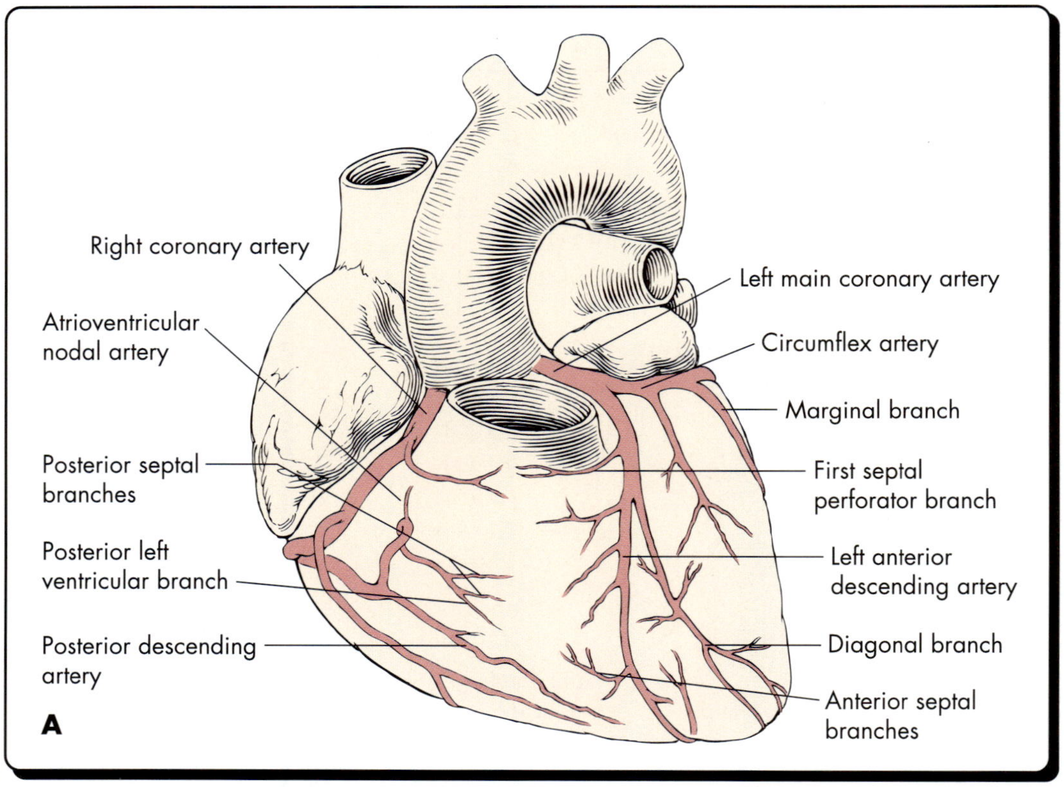

Figure 5-4. Anatomy of the coronary arteries. **A**, Frontal view of the heart. The coronary arteries arise from the left and right sinuses of valsalva above the aortic valve leaflets in the aortic root. Close to its origin, the left main coronary artery divides into the anterior descending and circumflex arteries, which lie in the anterior interventricular and left atrioventricular grooves, respectively. The right coronary artery follows the right atrioventricular groove and, in most cases, continues along the posterior interventricular groove as the posterior descending artery. Branches of the left anterior descending artery, called diagonals, supply the anterior and lateral walls of the left ventricle. Branches of the circumflex artery, called obtuse marginals, supply the lateral wall and portions of the posterior aspect of the left ventricle. The right coronary artery supplies the right ventricle and the posterior and inferior (diaphragmatic) walls of the left ventricle. The interventricular septum receives perforating branches from the right coronary artery via the posterior descending artery and left coronary artery via the left anterior descending artery. The sinoatrial and atrioventricular nodes are supplied by branches of the right coronary artery.

(*Continued on next page*)

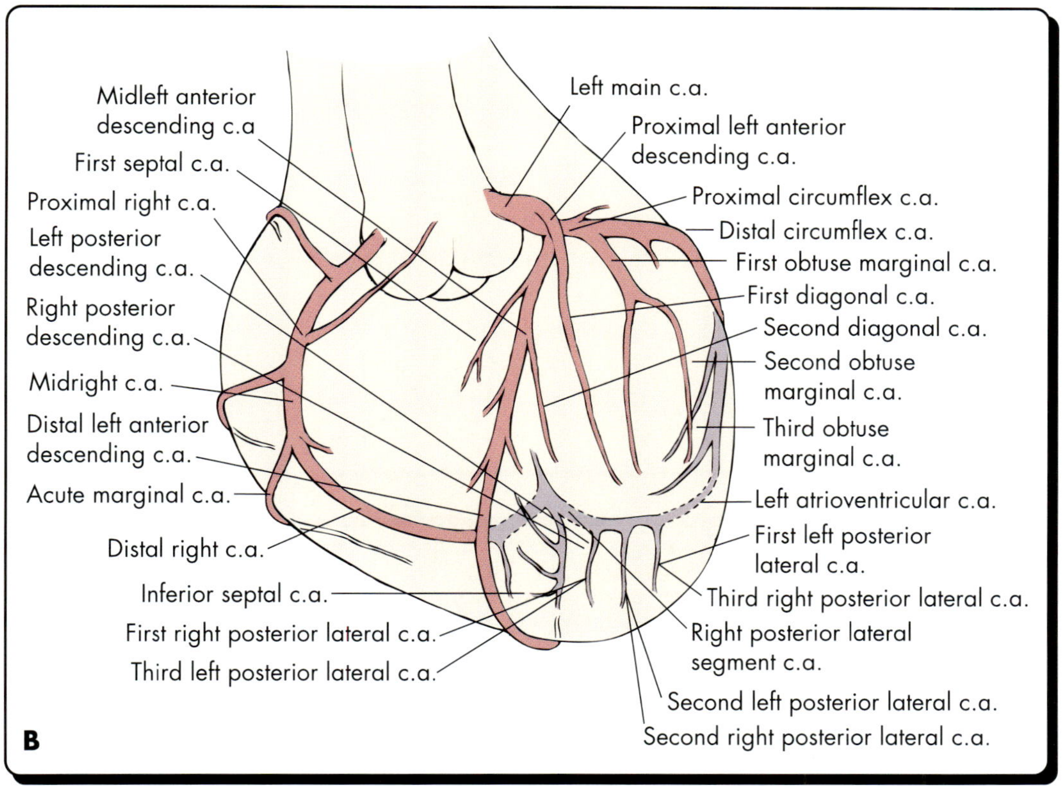

Figure 5-4. (*Continued*) B, The coronary artery visualized at angiography, as defined by cooperating centers in the Coronary Artery Surgery Study. (Part B *from* The National Heart, Lung, and Blood Institute [3].)

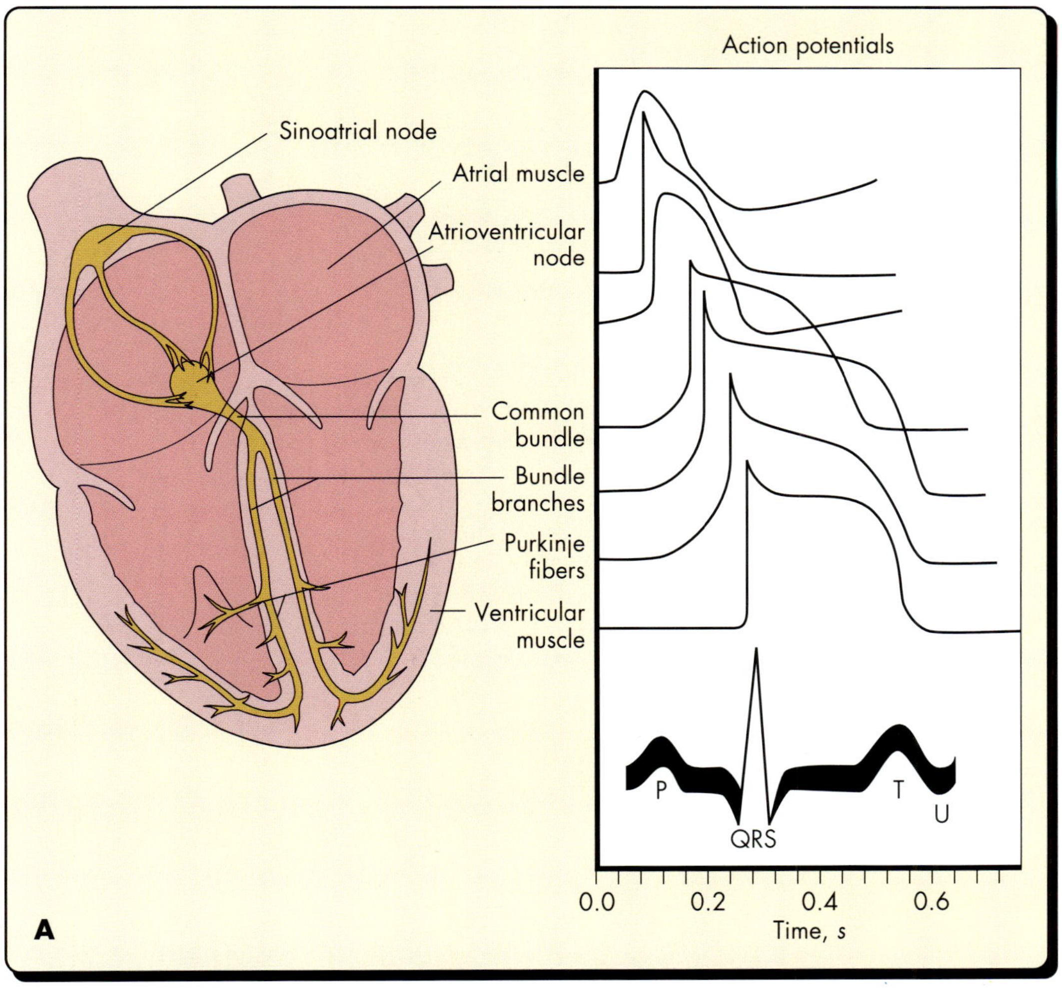

Figure 5-5. Cardiac action potentials. A, Characteristic cardiac action potentials recorded from different portions of the heart and its conduction system. The conduction system within the heart is comprised of specialized nerve cells that convey electrical impulses to the myocardium in a rapid, coordinated manner. The sinoatrial node, located near the junction of the superior vena cava and the right atrium, is the predominant pacemaker of the heart. An intrinsic automatic depolarization is propagated along interatrial pathways to the left atrium and toward the atrioventricular node, which lies near the interatrial septum above the tricuspid valve. The depolarization is propagated through the atrioventricular node to the conducting pathways in the ventricles. The fibrous atrioventricular skeleton electrically isolates the atria and ventricles, and thus, the atrioventricular node is the only conduction pathway between atria and ventricles. Depolarization is sufficiently delayed within the atrioventricular node to allow the atria to contract before the ventricles. Depolarization then travels to the bundle of His, which divides into bundle branches within the ventricles. The larger left bundle perforates the interventricular septum, then bifurcates into anterior and posterior fascicles, which supply the left ventricle. The right bundle follows the septum and traverses the moderator band, a muscular bridge or trabeculation, to supply the right ventricle. The coordinated movement of the action potentials along the conduction system to the myocardium is summarized in the familiar surface electrocardiogram.

(*Continued on next page*)

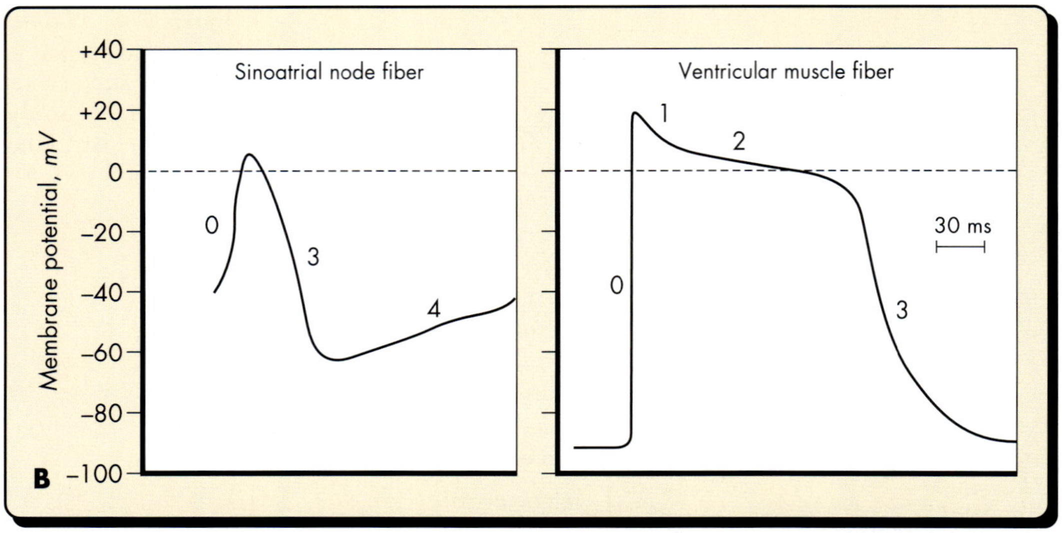

C. CARDIAC ACTION POTENTIAL

Phase	Name	Event	Cellular Ion Movement
0	Upstroke	Activation (opening) of fast Na^+ channels and decreased permeability to K^+	Na^+ in
1	Early rapid repolarization	Inactivation of Na^+ channel and transient increase in K^+ permeability	K^+ out
2	Plateau	Activation of slow Ca^{++} channels	Ca^{++} in
3	Final repolarization	Inactivation of Ca^{++} channels and increased permeability to K^+	K^+ out
4	Resting potential, or	Normal permeability restored (atrial and ventricular cells)	K^+ out
	Diastolic repolarization	Intrinsic slow “leakage” of sodium and possibly Ca^{++} into cells that spontaneously depolarize	Na^+ in ? Ca^{++} in

Figure 5-5. (*Continued*) B, Action potential morphology in pacemaker and ventricular myocardial cells. The cardiac action potentials in the sinoatrial cells (*left*) have a different morphology as compared with atrial and ventricular muscle (*right*). Note the slow upward phase 4 spontaneous depolarization in the sinoatrial node tracing. This accounts for the automaticity of the sinoatrial node.

C, The four phases of the cardiac action potential and their associated cellular ion movements. The phases of the action potentials reflect the changes in ion channel states with resultant ion flux. Rapid depolarization in phase 0 follows increased permeability to sodium. Repolarization in phases 1 through 3 relect slower movement of potassium and calcium via slower channels. Phase 4 reflects the return to baseline resting potential.(Parts B and C *from* Morgan and Mikhail [4]; with permission.)

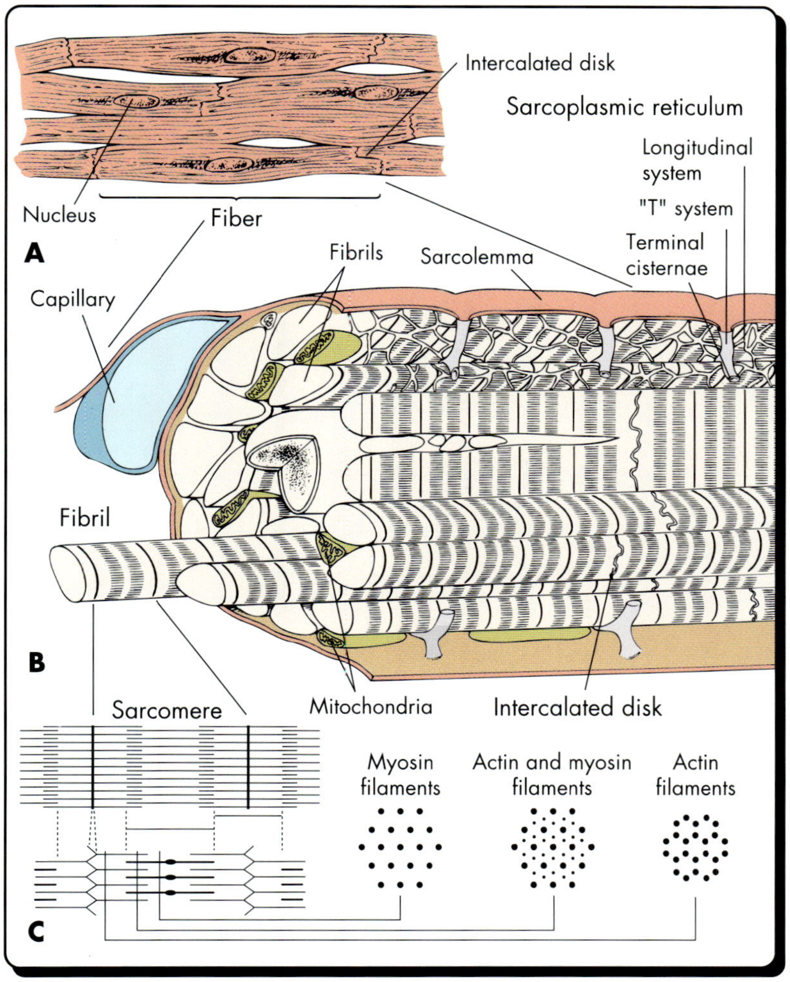

Figure 5-6. Microscopic structure of cardiac muscle. A, The myocardium is composed of a syncytium of discrete muscle cells arranged as fibers. Intercalated discs joining adjacent cells act as low-resistance pathways for propagation of the coordinated excitation-contraction wave. B, Within the muscle fiber is a network of longitudinally arranged myofibrils containing the contractile filaments, actin and myosin. The myofibrils are surrounded by an anastomosing network of tubules, the sarcoplasmic reticulum. The cell membrane, or sarcolemma, has tubular invaginations, the transverse tubules, which course into the interior of the myocardial cells adjacent to dilated sections of the sarcoplasmic reticulum, called terminal cisternae. C, The myofilaments are arranged in overlapping bands (*left*) that produce distinctive patterns on microscopy. Cross sections through the sarcomere at various points (*right*) reveal the arrangement of the myofibrils.

CARDIAC PHYSIOLOGY

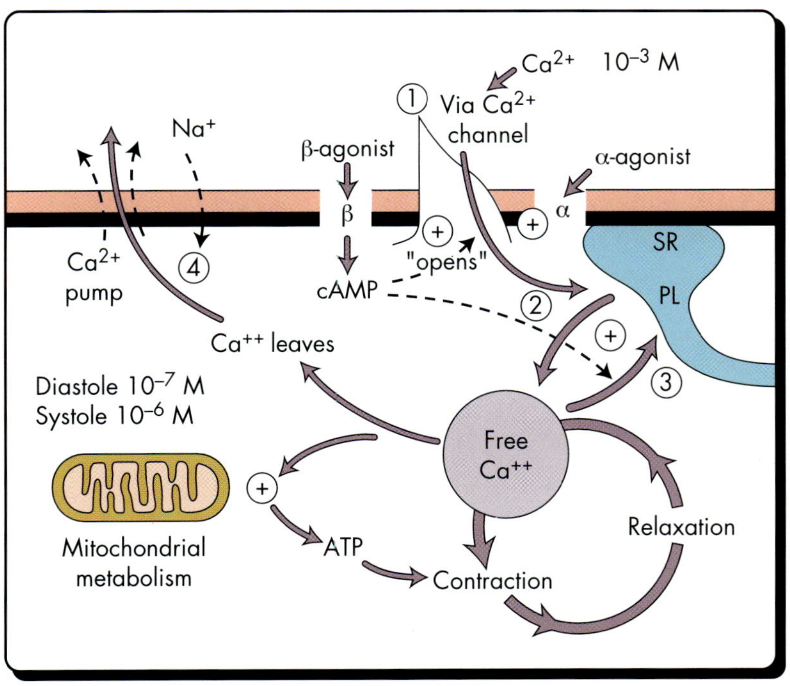

Figure 5-7. Calcium flux in the myocardium. During the cardiac cycle, the action potential travels along the sarcolemma, leading to depolarization of this membrane and movement of sodium and calcium into the cells. The action potential traversing the T-tubule apparatus and terminal cisternae leads to the release of calcium from the sarcoplasmic reticulum. Calcium movement at several sites during excitation-contraction participates in muscle contraction and relaxation (*circled numbers*): (1) Inward calcium movement across the sarcolemma during depolarization. (2) Calcium release from stores within the sarcoplasmic reticulum. The increase in intracellular calcium (10^{-7} M to 10^{-6} M) promotes the interaction of actin and myosin, the contractile components of the myofibrils. Rapid repetitive cross-bridging between actin and myosin causes shortening of the muscle cell. (3) Re-uptake of calcium into the sarcoplasmic reticulum via an energy-dependent ion pump. Energy-dependent relaxation of the myofibril cross-linking follows. (4) Extrusion of calcium from the cell by facilitated exchange with sodium. (5) Active transport via an energy-dependent pump (not shown). α—α-adrenergic receptor; ATP—adenosine triphosphate β—β-adrenergic receptor; cAMP—cyclic adenosine monophosphate; PL—phospholamban SR—sarcoplasmic retriculum. (Copyright © LH Opie [5]; with permission.)

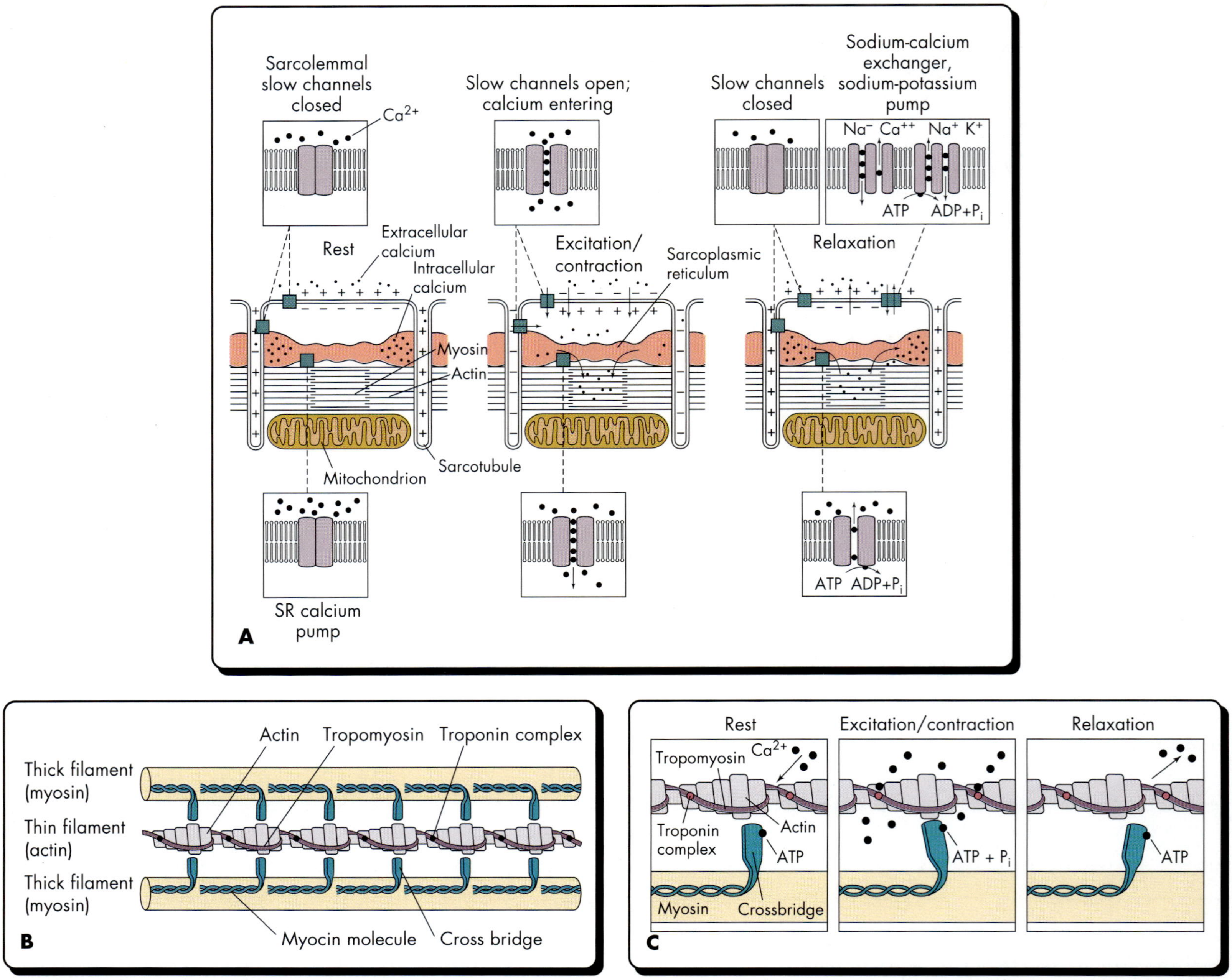

Figure 5-8. Excitation-contraction coupling and the interaction between actin and myosin. **A**, Calcium channel states during rest, excitation-contraction, and relaxation. At rest, the sarcolemmal and sarcoplasmic calcium channels are closed. Electrical depolarization leads to opening of these calcium channels, and intracellular calcium concentration increases 100-fold. During relaxation, the slow calcium channels close; however, calcium is removed from the intracellular space via facilitated and active exchange at the sarcolemma as well as active transport into the sarcoplasmic reticulum.

B, Structure of the actin-myosin complex at rest. The troponin and tropomyosin complexes cover active binding sites on actin and prevent cross-bridging.

C, Conformational changes in the tropomyosin-troponin complex during rest, excitation-contraction, and relaxation. Calcium binds to troponin, causing a conformational change in tropomyosin that facilitates cross-linking of actin and myosin. The myofilaments move relative to one another, shortening the length of the sarcomere. High-energy adenosine triphosphate (ATP) is necessary for the cross-linking, movement, and dissociation of the myofilaments. ADP—adenosine diphosphate; P_i—inorganic phosphate; SR—saracoplasmic reticulum. (*Adapted from* Morgan and Mikhail [4].)

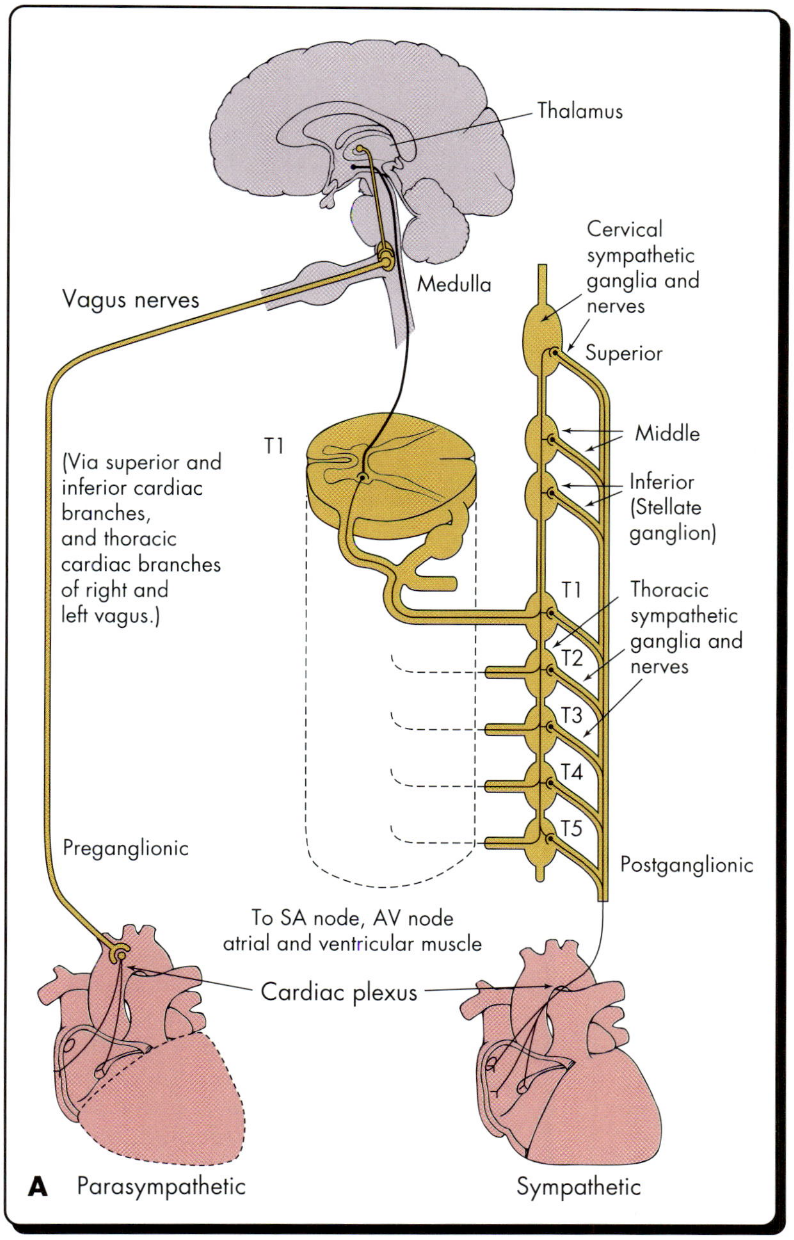

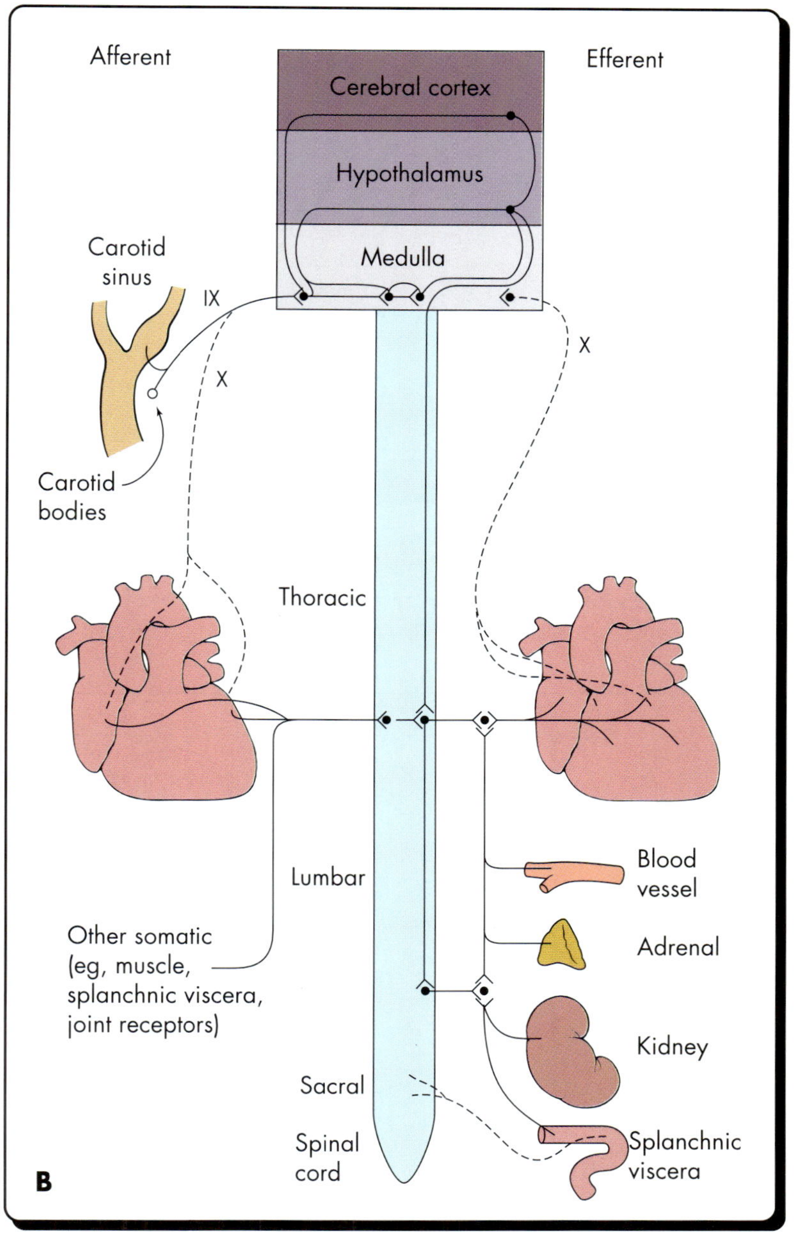

Figure 5-9. A, Efferent autonomic nerve supply to the heart. Parasympathetic fibers travel from the medulla via the vagus nerve and terminate in the sinoatrial (SA) node, the atrioventricular node (AV) and cardiac atria. Stimulation leads to the release of acetylcholine and results in decreased heart rate and prolonged conduction time. Sympathetic fibers travel via the sympathetic chain from the first four thoracic segments and innervate the SA node, AV node, atria and ventricles. Sympathetic stimulation causes release of norepinephrine, increases heart rate and contractility, and speeds conduction time. Autonomic innervation of the peripheral vasculature (not shown) produces vasoconstriction with sympathetic stimulation and vasodilation with parasympathetic stimulation.

B, Neural connections for circulatory control. Afferent fibers are depicted to the left, efferent fibers to the right. Afferent input to the central nervous system from baroreceptors located in the carotid sinus, great vessels, and cardiac chambers are carried by the ninth and tenth cranial nerves. Efferent outflow in the baroreceptor reflex arc is carried to the heart by the vagus nerve for parasympathetic regulation, and the first four thoracic segments via the sympathetic chain for sympathetic regulation. Additional sympathetic outflow through the entire thoracolumbar chain innervates the kidneys and adrenals, and causes vasoconstriction of the vasculature. Parasympathetic outflow to the periphery is provided by the tenth cranial nerve and the sacral outflow of the spinal cord. (Part A *adapted from* Johnson [6].)

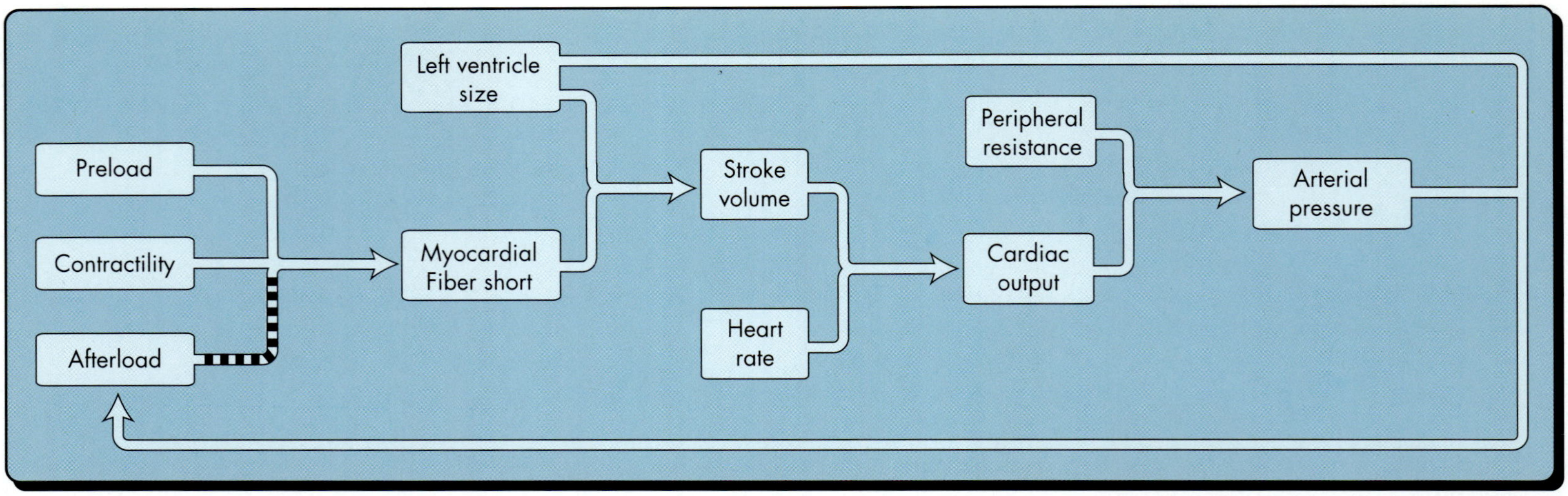

Figure 5-10. Determinants of cardiac performance and blood pressure. *Solid lines* indicate that direct relationships exist between variables. For example, increased stroke volume or increased heart rate result in increased cardiac output. The *dashed line* indicates that an inverse relationship exists between afterload and myocardial fiber shortening. Left ventricular afterload is best estimated by the systolic wall stress, which is directly proportional to both ventricular size and systolic arterial pressure according to the LaPlace relationship. (*Adapted from* Braunwald [7].)

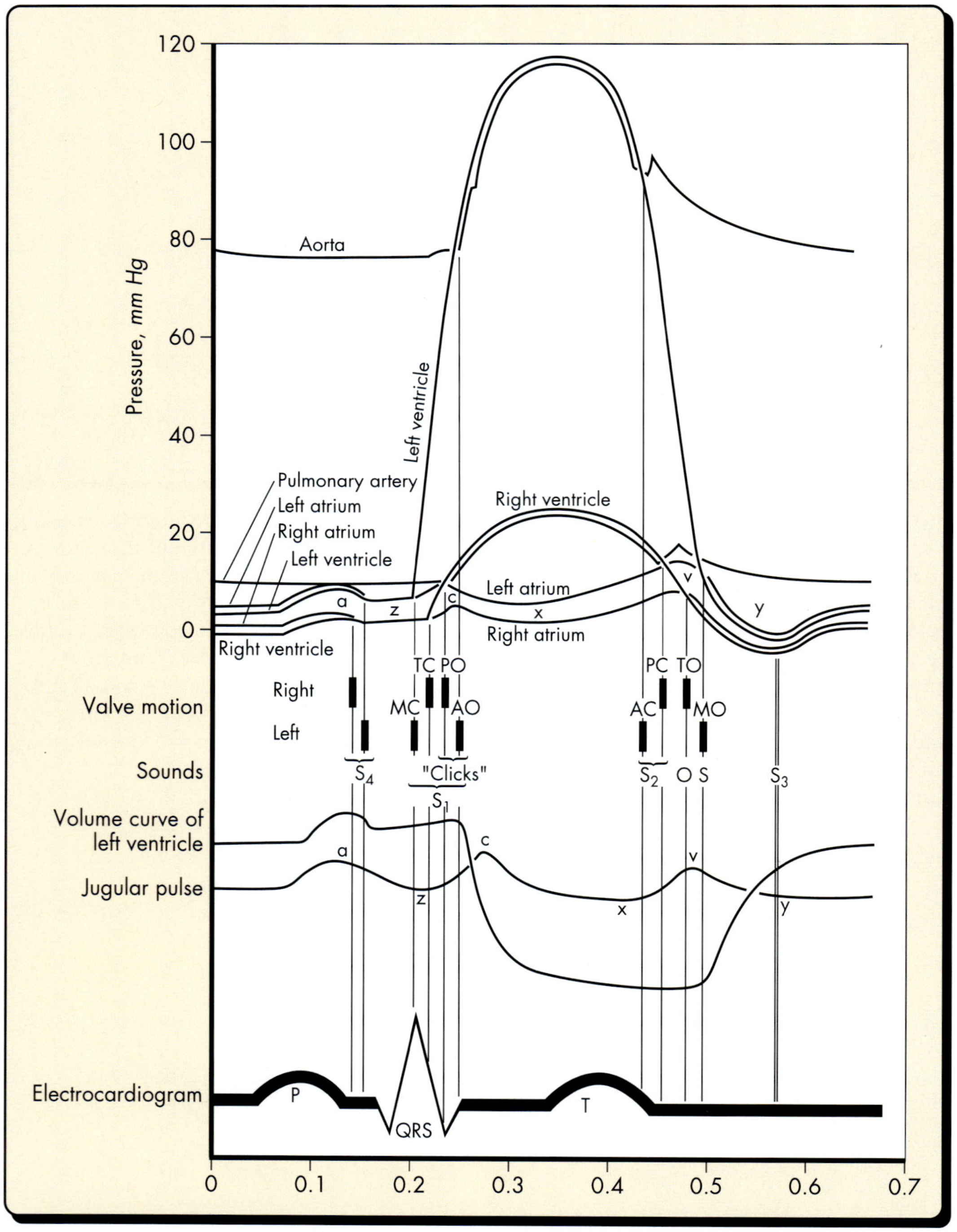

Figure 5-11. The cardiac cycle. The right-sided pressure waveforms (right atrium, ventricle, and pulmonary artery) are similar to the left-sided waveforms (left atrium, ventricle, and aorta) but reflect the low-pressure pulmonary circuit. The right and left atrial and the jugular pulse tracings inscribe similar waves during the cardiac cycle. The *a wave* marks atrial contraction after the electrocardiographic *p wave* (end-diastole). The *c wave* follows atrioventricular valve closure with the onset of isovolumic contraction (early systole). The *x descent* (midsystole) is associated with ventricular ejection and atrial relaxation. The *v wave* (late systole) marks atrial filling with the atrioventricular valves closed. The *y descent* (early diastole) corresponds to atrioventricular valve opening and rapid ventricular filling. Note the long isovolumic phases for the left (systemic) circuit (valve motion: *MC-AO*, *AC-MO*) compared with the right (pulmonic) circuit (valve motion: *TC-PO*, *PC-TO*). AC—aortic component of the second heart sound; AO—aortic valve opening; MC—mitral component of the first heart sound; MO—mitral valve opening; OS—opening snap of atrioventricular valves; PC—pulmonic valve component of the second heart sound; PO—pulmonic valve opening; TC—tricuspid component of the first heart sound; TO—tricuspid valve opening. (*Adapted from* Hurst [8]; with permission.)

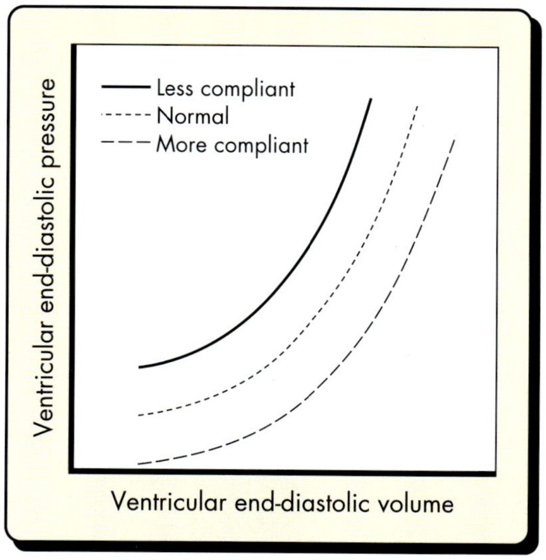

Figure 5-12. Normal and abnormal myocardial compliance relationship. The relationship between end-diastolic pressure and volume is compliance. Decreased compliance is the result of wall thickening (*eg*, hypertrophy) or stiffness (*eg*, ischemia). The right ventricle, with its thinner wall, is usually more compliant than is the left ventricle. (*From* Morgan and Mikhail [4]; with permission.)

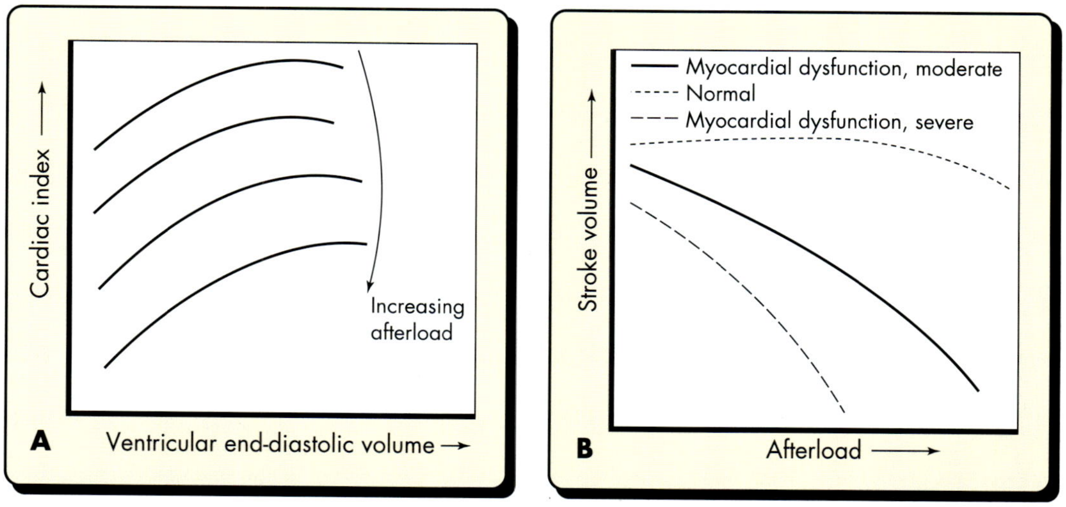

Figure 5-13. The relationship between afterload and cardiac output. Afterload is the impedence to ventricular ejection from systolic ventricular wall stress. **A**, A series of four ventricular function curves are shown. As afterload increases, cardiac output decreases for any level of ventricular end-diastolic volume. **B**, The impact of increasing afterload in reducing stroke volume is greater as intrinsic myocardial function deteriorates. Whereas an increase in afterload has little influence on stroke volume in a patient with normal ventricular function, the same increase in afterload reduces stroke volume markedly when there is severe myocardial dysfunction. (*From* Morgan and Mikhail [4]; with permission.)

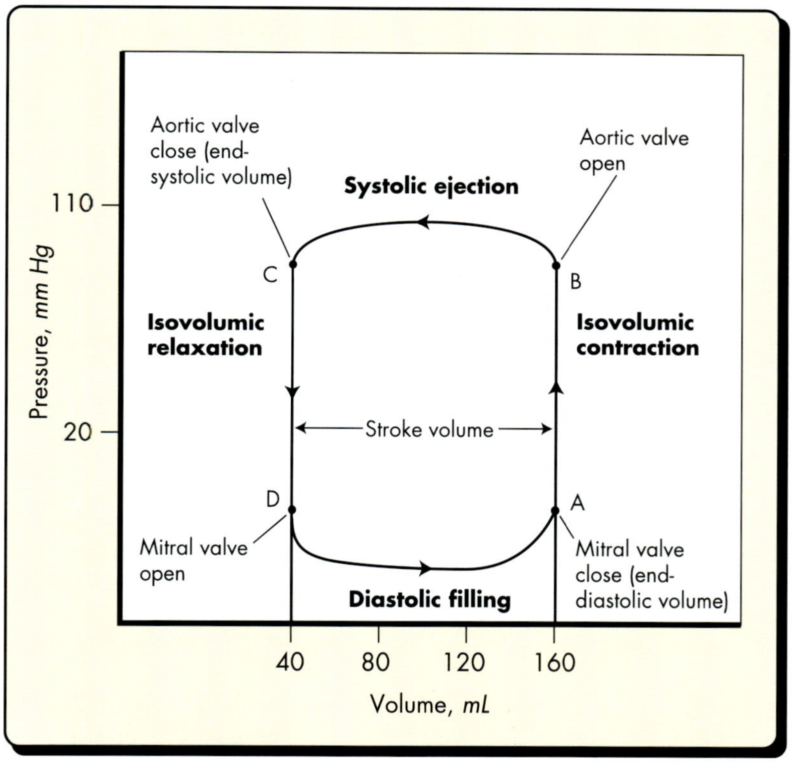

Figure 5-14. The relationship between left ventricular pressure and volume during a single cardiac cycle. Segment DA represents diastolic ventricular filling with the aortic valve closed and the mitral valve open. Segment AB begins with the closure of the mitral valve and describes isovolumic contraction, the onset of systole. Segment BC continues systole with the opening of the aortic valve and ventricular ejection. Segment CD begins diastole as the aortic valve closes and isovolumic relaxation occurs. Point A is end-diastole and point C is end-systole. The stroke volume can be calculated as the difference in ventricular volume between end-diastole and end-systole (EDV-ESV). The ejection fraction is the ratio of stroke volume and end-diastolic volume [(EDV-ESV)/ EDV]. The area circumscribed by the pressure-volume loop represents external work performed by the ventricle. (*From* Barash and Kopriva [9]; with permission.)

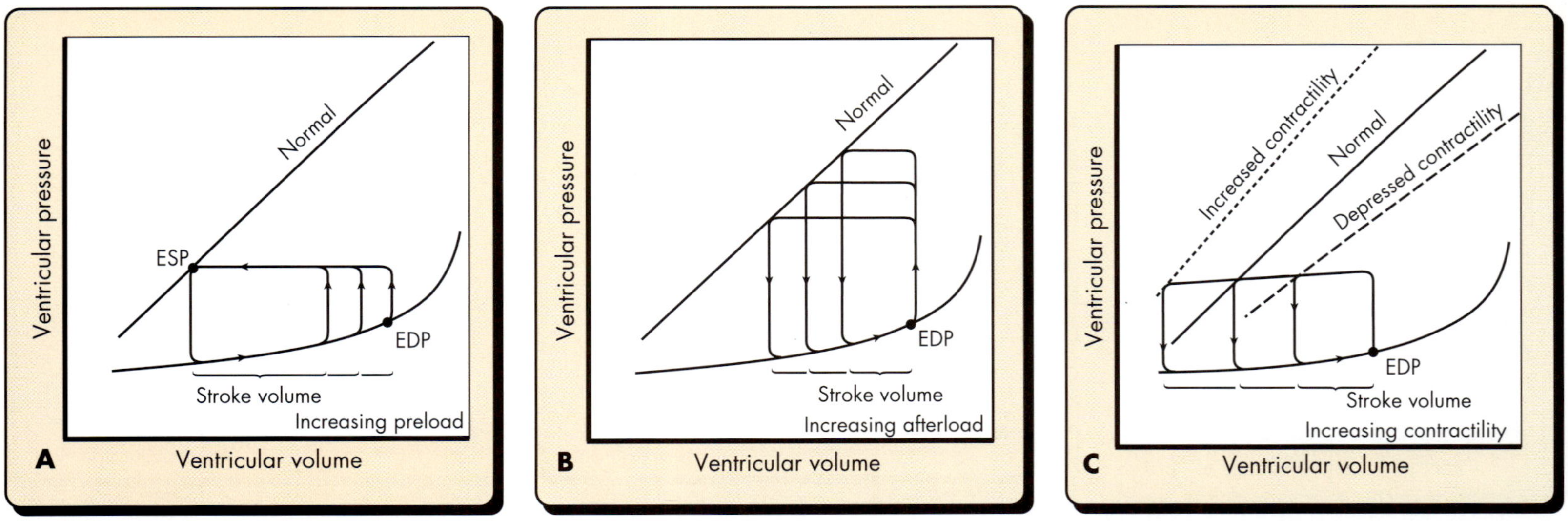

Figure 5-15. Ventricular pressure-volume diagrams. In this model of left ventricular function, preload (ventricular volume) is plotted on the x axis and afterload (ventricular pressure) is plotted on the y axis. The end-systolic pressure (ESP) line defines the contractile state of the ventricle. For any given level of ventricular volume and systolic pressure, the ventricle will eject a stroke volume down to the ESP line. **A**, Increasing preload with contractility and afterload constant. The stroke volume increases as the end diastolic volume increases. **B**, Increasing afterload with preload and contractility constant. The stroke volume decreases with increasing afterload. **C**, Increasing contractility with preload and afterload constant. Increasing contractility increases the stroke volume, and decreasing contractility decreases the stroke volume. EDP—end-diastolylic pressure. (*From* Morgan and Mikhail [4]; with permission.)

CARDIOVASCULAR PHARMACOLOGY

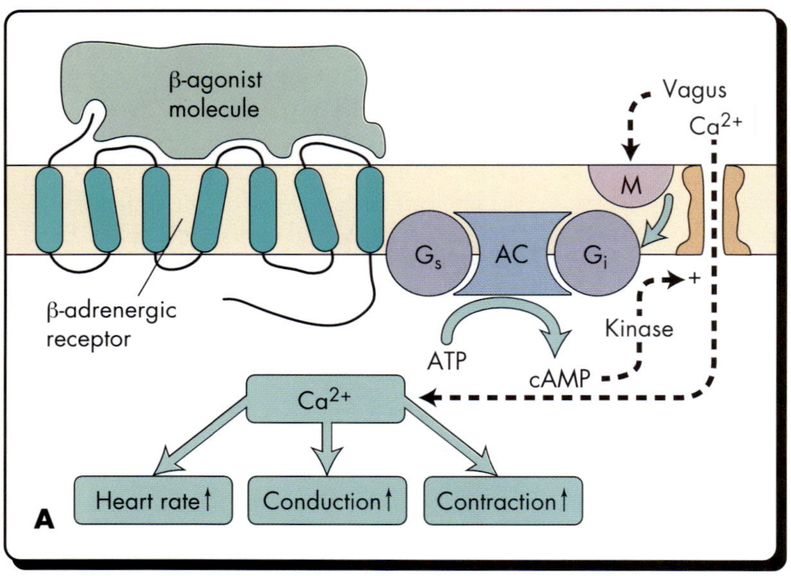

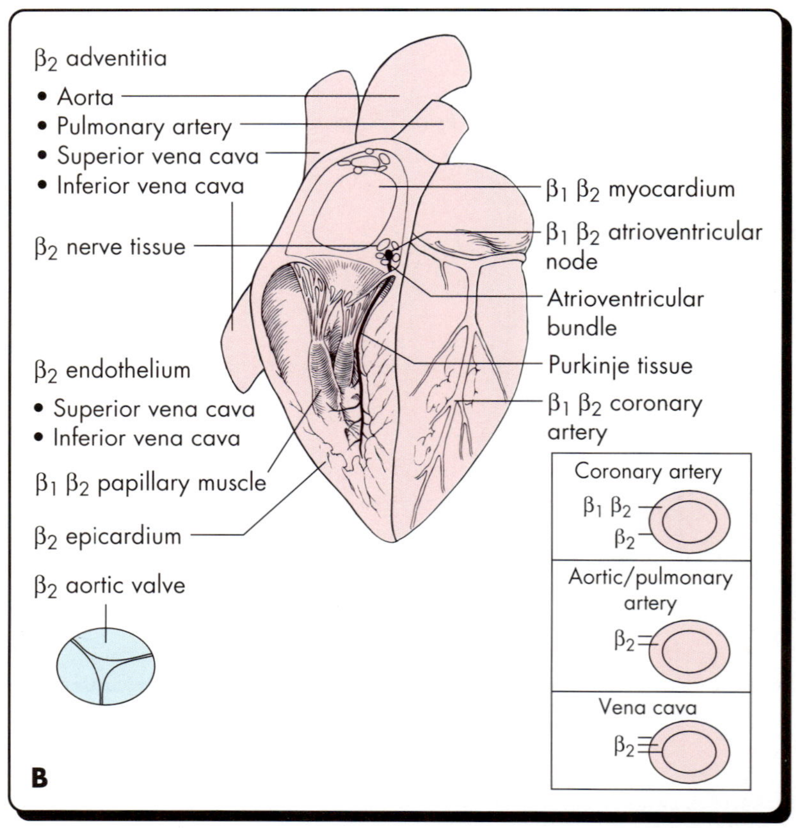

Figure 5-16. The cardiac β-adrenoceptor and signaling system. **A**, The beta-agonist molecule interacts with the β-receptor, whose molecular structure has been revealed and the amino acid sequence characterized. In the presence of the stimulator form of the G-protein (G_S), adenylate cyclase (AC) converts adenosine phosphate (ATP) to cyclic adenosine monophosphate (cAMP) that, acting via a protein kinase, enhances phosphorylation of the calcium channel and permits more calcium to enter through the calcium channel during voltage-induced depolarization. Such calcium releases much more from the sarcoplasmic reticulum (calcium-induced calcium release) to increase cytosolic calcium, heart rate, conduction, and contraction as well as the rate of relaxation (the latter via phosphorylation of the protein phospholamban in the sarcoplasmic reticulum).

B, Summary of the locations of the β_1- and β_2-adrenoceptors in rats, guinea pigs, dogs, and the human heart as determined by autoradiography. The β_1- and β_2-adrenoceptors are located on myocardium and specialized conducting tissue. A greater density of beta$_2$-adrenoceptors are located on the arterioventricular node, bundle of His, and left and right bundle branches in comparison with surrounding myocardium in guinea pigs. In addition, beta$_2$-adrenoceptors are located on blood vessels, nerve tissue, epicardium, and the aortic valve. AC—adenyl cyclase; CNS—central nervous system: G_i—inhibitory form of G protein; G_s—stimulatory form of G Protein; M—muscarinic receptor. (Part A copyright © LH Opie [5]; with permission; part B *adapted from* Kaplan [10].)

β-ADRENERGIC BLOCKING AGENTS

Name	Receptor Activity	Half-Life	Intrinsic sympathomimetic activity	Elimination
Acebutolol	B1	3–13 h	+	Hepatic/renal
Atenolol	B1	6–9 h	0	Renal
Betaxolol	B1	14–22 h	0	Hepatic/renal
Bisoprolol	B1	9–12 h	0	Renal
Esmolol	B1	9 min	0	Ester hydrolysis
Metoprolol	B1	3–4 h	0	Hepatic
Carteolol	B1, B2	6 h	++	Renal
Nadolol	B1, B2	14–24 h	0	Renal
Penbutolol	B1, B2	26 h	+	Renal
Pindolol	B1, B2	3–4 h	+++	Hepatic/renal
Propranolol	B1, B2	3–6 h	0	Hepatic
Sotalol	B1, B2	12 h	0	Renal
Timolol	B1, B2	3–4 h	0	Hepatic
Labetalol	B1, B2, A1	6–8 h	0	Hepatic/renal

Figure 5-17. B-adrenergic antagonists. B1 selective agents exhibit some B2 activity at higher levels. A1—α-1; B1—β-1; B2—β-2; 0–+++—no effect to most effect.

VASOPRESSORS AND INOTROPIC AGENTS

Agent	Bolus	Infusion Rate	Action: Direct Adrenergic Agonist α	Action: Direct Adrenergic Agonist β	Action: Indirect Adrenergic Agonist	Action: Phosphodiesterase Inhibition
Epinephrine	2–10 μg	1–2 μg/min	++	++++		
		2–10 μg/min	+++	++++		
		>10 μg/min	++++	+++		
Norephinephrine		2–16 μg/min	++++	+++		
Isoproterenol	1–4 μg	1–5 μg/min		++++		
Dobutamine		2–20 μg/kg/min	+	++++		
Dopamine		2–10 μg/min	+	++	+	
		10–20 μg/kg/min	++	+++	+	
		>20 μg/kg/min	+++	++	+	
Ephedrine	5–25 mg		+	++	+	
Metaraminol	100 μg	40–400 μg/min	+++	++	+	
Phenylephrine	50–200 μg	10–50 μg/min	++++			
Methoxamine	2–10 mg		++++			
Amrinone	0.5–1.5 mg/kg	5–10 μg/kg/min				+

Figure 5-18. Intravenous vasopressors and inotropic drugs. +–++++—mild effect to most effect. (*From* Schwinn [11]; with permission.)

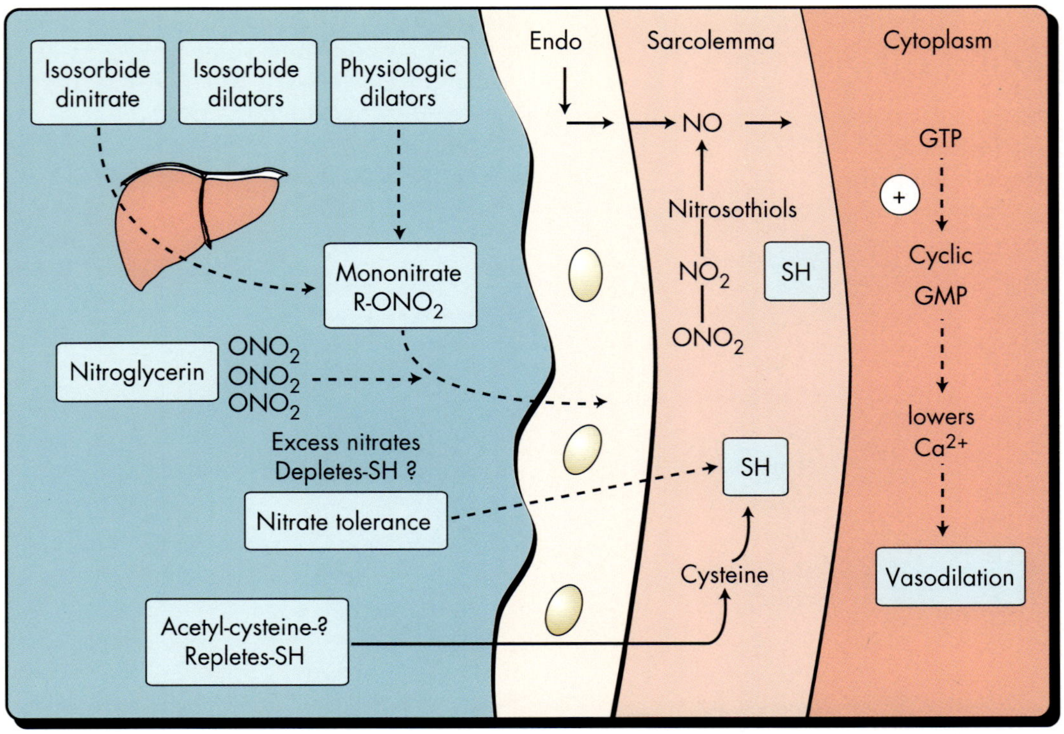

Figure 5-19. Mechanism of vasodilation by nitrates. Effects of nitrates in generating nitric oxide (NO) and stimulating guanylate cyclase to cause vasodilation. Note the role of the cysteine cascade in stimulating guanylate cyclase. Previously, sulfhydryl (SH) depletion was thought to explain nitrate tolerance. Note that mononitrates bypass hepatic metabolism. GMP—guanosine monophsophate; GTP—guanosine triphosphate. (Copyright © LH Opie [5]; with permission.)

VASODILATOR AND VENODILATOR DRUGS

Drug (Trade Name)	Vasodilation	Venodilation	Mechanism of Action	Drug Doses and Suggested IV Infusion Schemes*
Sodium nitroprusside	++++	++	Activation of NO	Drip: 50 mg/250 mL D5W (200 μg/mL), start at 0.5 μg/kg/min; titrate to effect Cyanide toxicity:5 mg/kg over 1–3 h = max acute dose 0.5 mg/kg/hr = max chronic dose (8 μg/kg/min)
Hydralazine	++++	+	Activation of NO	Bolus: 2.5–5 mg boluses, titrate to effect on blood pressure, lasts approx 2–4 h rare side effect = lupus-like syndrome
Trimethaphan	+++	+++	Ganglionic blockade	Drip: 500 mg/500 mL D5W (1 mg•mL^{-1}), start at 0.5 μg/kg/min and titrate to effect Bolus: 1 mg•mL^{-1}, 1–2 mg IV bolus (duration approx 2 min)
Pentolinium	+++	+++	Ganglionic blockade	Bolus: 10 mg•mL^{-1}, 0.03–0.1 mg/kg IV bolus
Phentolamine	++	+	αAR antagonist	Bolus: 5 mg IV bolus for hypertension 5–10 mg in 10 mL saline injected locally for catecholamine extravasation
Diazoxide	++++	—	Direct smooth muscle relaxation	Bolus: 300 mg/20 mL (15 mg•mL^{-1}), 150–300 mg rapid IV bolus
Nitroglycerin	+	++++	Activation of NO	Drip: 50 mg/250 mL D5W (200 μg/mL), start at 0.5 μg/kg/min and titrate to effect

*Doses should always be checked on individual package inserts before administering drug.

Figure 5-20. Vasodilator and venodilator drugs. Comparison of vasodilator drugs reveals selectivity for arterial and venous vascular beds. The mechanism of action of these drugs involves activation of nitric oxide at the cellular level or ganglionic blockade.

Treatment of cyanide toxicity: (1) Suspect it (especially when metabolic acidosis is present)! (2) Discontinue sodium nitroprusside. (3) If hemodynamics are stable, administer the specific cyanide antagonist thiosulfate (150 mg•kg^{-1} intravenously over 15 min; thiosulfate is a sulfur donor, and therefore, it converts cyanide to thiocyanate). (4) Alternative therapy when hemodynamics are unstable is slow intravenous infusion of sodium nitrate, 5 mg•kg^{-1} (converts hemoglobin to methemoglobin, which acts as an antiodote to cyanide by converting cyanide to cyanmethemoglobin). —no effect; +–++++mild to most effect; D5W—dextrose 5% in water; IV—intravenous; max—maximum; NO— nitric oxide. (*From* Schwinn [11]; with permission.)

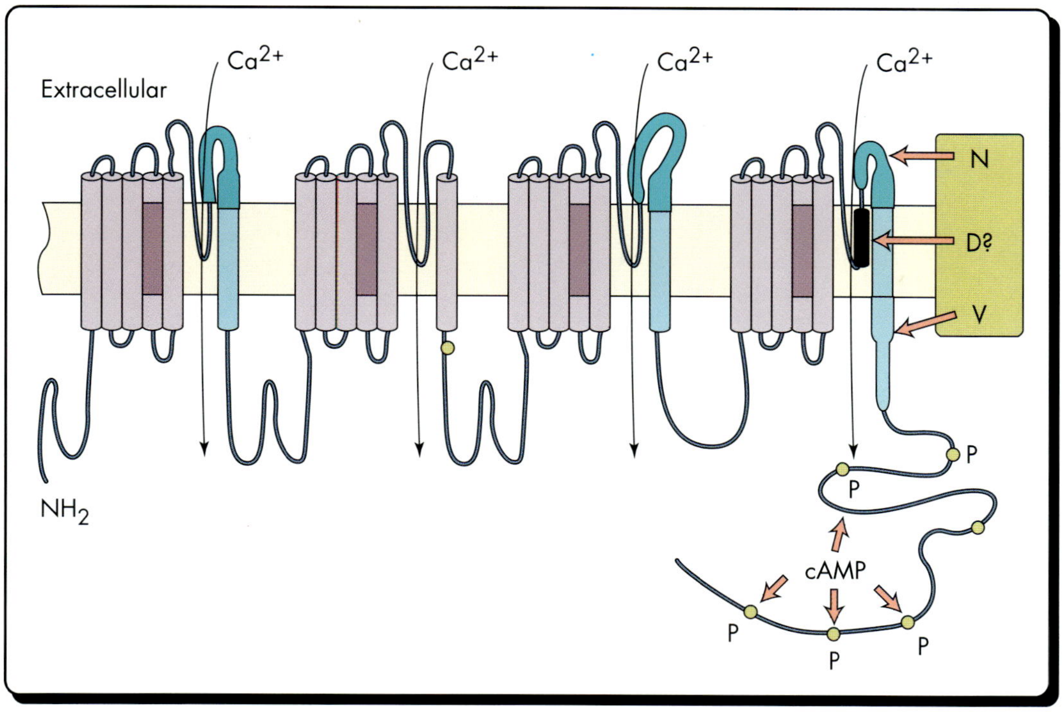

Figure 5-21. Calcium channels. Proposed molecular model of calcium channel - subunit with binding sites for nifedipine (N), diltiazem (D), and verapamil (V). It is thought that all DHPs bind to the same site as does nifedipine. *Arrows* radiating from cyclic adenosine monophosphate (cAMP) indicate sites of phosphorylation (P) that act to increase the opening probability of the calcium channel. Note the entry of calcium ions (Ca^{++}) through the pore between segments five and six of each of the four domains. NH_2—amino terminus. (Copyright © LH Opie [5]; with permission.)

CALCIUM CHANNEL ANTAGONISTS

Name	Nifedipine	Verapamil	Diltiazem	Nicardipine	Nimodipine	Isradipine	Felodipine	Amlodipine
Class	D	P	B	D	D	D	D	D
Half-life	2–5	5–18	3–5	8	2–6	8	11–16	30–50
Elimination	Hepatic	Hepatic	Hepatic/renal	Hepatic	Hepatic	Hepatic	Hepatic	Hepatic
Heart rate	+/NE	NE	NE	+/NE	+/NE	NE	+/NE	+/NE
Vasodilation	+++	++	++	+++	+++	+++	+++	+++
Contractility	NE	↓	↓	NE	↓	NE	NE	NE
Atrioventricular node conduction	NE	↓↓	↓	NE	↓	NE	NE	NE

Figure 5-22. Calcium channel antagonists. Cardiovascular effects of selected calcium channel antagonists. Half-lives are given in hours. ↓—decrease; +–+++—mild effect to most effect. B—benzothiazepine; D—dihydropyridine; NE—no effect; P—phenylalkylamine.

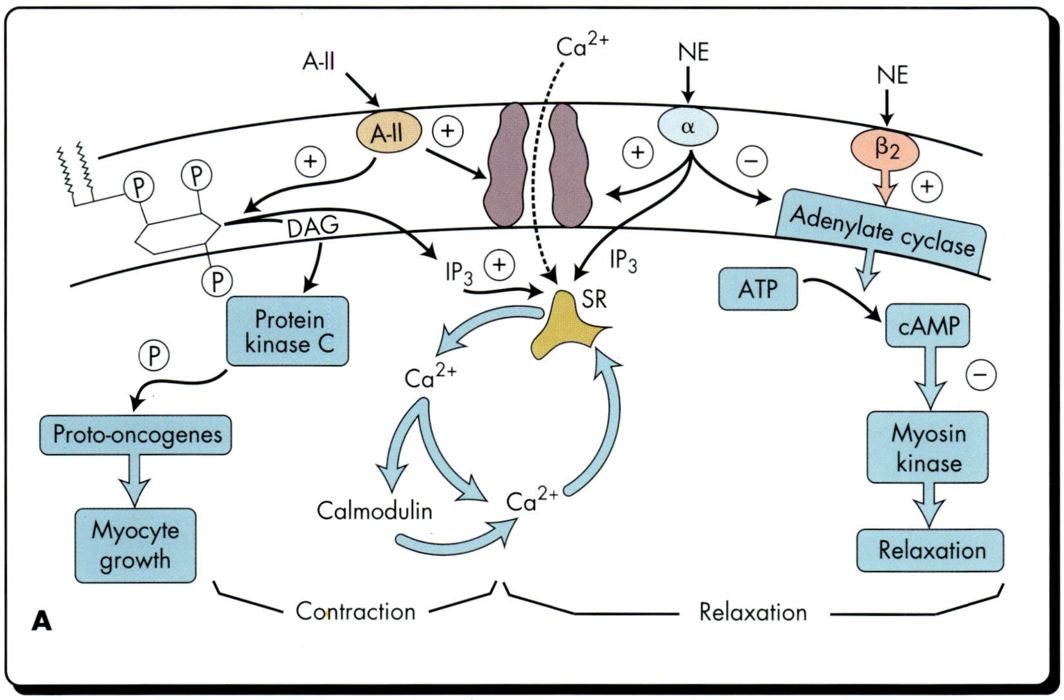

Figure 5-23. Angiotensin-converting enzyme (ACEs). **A**, Vascular angiotensin-II receptors (A-II). Proposed messengers of vascular A-II receptor stimulation. A phosphodiesterase (phospholipase C) splits phosphatidylinositol into two messengers: inositol trisphosphate (IP_3) and diacylglycerol (DAG). IP_3 promotes the release of calcium from the sarcoplasmic reticulum (SR), and DAG activates protein kinase C. The latter stimulates mycocyte growth. Activity of the A-II receptor also helps to open the calcium channel, possibly by G-proteins (G). Norepinephrine (NE) vasodilates by β_2-adrenergic stimulation and vasoconstricts via α-adrenergic activity.

(*Continued on next page*)

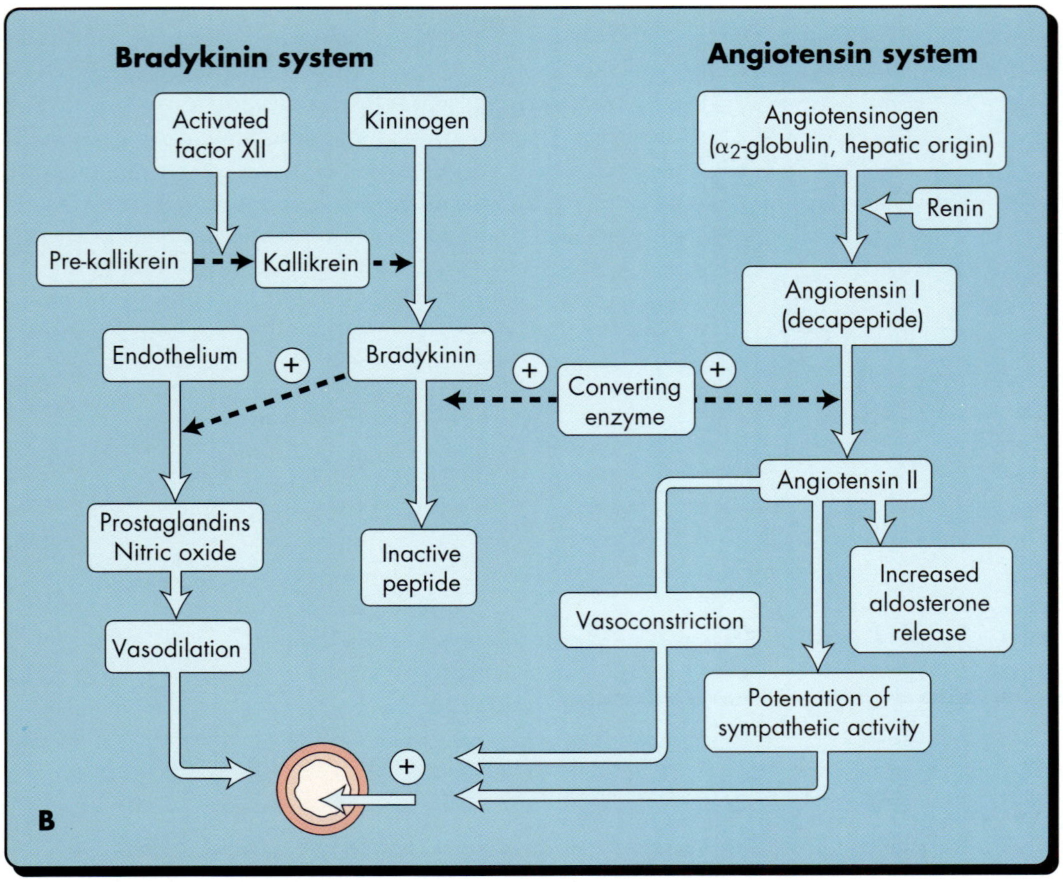

Figure 5-23. (*Continued*) B, ACE inhibitors have dual vasodilatory actions, chiefly on the renin-angiotensin system with ancillary effects on the breakdown of bradykinin. The result of the former action is the inhibiton of the vasoconstrictory systems, and the result of the latter is the formation of vasodilatory nitric oxide and prostacyclin. These effects of bradykinin may protect the endothelium. ATP—adenosine triphosphate; cAMP, cyclic adenosine monophosphate; P—phosphorylation; +—promotes activity; -—inhibits activity. (Copyright © LH Opie [5]; with permission.)

ANGIOTENSIN CONVERTING ENZYME INHIBITORS

Drug	Mechanism of Action	Total Daily Dose	Half-life, *h*	Duration of Action, *h*
Alacepril	ACE inhibitor	50 mg orally		6–10
Captopril	ACE inhibitor	25–100 mg orally div bid or tid	1.7	6–10 (active metabolites)
Enalapril	ACE inhibitor	2.5–40 mg orally div qd or bid	11.0	18–30 (active metabolites)
Enalaprilat	Active metabolite (diacid) of enalapril (ACE inhibitor)	1.25 mg q 6 h (IV) administered over 5 min		Clinical response seen within 15 min
Lisinopril	ACE inhibitor	10–40 mg qd orally	12.6	18–30 (no active metabolites)
Pentopril	ACE inhibitor	750 mg orally		10–18
Quinapril	ACE inhibitor Vascular converting enzyme inhibitor	10–80 mg qd orally	1.0	10–16 (active metabolites)
Ramipril	ACE inhibitor	20 mg orally		24–60

Figure 5-24. Angiotensin-converting enzyme (ACE) inhibitors. (*From* Schwinn [11]; with permission.)

REFERENCES

1. Mangano DT, Goldman L: Preoperative assessment of patients with known or suspected coronary disease. *New Engl J Med* 1995, 333:1750–1756.
2. Bullock J, Boyle J, Wang MB: *Physiology*. Media, PA: Harwal Publishing, 1984:94.
3. The National Heart, Lung, and Blood Institute Coronary Artery Surgery Study (CASS). *Circulation* 1981, 62(suppl):1–1.
4. Morgan GE, Mikhail MS: *Clinical Anesthesiology*. Norwalk, CT: Appleton & Lange. 1992:287–350.
5. Opie LH: *Drugs for the Heart*, edn 4. Philadelphia, WB Saunders, 1995:3–53.
6. Johnson Jr, M: In *The Heart, Arteries and Veins*, edn 6. Edited by Hurst JW. New York: McGraw-Hill, 1986:24.
7. Braunwald E: Regulation of the circulation. *N Engl J Med* 1974, 290:1124.
8. Hurst JW. *The Heart, Arteries and Veins* edn 6. New York: McGraw-Hill, 1986: plate 1.
9. Barash PG, Kopriva CJ: Cardiac Pump Function and How to Monitor It. In *Manual of Cardiac Anesthesia*, edited by Thomas SJ. New York: Churchill Livingstone, 1984:7.
10. Kaplan JA (ed). *Cardiac Anesthesia*, edn 3. Philadelphia: WB Saunders, 1993:101.
11. Schwinn DA: Cardiac Pharmacology. In *Cardiac Anesthesia: Principles and Clinical Practice*. Edited by Estafanous FG, Barash PG, Reves JG. Philadelphia: JB Lippincott, 1994:21–60.

6

The Lung During Anesthesia and in Adverse Environments

Bryant W. Stolp and Richard E. Moon

The effects of anesthetics on the respiratory system were first reported in the nineteenth century, when it was observed that deep levels of anesthesia were accompanied by depression of respiratory movements and cyanosis. In the early days of surgical anesthesia the acute respiratory effects often limited the usefulness of certain classes of drugs, particularly the narcotics. The advent of airway protection, mechanical ventilation, muscle relaxants and monitoring techniques such as pulse oximetry and capnography have minimized the risk of anesthetic side effects during surgery. However, perioperative respiratory complications continue to occur, particularly in the postoperative period. More recent investigations demonstrating the effects of both anesthesia and surgery on lung volume, diaphragm function, lung mechanics control of breathing, the development of atelectasis, and the role of receptors in the control of airway and vascular smooth muscle, have led to a better understanding of the mechanisms of these perioperative complications.

While the effects of hypoxia, increased airway resistance, and intravenous fluid administration are of immediate concern in clinical medicine, there has been a parallel history of investigation into lung physiology in humans exposed to high altitude, diving, and water immersion. The two topics have therefore been combined in this chapter.

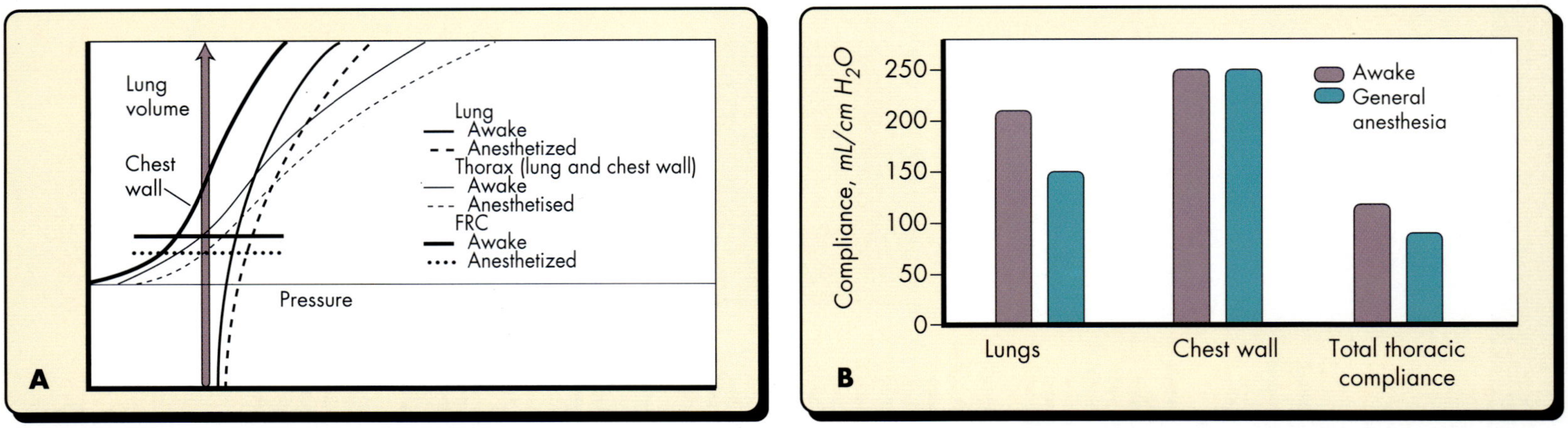

Figure 6-1. Effect of anesthesia on pressure-volume relationships (statics) of the respiratory system. The effects of anesthesia on pulmonary statics can be explained by examining the pressure-volume relationships of the lung and chest wall (**A**). The volume of the respiratory system is dependent upon the balance between these two components. At end-expiratory lung volume (FRC) the recoil pressure of the lung is equal in magnitude but opposite in direction to the outward recoil pressure of the chest wall. Anesthesia appears to exert its predominant effect on the lung, which becomes less compliant.

In addition to the reduction in FRC, induction of anesthesia is accompanied by a decrease in thoracic compliance, apparently caused by a 25% to 30% reduction in compliance of the lung (**B**). Resting lung volume is determined by a balance of forces between the chest wall (which at resting end-expiration tends to expand outward) and the lung (which tends to collapse). It has been hypothesized that anesthesia causes a change in pulmonary elasticity such that lung compliance is reduced. However, a reduced lung compliance could theoretically also be the result of a lung volume reduction due to a stiffer chest wall [1]. Atelectasis, distortion of the shape of the lung due to altered chest wall properties, a change in gas distribution, or alteration of surfactant properties (either from a reduction in lung volume or a physical effect of anesthetic gases) have all been suggested as reasons for the reduced lung compliance [2]. Although anesthesia may induce some reduction in outward chest wall recoil (shift of the pressure-volume curve of the chest wall to the right) [3] the effect of anesthesia on the compliance of the chest wall appears to be minimal.

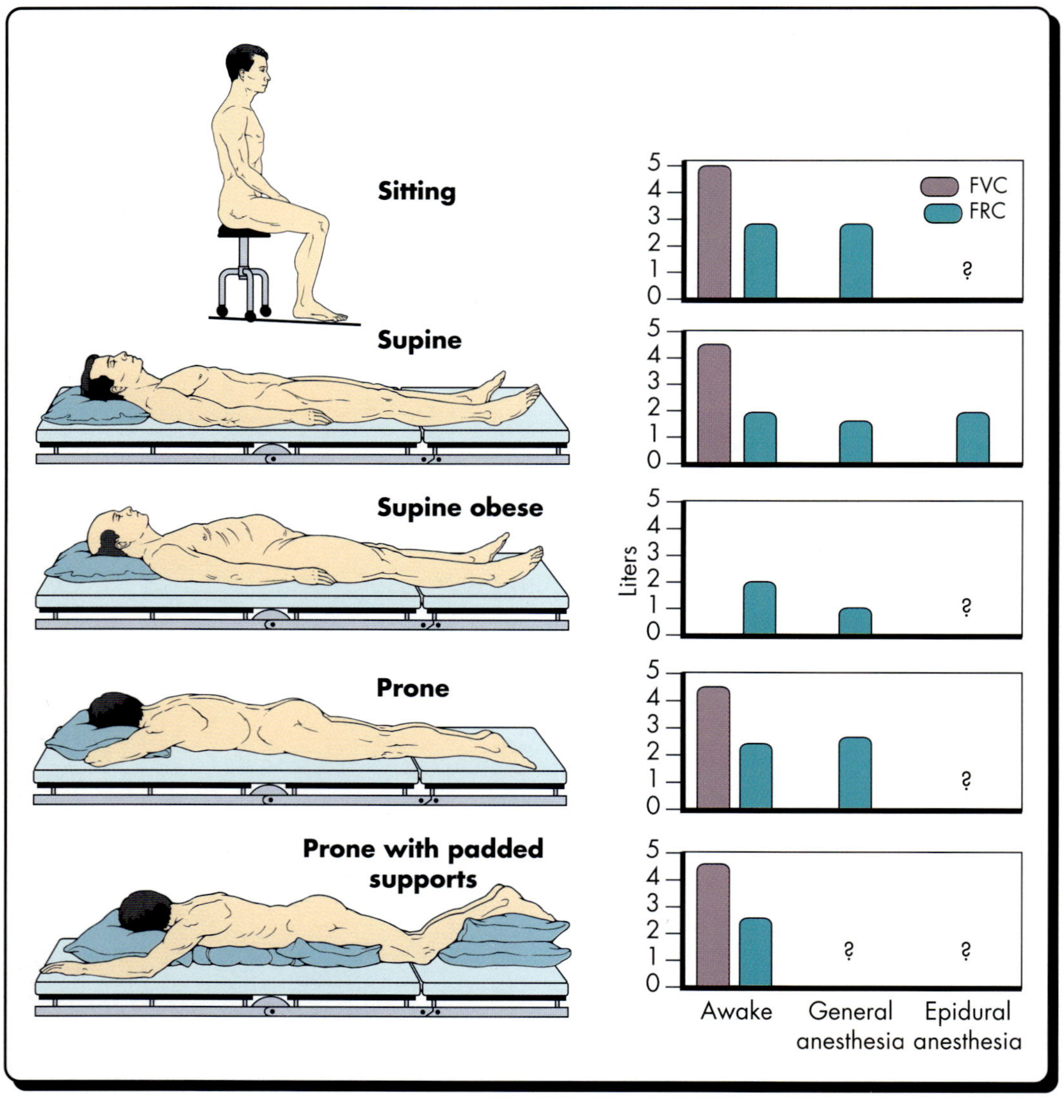

Figure 6-2. Effect of body position and anesthesia on lung volumes. Except for the sitting position, in which anesthesia does not cause appreciable change in lung volume, there is an average 20% reduction in functional residual capacity (FRC) after induction of general anesthesia (greater decline with obesity, less in prone position). Possible mechanisms could include a reduction of the thoracic dimensions, an increase in lung tissue or blood volume, and airway closure, thus rendering some gas inaccessible ("trapped gas") to tidal ventilation.

An increase in trapped gas has been measured [4]; however, studies using plethysmography, in which trapped gas is included in the volume measurement, suggest that trapped gas is not a significant component of the anesthesia-induced reduction in lung volume. Studies using three-dimensional fast-computed tomography suggest that a reduction in transverse cross sectional area and, less consistently, cephalad shift of the diaphragm, are primarily responsible. A redistribution of blood from the periphery to the thorax has been suggested as an additional cause of the gas volume reduction [5,6]. However measurement of thoracic blood volume has revealed a reduction [7,8]. In fact it appears that general anesthesia induces a redistribution of blood from the extremities and thorax into the abdomen. After a few minutes of anesthesia these changes are compounded by atelectasis in dependent areas of lung [9,10]. Observations during spinal anesthesia indicate a fall in lung volumes, including FRC [11]. However, induction of thoracic epidural anesthesia results in no significant change in FRC [12]. See data from the literature [2,12–16]. FVC—forced vital capacity.

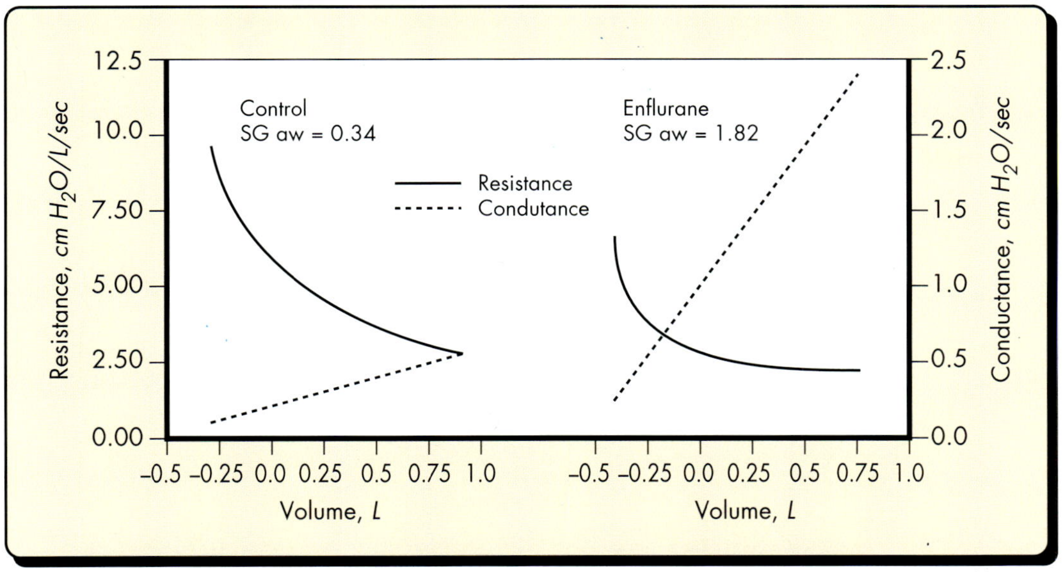

Figure 6-3. Effect of anesthesia on flow-volume relationships (dynamics) of the respiratory system. The major effect of anesthesia on airways resistance is via two opposing mechanisms. A reduction in lung volume tends to reduce airway diameter and thus causes an increase in airways resistance. Because of the increase in lung retractile force (which tends to increase airway diameter) after induction of anesthesia, this volume effect is less than it would be for a comparable reduction in lung volume for an awake person. On the other hand, volatile anesthetics cause bronchodilatation.

In addition to bronchoconstriction, decreased retractile force, mechanical displacement or kinking of an artificial airway, and accumulation of secretions within the tracheobronchial tree can all increase airway resistance. Studies in which resistance was measured awake and after induction of general anesthesia have reported values of 2.5–9.0 cm H_2O/L sec (awake) and 3.9–7.7 cm H_2O/L sec anesthetized. The reported variable and contradictory effects of anesthesia on airways resistance are probably from failure to account for lung volume and other confounding effects such as circulating catecholamines and mucus accumulation. Jordan *et al.* [17] have used specific conductance (resistance^{-1} x volume^{-1}) to demonstrate that, when corrected for lung volume, the net effect of enflurane and halothane (halothane not shown) is to reduce airway resistance. Resistance is measured at various lung volumes and, after correcting for upper airway resistance conductance (Gaw), is a linear function of lung volume. Specific conductance (sGaw) is then readily calculated as the slope of the line.

Pulmonary statics and dynamics during anesthesia have been reviewed by Don [18] and Rehder [2].

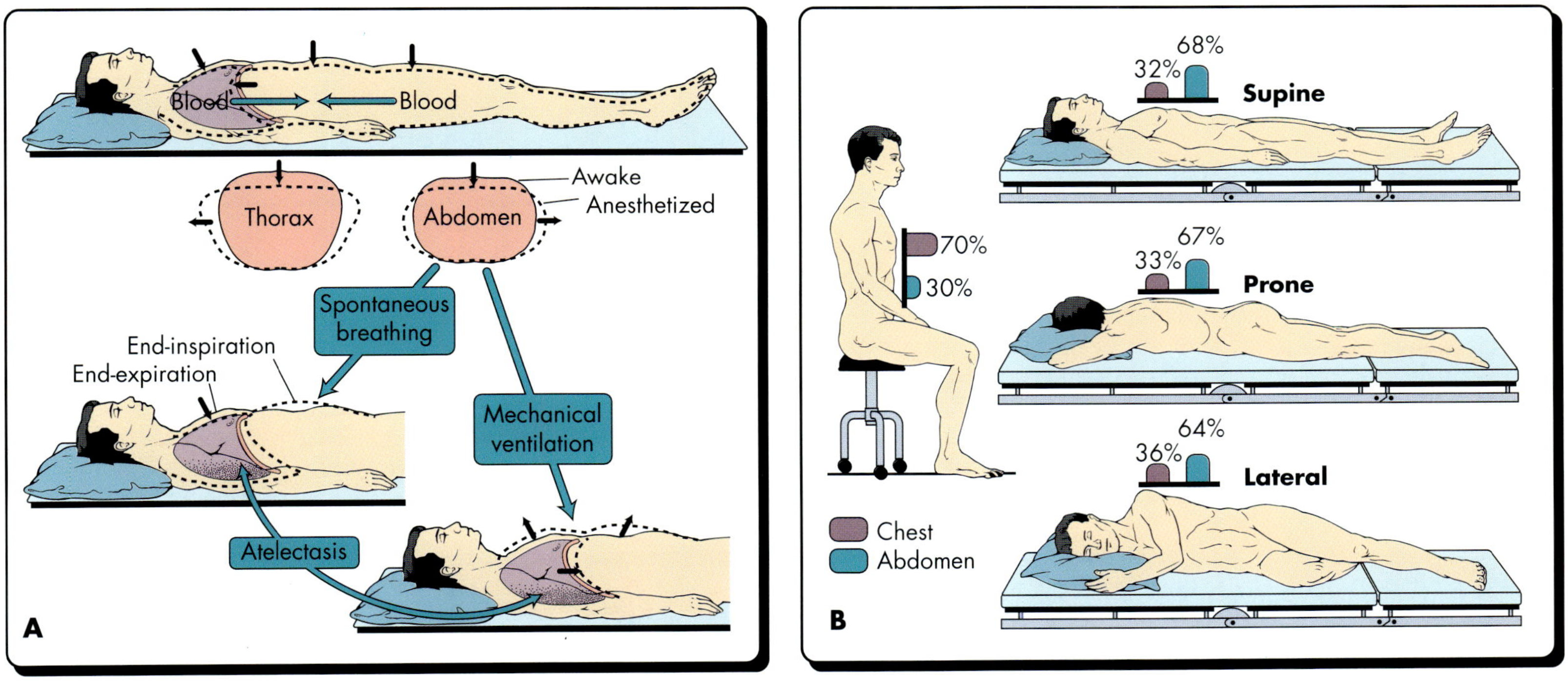

Figure 6-4. A and B, Effect of body position and anesthesia on partitioning of ventilation and chest wall movement. The figure shows the percent contribution of changes in cross sectional area of the rib cage and abdomen during tidal breathing [19].

Induction of anesthesia causes cephalad movement of the diaphragm and decrease of the antero-posterior diameter of both thorax and abdomen, while the lateral diameter of both thorax and abdomen increases. Volatile anesthetics preferentially inhibit the neurones that innervate intercostal muscles, thus in a patient anesthetized with volatile anesthetics who is breathing spontaneously during inspiration there is usually paradoxical inward motion of the thorax.

After induction of general anesthesia and initiation of mechanical ventilation the cephalo-cranial motion of the diaphragm changes from predominantly posterior movement to a more uniform or anterior motion [20,21].

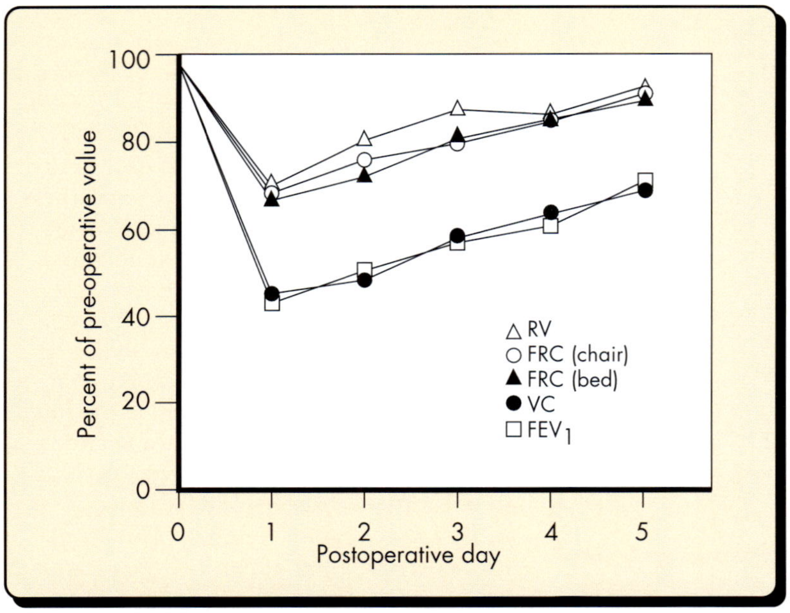

Figure 6-5. Postoperative changes in lung volumes. Postoperatively, the functional residual capacity (FRC) reduction due to anesthesia recovers almost completely, but effects of surgery become apparent. After abdominal surgery, for example, there is an immediate reduction in vital capacity, mediated by pain, reduced diaphragmatic contractility, altered lung compliance due to atelectasis [22], and probably reduced abdominal compliance. Following the drop in vital capacity there is a delayed postoperative drop in FRC, which peaks on the day after operation [23,24]. The FRC depends on the body position in which it is measured. While sitting in a chair, the FRC is 14% to 17% higher than in bed. Data shown are from 28 patients after elective upper abdominal surgery [25]. FEV_1—volume of gas exhaled from total lung capacity in 1 sec during an FVC maneuver; FVC—forced vital capacity; RV—residual volume; VC—vital capacity.

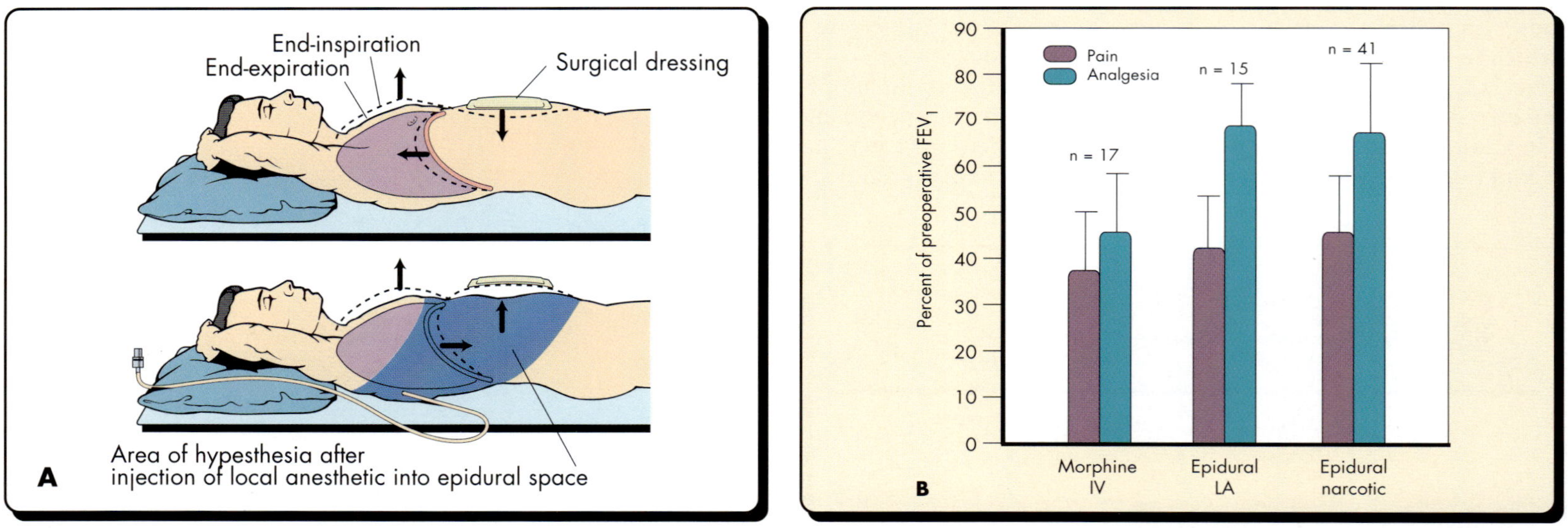

Figure 6-6. Postoperative analgesia. After abdominal and thoracic surgery, respiratory variables such as FVC, FEV_1, and MVV are reduced because of pain, altered chest wall mechanics, and impaired diaphragm contractility [26,27]. After upper abdominal surgery, during inspiration the diaphragm can move paradoxically cephalad (**A**). This can be observed clinically as an inward movement of the anterior abdominal wall. Epidural administration of local anesthetics or narcotics improves respiratory function to a greater degree than systemic narcotic administration. The bar graphs in **B** are from 66 patients after thoracic or upper abdominal surgery [28]. FEV_1—volume of gas exhaled from total lung capacity in 1 sec during an FVC maneuver; FVC—forced vital capacity.

In addition to relieving postoperative pain, blockade of the appropriate thoracic dermatomes by epidural administration of local anesthetic after upper abdominal surgery appears to improve diaphragm function [29].

PULMONARY GAS EXCHANGE

Figure 6-7. (*Opposite page*) Control of bronchomotor tone. Contraction of bronchial smooth muscle is initiated by entry of calcium into the cell either from the extracellular fluid or from the sarcoplasmic reticulum. Calcium enters the cytosol via calcium channels, which can be opened by rapid reduction (depolarization) of the negative intracellular potential (voltage gated channels: VDCC) or by stimulation of specific receptors (receptor gated channels: RDCC). Elevation of cytoplasmic calcium activates smooth muscle contraction in both bronchi and vessels. Calcium usually acts on its target effectors bound to a calcium binding polypeptide, calmodulin, each molecule of which has binding sites for four calcium ions.

The negative intracellular potential is maintained in part by efflux of potassium through potassium channels.

Bronchoconstriction and bronchodilatation also occur via G protein–coupled receptor mediated mechanisms. Stimulatory or inhibitory membrane-bound G-proteins (Gs, Gi) are so named because they bind guanine nucleotides, either guanine diphosphate (GDP) or guanine triphosphate (GTP). G proteins contain three polypeptide subunits (G_α, G_β, G_γ). Binding of a ligand to its receptor increases the affinity of the receptor for its G protein, to which it then binds, causing the G_α subunit to exchange its bound GDP for GTP, resulting in activation. The activated G_α then dissociates from its receptor and from the other two subunits, allowing it to activate an effector molecule such as an enzyme (*eg*, adenylyl cyclase) or an ion channel. A more detailed discussion of G proteins can be found in Karp [30].

Efferent preganglionic parasympathetic neurons release acetylcholine, which then causes postganglionic neuron depolarization via nicotinic (N) and M_1 muscarinic receptors. Postganglionic neurons may also be influenced by other neurotransmitters secreted within the parasympathetic ganglia, such as substance P and neurokinin A (which augment depolarization) and norepinephrine and neuropeptide Y (which inhibit depolarization) [31].

(*Continued on next page*)

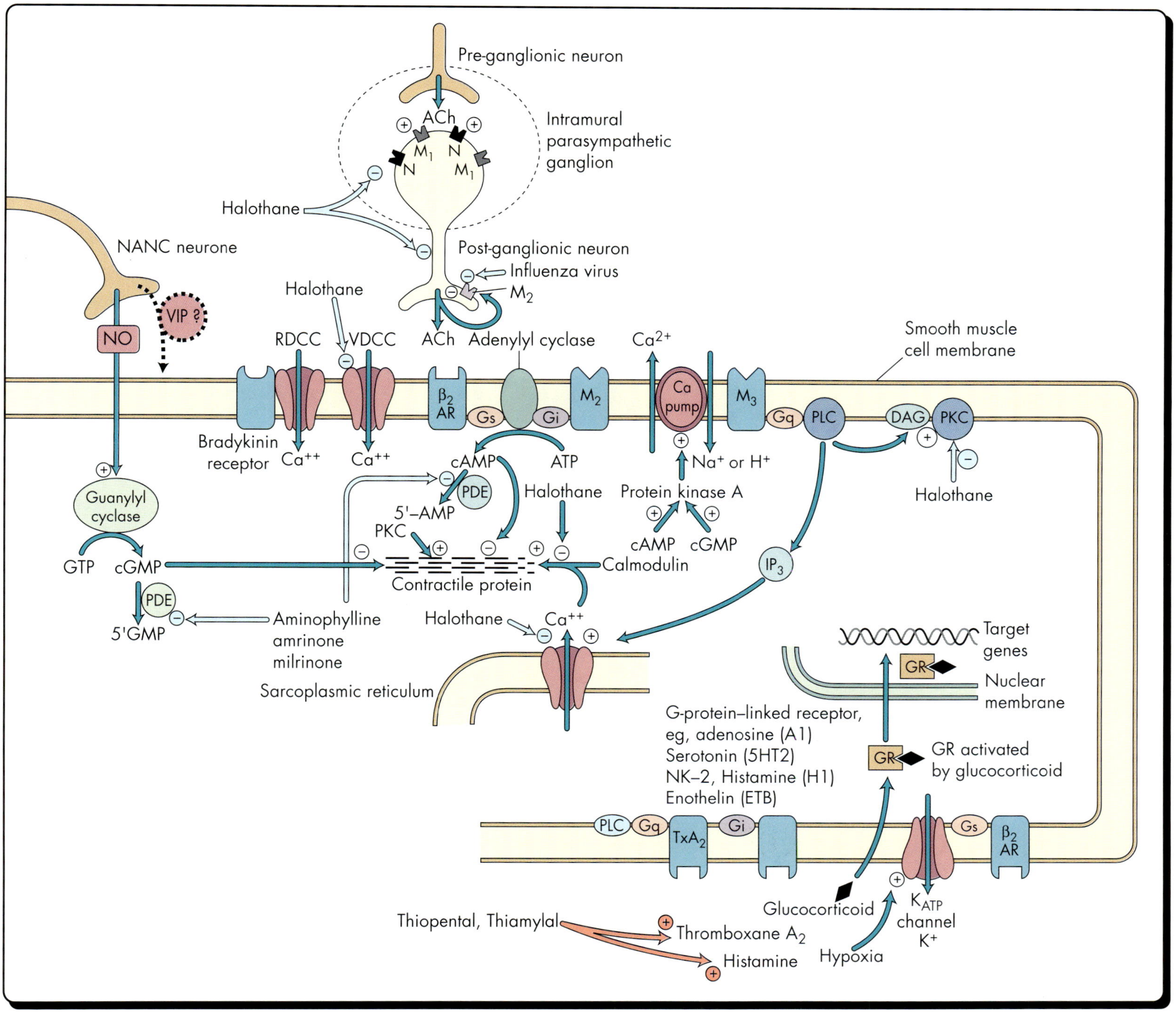

Figure 6-7. (*Continued*) Postganglionic neurons then release acetylcholine in proximity to the airway smooth muscle cell, allowing it to occupy muscarinic receptors, causing inhibition of bronchodilatation (via M_2 receptors, which inhibit adenylyl cyclase via an inhibitory G protein) and bronchoconstriction and glandular secretion (via M_3 receptors). M_3 muscarinic receptors also activate phospholipase C (PLC) to release two second messengers: inositol 1,4,5-triphosphate (IP_3) and diacylglycerol (DAG). IP_3 causes release of calcium from the sarcoplasmic reticulum, while DAG activates protein kinase C (PKC), which in turn activates contractile protein. Auto-inhibition of postganglionic neuronal depolarization occurs via M_2 receptors, a process which, in turn, is inhibited by influenza virus.

One mechanism of bronchomotor tone inhibition is provided by nonadrenergic, noncholinergic (NANC) nerves, of which the neurotransmitter is believed to be nitric oxide (NO) or vasoactive intestinal peptide (VIP) [32]. There is evidence that inhaled NO can attenuate methacholine-induced bronchoconstriction in humans [33].

The brochoconstricting effect of thiobarbiturates appears to be from release of the bronchoconstrictor prostaglandin, thromboxane [34,35], possibly from the endothelium. Histamine release may also contribute.

Volatile anesthetics reduce the influx of calcium via VDCC [36], attenuate the force developed when intracellular calcium interacts with contractile proteins [37], and reduce the binding of calcium to calmodulin [38]. PKC, which sensitizes contractile proteins to calcium, is inhibited by volatile anesthetics [36]. The volatile anesthetics reduce the excitability of the nicotinic receptors of the parasympathetic ganglia, inhibit the post-synaptic neuron and possibly also inhibit interaction of ACh with smooth muscle cholinergic receptors [39]. Halothane also, to a minor degree, increases intracellular cAMP [36].

The effects of glucocorticoids on bronchomotor tone in disease states such as asthma are probably due to their effects on inflammatory processes. Glucocorticoids exert their effects by binding to specific cytoplasmic receptors (glucocorticoid receptors, GR). Activated GR then crosses the nuclear membrane and binds to specific DNA sequences, causing transcription of specific target genes to be up- or down-regulated. For example, glucocorticoids have been shown to increase the expression of beta adrenergic receptors [40]. Mechanisms of glucocorticoid action on bronchial smooth muscle have been reviewed by Bloom and Miesfeld [41].

While the epithelium may release some mediators, the major effect of ligands on bronchomotor tone is via a direct effect on smooth muscle cells.

A. EFFECTS OF AGONISTS ON PULMONARY VASCULAR RESISTANCE

Increase	Decrease
α_1-adrenergic agonists	Acetylcholine
α_2-adrenergic agonists	Adenosine (via A_2 receptors)
Almitrine	ANF
Angiotensin-II	β_2-adrenergic agonists
Endothelin (via ET_A and ET_B receptors)	Bradykinin
PAF (high dose)	Calcium channel blockers
Serotonin	Carbon monoxide (CO)
Histamine (via H_1 receptors)	Histamine (via H_2 receptors)
↑ [H^+]	Hydralazine
↓ PO_2	Nitrates
	Nitric oxide (NO)
	Nitroprusside
	PAF (low dose)
	PGI_2, PGE_1 (via EP_2 receptors), iloprost, epoprostenol
	Phosphodiesterase inhibitors (*eg*, amrinone)
	VIP
	Volatile anesthetics

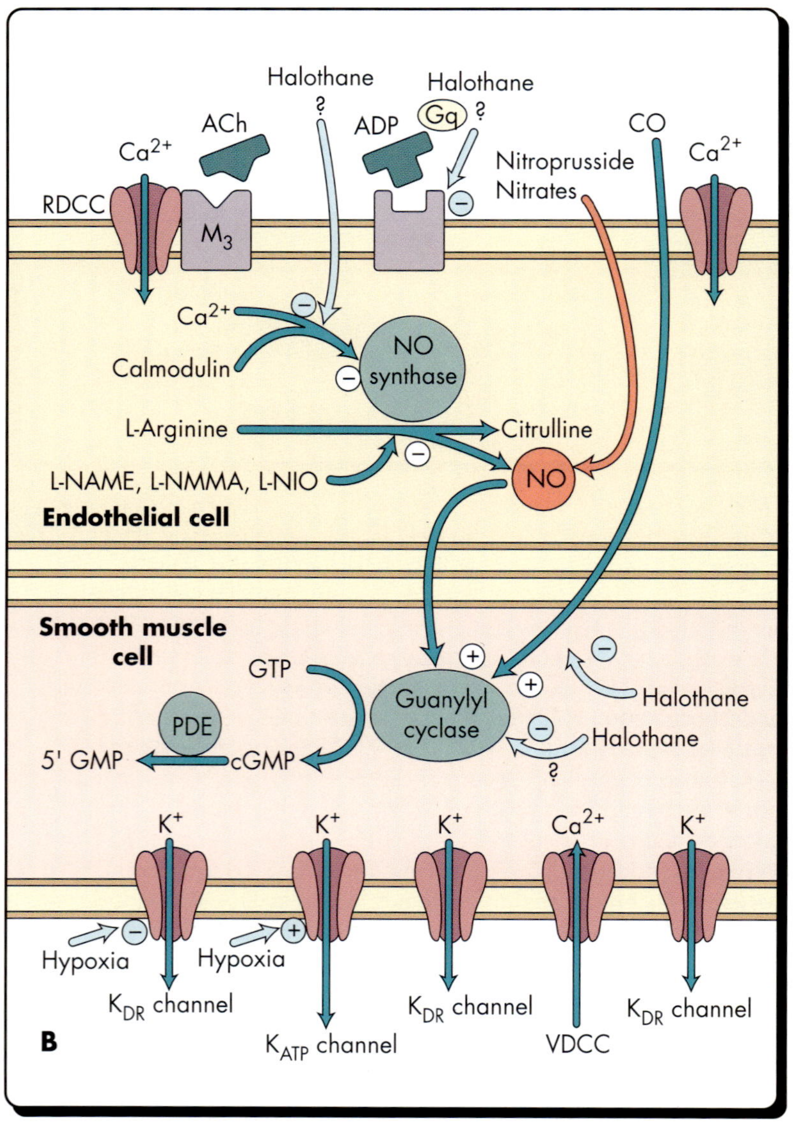

Figure 6-8. Control of pulmonary vascular tone. Pulmonary vascular tone is modulated by exogenous catecholamines and a variety of mediators derived from the endothelium, including constrictors (endothelin, thromboxane A_2, oxygen free radicals) and dilators (nitric oxide [NO], EDHF, and prostacyclin) (**A** and **B**). Unlike bronchial smooth muscle, with which ligands interact directly, vascular smooth muscle is modulated predominantly by the endothelium. Ligands bind to receptors on the endothelium, which then controls vascular smooth muscle tone by releasing contractile or relaxing mediators.

Vascular smooth muscle contracts when calcium enters the cytosol, either from the extracellular fluid or the sarcoplasmic reticulum (not shown), causing activation of contractile proteins, possibly with the participation of microtubules [1,42].

The most potent of the dilating mediators is NO. Binding of ligands to specific membrane receptors on the endothelial cell acts via receptor-dependent calcium channels or G-protein-coupled receptors to increase cytosolic calcium and calcium-calmodulin interaction, which then activates nitric oxide synthase. This enzyme then catalyzes the conversion of L-arginine to citrulline, in the process releasing NO. NO is the predominant dilating factor (endothelium-derived relaxing factor, EDRF), which diffuses from the endothelial cell into the cytoplasm of the vascular smooth muscle cell, activating guanylyl cyclase. The resulting production of cGMP causes relaxation of vascular smooth muscle. Toxic concentrations of carbon monoxide act in a similar manner to NO, causing stimulation of guanylyl cyclase, and hence increasing the production of cGMP.

When administered therapeutically by inhalation, low concentrations (1–50 ppm) of NO can reverse pulmonary hypertension. Because inhaled NO is only delivered to ventilated gas exchange units, unlike systemically administered pulmonary vasodilators, it does not impair regional ventilation/perfusion matching. Moreover, NO is rapidly inactivated by hemoglobin and therefore does not cause systemic vasodilatation. It has been used to improve oxygenation in diffuse lung disease such as acute respiratory distress syndrome (ARDS) and high altitude pulmonary edema [43–46]. Vasodilators such as nitroprusside and nitrates both act on vascular smooth muscle by releasing NO [47].

An additional smooth muscle relaxing factor produced by the endothelium is endothelium-derived hyperpolarizing factor (EDHF) [48], which increases potassium permeability of the smooth muscle membrane. It is hypothesized that EDHF is an epoxyeicosatrienoic acid synthesized by a cytochrome-P450–dependent oxygenase [49].

Pulmonary and systemic vessels act in a similar manner, with the major difference being the response to hypoxia, which causes dilatation in systemic vessels and constriction in pulmonary vessels. Hypoxic pulmonary vasoconstriction (HPV) is responsible for regional matching of ventilation and perfusion, in which blood is diverted away from poorly ventilated (and hence hypoxic) gas exchange units. HPV appears to be primarily mediated by potassium channels. Outward movement of potassium ions through specific ion channels helps maintain smooth muscle cell negative polarization. Hypoxia inhibits direct rectifier potassium (K_{DR}) channels, thereby causing membrane depolarization (the predominant effect in pulmonary vessels) and stimulation of ATP-sensitive potassium (K_{ATP}) channels (which predominate in systemic vessels) [50].

Anesthetic agents tend to dilate pulmonary vessels and counteract hypoxic pulmonary vasoconstriction [51]. Exact mechanisms are not fully elucidated, but probably include attenuation of receptor-ligand–mediated increase in cytosolic calcium [52] and interference with calcium-calmodulin binding [38]. Volatile anesthetics have been shown to block calcium influx through channels in vascular smooth muscle cells [53]. Vasodilatation by volatile anesthetics does not appear to involve membrane bound receptors or the vascular endothelium [54,55]. The effects of anesthetics on vessels have been reviewed by Johns [56] and Bosnjak [57].

Although their predominant effect is to relax vascular tone, volatile anesthetics can in fact inhibit endothelium-dependent relaxation by interfering with interactions between agonist and receptor and between muscarinic receptors and their G proteins. CO-induced relaxation of vascular smooth muscle is also inhibited by both halothane and isoflurane [58]. EDHF—endotheliam-derived hyperpolarization factor; EDRF—endotheliam-derived relaxing factor; L-NAME—N^G-L-arginine methyl ester; L-NMMA—N^G-monomethyl L-arginine; L-NIO—N-imino-L-ornithine.

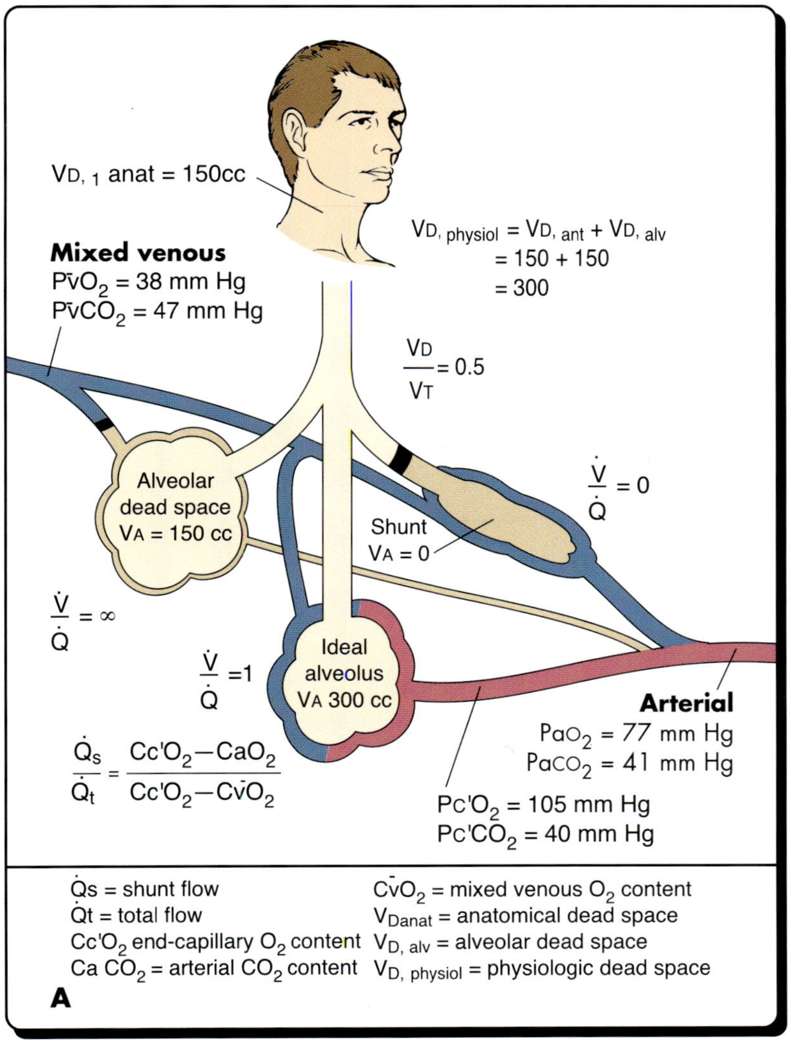

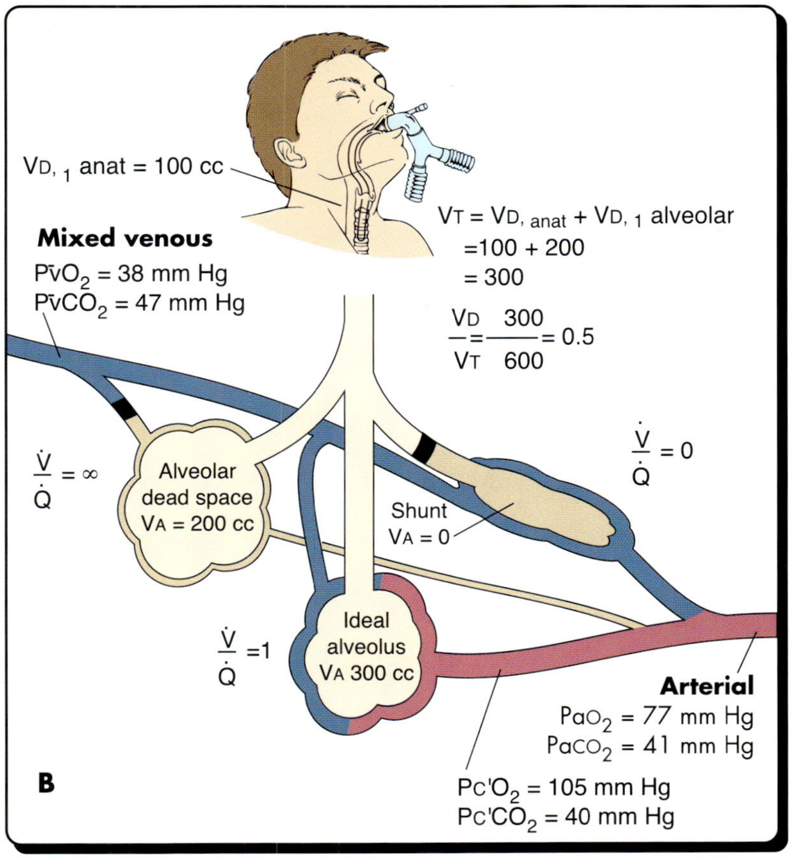

Figure 6-9. Pulmonary gas exchange during anesthesia. The effects of anesthesia on pulmonary gas exchange can be considered in terms of its effect on alveolar gases and the relationship between alveolar and arterial gases. The alveolar gas equation for oxygen is as follows: $PaO_2 = PIO_2 - PaCO_2\ [FIO_2 + (1 - FIO_2)/R]$, where PaO_2 = alveolar PO_2, $PaCO_2$ = alveolar PCO_2, $PIO_2 = FIO_2\ (Pbar - PH_2O)$, R = respiratory quotient $= \dot{V}CO_2/\dot{V}O_2$, $\dot{V}O_2$ = oxygen consumption rate, $\dot{V}CO_2$ = carbon dioxide production rate, PH_2O = saturated water vapor pressure at body temperature, Pbar = barometric pressure, FIO_2 = inspired O_2 concentration, and $PIO_2 = PO_2$ of inspired gas. The corresponding alveolar gas equation for CO_2 is $PaCO_2 = k\ \dot{V}CO_2/\dot{V}A$, where $\dot{V}A$ = alveolar ventilation and k is a constant (approximately 0.863 when $\dot{V}CO_2$ and $\dot{V}A$ are L/min). Inspection of these equations reveals that alveolar hypoxia may be caused by two major factors: low inspired PO_2 and high PCO_2 (relative hypoventilation). Anesthesia tends to depress respiratory drive, causing hypoventilation. Reduction of arterial PO_2 out of proportion to alveolar PO_2 (increased A-a gradient) may be caused by ventilation/perfusion mismatching, right-to-left shunt and diffusion impairment (which has never been demonstrated as a cause of hypoxemia in resting humans).

A, Pulmonary gas exchange can be conveniently modeled using a three-compartment representation of the lung. Arterial and mixed venous gas tensions for an ideal compartment where alveolar ventilation is exactly matched to perfusion ($\dot{V}/\dot{Q} = 1$), an alveolar dead space compartment ($V_{D,\ alv}$) where ventilated alveoli are not perfused ($\dot{V}/\dot{Q} = \infty$), and a shunt compartment ($\dot{Q}_s$) with perfusion of an unventilated alveoli ($\dot{V}/\dot{Q} = 0$) are shown for a spontaneously breathing, awake subject. (note: $V_{D,\ physiol}$ is physiological dead space and V_D/V_T is the dead space to tidal volume ratio).

B, Pulmonary gas exchange in an intubated, anesthetized, and mechanically ventilated patient.

General anesthsia results in (1) increased alveolar dead space from redistribution of blood flow and ventilation and (2) increased venous admixture. The increase in alveolar dead space is augmented by mechanical ventilation, which causes airway distension (increased $V_{D,anat}$) and causes gas to be distributed preferentially to non-dependent areas of the lung (i.e. away from blood flow which tends to be preferentially distributed to depedent areas). The increase in $V_{D,anat}$ caused by distension of airways is partially compensated for by reductions in anatomical dead space which result from the endotracheal tube. Increased venous admixture is caused by compression atelectasis, ventilation-perfusion mismatching and, during administration of high concentrations of volatile anesthetics, inhibition of hypoxic pulmonary vasoconstriction.

PEEP has been shown to decrease atelectasis but does not consistently improve oxygenation in patients undergoing general anesthesia. The reduction in shunt that can be attributed to PEEP appears to be offset by simultaneous reductions in cardiac output and mixed venous oxygen content [61].

Inhibition of the hypoxic pulmonary vasoconstriction (HPV) has been demonstrated for inhalational anesthetics but not intravenous anesthetic agents [62]. This effect can contribute to worsening pulmonary gas exchange. Although there have been conflicting results of *in vitro* versus *in vivo* studies on the degree of HPV inhibition by inhalational agents, Marshall and Marshall [63] showed that the variability was related to the anesthetic depressant effects on cardiac output. For a constant oxygen consumption, a decrease in cardiac output results in a decreased mixed venous PO_2, thus enhancing HPV. The net result therefore is related to a balance between the inhalational agent's depressant effect on HPV and the resultant enhancement of HPV reflex in response to the depression in cardiac output and mixed venous oxygen. At a MAC of 1.3 the HPV is attenuated by approximately 30% with no significant difference noted among the volatile agents.

Spinal anesthesia is not usually associated with alterations in arterial blood gases, as the accessory muscles of inspiration and diaphragm are innervated by craniocervical nerves with little resultant decrement from high spinal blocks [11,64]. Loss of the anterior abdominal muscles from high spinal anesthesia results in a reduction of maximum breathing capacity, expiratory flows, and pressures. Alterations in patterns of breathing that result from spinal anesthesia have not been systematically evaluated as to their effect on respiratory gas exchange, distribution of ventilation, or ventilation-perfusion matching [11,65]. Hypoxic pulmonary vasocontriction is not impaired during spinal anesthesia.

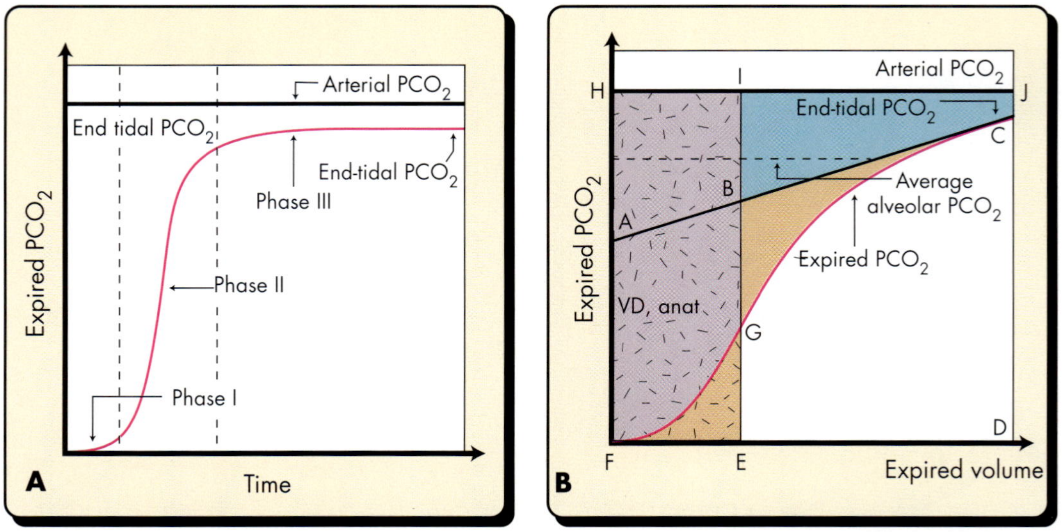

Figure 6-10. Expired carbon dioxide monitoring. Multi-breath measurement of pulmonary dead space/tidal volume ratio can be calculated from the alveolar and mixed expired P_{CO_2} as follows: $V_D/V_T = 1 - P_ECO_2/P_ACO_2$ (Bohr equation). Alveolar P_{CO_2} can be obtained from the capnograph tracing as end-tidal P_{CO_2}. If arterial PCO_2 (Pa_{CO_2}) is available one can make the following assumption: $P_ACO_2 = Pa_{CO_2}$ (Enghoff modification). The dead space measured by this method (physiologic dead space) includes both anatomic dead space (upper airway, trachea, and bronchi) and "alveolar" dead space [66] caused by hypoperfusion of ventilated lung units, or gas exchange units with high ventilation/perfusion ratios. Using this method of measurement Campbell has shown that mechanical ventilation increases dead space [67].
The usual capnograph displays expired P_{CO_2} *versus* time (**A**). Most of the tidal volume is exhaled in the initial portion of exhalation, thus in the conventional capnograph tracing there is minimal change in expired CO_2 during the alveolar plateau (phase III). Alternatively, if expired CO_2 is plotted *versus* exhaled volume (**B**), additional information can be obtained. It is in fact possible to use this plot to calculate anatomic dead space ($V_{D,\ anat}$), as shown in the figure, using a technique similar to the one originally described by Fowler [68]. Fletcher *et al.* [68] have further analyzed the expired CO_2 waveform and shown that, by using the arterial P_{CO_2}, one can also calculate physiologic dead space ($V_{D,\ physiol}$). This technique has been applied by Breen *et al.* [69], who have demonstrated the feasibility of using digitized data to calculate average alveolar CO_2 and dead space. Line AC is drawn by extrapolation of the best fit to the end-expiratory plateau. Line BE is then situated such that areas FEG and GBC are equal. Anatomic dead space is then defined as the volume represented by area EFHI. The remaining volume (DEIJ) represents alveolar gas, which has an average P_{CO_2} represented by that portion of the alveolar gas that contains no CO_2 (area BCJI). Physiologic dead space (= $V_{D,\ anat} + V_{D,\ physiol}$) is therefore the sum of the cross-hatched and dotted areas.

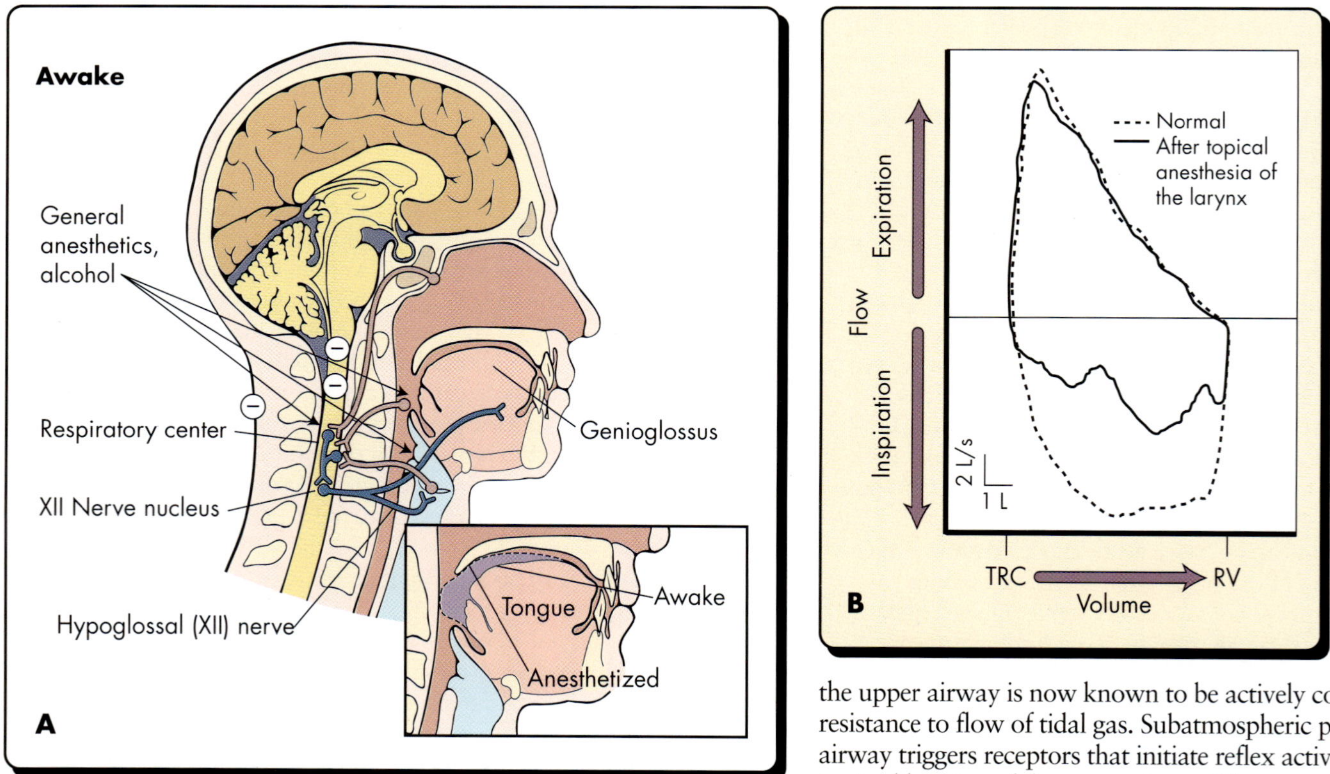

Figure 6-11. A and B, Upper airway effects of anesthesia. Phasic inspiratory neuronal activity is provided to the diaphragm, intercostal muscles and dilator muscles of the upper airway, particularly the genioglossus, geniohyoid, and laryngeal abductors (posterior cricoarytenoid muscles). Originally believed to be a passive conduit, the caliber of the upper airway is now known to be actively controlled to minimize the resistance to flow of tidal gas. Subatmospheric pressure in the upper airway triggers receptors that initiate reflex activation of muscles, resulting in dilatation of the upper airway. The presence of such reflexes can be demonstrated by applying topical anesthesia to the larynx and observing the effects on the flow volume loop, in which expiratory flow is unaltered by topical anesthesia, but inspiratory flow is significantly decreased [70]. The reflex is also inhibited by sleep, alcohol ingestion, and general anesthesia, which can result in airway obstruction [70–72].

Figure 6-12. Control of ventilation. The rhythmic pattern of respiration originates from the complex interaction of at least six groups of neurons located in the brain stem [73]. Their complex wiring in parallel networks provides a redundant system that is responsible for a respiratory cycle that can be divided into three phases. The inspiratory phase is preceded by dilatation of the pharyngeal muscles and consists of a sudden discharge followed by a ramp increase in motor discharge to the inspiratory musculature. The post-inspiratory or expiratory phase I is characterized by a braking or slowing of the expiratory flow rate which results from a decrease in the motor discharge to the inspiratory muscles. This phase does not occur under general anesthesia or during mechanical ventilation of a paralyzed patient. The third or final phase of the respiratory cycle is the expiratory phase II and is characterized by an absence of inspiratory motor activity. Expiratory muscle activity may also be silent at rest in the supine position during this phase.

Interconnections between the dorsal and ventral respiratory neurons in the medulla are responsible for both the timing as well as expiratory functions of the respiratory cycle (**A**). The dorsal respiratory group near the tractus solitaris is primarily concerned with respiratory timing and is connected to upper motor neurons passing to the inspiratory anterior horn cells of the opposite side. The ventral respiratory group primarily controls expiratory muscles of the opposite side and dilator functions of the larynx, pharynx, and tongue but also controls some contralateral inspirtory nerves [61].

The pattern of firing of the three types of neurons in the pontine pneumotaxic center appear to be involved in the fine tuning and control of the respiratory rhythm. Within limits of arterial blood gas tensions, breathing pattern can be modified both voluntarily from signals originating in cortical areas and in response to suprapontine reflexes such as sneezing, coughing, and swallowing.

Integration of the three groups of neurons involved in respiratory control takes place at the level of the anterior horn cell [74] and at the pontomedullary level [75] (**B, upper right**). (*Continued on next page*)

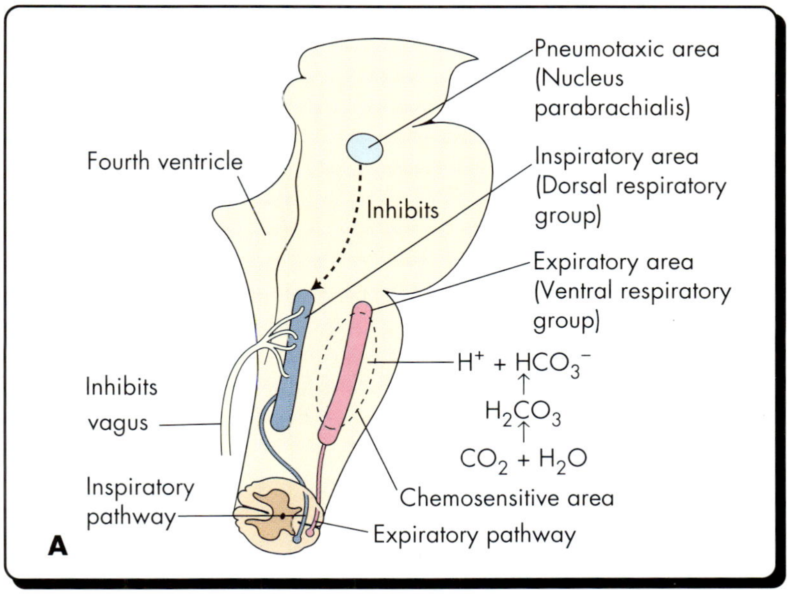

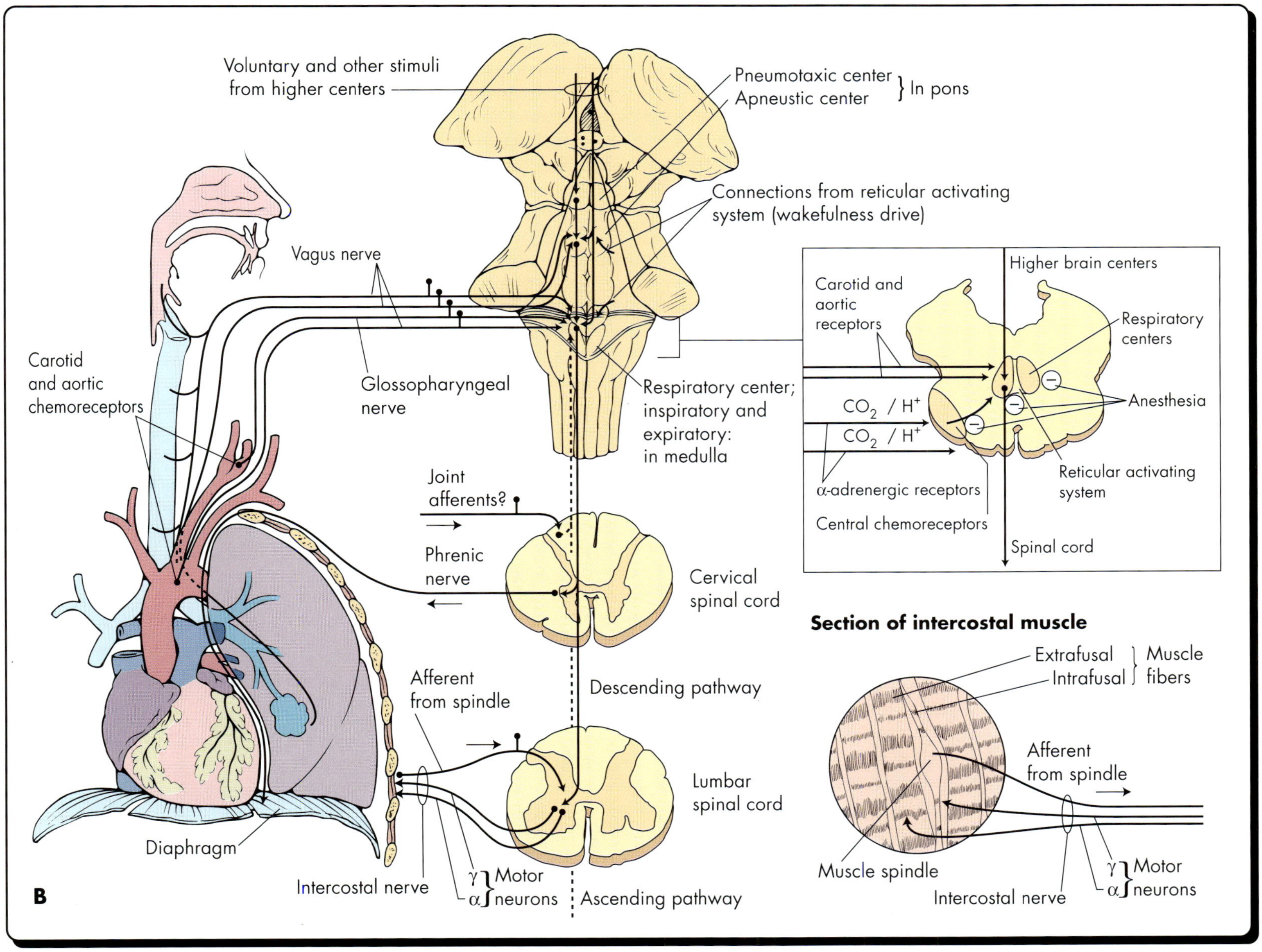

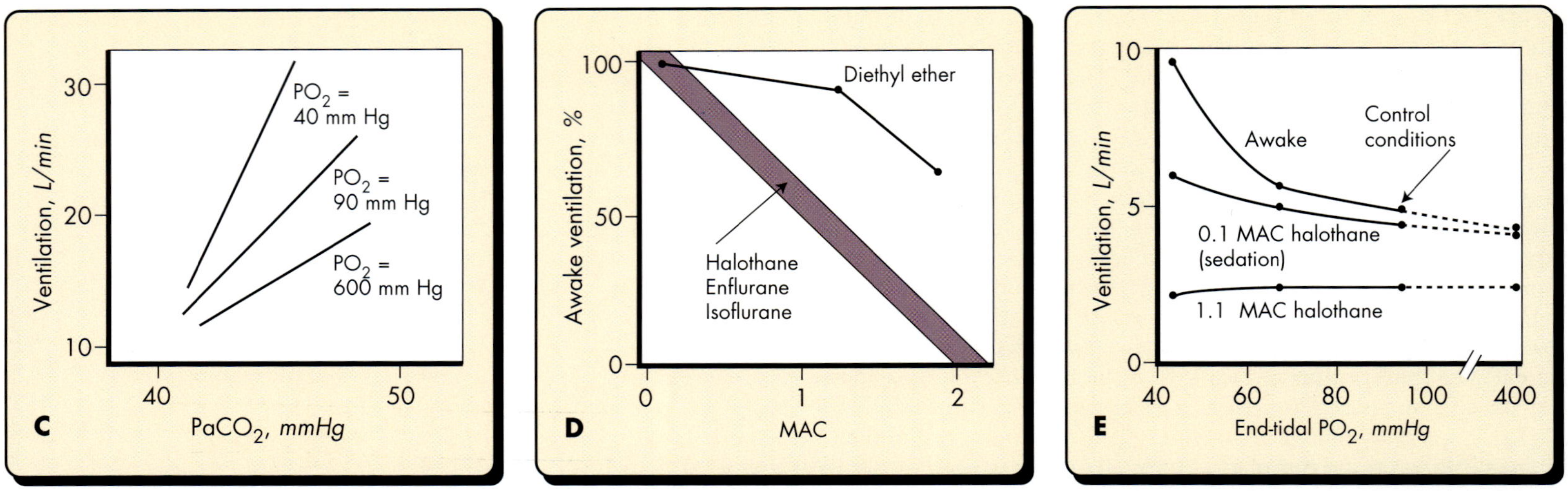

Figure 6-12. (*Continued*) The first group from the dorsal and ventral respiratory areas of the medulla descends in the ventrolateral quadrant of the spinal cord and is involved in the involuntary generation of rhythmic breathing. The second group is contained in the dorsolateral and ventrolateral quadrants of the cord and is important in the voluntary control of breathing. The third group does not descend in a single spinal tract and is involved in the involuntary control of non-rhythmic breathing.

Respiratory muscle tension is controlled by a servo mechanism involving the alpha and gamma motor neurons of the muscle spindles (*panel B, lower right*). This feedback control mechanism is more important in the control of the intercostal muscles than in the diaphragm [76] and provides for fine control of respiratory muscle contraction as well as a mechanism to rapidly respond to changes in airway resistance. Muscle contraction may be controlled either by efferents travelling solely in the gamma fibers or from discharge of the alpha and gamma motor neurons [61] and requires intact dorsal roots.

The peripheral chemoreceptors respond rapidly to decreased arterial PO_2, increased PCO_2, and decreased pH (*panel B, left side*). The paired carotid bodies are located at the bifurcation of the carotid artery. They have a very high metabolic rate and a high rate of perfusion and are primarily responsible for the respiratory responses to changes in arterial blood gas tensions due to rapid sensing of small arterial-venous oxygen tension differences in the blood flowing through them [77–79].

Increased output from the afferent nerves of the carotid bodies results from a decreased PO_2 (not content), decreased arterial pH, respiratory oscillations of PCO_2, increased blood temperature, hypoperfusion and/or hypotension of the carotid bodies, and chemical stimulants. The mechanism of action for increased output in the carotid sinus nerve has been attributed to release of a number of neurotransmitters from the Type I or glomus cells including dopamine, noradrenaline, acetylcholine, substance P and enkephalins due to a metabolic response to hypoxia [78] as well as to the presence of a specialized carotid body cytochrome with an unusually high P_{50} which would be exquisitively sensitive to small changes in arterial PO_2 [80].

The majority of the body's ventilatory response to carbon dioxide originates in the central medullary chemoreceptors near the origins of the glossopharyngeal nerve and the vagus nerve in a highly vascularized area crossed by the anterior inferior cerebellar arteries. Increases in $PaCO_2$ cause a similar increase in CSF PCO_2, which results in a decrease in CSF pH and an increase in neuronal output possibly mediated through enzymatic inhibition of acetylcholine metabolism [81] or a mechanism that senses transmembrane pH gradient. Sustained increases in $PaCO_2$ result in compensatory changes in CSF bicarbonate concentration in parallel with the arterial bicarbonate concentrations as blood pH is normalized and result in an attentuation of the ventilatory response.

The assessment of respiratory drive is conventionally performed by measuring the increase in ventilation in response to hypoxia at constant Pco_2 or to hypercapnia at constant PO_2. The ventilatory response to hypoxia is nonlinear and highly variable among individuals. The ventilatory response to hypercapnia is typically linear and shows much less individual variability than the hypoxic response but is modulated by changes in inspired oxygen tension (**C**).

Inhalational anesthetics depress respiration (**D**. Inhalational anesthetics and nitrous oxide have been reported to markedly attenuate the ventilatory drive to hypoxia at levels as low as 0.1 MAC (**E** [82]). The magnitude of this effect is agent specific and recently has been shown for isoflurane to have no effect on the ventilatory response to mild isocapnic hypoxia nor to mild hypercapnic hypoxic challenge at an end-tidal isoflurane concentration of 0.2% [83]. They report a parallel 60-70% reduction in ventilatory response to both of these ventilatory challenges at end-tidal isoflurane concentrations of 1.0% and 1.4%. The anesthetic implications of attenuation of hypoxic ventilatory response include an inability of an anesthetized patient to increase a low arterial PaO_2 through hyperventilation. Further, pulmonary patients with preexisting attentuation of their CO_2 drive to breathe, may stop breathing after induction of anesthesia if their hypoxic ventilatory drive is also abolished. Patients are at risk during the post-operative period when trace amounts of residual inhalational agents may significantly impair normal hypoxic ventilatory drive.

(*Continued on next page*)

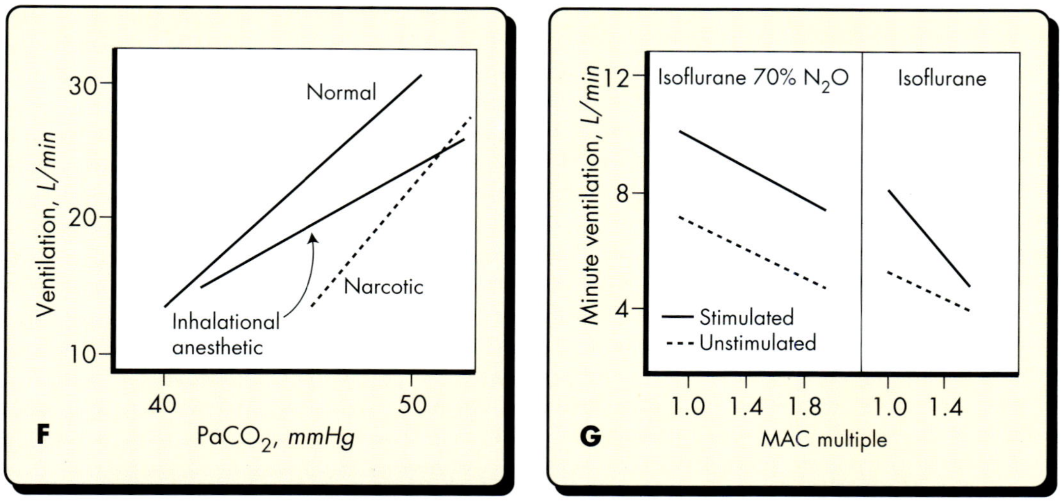

Figure 6-12. (*Continued*) All inhalational anesthetic agents decrease the slope of the PCO_2/ventilation response curve to varying degrees with obliteration of the response at deeper levels of anesthesia (F) [61]. Use of N_2O with a volatile agent compared to an equi-MAC dose of volatile agent alone results in less ventilatory depression (G). In addition, anesthetized patients lose their CO_2 drive to breathe when arterial tensions of CO_2 are decreased to levels below the apneic threshold. Surgical stimulation has been shown by Eger *at al.* 1972 to increase ventilation during spontaneous respiration regardless of the depth of anesthesia (G). Barbiturates have little depressive effects at low doses but diminish the response at anesthetic concentrations. Ketamine has little effect of the PCO_2/ventilation response curve. Opiates seem to diminish the ventilatory response to carbon dioxide primarily as a result of decreases in the respiratory rate (*panel F*).

Epidural and spinal anesthesia usually do not significantly affect arterial blood gases, however high thoracic blockade has been shown to depress the ventilatory response to CO_2, presumably due to mechanical impairment of chest wall function induced by blockade of intercostal nerve segments [84].

THE LUNG IN ADVERSE ENVIRONMENTS

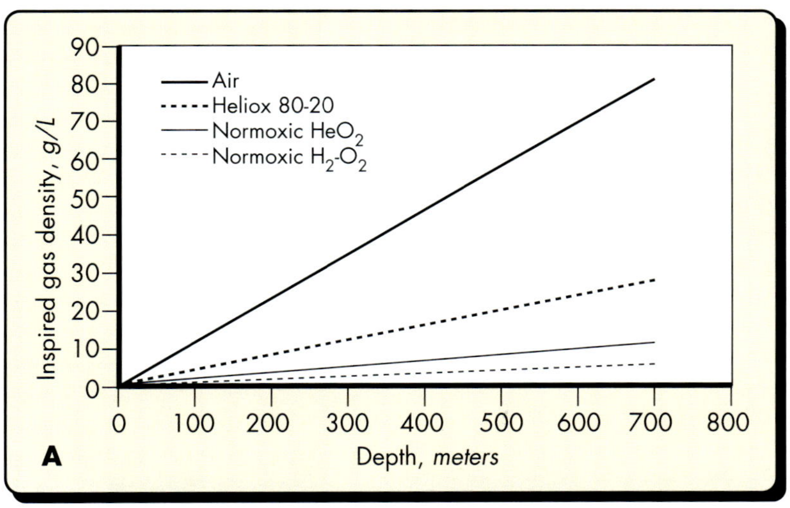

Figure 6-13. Diving (A–D). Descent into water exposes the body to increasing hydrostatic pressure such that each 10 m of sea water is equivalent to 1 atm of pressure (760 mm Hg). This pressure increase causes a reduction in volume of closed gas spaces, including the lungs. Head-out immersion causes an immediate 10% reduction in total lung capacity because of the slight increase in external hydrostatic pressure and redistribution of blood from the legs into the thorax (see discussion that follows and *panel C*).

(*Continued on next page*)

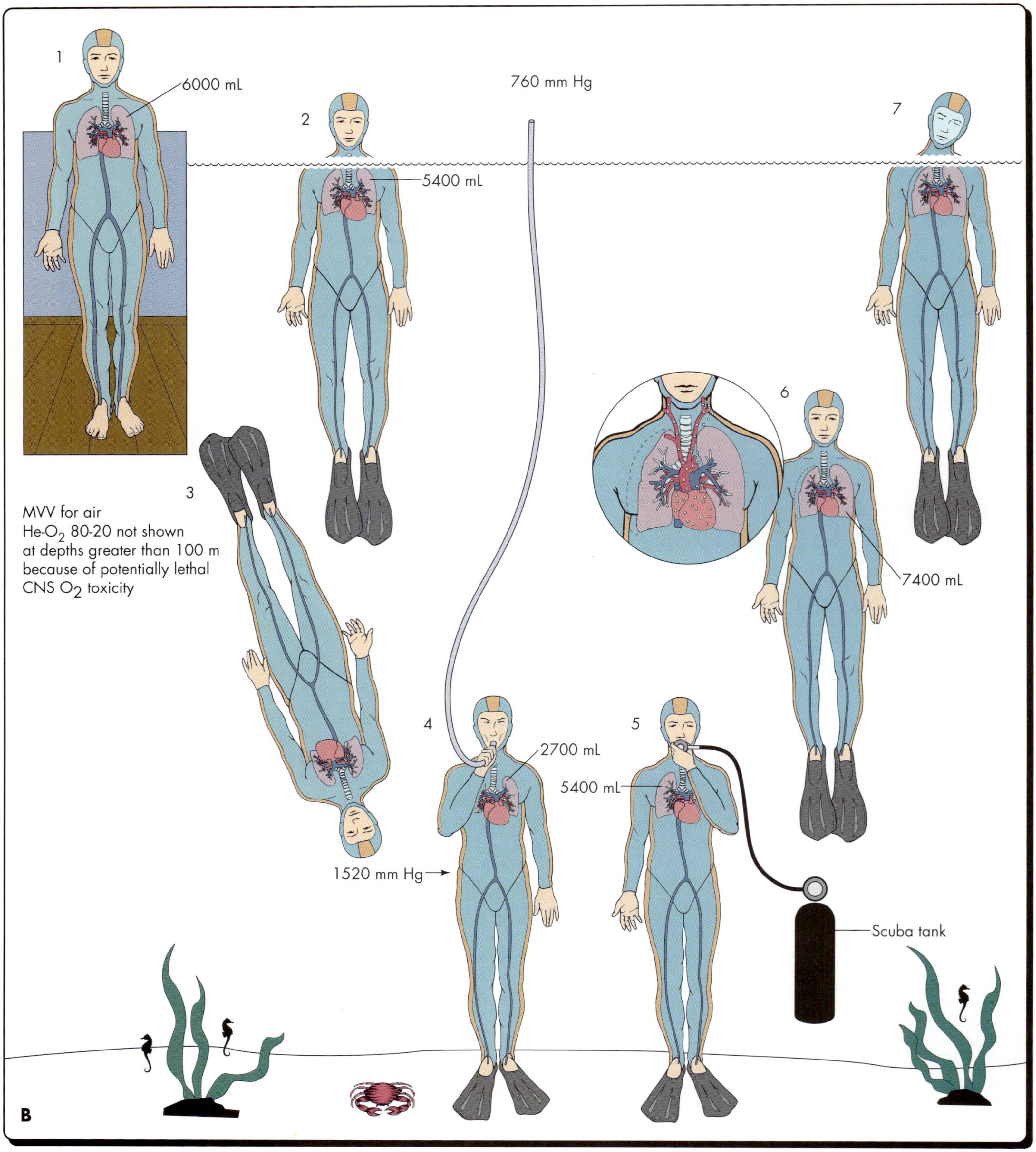

Figure 6-13. (*Continued*) Breath-hold diving to a depth of 10m (*panel B*) further reduces lung volume by an additional 50% (Boyle's law). Except at extremely shallow depths, attempting to breathe underwater while connected to the surface by a snorkel is unsuccessful because of the inability of the inspiratory muscles to overcome the hydrostatic pressure of the water column. Therefore, in order to restore lung volume, gas must be supplied to the diver at a pressure close to his ambient pressure (scuba apparatus). A subsequent ascent without exhaling may cause pulmonary barotrauma (pneumothorax, pneumomediastinum, or arterial gas embolism).

(*Continued on next page*)

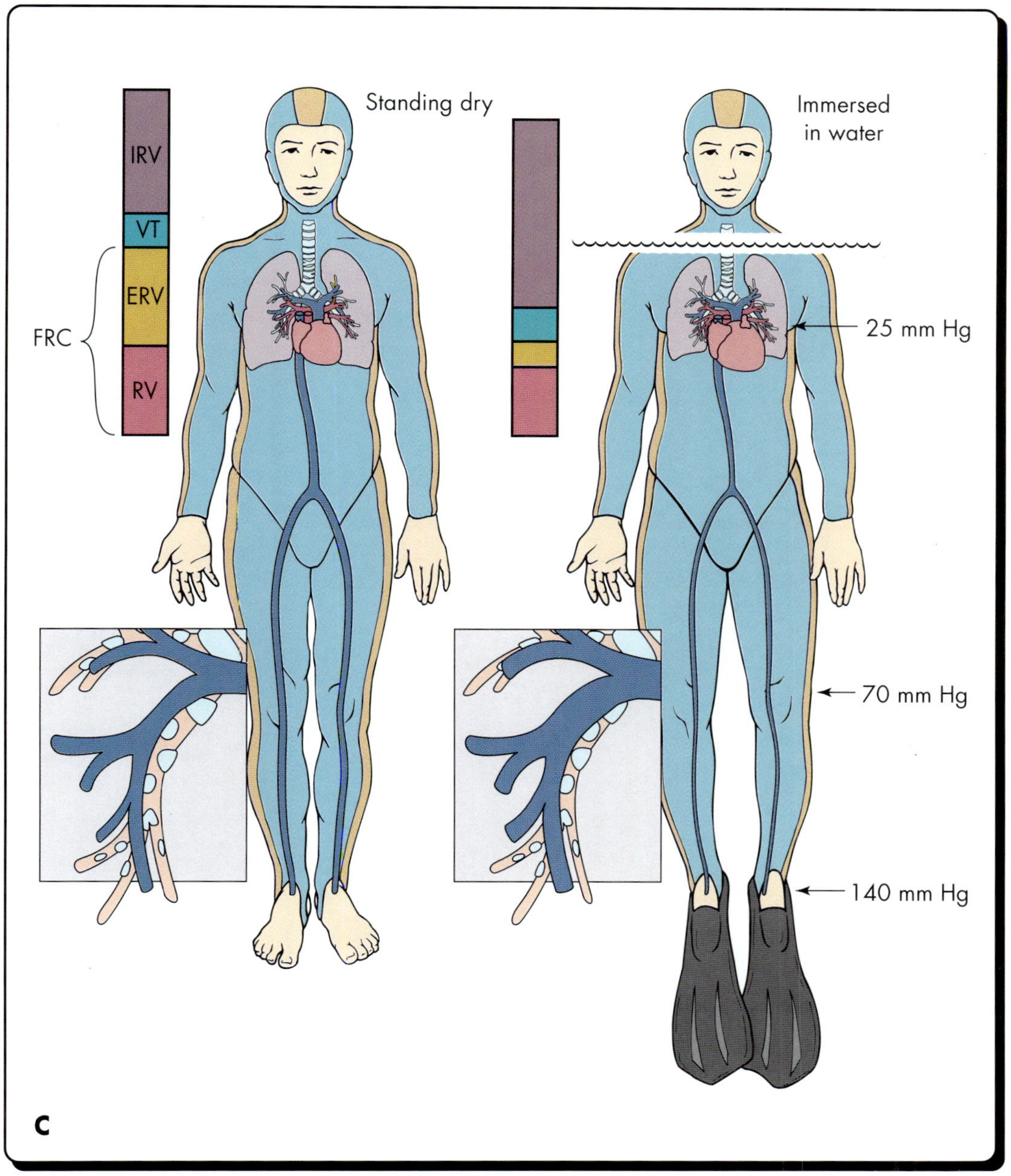

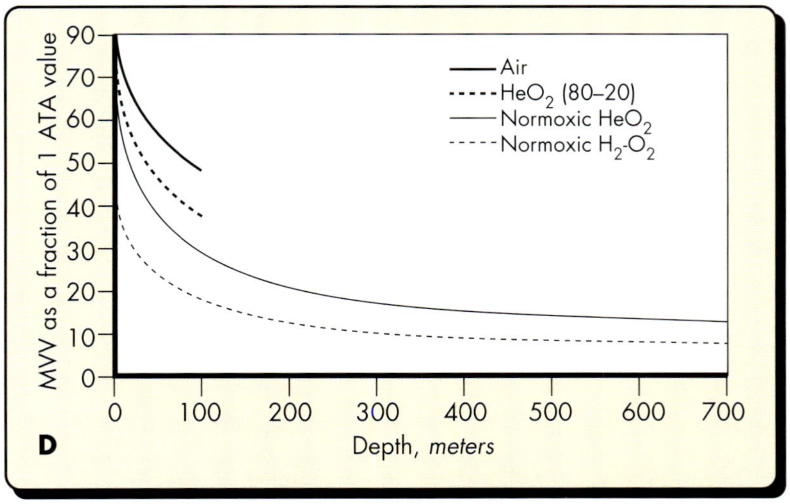

Figure 6-13. (*Continued*) The effects of diving on the lung are fourfold: (1) the effect of immersion in water causing reduced lung volumes and a static inspiratory load (*panel C*); (2) the effects of increased airway resistance caused by the greater gas density (**A**), which increases in direct proportion to the ambient pressure, reducing ventilatory capacity (MVV) as shown in *panel D*; (3) pulmonary barotrauma caused when pulmonary overexpansion due to breath holding during ascent forces gas into the pulmonary vessels (arterial gas embolism); (4) the effect of impingement on the pulmonary capillaries of venous gas bubbles formed due to inert gas supersaturation, causing pulmonary edema due to an increase in capillary permeability [28,86].

Immersion causes an immediate transfusion of 0.5–0.7 L of blood into the thorax as blood that normally pools in the legs is redistributed [87]. This causes an increase in pulmonary capillary volume, and more uniform perfusion of the lung and reduced lung volume (*panel C*). Bronchi then become smaller, causing an increase in airway resistance. The vessel engorgement also reduces lung compliance. These changes tend to be compounded in cold water, in which there is greater redistribution of blood from the periphery due to active vasoconstriction. Because of this central redistribution of blood, immersion in water can precipitate heart failure in individuals with impaired left ventricular performance.

In addition, immersion subjects the thorax and abdomen to increased hydrostatic pressure, tending to increase the static load on the inspiratory muscles. These two effects result in a decrease in pulmonary gas volumes, an increase in airways resistance and a slightly reduced MVV [88].

Immersion tends to increase the volume at which airway closure occurs, particularly in older individuals [89,90], although in healthy individuals this has very little effect on pulmonary gas exchange [89]. In COPD, upright immersion results in a decrease of arterial PO_2, although limited numbers of observations suggest that while swimming in the prone position, oxygenation reverts toward normal [91].

While the effects of immersion on the normal lung have been well described, there has been very little investigation of its effects on diseased lung. The relatively few observations that have been published suggest that closing volume is frequently greater than FRC, and upright immersion enhances pre-existing arterial hypoxemia [91].

The introduction of extracorporeal lithotripsy in the 1980s made the physiology of immersion of immediate interest to anesthesiologists. In addition to its effects on blood redistribution, immersion in the lithotripsy bath after epidural anesthesia increases ventilatory frequency and decreases tidal volume, and appears to augment the respiratory depressant effects of benzodiazepines [28].

The density effect is such that airway resistance is increased in approximate proportion to the square root of the gas density. MVV is reduced in proportion to density^{-k}, where k is a constant (0.3–0.4) [92].

Humans have breathed gas up to nearly 25 times the density of air. Despite the increase in resistive load, gas exchange is reasonably well maintained. Arterial oxygenation is somewhat more efficient, in fact, while CO_2 elimination is mildly impaired. The net effect is a reduction in alveolar-arterial PO_2 gradient and an increase in physiologic dead space [88,92,93].

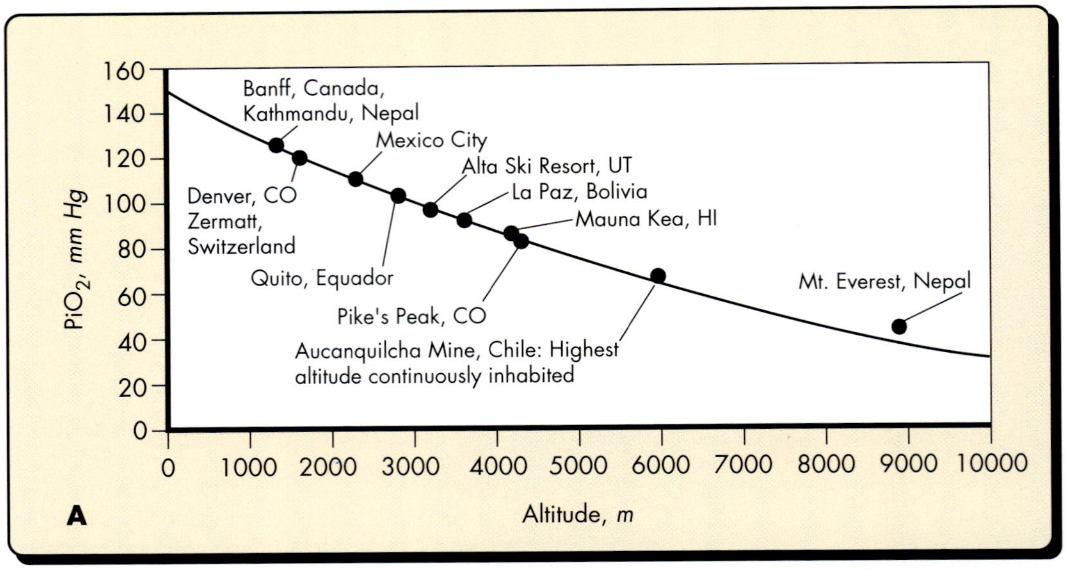

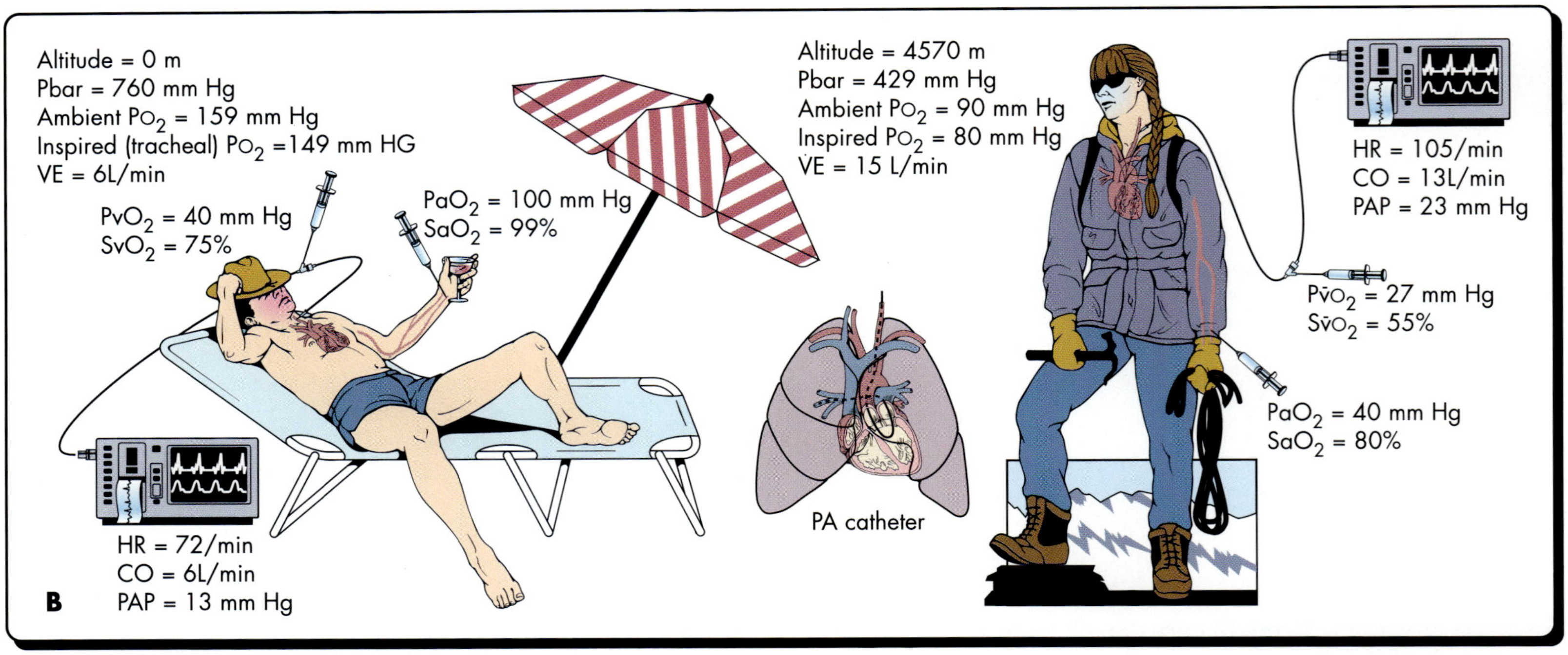

Figure 6-14. Altitude exposure. The most significant effect of altitude exposure is hypoxia. This causes pulmonary hypertension and, in some individuals, high altitude pulmonary edema (HAPE) [94]. The genesis of HAPE is not fully understood, but may be in part related to high intravascular pressures, as suggested by a propensity for individuals with unilateral absence of the pulmonary artery to experience HAPE in the opposite lung [95]. However, the edema fluid in HAPE is higher in protein than is usually observed in hydrostatic pulmonary edema, indicating a possible disruption of alveolar-capillary integrity [96]. It has been suggested that increased cardiac output and pulmonary hypertension may induce "stress failure" of the pulmonary capillaries, allowing both fluid and proteins to leak into the interstitium and alveoli [97]. Atmospheric PO_2 as a function of altitude is shown in **A. B,** The cardiopulmonary effects of a direct ascent to an altitude of 4500 m (15,000 ft). The reduced arterial oxygen content is accompanied by hyperventilation, hypocapnia, and an increase in cardiac output and pulmonary hypertension.

REFERENCES

1. Caro CG, Butler J, DuBois AB: Some effects of restriction of chest cage expansion on pulmonary function in man: an experimental study. *J Clin Invest* 1960, 39:573–583.
2. Rehder K, Marsh HM: Respiratory mechanics during anesthesia and mechanical ventilation. In *Handbook of Physiology*, vol. III. Macklem PT, Mead J, eds. Bethesda, MD: American Physiological Society; 1986:737–752.
3. Rehder K, Mallow JE, Fibuch EE, *et al.*: Effects of isoflurane anesthesia and muscle paralysis on respiratory mechanics in normal man. *Anesthesiology* 1974, 41:477–485.
4. Don HF, Wahba WM, Craig DB: Airway closure, gas trapping, and the functional residual capacity during anesthesia. *Anesthesiology* 1972, 36:533–539.
5. Hedenstierna G, Johansson H, Linde B: Central blood pooling as an explanation for lowered FRC during anaesthesia? Thigh volume measurements by plethysmography. *Acta Anaesth Scand* 1982, 26:633–637.
6. Krayer S, Rehder K, Beck KC, *et al.*: Quantification of thoracic volumes by three-dimensional imaging. *J Appl Physiol* 1987, 62:591–598.

7. Hedenstierna G, Strandberg A, Brismar B, *et al.*: Functional residual capacity, thoracoabdominal dimensions, and central blood volume during general anesthesia with muscle paralysis and mechanical ventilation. *Anesthesiology* 1985, 62:230–233.
8. Warner DO, Warner MA, Ritman EL: Atelectasis and chest wall shape during halothane anesthesia. *Anesthesiology* 1996, 85:49–59.
9. Tokics L, Hedenstierna G, Strandberg A, *et al.*: Lung collapse and gas exchange during general anesthesia: effects of spontaneous breathing, muscle paralysis and positive end-expiratory pressure. *Anesthesiology* 1987, 66:157–167.
10. Warner DO, Warner MA, Ritman EL: Human chest wall function while awake and during halothane anesthesia. I. Quiet breathing. *Anesthesiology* 1995, 82:6–19.
11. Greene NM: Physiology of Spinal Anesthesia. Baltimore, MD: Williams & Wilkins; 1981.
12. McCarthy GS: The effect of thoracic extradural analgesia on pulmonary gas distribution, functional residual capacity and airway closure. *Br J Anaesth* 1976, 48:243–248.
13. Coonan TJ, Hope CE: Cardio-respiratory effects of change of body position. *Can Anaesth Soc J* 1983, 30:424–437.
14. Damia G, Mascheroni D, Croci M, Tarenzi L: Perioperative changes in functional residual capacity in morbidly obese patients. *Br J Anaesth* 1988, 60:574–578.
15. Mahajan RP, Hennessy N, Aitkenhead AR, Jellinek D: Effect of three different surgical prone positions on lung volumes in healthy volunteers. *Anaesthesia* 1994, 49:583–586.
16. Pelosi P, Croci M, Calappi E, *et al.*: The prone positioning during general anesthesia minimally affects respiratory mechanics while improving functional residual capacity and increasing oxygen tension. *Anesth Analg* 1995, 80:955–960.
17. Jordan C, Lehane JR, Jones JG, *et al.*: Specific conductance using forced airflow oscillation in mechanically ventilated human subjects. *J Appl Physiol* 1981, 51:715–724.
18. Don H: The mechanical properties of the respiratory system during anesthesia. *Int Anesthesiol Clin* 1977, 15:113–136.
19. Lumb AB, Nunn JF: Respiratory function and ribcage contribution to ventilation in body positions commonly used during anesthesia. *Anesth Analg* 1991, 73:422–426.
20. Froese AB, Bryan AC: Effects of anesthesia and paralysis on diaphragmatic mechanics in man. *Anesthesiology* 1974, 41:242–255.
21. Reber A, Enberg G, Sporre B, *et al.*: Volumetric analysis of aeration in the lungs during general anaesthesia. *Br J Anaesth* 1996, 76:760–766.
22. Strandberg A, Tokics L, Brismar B, *et al.*: Atelectasis during anaesthesia and in the postoperative period. *Acta Anaesth Scand* 1986, 30:154–158.
23. Ali J, Weisel RD, Layug AB, *et al.*: Consequences of postoperative alterations in respiratory mechanics. *Am J Surg* 1974, 128:376–382.
24. Craig DB: Postoperative recovery of pulmonary function. *Anesth Analg* 1981, 60:46–52.
25. Meyers JR, Lembeck L, O'Kane H, Baue AE: Changes in functional residual capacity of the lung after operation. *Arch Surg* 1975, 110:576–583.
26. Ford GT, Whitelaw WA, Rosenal TW, *et al.*: Diaphragm function after upper abdominal surgery in humans. *Am Rev Respir Dis* 1983, 127:431–436.
27. Simonneau G, Vivien A, Sartene R, *et al.*: Diaphragm dysfunction induced by upper abdominal surgery. Role of postoperative pain. *Am Rev Respir Dis* 1983, 128:899–903.
28. Bromage PR, Camporesi E, Chestnut D: Epidural narcotics for postoperative analgesia. *Anesth Analg* 1980, 59:473–480.
29. Mankikian B, Cantineau JP, Bertrand M, *et al.*: Improvement of diaphragmatic function by a thoracic extradural block after upper abdominal surgery. *Anesthesiology* 1988, 68:379–386.
30. Karp G: Cell and Molecular Biology. New York: John Wiley & Sons; 1996.
31. Baraniuk JN: Muscarinic receptors. In *Pulmonary and Critical Care Pharmacology and Therapeutics*. Leff AR, ed. New York: McGraw-Hill; 1996:97–104.
32. Diamond L, Altiere RJ: The airway nonadrenergic, noncholinergic inhibitory nervous system. In *Pulmonary and Critical Care Pharmacology and Therapeutics*. Leff AR, ed. New York: McGraw-Hill; 1996:111–117.
33. Högman M, Frostell CG, Hedenström H, Hedenstierna G: Inhalation of nitric oxide modulates adult human bronchial tone. *Am Rev Respir Dis* 1993, 148:1474–1478.
34. Curry C, Lenox WC, Spannhake EW, Hirshman CA: Contractile responses of guinea pig trachea to oxybarbiturates and thiobarbiturates. *Anesthesiology* 1991, 75:679–683.
35. Lenox WC, Mitzner W, Hirshman CA: Mechanism of thiopental-induced constriction of guinea pig trachea. *Anesthesiology* 1990, 72:921–925.
36. Yamakage M: Direct inhibitory effects of halothane on canine smooth muscle contraction. *Anesthesiology* 1992, 77:546–553.
37. Jones KA, Wong GY, Lorenz RR: Effects of halothane on the relationship between cytosolic calcium and force in airway smooth muscle. *Am J Physiol* 1994, 266:L199–L204.
38. Levin A, Blanck TJJ: Halothane and isoflurane alter the Ca^{2+} binding properties of calmodulin. *Anesthesiology* 1995, 83:120–126.
39. Brichant J-F, Gunst SJ, Warner DO, Rehder K: Halothane, enflurane, and isoflurane depress the peripheral vagal motor pathway in isolated canine tracheal smooth muscle. *Anesthesiology* 1991, 74:325–332.
40. Collins S, Caron MG, Lefkowitz RJ: Beta-adrenergic receptors in hamster smooth muscle cells are transcriptionally regulated by glucocorticoids. *J Biol Chem* 1988, 263:9067–9070.
41. Bloom JW, Miesfeld RL: Molecular mechanisms of Glucocorticoid action. In Lung Biology in Health and Disease, vol. 86. Szefler SJ, Leung DYM, eds. New York: Marcel Dekker; 1996:255–284.
42. Sheridan BC, McIntyre RC Jr, Meldrum DR, *et al.*: Microtubules regulate pulmonary vascular smooth muscle contraction. *J Surg Res* 1996, 62:284–287.
43. Bigatello LM, Hurford WE, Kacimarek RM, *et al.*: Prolonged inhalation of low concentrations of nitric oxide in patients with severe adult respiratory distress syndrome. *Anesthesiology* 1994, 80:761–770.
44. Gerlach H, Falke KJ: Low levels of inhaled nitric oxide in acute lung injury. In *Lung Biology in Health and Disease*, vol. 98. Zapol WM, Bloch KD, eds. New York: Marcel Dekker; 1997:271–283.
45. Head CA, Kacmarek RM, Wain JC: Nitric Oxide and Lung Transplantation. In *Lung Biology in Health and Disease*, vol. 98. Zapol WM, Bloch KD, eds. New York: Marcel Dekker; 1997:393–409.
46. Scherrer U, Vollenweider L, Delabays A, *et al.*: Inhaled nitric oxide for high-altitude pulmonary edema. *New Engl J Med* 1996, 334:624–629.
47. Anderson TJ, Meredith IT, Ganz P: Nitric oxide and nitrovasodilators: similarities, differences, and potential interactions. *J Am Coll Cardiol* 1994, 24:555–566.
48. Wylam ME: Pulmonary Vascular Pharmacology. In *Pulmonary and Critical Care Pharmacology and Therapeutics*. Leff AR, ed. New York: McGraw-Hill; 1996:209–227.
49. Hecker M, Bara AT, Bauersachs J, Busse R: Characterization of endothelium-derived hyperpolarizing factor as a cytochrome P450-derived arachidonic acid metabolite in mammals. *J Physiol (Lond)* 1994, 481:407–414.
50. Weir EK, Archer SL: The mechanism of acute hypoxic pulmonary vasoconstriction: the tale of two channels. *FASEB J* 1995, 9:183–189.
51. Eisencraft JB: Effects of anaesthetics on the pulmonary circulation. *Br J Anaesth* 1990, 65:63–78.
52. Ozhan M, Sill JC, Atagunduz P: Volatile anesthetics and agonist-induced contractions in porcine coronary artery smooth muscle and Ca^{2+} mobilization in cultured immortalized vascular smooth muscle cells. *Anesthesiology* 1994, 80:1102–1113.
53. Buljubasic N, Flynn NM, Marijic J, *et al.*: Effects of isoflurane on K^+ and Ca^{2+} conductance in isolated smooth muscle cells of canine cerebral arteries. *Anesth Analg* 1992, 75:590–596.
54. Brendel JK, Johns RA: Isoflurane does not vasodilate rat thoracic aortic rings by endothelium-derived relaxing factor or other cyclic GMP-mediated mechanisms. *Anesthesiology* 1992, 77:126–131.

7

Cerebral Anatomy and Physiology

Johnny E. Brian, Jr., and David Warner

Patients who present for intracranial surgery usually have derangements of cerebral anatomy and physiology that impact their anesthesia care. An understanding of how such derangements affect patients is key to providing care in a rational fashion. In this chapter, we present an overview of functional cerebral anatomy, physiology, and pharmacology that will allow the reader to develop insights into the central nervous system. Basic knowledge of cerebral anatomy will allow the neurologic examination to be correlated with preoperative central nervous system lesions and new postoperative deficits anticipated. Preexisting or new neurologic deficits may significantly influence postoperative management. Anesthesia for neurosurgery revolves around control of cerebral blood flow, cerebral blood volume, and intracranial pressure. Under normal circumstances, cerebral blood flow is finely regulated by a number of influences. However, cerebral blood flow may be reduced in patients with intracranial pathology, predisposing these patients to neurologic injury. Derangement of intracranial pressure dynamics is common in patients undergoing intracranial surgery. Marked elevation of intracranial pressure may severely compromise patients, and relatively simple interventions may significantly improve cerebral well being. Finally, anesthetics may affect control of cerebral blood flow and alter intracranial dynamics. Optimal anesthetic care of neurosurgical patients requires an integrative understanding of cerebral anatomy and physiology and how disease and anesthetics may act to compromise the well being of the central nervous system.

CEREBRAL BLOOD FLOW

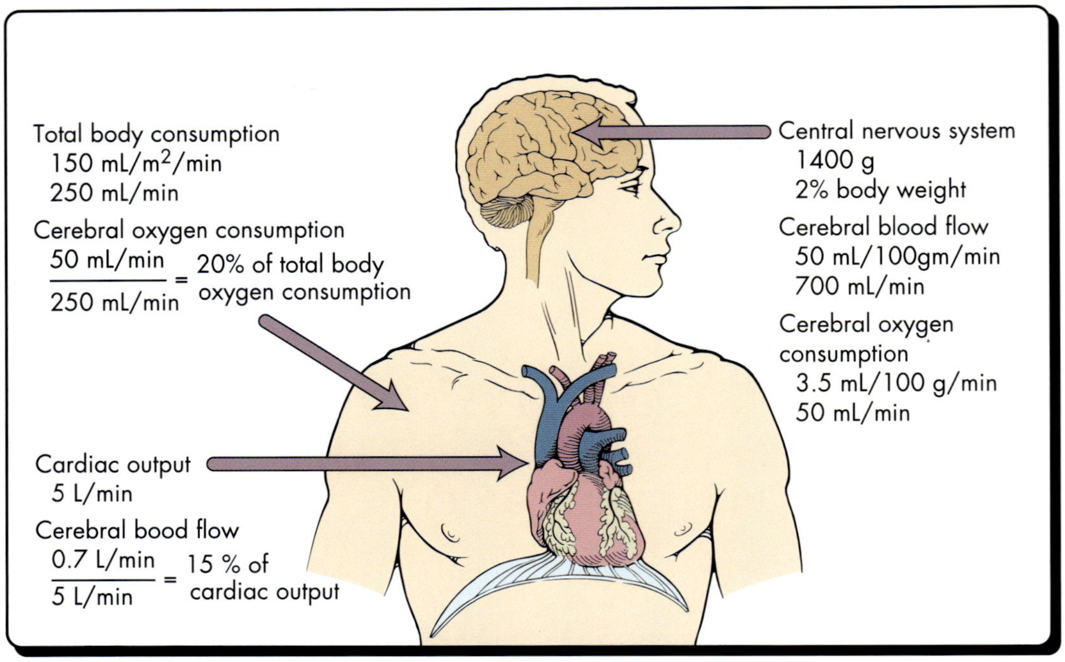

Figure 7-1. Cerebral blood flow. In awake humans under normal conditions cerebral blood flow averages 50 mL/100 g of brain tissue/min (cerebral blood flow is most commonly expressed as flow per weight of brain tissue per minute to allow comparisons among brain areas, across species and time) [1,2]. The central nervous system represents about 2% of body weight, but because of its high metabolic state, it receives 15% of cardiac output and uses 20% of total body oxygen consumption. To utilize 20% of total body oxygen consumption from 15% of the cardiac output, the brain extracts oxygen to a lower venous hemoglobin saturation. Cerebral venous oxygen saturation is approximately 65%, whereas normal mixed venous oxygen saturation is approximately 75%.

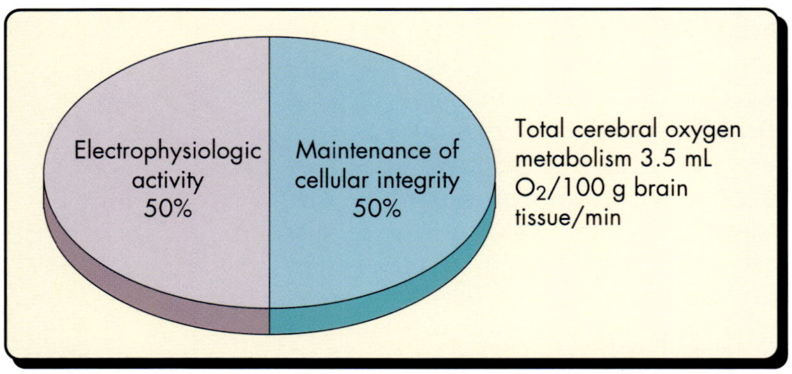

Figure 7-2. Cerebral metabolism and electrophysiologic activity. In the brain, a significant amount of energy expenditure is directed toward the electrophysiologic activities of neurons. Approximately one half of the total energy consumed in the brain is used by neurons during depolarization and repolarization [3]. The remainder of energy consumption in neurons and other brain cells is directed toward maintenance of cellular homeostasis. When a cerebral metabolic suppressant such as thiopental is administered, only the portion of energy directed to generation of electrical activity is reduced. When sufficient thiopental has been administered to render the electroencephalogram (EEG) isoelectric, electrical activity in the brain has been fully suppressed and metabolic requirements in the brain have been reduced by approximately one half. Once the EEG is isoelectric, further administration of thiopental does not further reduce metabolic requirements.

REGIONAL CEREBRAL BLOOD FLOWS

Brain Area	Cell Types	CBF	$CMRO_2$
Cortical blood flow (gray matter)	Neuron cell bodies, astrocytes, oligodendrocytes, microglia	80 mL/100 gm/min	4 mL/100 gm/min
Subcortical blood flow (white matter)	Axon processes of neurons, astrocytes, oligodendrocytes, microglia	20 mL/100 gm/min	1 mL/100 gm/min

Figure 7-3. Regional cerebral blood flows. Cerebral blood flow (CBF) and metabolism (cerebral metabolic rate of oxygen consumption; $CMRO_2$) are inhomogeneous with significant regional differences. In general, flow follows metabolism and more highly metabolic areas receive higher flow. The cerebral cortex is composed of gray matter where neuronal cell bodies are located. Most of the metabolism of neurons, including synthesis of peptide neurotransmitters, occurs in the neuron cell body. Because neuron cell bodies are highly metabolically active, gray matter blood flow is greater than average brain blood flow [2]. White matter is composed of axons of neurons as well as supportive cells and receives less blood flow, as it is less metabolically active.

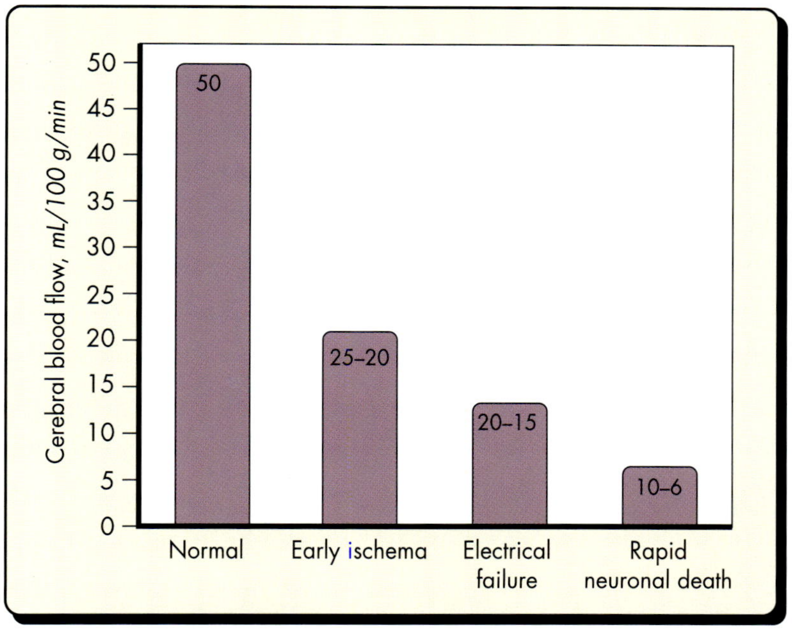

Figure 7-4. Cerebral blood flow and ischemic thresholds. When cerebral blood flow is reduced, oxygen extraction is initially increased to maintain constant oxygen delivery. However, when cerebral blood flow is reduced to 25–20 mL/100 g/min, maximal oxygen extraction is achieved, and oxygen delivery begins to fail. At this flow level, the first evidence of cerebral ischemia appears. Awake humans demonstrate signs and symptoms of cerebral ischemia, including somnolence, nausea, and impaired mentation. In normal, awake humans, to reduce cerebral blood flow to the cerebral ischemic threshold, mean arterial pressure has to be reduced to 30–35 mm Hg [4]. In both animals and humans, when cerebral blood flow declines to 25–20 mL/100 g/min, electroencephalographic (EEG) and evoked responses are present but depressed, which also suggests early ischemia. When cerebral blood flow declines below 20 mL/100 g/min, electrical failure occurs and EEG and somatosensory evoked responses are lost. At this flow level, neurons do not immediately die but may survive for hours after electrical failure. These neurons are receiving some nutrient supply and may be able to maintain their cellular functions at the cost of shutting off generation of electrical activity. Brain tissue with flows in the range of 10–20 mL/100 g/min is the "ischemic penumbra," and if flow is reestablished, function may return to these neurons. However, if flow remains at 10–20 mL/100 g/min for some time, neurons will eventually die. The lower the flow, the more rapid the neuronal death. When blood flow falls to very low levels (under 10 mL/100 g/min), neurons die within minutes. The flow values in this graph represent a composite of data from studies in both awake and anesthetized animals and humans [1,4,5].

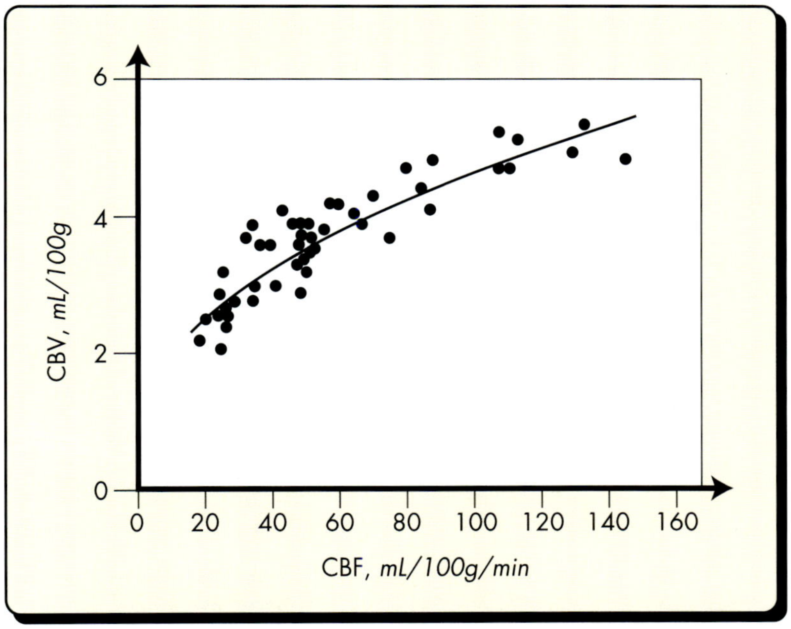

Figure 7-5. Cerebral blood flow and blood volume. Cerebral blood flow (CBF) and cerebral blood volume (CBV) are linearly related, and when cerebral blood flow increases, so does blood volume [6]. Blood vessels dilate to increase flow, leading to increased blood volume. Blood volume changes less than blood flow, and the relative change in volume is approximately one half of the relative change in flow. Although cerebral blood flow is measured much more often than cerebral blood volume (because of technical difficulties with measurement of volume), it is blood volume that is important in determining intracranial pressure. In patients with increased intracranial pressure, increased cerebral blood flow increases cerebral blood volume and may further elevate intracranial pressure. (*Adapted from* Grubb and coworkers [6]; with permission.)

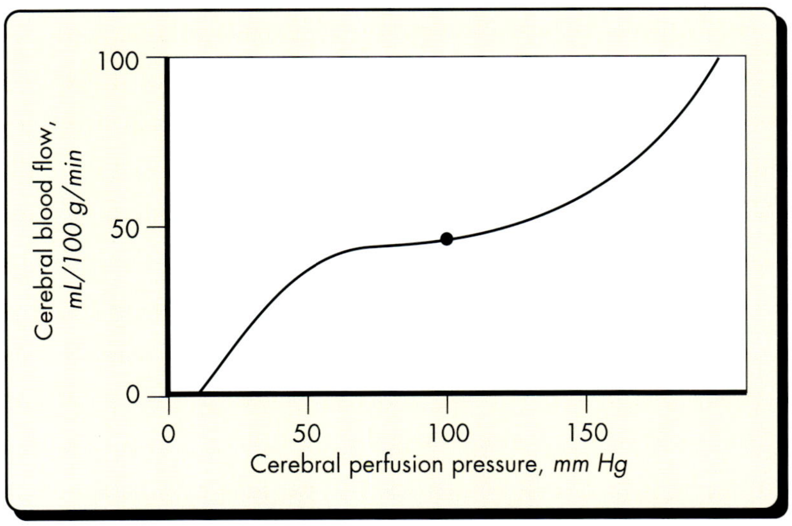

Figure 7-6. Cerebral autoregulation. Cerebral autoregulation maintains cerebral blood flow relatively constant between cerebral perfusion pressures of 50 and 150 mm Hg. Cerebral perfusion pressure (CPP) is calculated by subtraction of intracranial pressure (ICP) from mean arterial pressure (MAP): CPP = MAP - ICP. The autoregulatory curve is most often depicted with a flat midportion with sudden transitions at 50 and 150 mm Hg. However, in reality, there is some slope to the midportion of the curve, and the transitions at either end of the curve are not acute [1]. Studies from humans suggest that in the "flat" midportion of the curve, there is a 2% to 7% change in flow per 10 mm Hg change in CPP [4]. Blood flow to the brain stem autoregulates to both higher and lower pressures than the cerebrum [7]. When cerebral perfusion pressure exceeds the upper limit of autoregulation, the blood–brain barrier may be disrupted, leading to cerebral edema [8]. Cerebral autoregulatory curves are constructed from study of a number of subjects, and cerebral autoregulatory ability may vary widely in individual patients. The curve in this figure is idealized from review of a number of studies in animals and humans [1,4,9,10].

FACTORS THAT CAN IMPAIR CEREBRAL AUTOREGULATION

Head injury
Hypercapnia
Hypertension
Hypoxia/ischemia
Hypothermia
Intracranial tumors
Subarachnoid hemorrhage
Volatile anesthetics

Figure 7-7. Factors that can impair cerebral autoregulation. Cerebral autoregulation is relatively easy to attenuate, and several factors either impair or abolish autoregulation. Cerebral insults such as closed head injury [11], subarachnoid hemorrhage [12], and cerebral hypoxia/ischemia [13] impair or abolish autoregulation, depending on the severity of the insult. Blood flow to intracranial tumors frequently is not autoregulated, and metabolites or pressure effect from the tumor mass may attenuate autoregulation in brain surrounding tumors [14]. Modest hypercapnia attenuates and marked hypercapnia ($PaCO_2$ 60–80 mm Hg) abolishes autoregulation [15]. Hypothermia (to 30°C) impairs autoregulation, and the degree of impairment depends on the method of arterial pH management [16]. Chronic hypertension results in a shift of the autoregulatory curve to the right [9]. Finally, volatile anesthetics produce a dose-dependent inhibition of cerebral autoregulation, with halothane and enflurane being more potent than isoflurane and desflurane [17–19]. It should be inferred from this that many patients presenting for intracranial surgery may not possess a fully functional autoregulatory response. In addition, when autoregulation is impaired, increased cerebral perfusion pressure results in increased cerebral blood volume and, possibly, increased intracranial pressure.

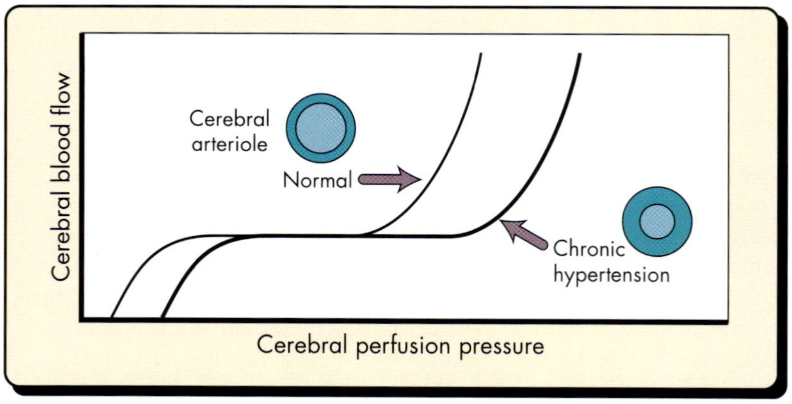

Figure 7-8. Autoregulation and chronic hypertension. Chronic untreated hypertension results in a rightward shift in the autoregulatory curve. The upper end of the curve is shifted further to the right than the lower end, resulting in a widened autoregulatory range. Morphologic and functional changes in cerebral arteries accompany the shift of the autoregulatory range [20]. With chronic hypertension, the lumen diamaeter of cerebral arteries is reduced and the arteries have less capacity to dilate [21]. The reduction in lumen size is caused by both increase in smooth muscle mass and remodeling of the artery wall, where smooth muscle cells migrate to increase overlap [21]. In hypertensive animal models, antihypertensive treatment for 8 to 10 weeks restores the autoregulatory range to normal [22]. In hypertensive rats, treatment with antihypertensives also reverses structural changes in cerebral arteries [23]. In humans, treatment of hypertension appears to restore the autoregulatory range to normal [10].

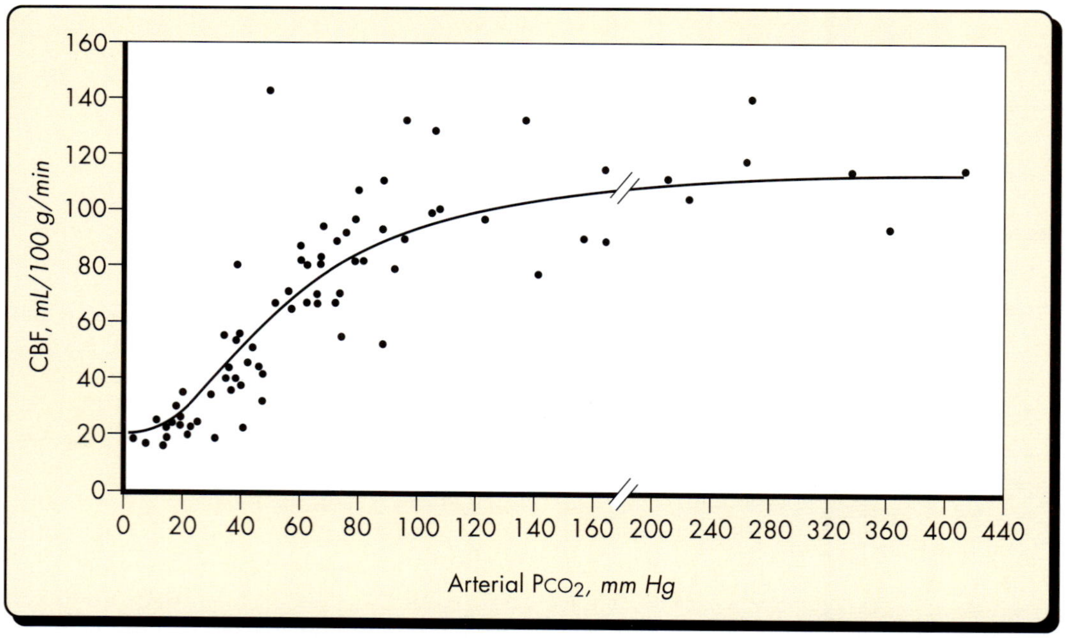

Figure 7-9. Carbon dioxide and cerebral blood flow (CBF). Carbon dioxide and CBF are linearly related between $PaCO_2$ values of 20 and 80 mm Hg, with flow changing about 2% for each 1 mm Hg change in carbon dioxide. Above and below these values, the slope of the response is reduced and a plateau is reached. The middle portion of this graph demonstrates a slope of 1.11 mL/ 100 g/min for each 1 mm Hg change in $PaCO_2$ [24]. When $PaCO_2$ is reduced to 25 mm Hg, cerebral blood flow is reduced to 20-25 mL/100 g/min, which is the threshold for early ischemic changes in the central nervous system. However, reduction of $PaCO_2$ to less than 25 mm Hg does not further reduce CBF. It is currently unclear whether hypocapnia alone can reduce CBF below the cerebral ischemic threshold in normal brain. It seems prudent, however, to avoid excessive hyperventilation. In addition, there is no advantage to severe hypocapnia, as reducing $PaCO_2$ to less than 25 mm Hg does not further reduce CBF. Above a $PaCO_2$ of 60–100 mm Hg, CBF does not further increase. Unlike autoregulation, the carbon dioxide responsivity of the cerebral circulation is relatively robust and difficult to attenuate or abolish. (*Adapted from* Reivich [24]; with permission.)

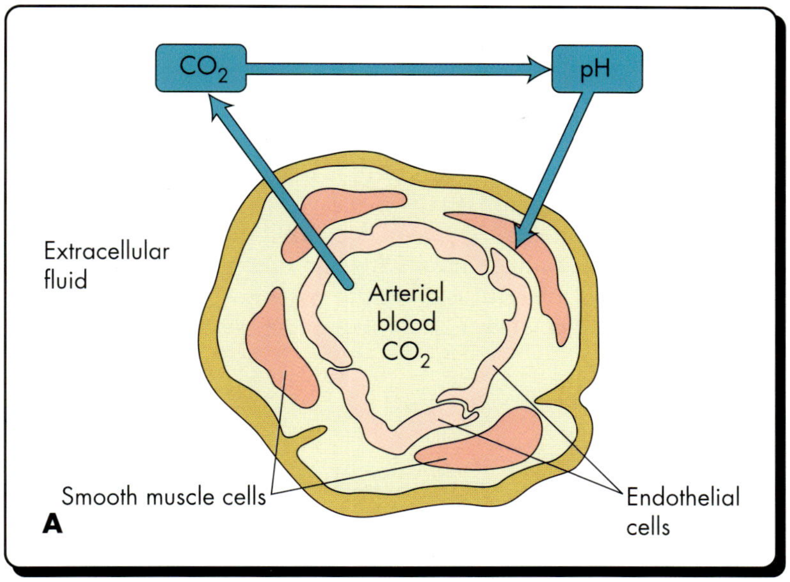

Figure 7-10. Carbon dioxide and cerebral arterioles. **A**, Changes in carbon dioxide tension alter cerebral vasomotor tone through alteration of perivascular extracellular pH [25]. The blood–brain barrier is freely permeable to carbon dioxide but is not permeable to fixed acids or bases. Changes in arterial carbon dioxide are rapidly reflected in brain extracellular PCO_2 and pH, leading to changes in cerebrovasomotor tone.

B. EFFECTS OF HYPOCAPNIA AND HYPERCAPNIA WITHOUT CHANGE IN PH

Arteriolar diameter (μ)	44.7 ± 10.1	42.7 ± 7.2	45.6 ± 10.6
CSF P_{CO_2} (mm Hg)	39.9 ± 1.2	15.2 ± 0.8	150.1 ± 1.2
CSF pH	7.32 ± 0.13	7.23 ± 0.12	7.25 ± 0.11

Experiments that altered brain extracellular carbon dioxide but kept extracellular pH constant have confirmed that extracellular pH and not PCO_2 is the controlling element. **B**, In the study by Kontos *et al.* [25], holding extracellular pH constant and varying carbon dioxide from 15 to 150 mm Hg did not alter brain vascular diameter (the measure of vascular tone used in this experiment), indicating that pH and not carbon dioxide is the controlling element. When systemic pH is altered, cerebral blood flow is unchanged as long as arterial carbon dioxide is held constant. However, systemic administration of sodium bicarbonate frequently increases $PaCO_2$, which will increase cerebral blood flow. In all of the studies cited, the blood–brain barrier was intact. However, if the blood–brain barrier is disrupted, fixed acids and bases can cross into the perivascular space of the brain, altering local pH and thereby cerebral blood flow. CSF—cerebrospinal fluid. PCO_2—partial pressure of CO_2. (*Adapted from* Kontos and coworkers [25]; with permission.)

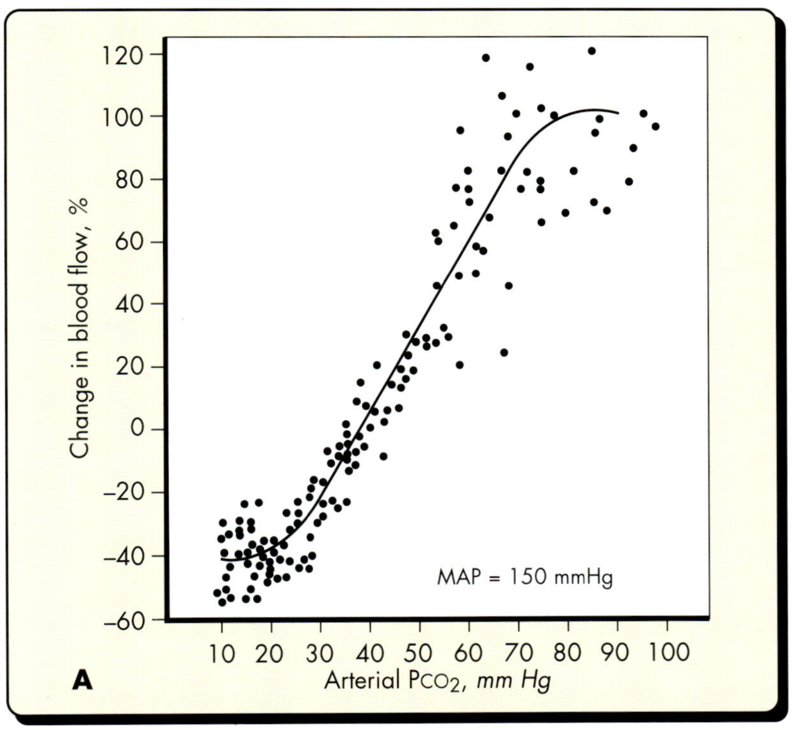

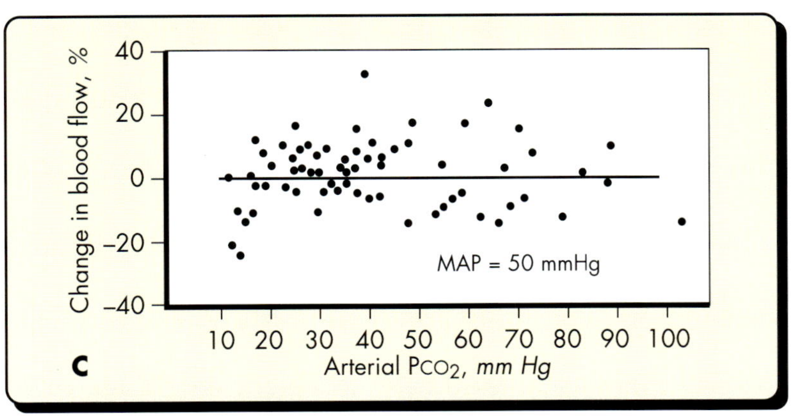

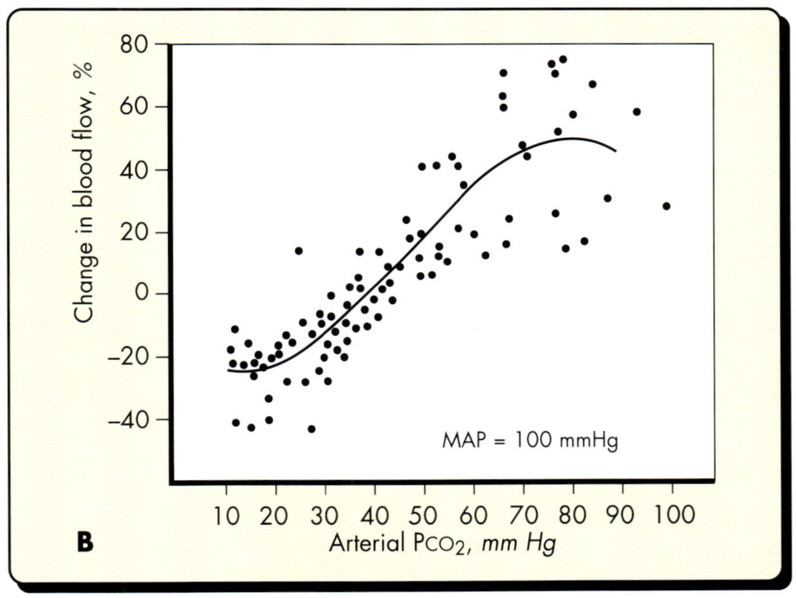

Figure 7-11. Carbon dioxide response and alteration of cerebral perfusion pressure. The slope of the carbon dioxide response curve is dependent on cerebral perfusion pressure (**A**). As perfusion pressure declines (**B**), the response of the cerebral vasculature to carbon dioxide is attenuated. At low perfusion pressure, the response of the cerebral circulation to carbon dioxide is lost entirely (**C**). P_{CO_2}—partial pressure of carbon dioxide. (*Adapted from* Harper and Glass [26]; with permission.)

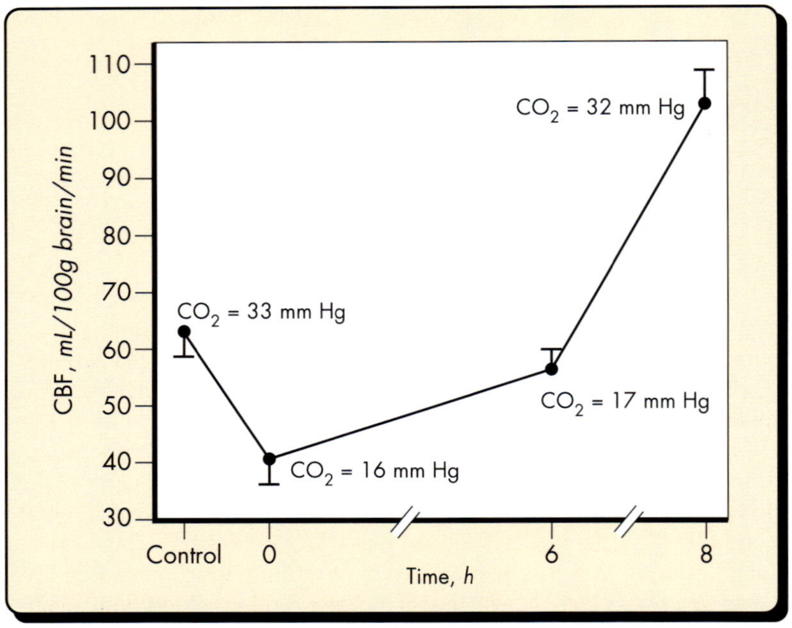

Figure 7-12. Effect of prolonged hyperventilation. With sustained hyperventilation, the reduction in cerebral blood flow (CBF) is relatively shortlived [27,28]. In a study performed in awake goats, hyperventilation initially reduced CBF. However, despite continued hyperventilation, by 6 hours CBF had returned almost to baseline [27]. When hyperventilation was terminated and arterial partial pressure of carbon dioxide ($PaCO_2$) allowed to return to control levels, significant cerebral hyperemia occurred. In awake humans, hyperventilation initially reduces CBF, but after 4 hours of sustained hyperventilation, CBF returns almost to baseline [28]. (*Adapted from* Albrecht and coworkers [27]; with permission.)

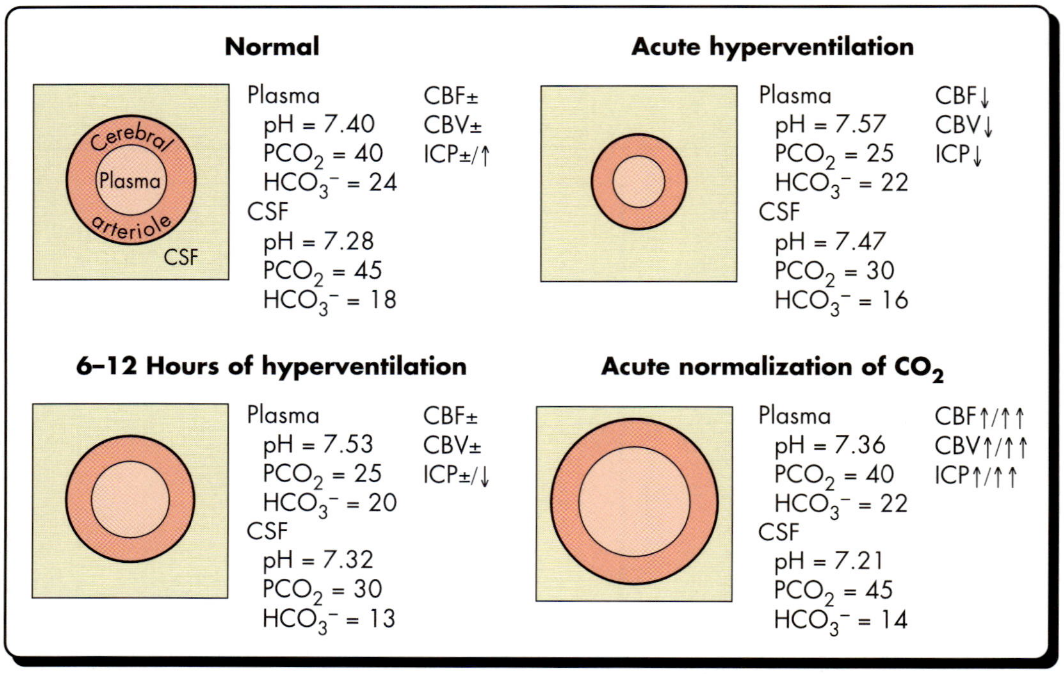

Figure 7-13. Cerebral arterioles, chronic hyperventilation, and extracellular pH. When the arterial partial pressure of carbon dioxide ($PaCO_2$) is reduced, extracellular perivascular pH is rapidly increased, resulting in constriction of cerebral arterioles. However, with sustained hypocapnia, local regulatory mechanisms in the brain begin to adjust extacellular pH back to normal within a short period of time. Extracellular fluid bicarbonate concentration is reduced to bring about the pH adjustment [29]. When extracellular pH has returned to normal, cerebral blood flow (CBF) has also returned to baseline despite continued hypocapnia. After re-equilibration of extracellular pH, acute termination of hyperventilation results in increased carbon dioxide and reduced pH of the extracellular fluid. Furthermore, because bicarbonate concentration in extracellular fluid is reduced during sustained hypocapnia, any given increase in $PaCO_2$ results in a relatively greater decrease in extracellular pH and a more marked elevation of CBF. These mechanisms probably account for the marked hyperemia seen when hyperventilation is terminated. (See Fig. 7-12.) Increased CBF also results in increased cerebral blood volume (CBV), which may lead to increased intracranial pressure (ICP). In patients who have been chronically hyperventilated, it is best to allow the $PaCO_2$ to slowly normalize to give the central nervous system time to readjust its pH and bicarbonate concentration, thus preventing any marked increase in CBV. (Values represent a composite of values available in the literature.) CSF—cerebrospinal fluid; HCO_3^-—bicarbonate ion, in meq/dL; PCO_2—partial pressure of carbon dioxide, in mm Hg.

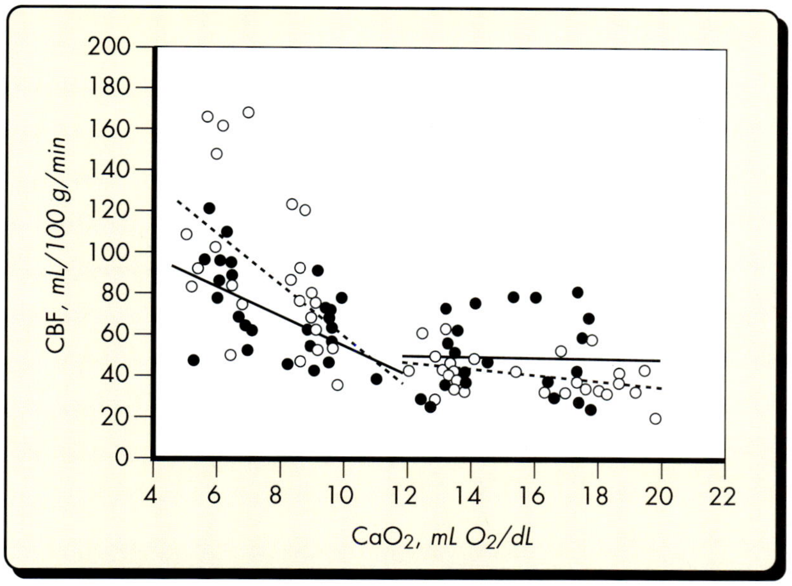

Figure 7-14. Hypoxia and cerebral blood flow (CBF). Under normal conditions, arterial oxygen tension has little influence on CBF. However, when arterial partial pressure of oxygen declines to less than approximately 50 mm Hg, cerebral blood flow increases to maintain oxygen delivery. A number of mechanisms appear to account for dilatation of cerebral arteries during hypoxia. A portion of the response appears to be intrinsic to the vessel, as isolated cerebral arteries respond to reduced oxygen tension with dilatation [30]. *In vivo* study of cerebral circulation suggests that activation of adenosine triphosphate–sensitive potassium channels is involved in hypoxic-induced dilatation of cerebral arterioles [31]. Other mechanisms proposed in hypoxic dilatation of cerebral arterioles include adenosine, pH, prostanoids, and excitatory amino acids [30]. Although hypoxia does not play a large role in normal regulation of the cerebral circulation, it appears that similar vasodilatation and increased CBF occur when oxygen delivery is reduced by hemodilution [32]. As shown in this example, when arterial oxygen content (CaO_2) was reduced below approximately 13 mL/dL by either hypoxia (*open circles*) or hemodilution (*closed circles*), CBF increased [32]. (*Adapted from* Todd and coworkers [32]; with permission.)

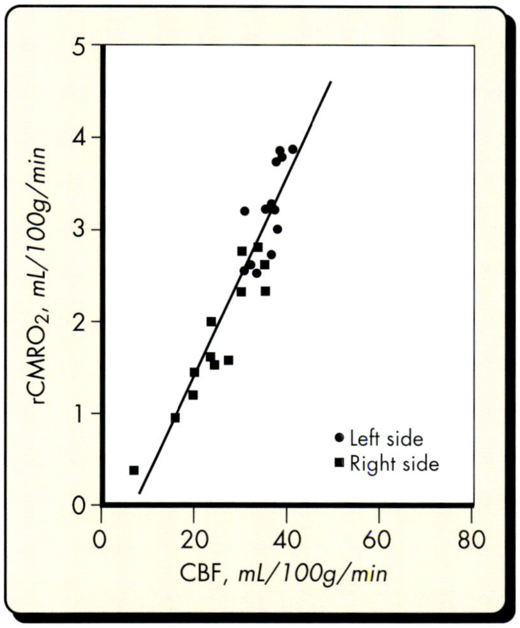

Figure 7-15. Flow-metabolism coupling in the brain. In brain, blood flow is closely linked to metabolism [33]. In humans, mental and physical activity produces discrete increases of flow to functionally appropriate areas of brain [34]. In this graph, cerebral blood flow (CBF) and metabolism were simultaneously measured in a patient who had suffered a right hemispheric infarction [33]. Lower blood flow values mirror the reduced metabolic state of the right hemisphere. Vasodilator compound(s) released from active neurons have been proposed as mediators of flow-metabolism coupling [1]. $rCMRO_2$—cerebral metabolic rate of oxygen consumption. (*Adapted from* Raichle and coworkers [33]; with permission.)

INTRINSIC VASOACTIVE COMPOUNDS IN BRAIN

Compound	Source	Action	Released during
Norepinephrine	Sympathetic perivascular neurons	Constriction	Hypertension [35]
Neuropeptide Y	Sympathetic perivascular neurons	Constriction	Cotransmitter with norepinephrine [35]
Endothelin	? Endothelium	Constriction	Subarachnoid hemorrhage [36]
	?	Dilatation (37)	? Stimuli
	Astrocytes [38]	?	
Calcitonin gene-related peptide (CGRP)	Perivascular sensory neurons	Dilatation	Hypotension [39] Inflammation [40]
Substance P	Perivascular sensory neurons	Dilatation	Inflammation [41]
Potassium	Astrocytes	Dilatation	Metabolic activation [42]
Nitric oxide	Endothelium	Dilatation	Tonic [43] ? Stimuli
	Parenchymal neurons	Dilatation	Increased metabolism [44]
	Astrocytes	Dilatation	? Stimuli [45]
	Nitronergic perivascular neurons	Dilatation [46]	? Stimuli
	Smooth muscle	Dilatation	? Inflammation [47]
Adenosine	?	Dilatation	Hypoxia [30]
Reactive oxygen species	Endothelium	Dilatation [48]	? Stimuli
Acetylcholine	Parasympathetic neurons	Dilatation [35]	? Hypoxia/ischemia [49]
Vasoactive intestinal peptide	Parasympathetic neurons	Dilatation [35]	? Hypoxia/ischemia [49]
Prostanoids	?	Constriction [50]	? Stimuli
	Astrocytes	Dilatation [51]	? Stimuli

Figure 7-16. Intrinsic vasoactive compounds in brain. Source, action, and circumstances of release are shown.

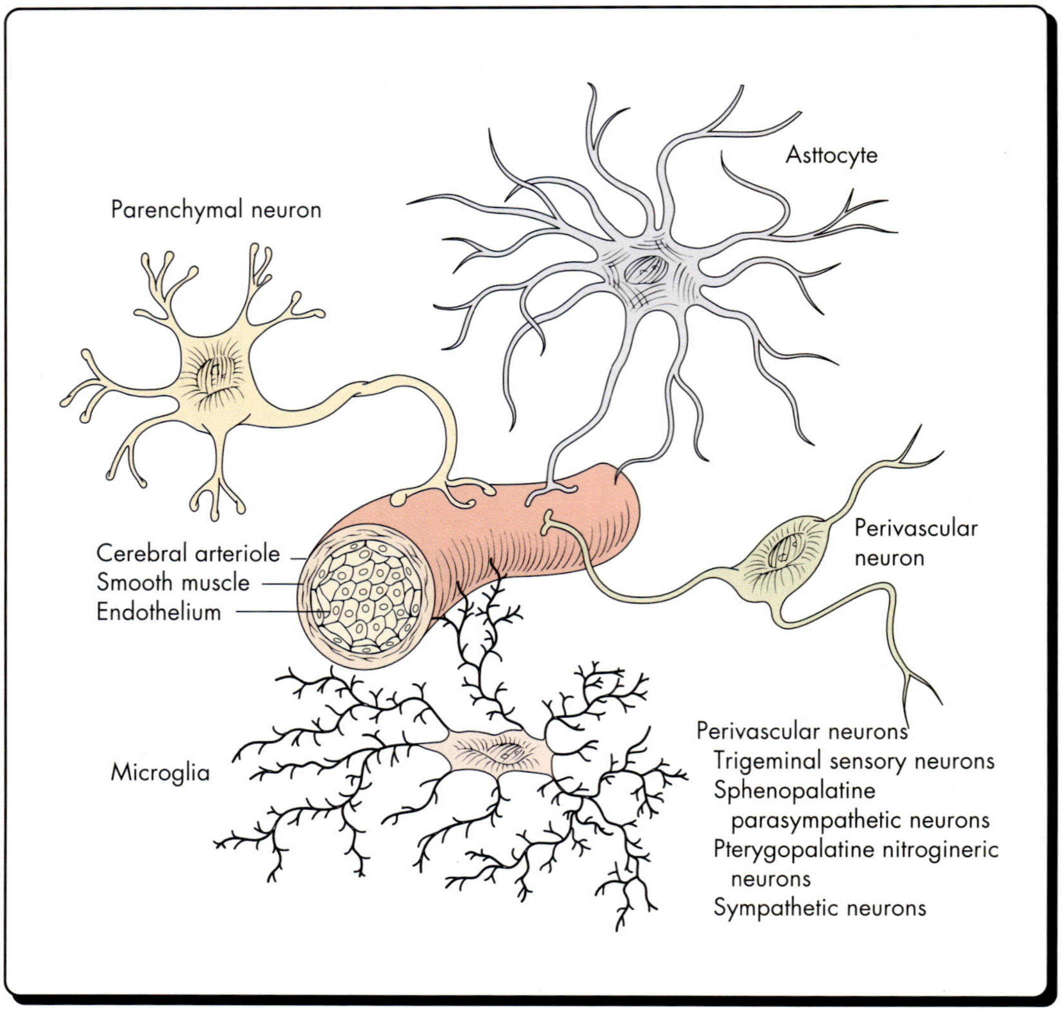

Figure 7-17. Anatomic sources of vasoactive compounds in brain. In brain, numerous cell types can release compounds that influence cerebral vascular tone. Cerebral vessels are innervated with a variety of perivascular nerves. Sympathetic nerves, arising from the ipsilateral superior cervical ganglia, release norepinephrine and neuropeptide Y [35]. Parasympathetic nerves arise in the sphenopalatine ganglia and release acetylcholine and vasoactive intestinal peptide (VIP) [52]. Nitrogineric nerves arise in the ipsilateral pterygopalatine ganglia and release nitric oxide when activated [53]. Sensory nerves arise in the ipsilateral trigeminal ganglia and release calcitonin gene-related peptide and substance P [54]. Astrocytes have foot processes on cerebral vessels and can release several vasoactive compounds, including nitric oxide, potassium, prostanoids, excitatory amino acids, and endothelin [42,51]. Parenchymal neurons may influence vascular tone in brain by release of nitric oxide and adenosine [55]. Microglia can release nitric oxide when activated by inflammatory stimuli. The vascular endothelium produces nitric oxide, endothelin, oxygen radicals, and prostanoids, all of which can affect vascular tone [36,48,56].

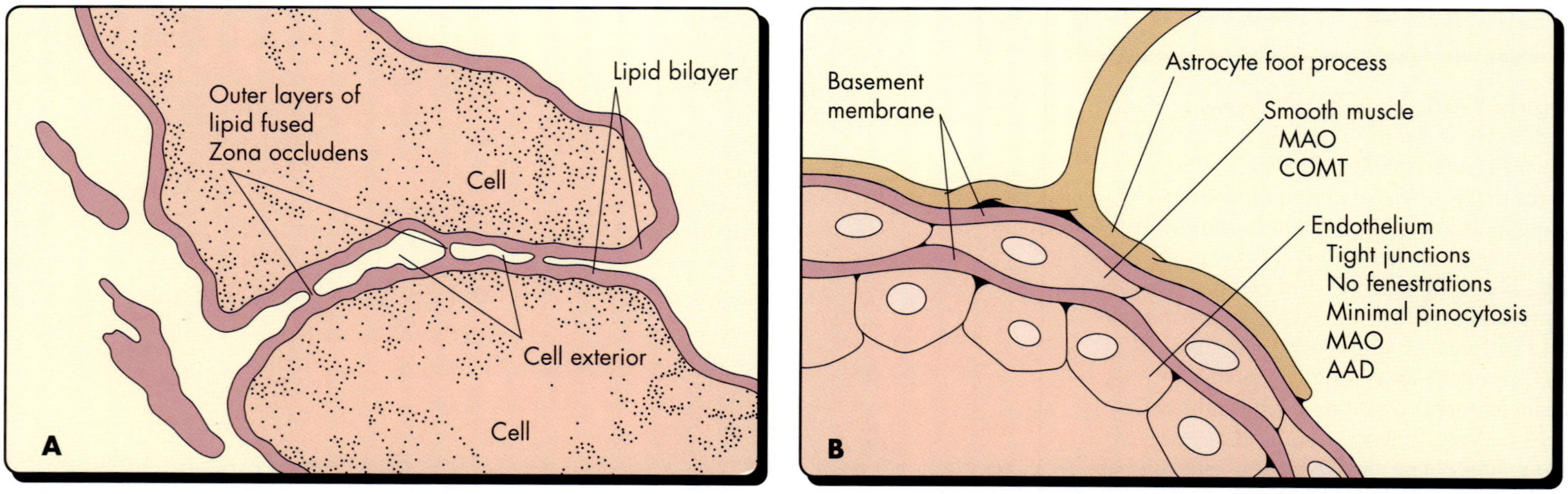

Figure 7-18. Blood–brain barrier. The blood–brain barrier isolates the brain from many circulating substances, allowing the internal environment of the brain to be more finely regulated. There are several elements to the blood–brain barrier, including both anatomic and metabolic components. **A**, In contrast to peripheral vascular endothelial cells, cerebral endothelial cells form "tight junctions" in which adjacent endothelial cells have outer leaflets of the plasma membranes fused (zona occludens). Cerebral endothelial cells lack the fenestrations found in peripheral vascular endothelial cells. Cerebral endothelial cells also exhibit minimal pinocytosis, which can transport solutes across the endothelium. The presence of tight junctions with the lack of fenestrations and pinocytosis prevents easy egress of large molecules and polar substances from the intravascular space [1]. **B**, In addition to the anatomic barrier, cerebral endothelial and smooth muscle cells also express high levels of several enzymes, which primarily prevent the passage of catecholamines into the brain. Smooth muscle cells express monoamine oxidase (MAO) and catechol-O-methyl transferase (COMT), and in capillaries and venules endothelial cells express MAO and aromatic L-amino acid decarboxylase (AAD) [1].

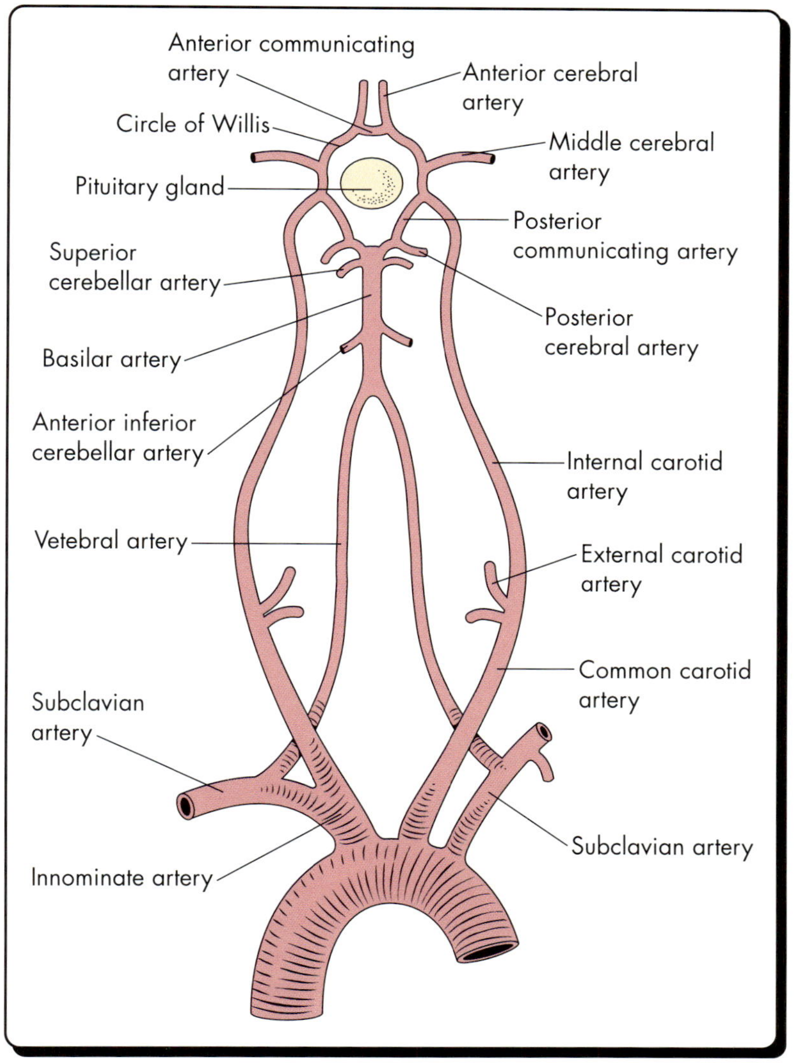

Figure 7-19. Blood supply to brain. Blood is supplied to the brain by the paired vertebral arteries that arise from the subclavian arteries and by the paired carotid arteries that arise from the aorta on the left and the innominate on the right. The vertebral arteries course through the foramina transversaria of the cervical vertebrae, entering the skull through the foramen magnum. At the caudal border of the pons the vertebral arteries unite to form the basilar artery. The basilar artery courses rostrally where it bifurcates to form the paired posterior cerebral arteries and the posterior communicating arteries. The internal carotid arteries enter the skull by the carotid foramina where they divide to give off the middle cerebral arteries, the anterior cerebral arteries and ophthalmic arteries (not shown). The anterior communicating artery connects the two anterior cerebral arteries. The circle of Willis is formed by the connection of the anterior cerebral arteries by the anterior communicating artery and the middle cerebral arteries and posterior cerebral arteries by the posterior communicating arteries. Normally, no blood flows through the communicating arteries because pressure is equal between the internal carotid arteries and the basilar artery. However, if pressure inequalities exist as a result of atherosclerosis, flow in communicating arteries may increase. Abnormalities of communicating arteries are common, and approximately 25% of patients have one or more communicating arteries absent or hypoplastic [57].

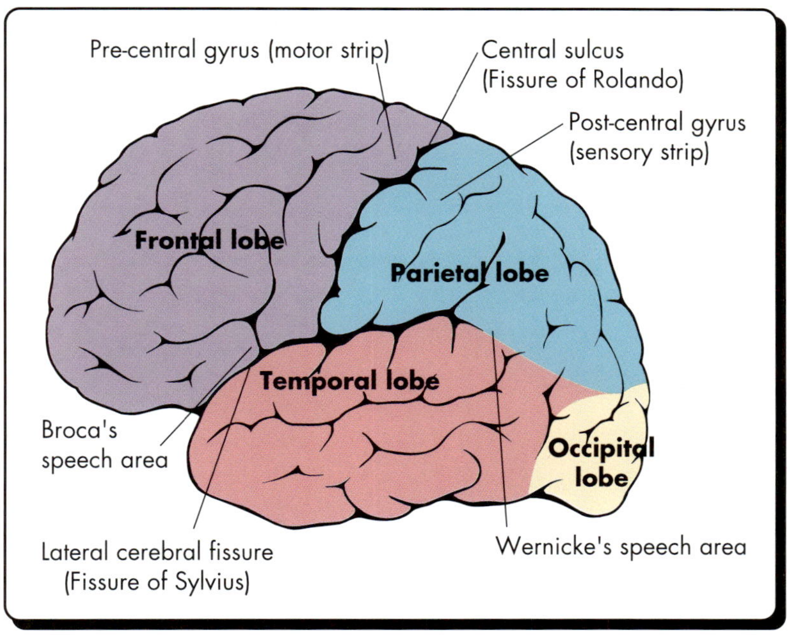

Figure 7-20. Lobes of the brain. The cerebrum is divided into four lobes, each of which has a distinctive function. The frontal lobe is the largest lobe, representing approximately one-third of the hemispheric surface of the brain. Extending posteriorly to the central sulcus (fissure of Rolando), the frontal lobe contains the motor cortex of the brain. The precentral gyrus is the motor strip, where the distribution of the motor components is in an anatomically consistent fashion. Anterior to the inferior portion of the motor strip is Broca's speech area, which controls motor components of speech. Lesions in Broca's area produce expressive aphasia. The frontal lobe is of primary importance in memory, personality, and mood. The parietal lobe extends from the central sulcus posteriorly to the parieto-occipital sulcus. The postcentral gyrus of the parietal lobe is the sensory cortex of the brain. As in the motor strip, distribution in the sensory strip is in an anatomically consistent fashion. The parietal lobe is important in integrating sensory inputs to allow discrimination based on shape, texture, size, and weight. The temporal lobe lies inferior to the lateral fissure (Sylvian fissure) and extends posteriorly to the parietal and temporal lobes. The temporal lobe of the dominant hemisphere is the primary site of language in the brain. Wernicke's speech area is located at the junction of the parietal and temporal lobes and is responsible for the integration of language input. Lesions in Wernicke's area produce receptive aphasia. Posteriorly and medially in the temporal lobe are the transverse gyri of Heschl, which are the auditory cortex of the brain (not shown). The most medial portion of the temporal lobe (the uncus) contains the olfactory cortex (not shown). The occipital lobe begins at the parieto-occipital sulcus and extends posteriorly, resting on the tentorium cerebelli. The occipital lobe contains the visual cortex and areas of brain that integrate the visual system.

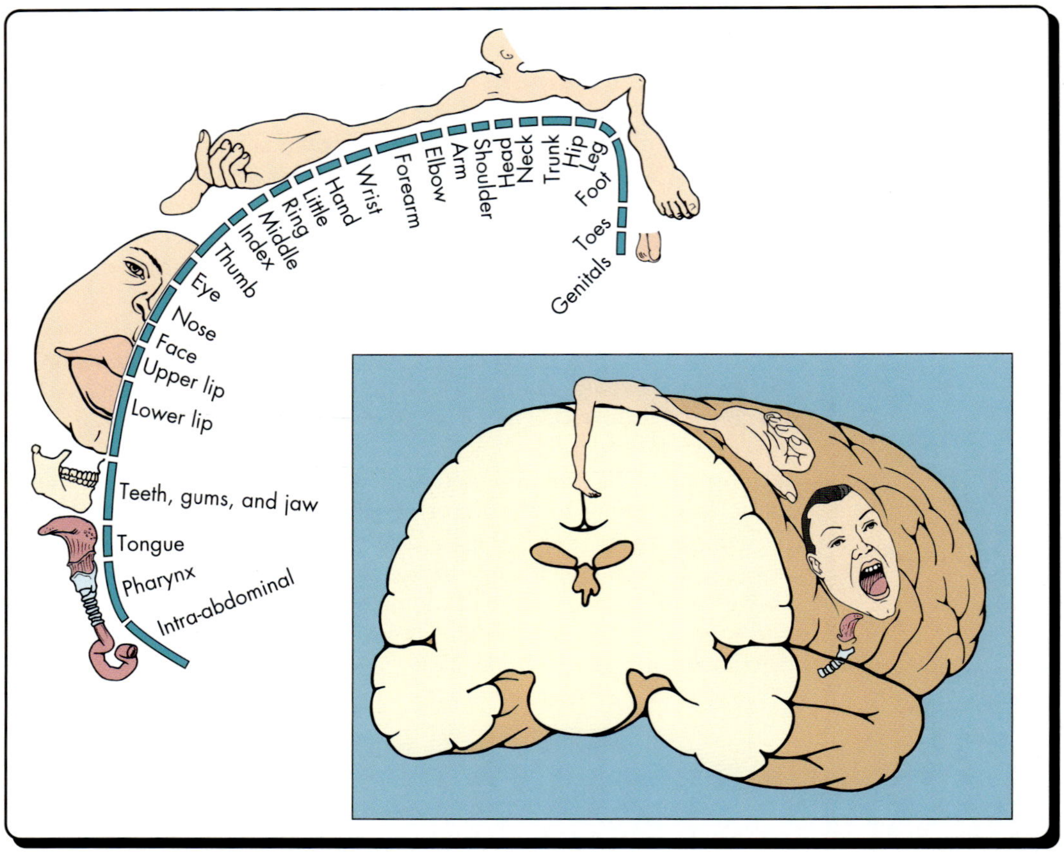

Figure 7-21. Sensory and motor distribution in brain. In both the motor strip (frontal lobe) and the sensory strip (parietal lobe), the distribution of innervation is in an anatomically consistent fashion. In addition, the proportion of cortical representation of a body area is related to its functional importance. Thus, the face and hand have very large areas of representation.

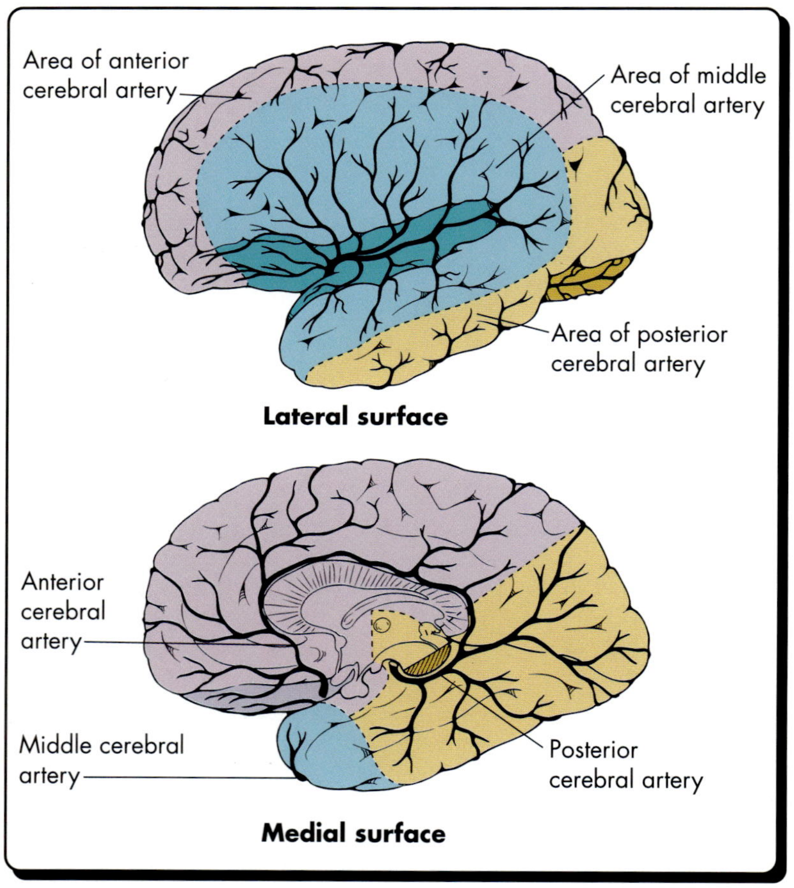

Figure 7-22. Vascular distribution to the cerebrum. The cerebrum is supplied by the anterior, middle, and posterior cerebral arteries. The anterior cerebral artery is derived from the internal carotid artery and supplies the medial portion of the frontal and parietal lobes. Thus, occlusion of the anterior cerebral artery causes dysfunction of the cortical area supplying primarily the lower extremity. The middle cerebral artery, also derived from the internal carotid artery, courses laterally to emerge in the Sylvian fissure, supplying a large area of the frontal, parietal, and temporal lobes. Occlusion of the middle cerebral artery causes dysfunction of cortical areas innervating the face and upper extremity. In addition, the middle cerebral artery of the dominant hemisphere supplies areas of brain involved in language and speech. The posterior cerebral artery, derived from the basilar artery, supplies the occipital lobe, where the visual systems of the brain are located.

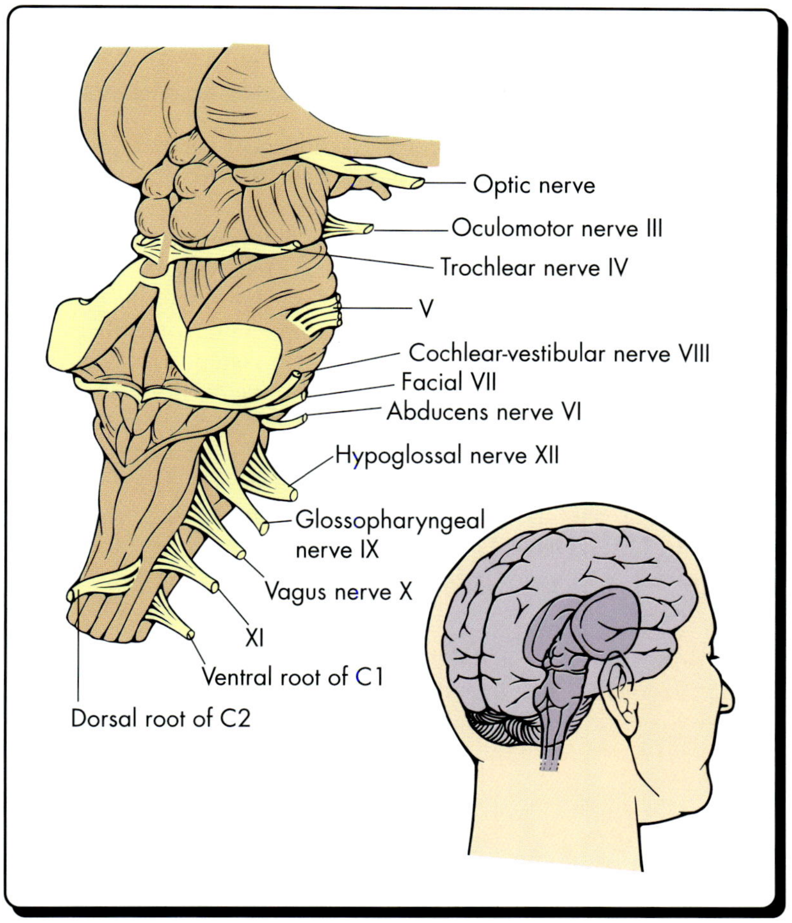

Figure 7-23. Posterior fossa anatomy. The posterior fossa extends from the tentorium cerebelli to the foramen magnum and contains the brain stem, pons, and cerebellum. The brain stem contains the cardiovascular and respiratory control centers as well as cranial nerves III–XII and their respective nuclei. The brain stem also contains all ascending sensory and descending motor pathways to the body. Compression of the brain stem by an expanding mass in the posterior fossa or by progressive transtentoral or cerebellar herniation leads to changes in hemodynamics, respiratory control, and motor and sensory function. Chronic compression of the brain stem as from Arnold-Chiari malformation or by slowly growing tumors can lead to dysfunction of airway motor and sensory innervation and an inability to protect the airway from aspiration. Cranial nerve IX (glossopharyngeal) conveys sensation from the upper pharynx and tongue. Cranial nerve X (vagus) conveys motor information to the soft palate, larynx, and pharynx as well as sensation from the larynx and trachea. Cranial nerve XII (hypoglossal) conveys motor information to the tongue. Patients with posterior fossa lesions should be carefully questioned regarding the ability to protect the airway, and the presence of a gag reflex documented. A patient who cannot protect their airway preoperatively will likely require postoperative tracheal intubation for airway protection. Compression of cardiovascular control centers in the brain stem leads to hypertension and bradycardia (Cushing response) as these control centers attempt to elevate mean arterial pressure and maintain cerebral perfusion. Compression of the respiratory control centers can lead to a variety of respiratory abnormalities, including Cheyne-Stokes ventilation (periodic hyperventilation followed by apnea), central hyperventilation, and Biot's ventilation (ataxic; irregularly irregular).

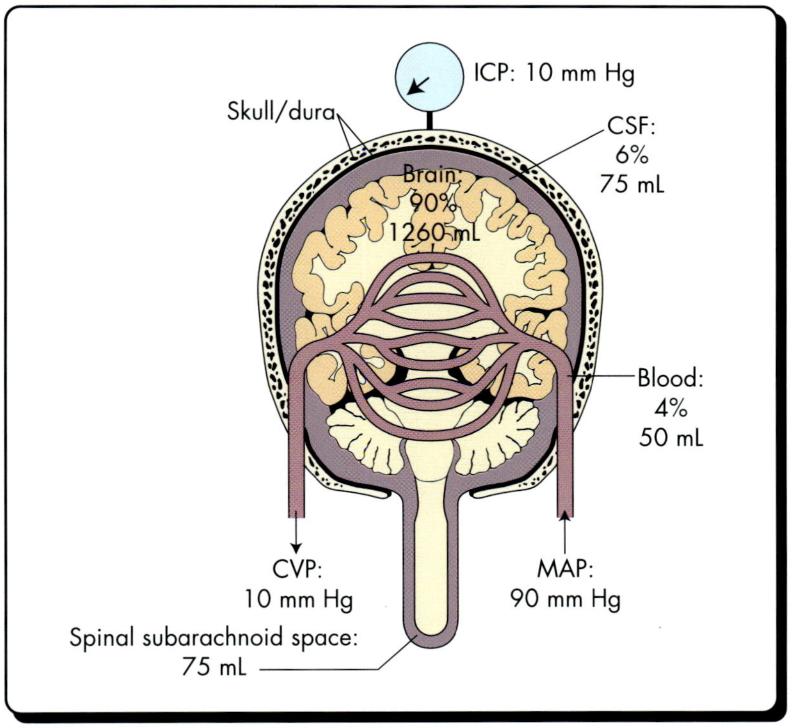

Figure 7-24. Intracranial contents. Intracranial space is occupied principally by brain matter, which constitutes 90% of the volume. Solid matter in brain accounts for only 12% of intracranial volume, and brain tissue water accounts for 78%. Cerebrospinal fluid (CSF) occupies 6% of intracranial volume and in adults amounts to approximately 75 mL. An equal amount of CSF resides in the spinal subarachnoid space. Blood occupies the least amount of intracranial volume, accounting for 4%, or 50 mL. During expansion of an intracranial mass lesion, displacement of cerebrospinal fluid from the intracranial to the subarachnoid space normally accounts for the majority of the compensation in volume. When this compensatory mechanism is exhausted (no more cerebrospinal fluid can be displaced) or if outflow of CSF into the spinal subarachnoid space is obstructed, intracranial pressure (ICP) begins to rise. Intracranial volume can be manipulated acutely by alteration of cerebral blood volume. Hyperventilation constricts cerebral blood vessels and reduces intracranial blood volume and intracranial pressure. Conversely, obstruction of venous outflow (jugular compression, coughing, head down) elevates cerebral blood volume and intracranial pressure. CVP—central venous pressure; MAP—mean arterial pressure.

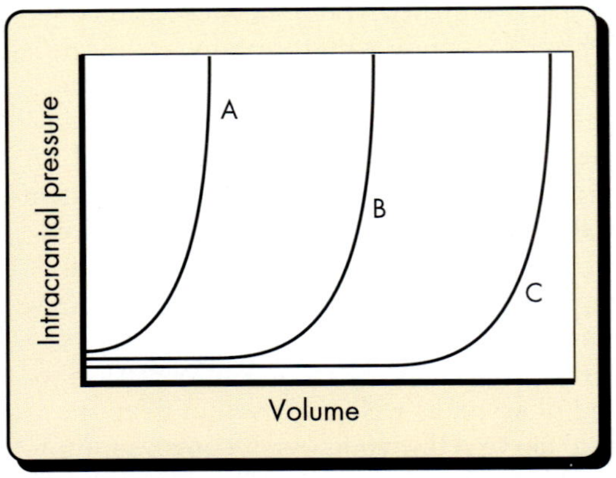

Figure 7-25. Intracranial elastance/compliance. Intracranial "compliance" curves typically depict a long, flat portion of the curve followed by an acute increase, as shown by *curve C*. Although such curves are traditionally labeled "compliance," in reality they are a measure of elastance (compliance measures change in volume/change in pressure, whereas elastance measures change in pressure/change in volume, as the curve depicts). Intracranial volume is fixed, and the increase in volume is not an increase in total intracranial volume but rather the increase in the volume of tumor, edema, or hemorrhage. The response of the intracranial pressure to increased volume depends on the magnitude and speed of the increase in volume as well as the ability of the patient to compensate for the increase. With slowly expanding masses, a curve similar to curve C may be expected as there is sufficient time for the brain to compensate by displacement of cerebrospinal fluid out of the intracranial space. However, when a mass rapidly increases in size, a curve similar to *curve A* can be expected, as there is insufficient time for compensatory displacement of cerebrospinal fluid out of the intracranial space. Intermediate responses, as depicted in *curve B*, are also possible. Because intracranial elastance is measured uncommonly, the precise pressure/volume curve for individual patients is rarely known.

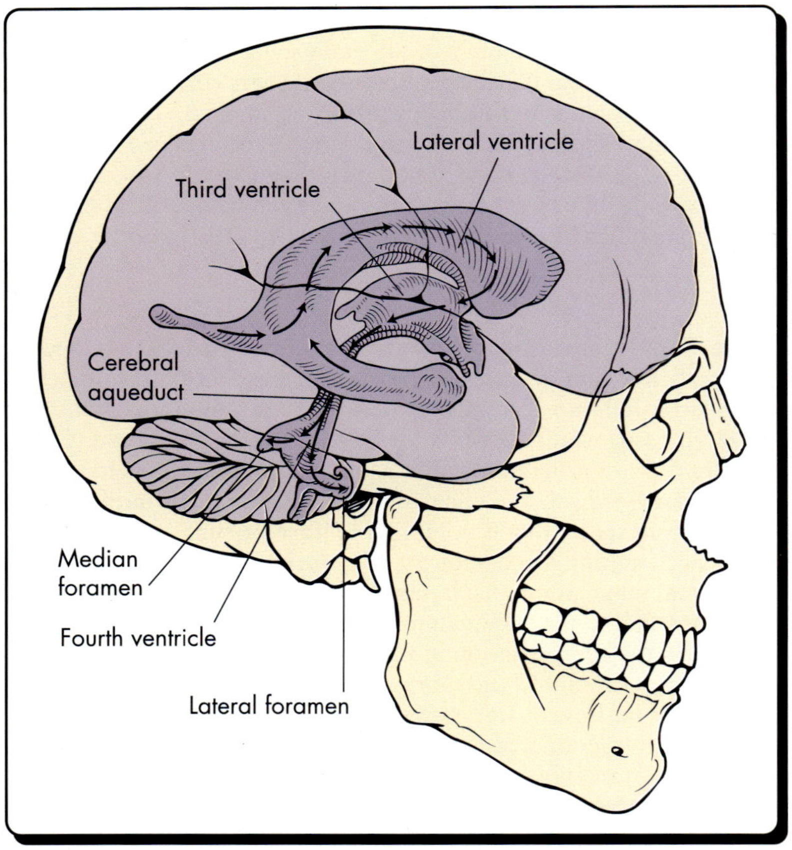

Figure 7-26. Cerebrospinal fluid (CSF) dynamics. CSF is produced by the choroid plexus in the lateral and fourth cerebral ventricles and circulates from the lateral ventricles to the third ventricle then through the cerebral aqueduct to the fourth ventricle, where it exits the brain by the foramina of Luschka (lateral) and Magendie (median). The CSF then circulates over the cortical surface of the brain where it is resorbed into the venous circulation by the arachnoid granulations. Adults produce approximately 0.35 mL/min of CSF, replacing the total CSF volume of 150 mL (intracranial plus subarachnoid) three to four times a day [58]. Egress of CSF from the brain can be impeded by compression of the aqueduct by a posterior fossa mass, resulting in noncommunicating hydrocephalus. In this situation, intracranial pressure can be reduced and the clinical condition of the patient improved by placement of a ventriculostomy and drainage of small amounts of CSF. Resorption of CSF can be impaired during inflammatory conditions such as infection or subarachnoid hemorrhage, leading to communicating hydrocephalus. Anesthetics can affect CSF production and resorption, but enflurane is the only one with a negative influence. Enflurane increases the rate of production of CSF and decreases the rate of resorption, leading to an accumulation of CSF and possibly increased intracranial pressure [59].

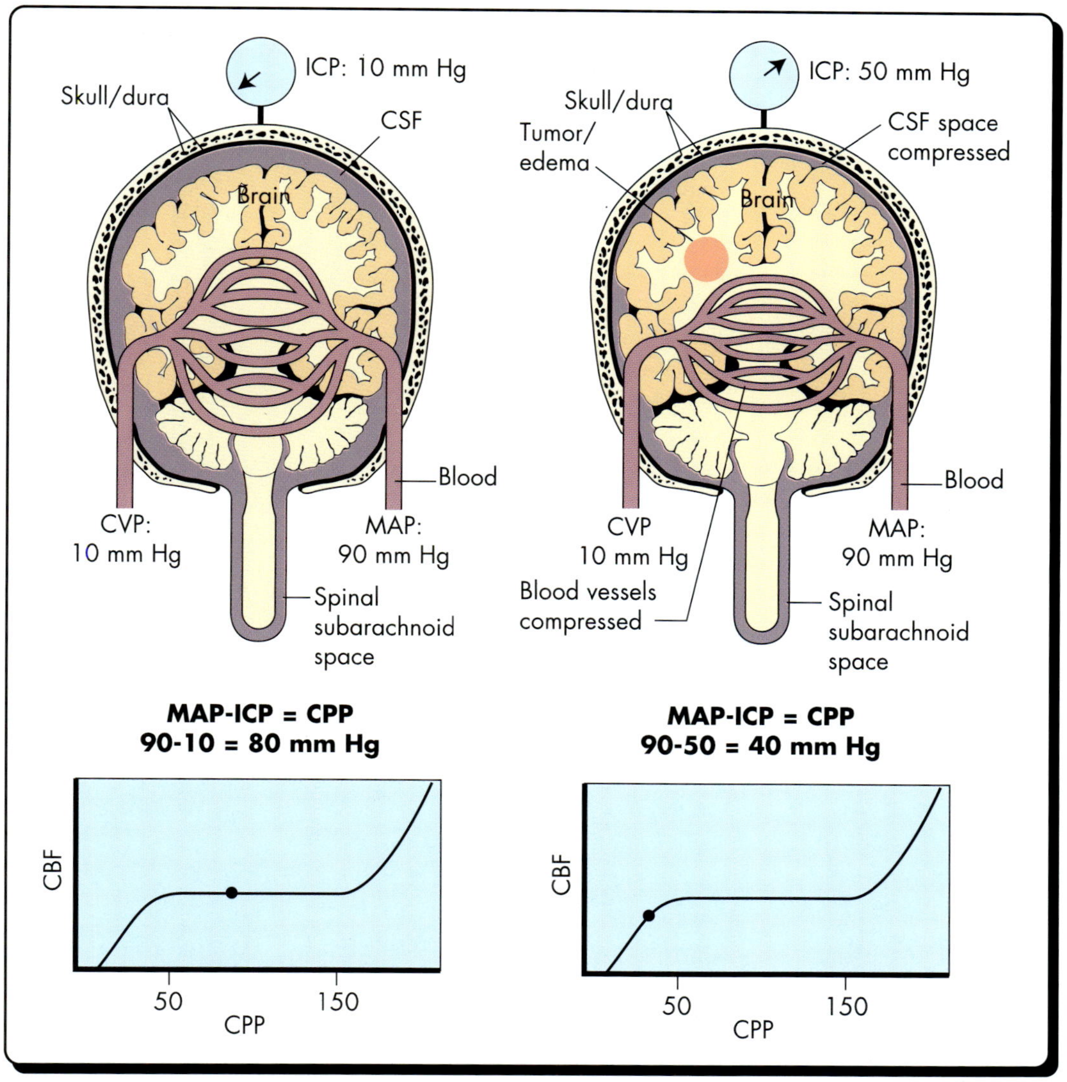

Figure 7-27. Role of intracranial pressure (ICP) in determination of cerebral perfusion pressure (CPP). Perfusion to the brain is determined not only by mean arterial pressure (MAP), but also by intracranial pressure. Autoregulation in brain does not discriminate between reduction in CPP by reduced mean arterial pressure or by increased ICP. In this example, elevation of the ICP to 50 mm Hg reduces CPP to 40 mm Hg, which is below the lower limit of autoregulation. However, ICP may not be uniform, and areas around expanding mass lesions are frequently subject to much higher local tissue pressures that may render these areas of the brain ischemic. CBF—cerebral blood flow; CSF—cerebrospinal fluid; CVP—central venous pressure.

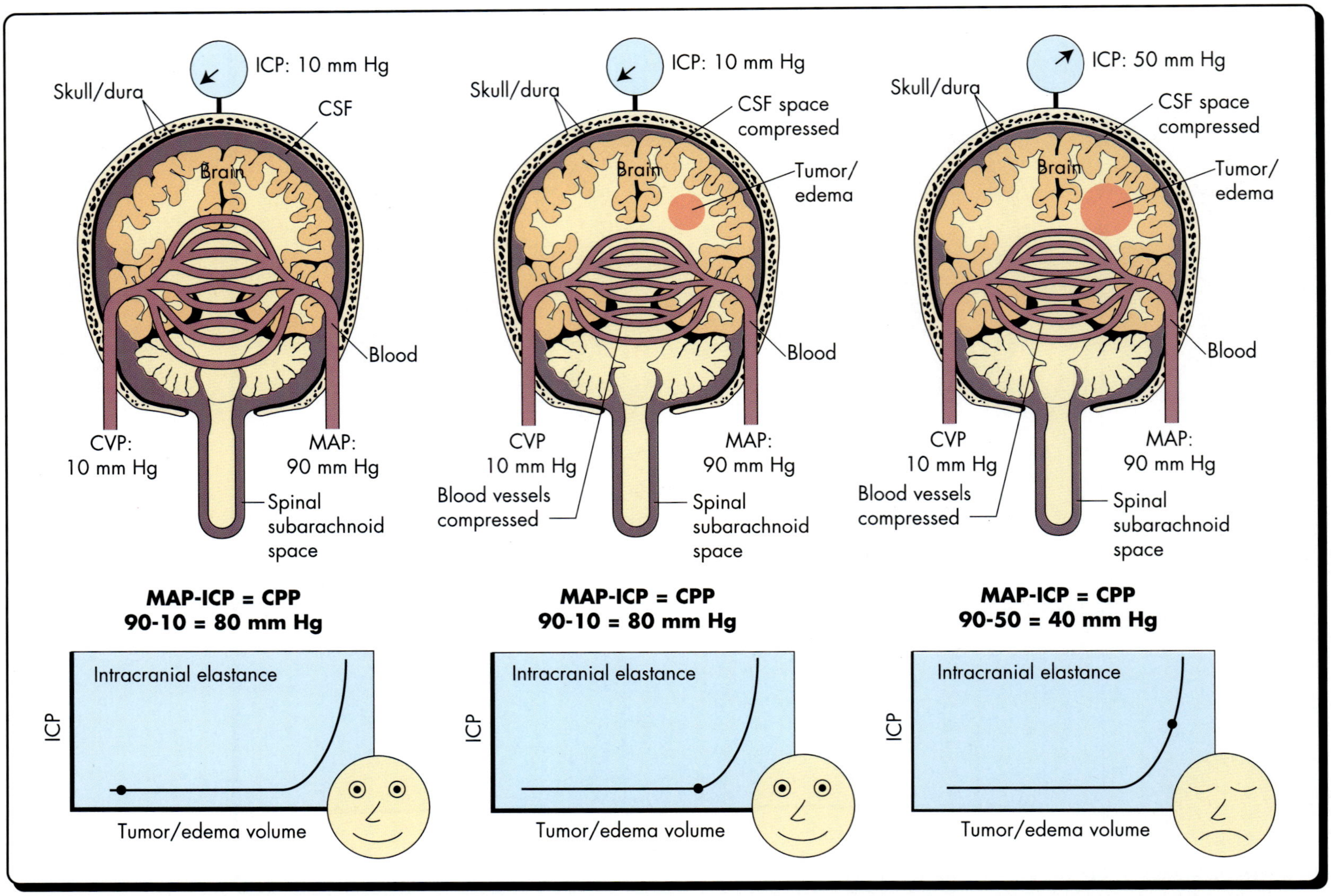

Figure 7-28. Intracranial pressure (ICP) and intracranial tumors. In patients with intracranial tumors, some of the intracranial space is occupied by the tumor mass, resulting in a compensatory decrease principally in cerebrospinal fluid (CSF) volume. Normal brain surrounding the tumor may demonstrate variable degrees of edema, which also increases the mass effect of the tumor. Depending on the speed at which the tumor grows, there is a variable time during which ICP remains normal while the patient remains on the "flat" portion of the pressure/volume curve. During this phase of tumor growth, patients may develop signs and symptoms of local compression or invasion of brain structures, but symptoms of increased intracranial pressure (headache, nausea, vomiting, lethargy, coma) are not yet present. As the tumor and edema increase in volume, compensatory responses are less able to maintain normal intracranial pressure. When patients are near the end of the flat portion of the pressure/volume curve, the supine position may decrease venous drainage and cause symptoms of increased ICP. Once the ICP begins to rise, compensatory responses have been exhausted and any further increase in intracranial volume cause a marked increase in ICP. When patients are on the upward portion of the curve, signs and symptoms of increased ICP are almost invariably present. CPP—cerebral perfusion pressures; CVP—central venous pressure; MAP—mean arterial pressure.

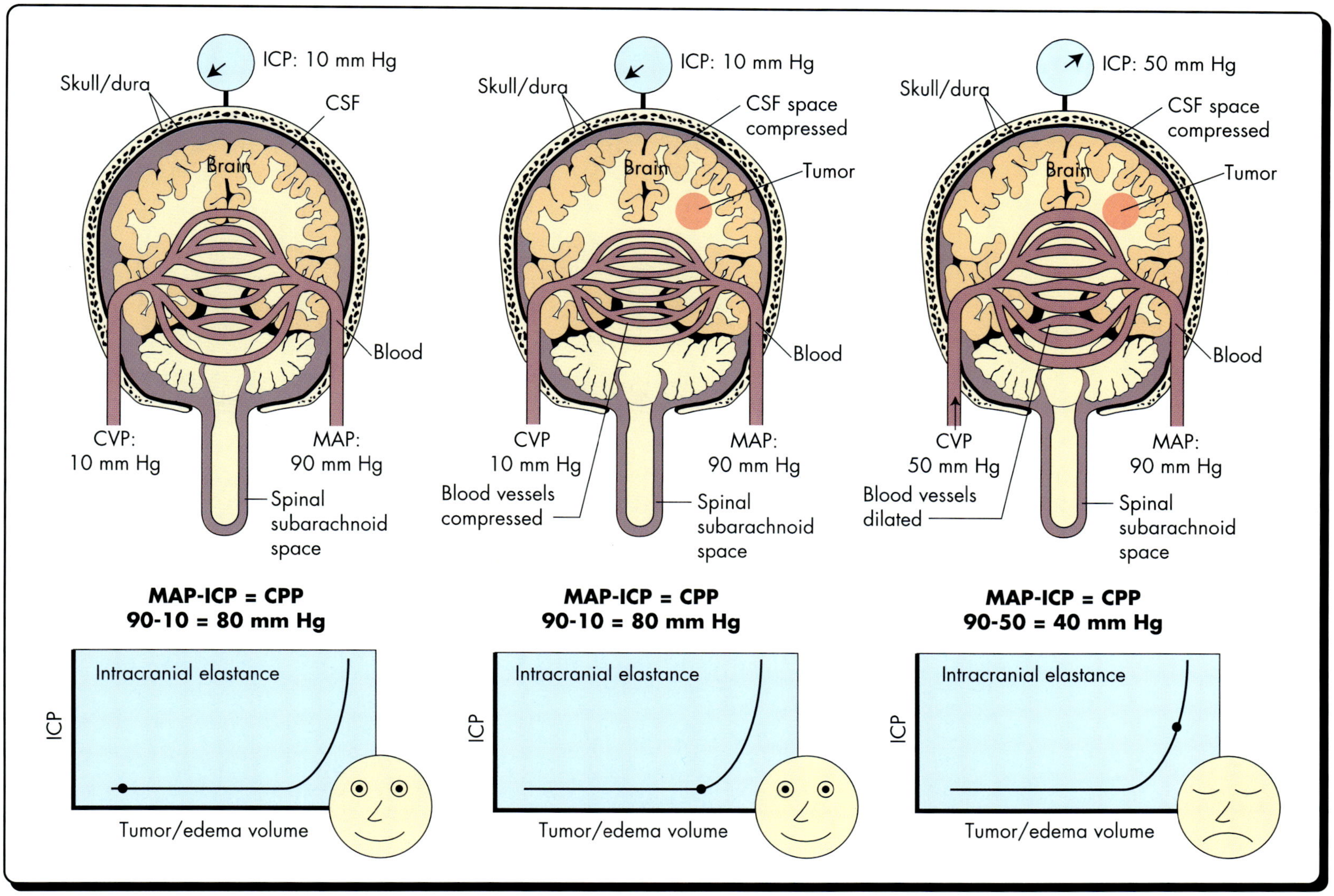

Figure 7-29. Intracranial pressure (ICP) and elevated venous pressure. The importance of maintenance of unimpeded venous drainage in controlling ICP cannot be overemphasized. In patients who have reduced intracranial compliance, increases in cerebral venous pressure may cause precipitous increases in ICP. Venous pressure may be increased by coughing, Valsalva maneuver, head down tilt, constricting ties, tubing or electrocardiogram (ECG) leads, or excessive rotation of the neck. Increased venous pressure increases venous blood volume in the skull and increases ICP. CPP—Cerebral perfusion pressure; CSF—cerebrospinal fluid; CVP—central venous pressure; MAP—mean arterial pressure.

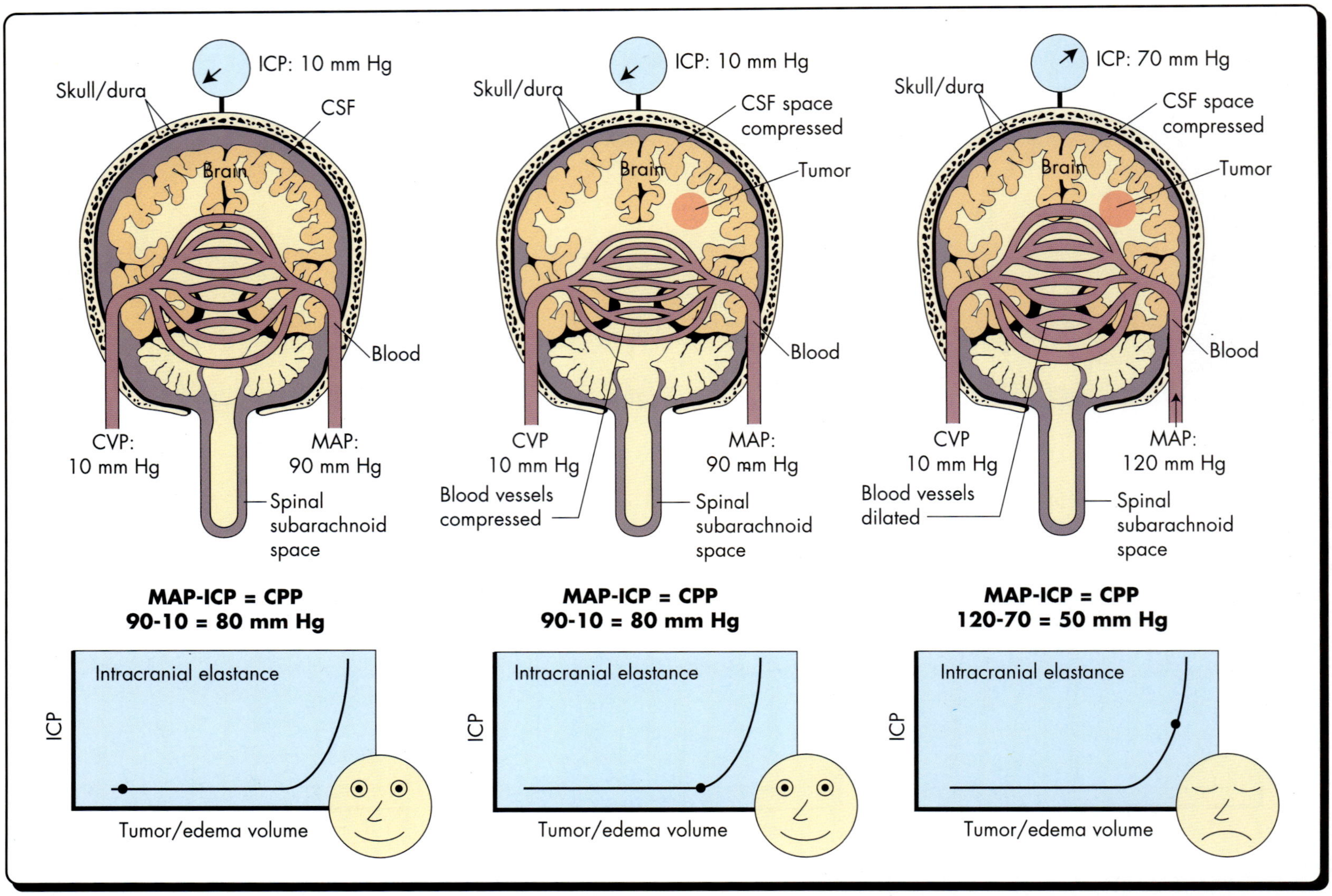

Figure 7-30. Cerebral blood flow, cerebral blood volume, autoregulation, and intracranial pressure (ICP). Most, if not all, patients presenting for neurosurgical procedures can be considered to have some defect in autoregulation. (See Fig. 7-9.) In patients with defective autoregulation and reduced intracranial compliance, increased blood pressure can lead to increased ICP. When cerebral blood vessels lack autoregulation, increased blood pressure increases blood flow and volume in these vessels. As in Figure 7-32, increased blood volume in a patient with reduced intracranial compliance results in increased ICP. CPP—cerebral perfusion pressure; CSF—cerebrospinal fluid; CVP—central venous pressure; MAP—mean arterial pressure.

EFFECTS OF ANESTHETICS

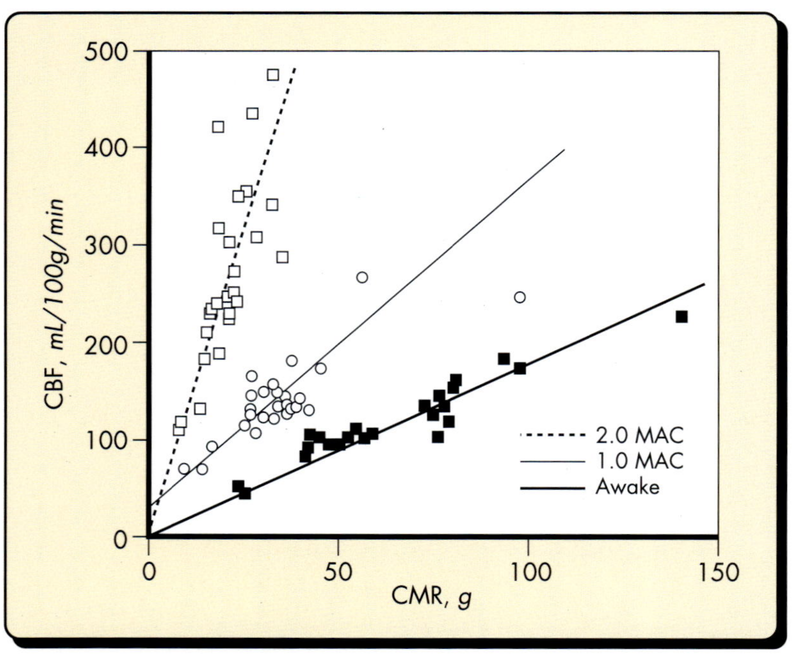

Figure 7-31. Anesthetics and flow-metabolism coupling. Anesthetic agents affect the coupled relationship between cerebral blood flow (CBF) and metabolism. In this figure, CBF (mL/100 g/min) and cerebral metabolic rate of glucose (CMRg; µmol/100 g/min) values are depicted from various regions of the brain in rats exposed to different concentrations of isoflurane. A linear relationship between flow and metabolism persists at each anesthetic concentration [60]. However, the ratio (slope) between flow and metabolism is altered in such a way that at increased concentrations of isoflurane, more flow is associated with any given CMRg value. Although it is a common miconsception that inhaled anesthetics "uncouple" CBF and metabolism, as can be seen from this figure, flow and metabolism remained coupled, although the slope of the relationship is altered. Furthermore, it can be inferred from this figure that as the concentration of isoflurane is increased, cerebral metabolism is suppressed (the curve shifts to the left on the graph). Anesthetic-induced reduction of cerebral metabolism can partially offset direct anesthetic-induced cerebral vasodilation. Thus, an anesthetic that suppresses cerebral metabolism, such as isoflurane, may produce less cerebral vasodilatation than nitrous oxide, which does not affect cerebral metabolism [61]. MAC—minimum alveolar concentration. (*Adapted from* Maekawa and coworkers [60]; with permission.)

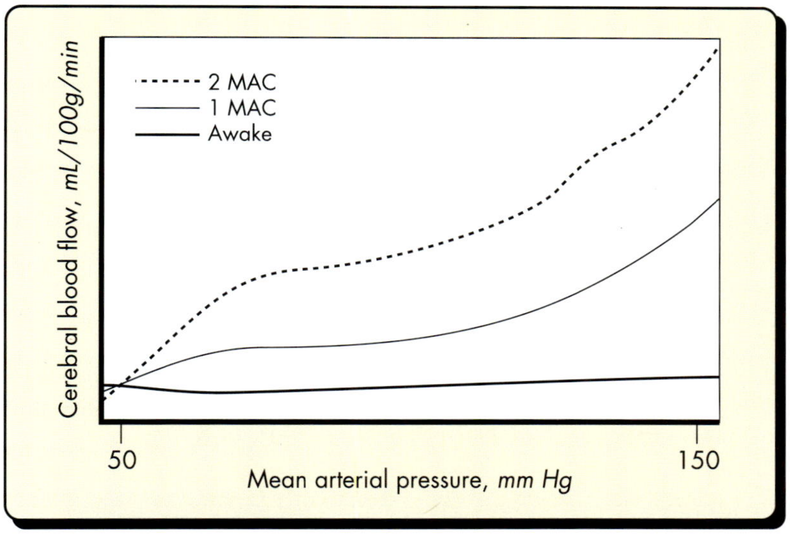

Figure 7-32. Volatile anesthetics and autoregulation. Volatile anesthetics impair autoregulation in a dose-dependent manner. Across a variety of species it has been found that little or no change occurs with inhaled anesthetic doses up to 0.5 MAC [17,62,63]. Increasing doses of inhaled anesthetic progressively render cerebral blood flow (CBF) pressure passive. In awake rats, cerebral blood flow remains relatively constant between 50 and 170 mm Hg. As the concentration of isoflurane is increased to 1 MAC and then 2 MAC, the "flat" portion of the curve is progressively eliminated and an increasingly positive slope develops. In contrast, intravenous anesthetics such as barbiturates and propofol have been shown to have little effect on autoregulation [19,64]. (*Data from* Hoffman and coworkers [63].)

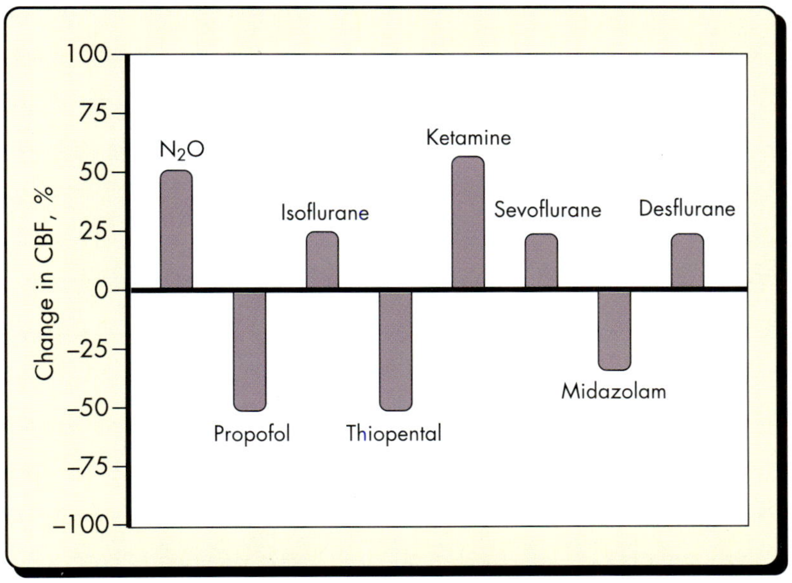

Figure 7-33. Anesthetics produce differential effects on cerebral blood flow (CBF). Volatile anesthetics increase CBF, although this effect may be attenuated by hyperventilation. A decrease in CBF typically occurs with intravenous anesthetics, although ketamine is a salient exception. For all anesthetics, the effect on CBF is dose-dependent. The net effect of the anesthetic on CBF is also a function of cerebral perfusion pressure and the integrity of autoregulation. An understanding of how anesthetics alter CBF is of importance in the care of patients with intracranial hypertension. Anesthetic agents are often selected because they are least likely to increase CBF. The applied logic is that agents that increase CBF do so by causing cerebral arterial dilation, which will then increase intracranial pressure. In most circumstances, this logic has been found to be true under experimental conditions. However, it ignores the effects of anesthetic agents on the venous circulation, which also contributes to intracranial blood volume. Further, increases in intracranial pressure caused by inhaled anesthetic agents are typically small, causing some to question whether it is always appropriate to avoid drugs that increase CBF when such agents may provide other beneficial effects [65].

REFERENCES

1. Heistad DD, Kontos HA: Cerebral Circulation. In *Handbook of Physiology*. Edited by Abboud F, Shephard J. Bethesda, MD: American Physiological Society; 1983:137–182.
2. Obrist WD, Thompson HK Jr, King CH, *et al.*: Determination of regional cerebral blood flow by inhalation of 133-xenon. *Circ Res* 1967, 20:124–135.
3. Michenfelder JD: The interdependency of cerebral functional and metabolic effects following massive doses of thiopental in the dog. *Anesthesiology* 1974, 41:231–236.
4. Finnerty FA Jr, Witkin L, Fazekas JF: Cerebral hemodynamics during cerebral ischemia induced by acute hypotension. *J Clin Invest* 1954, 33:1227–1232.
5. Powers WJ, Grubb RL Jr, Darriet D, *et al.*: Cerebral blood flow and cerebral metabolic rate of oxygen requirements for cerebral function and viability in humans. *J Cereb Blood Flow Metab* 1985, 5:600–608.
6. Grubb RL Jr, Raichle ME, Eichling JO, *et al.*: The effects of changes in $PaCO_2$ on cerebral blood volume, blood flow, and vascular mean transit time. *Stroke* 1974, 5:630–639.
7. Faraci FM, Baumbach GL, Heistad DD: Myogenic mechanisms in the cerebral circulation. *J Hypertens* 1989, 7(suppl 4):S61–S64.
8. Gross PM, Heistad DD, Strait MR, *et al.*: Cerebral vascular responses to physiological stimulation of sympathetic pathways in cats. *Circ Res* 1979, 44:288–294.
9. Harper SL: Antihypertensive drug therapy prevents cerebral microvascular abnormalities in hypertensive rats. *Circ Res* 1987, 60:229–237.
10. Strandgaard S, Olsen J, Skinhøj E, *et al.*: Autoregulation of brain circulation in severe arterial hypertension. *BMJ* 1973, 1:507–510.
11. DeWitt DS, Prough DS, Taylor CL, *et al.*: Regional cerebrovascular responses to progressive hypotension after traumatic brain injury in cats. *Am J Physiol* 1992, 263:H1276–H1284.
12. Rasmussen G, Hauerberg J, Waldemar G, *et al.*: Cerebral blood flow autoregulation in experimental subarachnoid haemorrhage in rat. *Acta Neurochir* 1992, 119:128–133.
13. Olsen TS, Larsen B, Herning M, *et al.*: Blood flow and vascular reactivity in collaterally perfused brain tissue: evidence of an ischemic penumbra in patients with acute stroke. *Stroke* 1983, 14:332–341.
14. Bedford RF, Morris L, Jane JA: Intracranial hypertension during surgery for supratentorial tumor: correlation with preoperative computed tomography scans. *Anesth Analg* 1982, 61:430–433.
15. Ekström-Jodal B, Häggendal E, Linder L-E, *et al.*: Cerebral blood flow autoregulation at high arterial pressures and different levels of carbon dioxide tension in dogs. *Eur Neurol* 1972, 6:6–10.

16. Verhaegen MJJ, Todd MM, Hindman BJ, *et al.*: Cerebral autoregulation during moderate hypothermia in rats. *Stroke* 1993, 24:407–414.
17. Miletich DJ, Ivankovich AD, Albrecht RF, *et al.*: Absence of autoregulation of cerebral blood flow during halothane and enflurane anesthesia. *Anesth Analg* 1976, 55:100–109.
18. Todd MM, Drummond JC: A comparison of the cerebrovascular and metabolic effects of halothane and isoflurane in the cat. *Anesthesiology* 1984, 60:276–282.
19. Strebel S, Lam AM, Matta B, *et al.*: Dynamic and static cerebral autoregulation during isoflurane, desflurane, and propofol anesthesia. *Anesthesiology* 1995, 83:66–76.
20. Baumbach GL, Faraci FM, Heistad DD: Effects of local reduction in pressure on endothelium-dependent responses of cerebral arterioles. *Stroke* 1994, 25:1456–1462.
21. Baumbach GL, Dobrin PB, Hart MN, *et al.*: Mechanics of cerebral arterioles in hypertensive rats. *Circ Res* 1988, 62:56–64.
22. Vorstrup S, Barry DI, Jarden JO, *et al.*: Chronic antihypertensive treatment in the rat reverses hypertension-induced changes in cerebral blood flow autoregulation. *Stroke* 1984, 15:312–318.
23. Hajdu MA, Heistad DD, Baumbach GL: Effects of antihypertensive therapy on mechanics of cerebral arterioles in rats. *Hypertension* 1991, 17:308–316.
24. Reivich M: Arterial PCO_2 and cerebral hemodynamics. *Am J Physiol* 1964, 206:25–35.
25. Kontos HA, Raper J, Patterson JL Jr: Analysis of vasoactivity of local pH, PCO_2 and bicarbonate on pial vessels. *Stroke* 1977, 8:358–360.
26. Harper AM, Glass HI: Effect of alterations in the arterial carbon dioxide tension on the blood flow through the cerebral cortex at normal and low arterial blood pressures. *J Neurol Neurosurg Psychiatry* 1965, 28:449–452.
27. Albrecht RF, Miletich DJ, Ruttle M: Cerebral effects of extended hyperventilation in unanesthetized goats. *Stroke* 1987, 18:649–655.
28. Raichle ME, Posner JB, Plum F: Cerebral blood flow during and after hyperventilation. *Arch Neurol* 1970, 23:394–403.
29. Arieff AI, Kerian A, Massry SG, *et al.*: Intracellular pH of brain: alterations in acute respiratory acidosis and alkalosis. *Am J Physiol* 1976, 230:804–812.
30. Pearce WJ: Mechanisms of hypoxic cerebral vasodilatation. *Pharmacol Ther* 1995, 65:75–91.
31. Taguchi H, Heistad DD, Kitazono T, *et al.*: ATP-sensitive K^+ channels mediate dilatation of cerebral arterioles during hypoxia. *Circ Res* 1994, 74:1005–1008.
32. Todd MM, Wu B, Makatabi M, *et al.*: Cerebral blood flow and oxygen delivery during hypoxemia and hemodilution: role of arterial oxygen content. *Am J Physiol* 1994, 267:H2025–H2031.
33. Raichle ME, Grubb RL Jr, Gado MH, *et al.*: Correlation between regional cerebral blood flow and oxidative metabolism. *Arch Neurol* 1976, 33:523–526.
34. Ingvar DH: Functional landscapes of the dominant hemisphere. *Brain Res* 1976, 107:181–197.
35. Branston NM: Neurogenic control of the cerebral circulation. *Cerebrovasc Brain Metab Rev* 1995, 7:338–349.
36. Clozel M, Watanabe H: BQ-123, a peptidic endothelin ET_A receptor antagonist, prevents the early cerebral vasospasm following subarachnoid hemorrhage after intracisternal but not intravenous injection. *Life Sci* 1993, 52:825–834.
37. Kitazono T, Heistad DD, Faraci FM: Dilatation of the basilar artery in response to selective activation of endothelin B receptors in vivo. *J Pharmacol Exp Ther* 1995, 273:1–6.
38. MacCumber MW, Ross CA, Snyder SH: Endothelin in brain: receptors, mitogenesis, and biosynthesis in glial cells. *Proc Natl Acad Sci U S A* 1990, 87:2359–2363.
39. Hong KW, Pyo KM, Lee WS, *et al.*: Pharmacological evidence that calcitonin gene-related peptide is implicated in cerebral autoregulation. *Am J Physiol* 1994, 266:H11–H16.
40. Brian JE Jr, Heistad DD, Faraci FM: Mechanisms of endotoxin-induced dilatation of cerebral arterioles. *Am J Physiol* 1995, 269:H783–H788.
41. Pfister H-W, Kümpfel T, Koedel U: Involvement of substance P in pial arteriolar vasodilatation during pneumococcal meningitis in the rat. *Neuroreport* 1995, 6:1301–1305.
42. Paulson OB, Newman EA: Does the release of potassium from astrocyte endfeet regulate cerebral blood flow? *Science* 1987, 237:896–898.
43. Brian JE Jr, Kennedy RH: Modulation of cerebral arterial tone by endothelium-derived relaxing factor. *Am J Physiol* 1993, 264:H1245–H1250.
44. Faraci FM, Breese KR: Nitric oxide mediates vasodilatation in response to activation of *N*-methyl-D-aspartate receptors in brain. *Circ Res* 1993, 72:476–480.
45. Murphy S, Simmons ML, Agullo L, *et al.*: Synthesis of nitric oxide in CNS glial cells. *Trends Neurosci* 1993, 16:323–328.
46. Nozaki K, Moskowitz MA, Maynard KI, *et al.*: Possible origins and distribution of immunoreactive nitric oxide synthase-containing nerve fibers in cerebral arteries. *J Cereb Blood Flow Metab* 1993, 13:70–79.
47. Ueno M, Lee TJ-F: Endotoxin decreases the contractile responses of the porcine basilar artery to vasoactive substances. *J Cereb Blood Flow Metab* 1993, 13:712–719.
48. Wei EP, Kontos HA: H_2O_2 and endothelium-dependent cerebral arteriolar dilation. *Hypertension* 1990, 16:162–169.
49. Kano M, Moskowitz MA, Yokota M: Parasympathetic denervation of rat pial vessels significantly increases infarction volume following middle cerebral artery occlusion. *J Cereb Blood Flow Metab* 1991, 11:628–637.
50. Mayhan WG, Faraci FM, Heistad DD: Responses of cerebral arterioles to adenosine 5prime-diphosphate, serotonin, and the thromboxane analogue U-4619 during chronic hypertension. *Hypertension* 1988, 12:556–561.
51. Murphy S, Rich G, Orgren KI, *et al.*: Astrocyte-derived lipoxygenase product evokes endothelium-dependent relaxation of the basilar artery. *J Neurosci Res* 1994, 38:314–318.
52. Hardebo JE, Arbab M, Suzuki N, *et al.*: Pathways of parasympathetic and sensory cerebrovascular nerves in monkeys. *Stroke* 1991, 22:331–342.
53. Yoshida K, Okamura T, Kimura H, *et al.*: Nitric oxide synthase-immunoreactive nerve fibers in dog cerebral and peripheral arteries. *Brain Res* 1993, 629:67–72.
54. Suzuki N, Hardebo JE, Owman C: Origins and pathways of cerebrovascular nerves storing substance P and calcitonin gene-related peptide in rat. *Neuroscience* 1989, 31:427–438.
55. Li J, Iadecola C: Nitric oxide and adenosine mediate vasodilation during functional activation in cerebellar cortex. *Neuropharmacology* 1994, 33:1453–1461.
56. Faraci FM, Brian JE Jr: Nitric oxide in the cerebral circulation. *Stroke* 1994, 25:692–703.
57. Alpers BJ, Berry RG, Paddison RM: Anatomical studies of the circle of Willis in normal brain. *Arch Neurol Psychiatry* 1959, 81:409–418.
58. Cutler RWP, Spertell RB: Cerebrospinal fluid: a selective review. *Ann Neurol* 1982, 11:1–10.
59. Artru AA: Reduction of cerebrospinal fluid pressure by hypocapnia: changes in cerebral blood volume, cerebrospinal fluid volume and brain tissue water and electrolytes. II. Effects of anesthetics. *J Cereb Blood Flow Metab* 1988, 8:750–756.
60. Maekawa T, Tommasino C, Shapiro HM, *et al.*: Local cerebral blood flow and glucose utilization during isoflurane anesthesia in the rat. *Anesthesiology* 1986, 65:144–151.
61. Hansen TD, Warner DS, Todd MM, *et al.*: Effects of nitrous oxide and volatile anaesthetics on cerebral blood flow. *Br J Anaesth* 1989, 63:290–295.
62. McPherson RW, Traystman RJ: Effects of isoflurane on cerebral autoregulation in dogs. *Anesthesiology* 1988, 68:493–499.
63. Hoffman WE, Edelman G, Kochs E, *et al.*: Cerebral autoregulation in awake versus isoflurane-anesthetized rats. *Anesth Analg* 1991, 73:753–757.
64. Donegan JH, Traystman RJ, Koehler RC, *et al.*: Cerebrovascular hypoxic and autoregulatory responses during reduced brain metabolism. *Am J Physiol* 1985, 249:H421–H429.
65. Todd MM, Warner DS, Sokroll MD, *et al.*: A prospective, comparative trial of three anesthetics for elective supratentorial craniotomy. *Anesthesiology* 1993, 78:1005–1020.

8

Neuromuscular Transmission

Stanley Feldman

Although Dale and Feldberg [1] and Dale *et al.* [2] working at University College in London in the 1930s proposed that the transmission between motor nerve and muscle involved the biotransmitter acetylcholine (ACh), it is only in the past 50 to 60 years that this hypothesis has been completely accepted. Much of the original evidence for chemically mediated transmission came from evidence that it could be blocked by curare [3], a substance known to prevent the action of ACh at nicotinic receptors [4]. It is now evident that ACh modulates and amplifies the effect of motor nerve activity turning the all-or-none response of individual muscle fibers into a modulated output capable of meeting the varied needs of muscle activity.

Motor nerve activity leads to the discharge of ACh into the synaptic junction. ACh reacts with receptors (AChRs) on the muscle (postsynaptic membrane) to produce a current that will initiate an action potential if a sufficient number of AChRs are simultaneously activated. The muscle action potential causes calcium to enter the sarcoplasmic reticulum of the muscle, triggering off a contraction. The junction between the motor nerve and the muscle is a specialized area of high metabolic activity and is vulnerable to physical and chemical events that affect neuromuscular transmission. Some of these effects may lead to neuromuscular block. In order to understand the events occurring in drug-induced neuromuscular block, it is essential to appreciate the complexities of neuromuscular conduction.

THE ANATOMY OF THE MOTOR NERVE

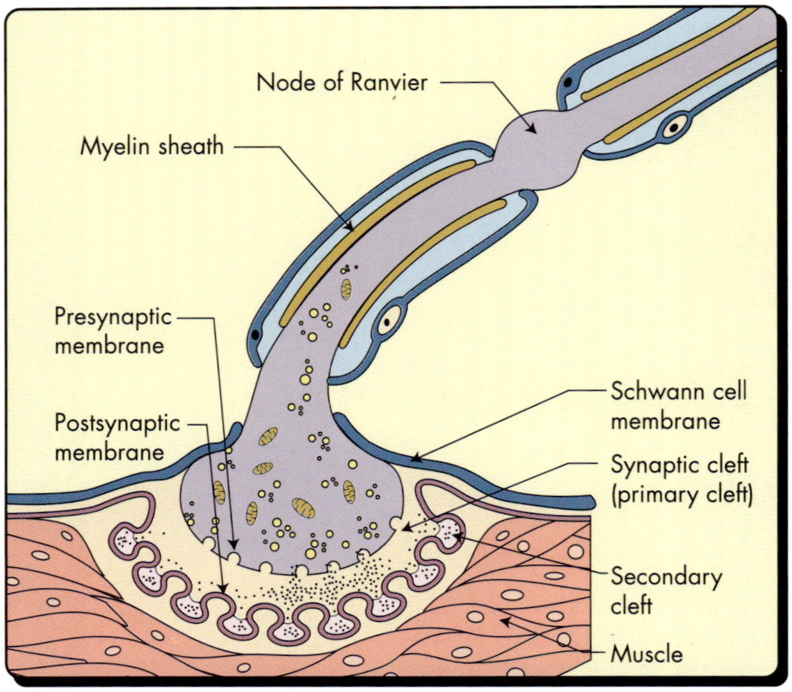

Figure 8-1. Myoneural junction. Motor nerves are the axons of ventral horn neurons in the spinal cord. They are large myelinated nerves (alpha up to 120 µm in diameter) that terminate at the myoneural junction. As the motor nerve approaches the muscle, it loses its myelin sheath and becomes enveloped in the Schwann cell membrane (contiguous with epimysium and perineural membrane).

The Schwann cells maintain the integrity of the myelin and are situated on the sheath. They secrete neurotrophic peptides and possibly ACh. The synaptic cleft between the presynaptic (motor nerve) membrane and the postsynaptic (muscle endplate) membrane contains mucopolysaccharide basement substance and long-tailed cholinesterase molecules. The myoneural junctions are situated on the surface of the muscle they innervate midway along the belly of the muscle fiber.

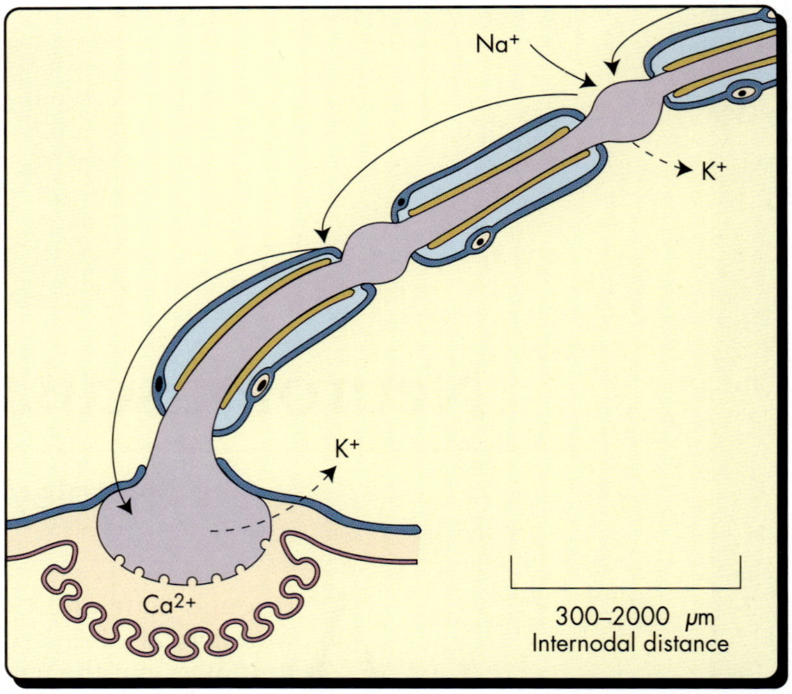

Figure 8-2. Saltatory conduction in motor nerves. The motor nerve transmits the action potential from one node of Ranvier to the next. Each node of Ranvier is free of the enveloping myelin sheath. The internodal distance varies between 300 and 2000 µm. The longer the internodal distance the faster the rate of conduction in the nerve.

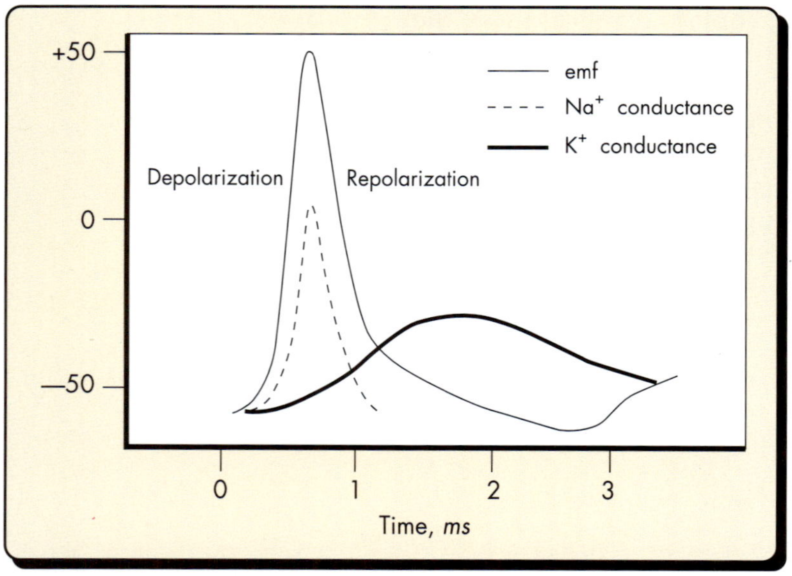

Figure 8-3. Ionic changes in motor nerve associated with an action potential. At each node of Ranvier a local current is established as a result of the rapid inflow of Na^+ followed by the outflow of K^+. The activity of the Na+ pump (blocked by tetrodotoxin) [5] and the K^+ pump (blocked by aminopyridine) [6] restores the ionic balance and produces repolarization. When the action potential reaches the nerve ending (presynaptic membrane), the outward passage of K^+ produces a slower inward movement of Ca^{2+}. Aminopyridine delays closure of the K^+ channel, which results in an increased Ca^{2+} flux into the axoplasm. emf—electromotive force, in mV.

THE MOTOR UNIT

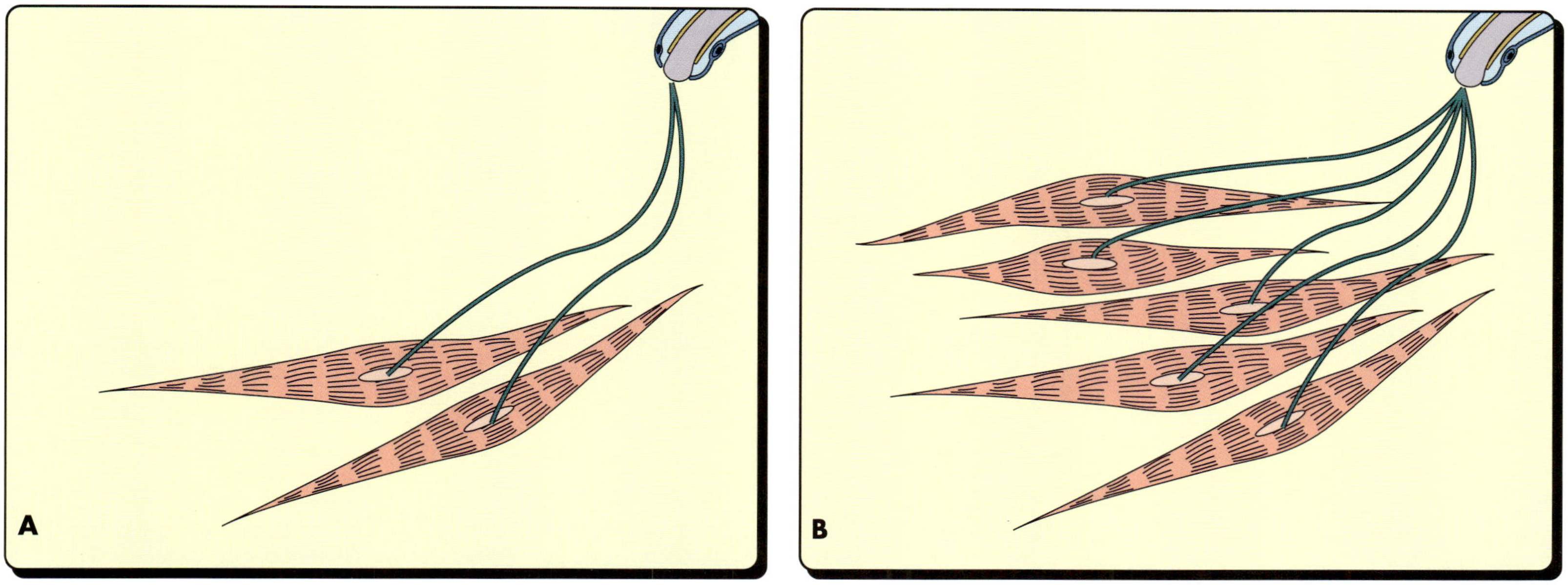

Figure 8-4. Motor units. A motor unit is made up of the motor nerve fibril and the muscle fibers it innervates. The number of muscle fibers in one motor unit determines the sensitivity of its response. The nerve fibril may innervate from two or three (**A**) to many hundreds (**B**) of muscle fibers. As all muscle fibers in one motor unit usually either contract or do not in response to a nerve action potential, it follows that only those motor units with few muscle fibers (*panel A*) are capable of the gradation of muscle response required for fine motor activity (*eg*, sewing, writing). Conversely, the motor response necessary in the postural muscles is best served by large motor units (*panel B*).

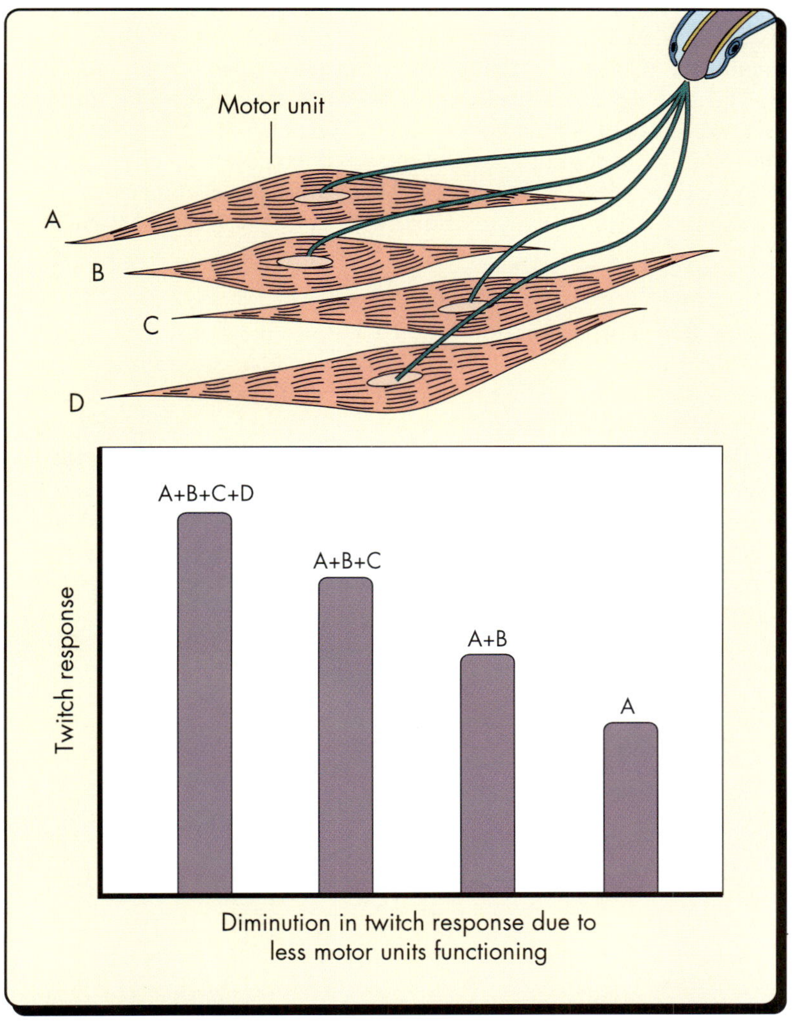

Figure 8-5. Refinement of motor activity. As each muscle fiber in a motor unit (**top**) either responds to motor nerve stimulation or fails to do so (all-or-none response)—and in health all the fibers in one motor unit usually respond together—it follows that when a diminishing muscle twitch is measured in response to motor nerve stimulation (indirect stimulation), this diminution (**bottom**) is due to fewer and fewer units responding and not to a reduction in the force of contraction of any individual fiber.

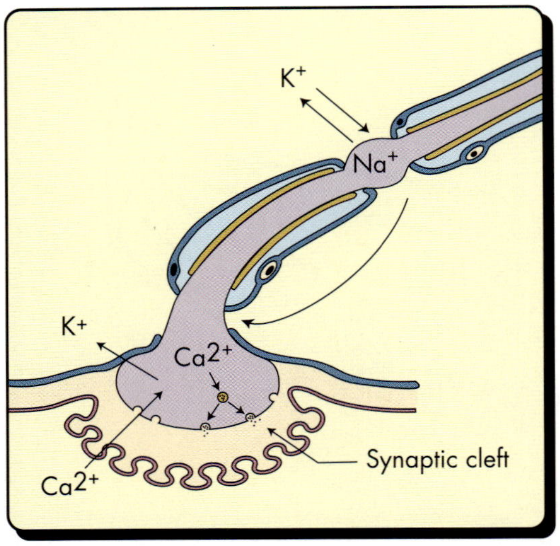

Figure 8-6. Events leading to acetylcholine release. Depolarization of the terminal nerve ending, the presynaptic membrane, causes Ca^{2+} to enter the axoplasm as K^+ leaves [7]. The Ca^{2+} triggers the release of ACh into the synaptic cleft, initiating the events leading to contraction of the muscle.

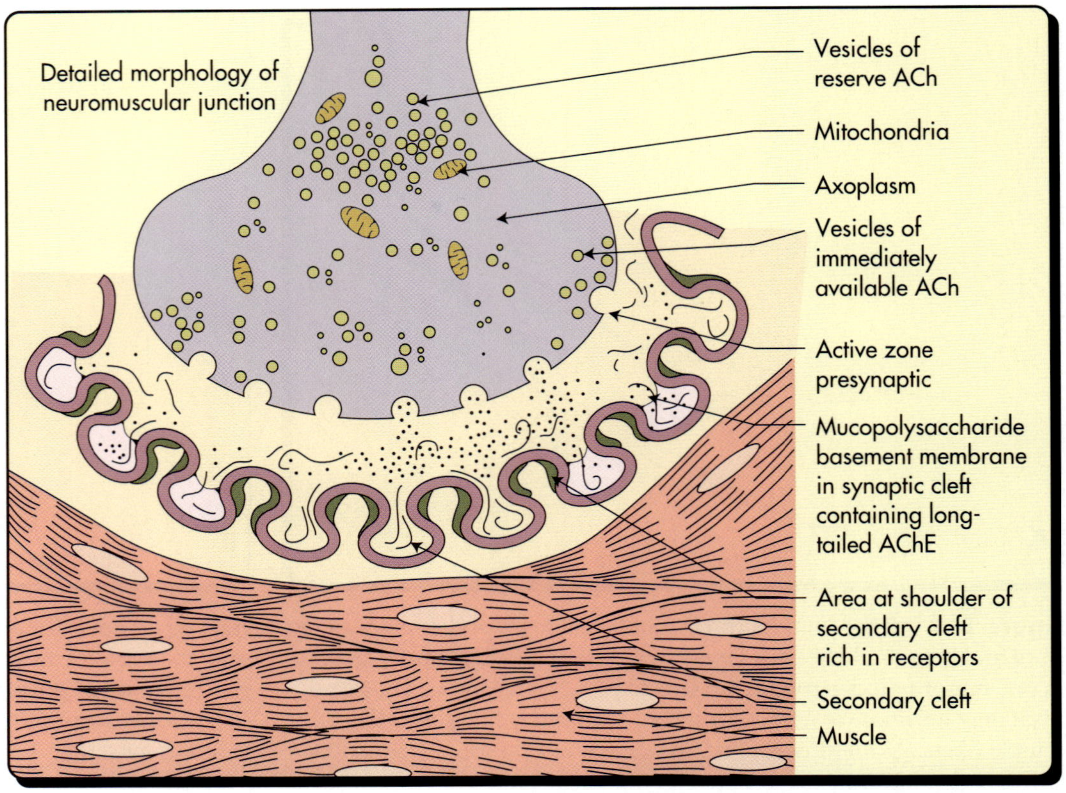

Figure 8-7. Detailed morphology of neuromuscular junction. Ach exists in the axoplasm in three forms: free molecules of ACh, ACh in vesicles of the reserve store (90% of all the ACh), or as immediately available ACh vesicles that are constantly recycled when there is minimal nerve activity [8]. The ACh vesicles release their content at the active zones on the presynaptic membrane. The molecules of ACh traverse the synaptic cleft to react with the ACh recognition sites on the AChRs on the shoulders of the secondary clefts. The cleft is filled with chains of mucopolysaccharide in which long-tailed cholinesterase molecules (AChE) are found. ACh leaving the AChR is hydrolyzed in < 1 ms by the AChE, producing choline and acetic acid.

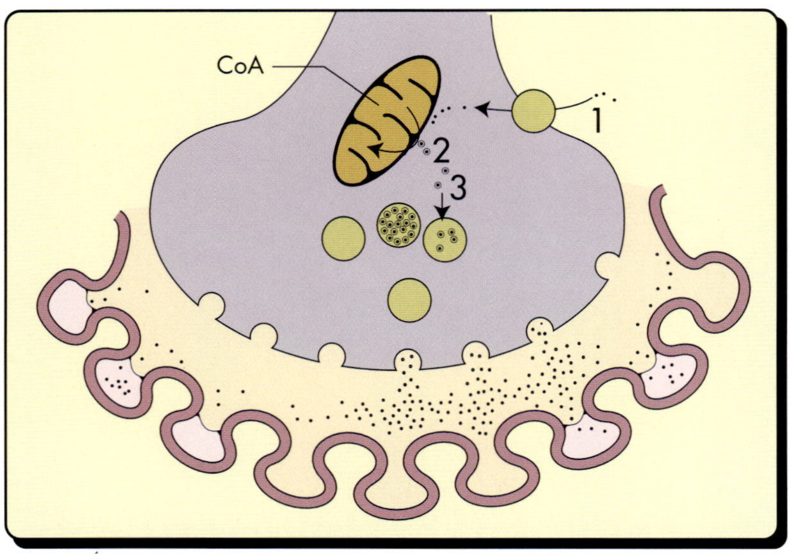

Figure 8-8. Formation of ACh. (*1*)Choline enters the cytoplasm of the motor nerve terminal. This requires an active carrier mechanism (inhibited by hemicholinium). About 50% of the choline is recycled from hydrolyzed ACh. (*2*) Choline is acetylated by acetylcoenzyme A (choline-O-acetyltransferase) at the mitochondria. (*3*) The molecules of ACh are concentrated in empty vesicles against a concentration gradient. This loading process requires an ATPase-dependent proton pump, which is depressed by vesamicol and tetraphenylboron. These drugs cause a slow rundown of transmitter release and neuromuscular block (9,10).

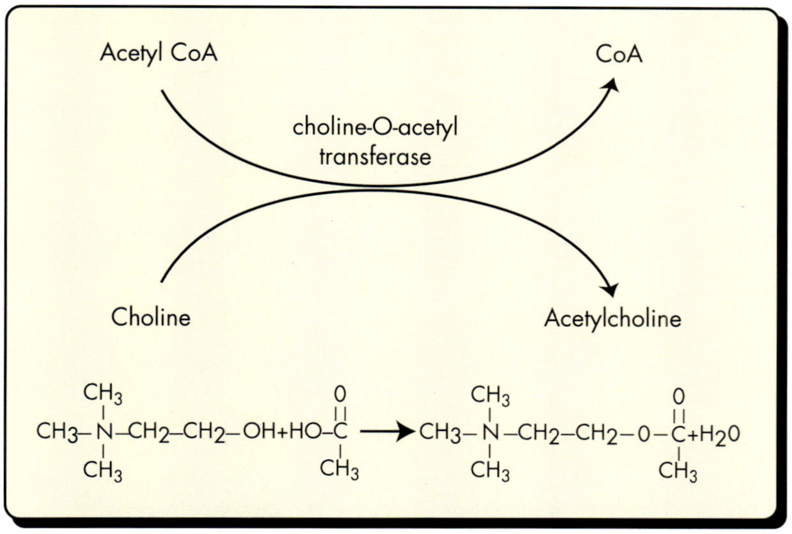

Figure 8-9. Formation of ACh. The formation of ACh requires a source of choline and the presence of choline-O-acetyltransferase (CoA).

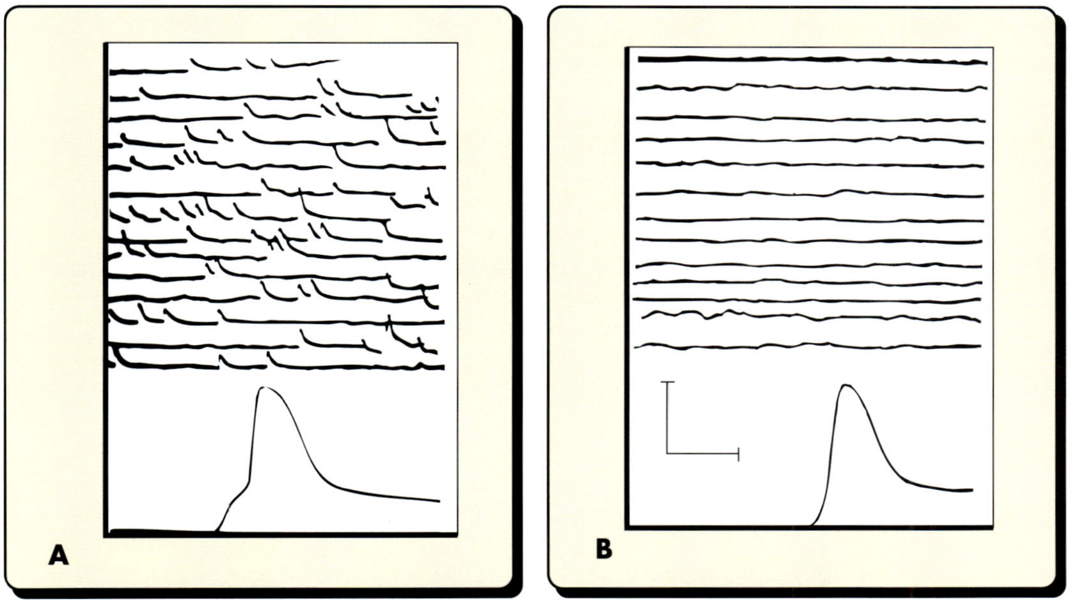

Figure 8-10. Endplate potentials. ACh is constantly "leaking" from the vesicles of the readily available pool in the nerve terminal in the absence of neural activity. This produces miniature endplate potentials on the postsynaptic membrane [11] (*upper traces* in **A**). Each miniature end plate potential is caused by the ACh content of one or two vesicles. If sufficient ACh releases to stimulate a critical number of ACh R, then it will trigger off an action potential (*lower trace* in *panel A*). Miniature end plate potentials are suppressed by curare (**B**).

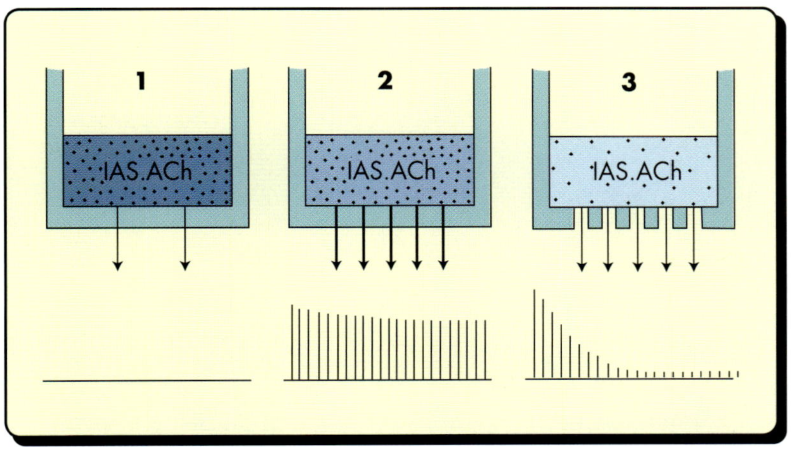

Figure 8-11. ACh "leak." At rest, the leak of ACh into the synaptic cleft is too small to produce a muscle response (*1*). During physiologic activity the motor nerves stimulate the muscle at tetanic rates of stimulation (> 10 Hz). The most sensitive motor units respond at lower rates of stimulation than the larger resistant units. At tetanic rates of stimulation it is necessary to mobilize the reserve stores of vesicular ACh if the output is to keep pace with the increased demands. The amount of ACh discharged into the synaptic cleft during each motor nerve depolarization depends on the presynaptic loading with immediately available ACh (IAS ACh) vesicles. The greater the concentration of immediately available ACh at the motor nerve ending, the greater the discharge into the synaptic cleft during depolarization (*2*). Failure of ACh mobilization to keep up with the loss of ACh causes a failure of transmission at the more resistant neuromuscular junctions and a decrease in the indirectly elicited twitch (*3*) (train-of-four fade) and tetanic fade. The normal small leak at ACh does not trigger off an action potential or muscle contraction (*1, lower trace*). Provided the immediately available store of ACh is maintained, tetanic stimulation will not produce fade (*2, lower trace*). Failure to mobilize reserve ACh causes tetanic fade (*3, lower trace*).

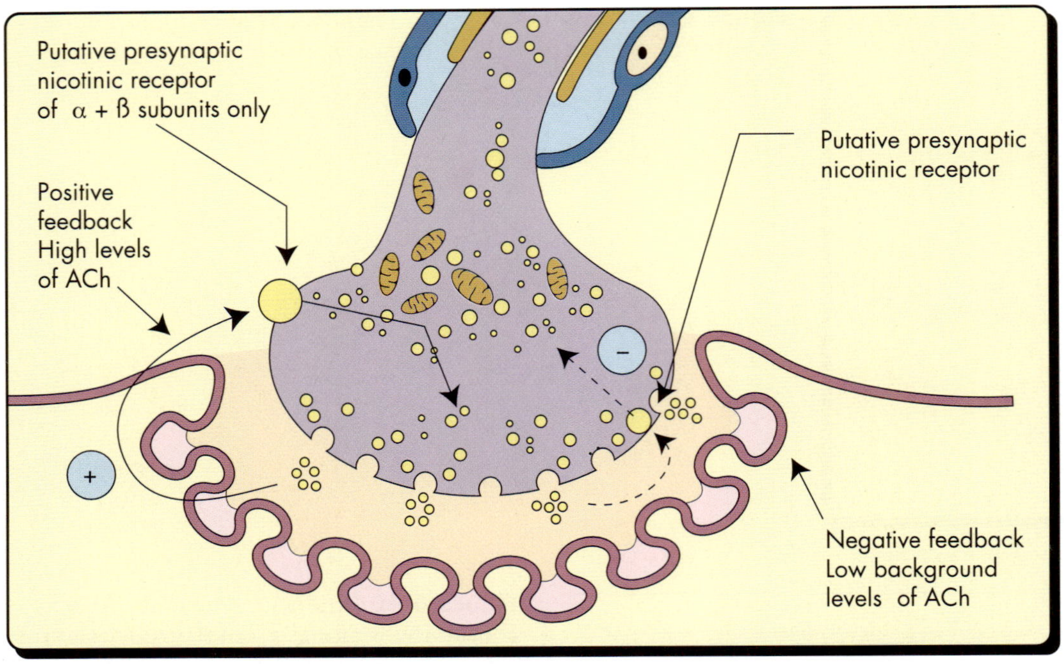

Figure 8-12. Positive and negative feedback at the presynaptic nicotinic receptors. To meet the increased demand for ACh during motor nerve activity, the reserve vesicular store of ACh must be mobilized. Calcium ions play an important role in this process [12,13]. An increase in Ca^{2+} in the axoplasm causes an enhanced rate of mobilization and release of vesicular ACh. It is believed that this is modulated by presynaptic nicotinic receptors, which can be blocked to a varying extent by most nondepolarizing neuromuscular blocking drugs. Activation of these receptors by ACh produces calcium influx and a positive feedback of ACh mobilization and release [13]. There is evidence that there is also a less important negative feedback mediated by low concentrations of ACh, such as that resulting from the constant leak of ACh in the absence of neural activity. This negative feedback is blocked by low concentrations of D-tubocurare [14]. The putative presynaptic nicotinic AChR are presumed to be composed of alpha and beta subunit pentamers only, as the genes for expression of gamma, delta, or epsilon subunits are not found in neural tissue.

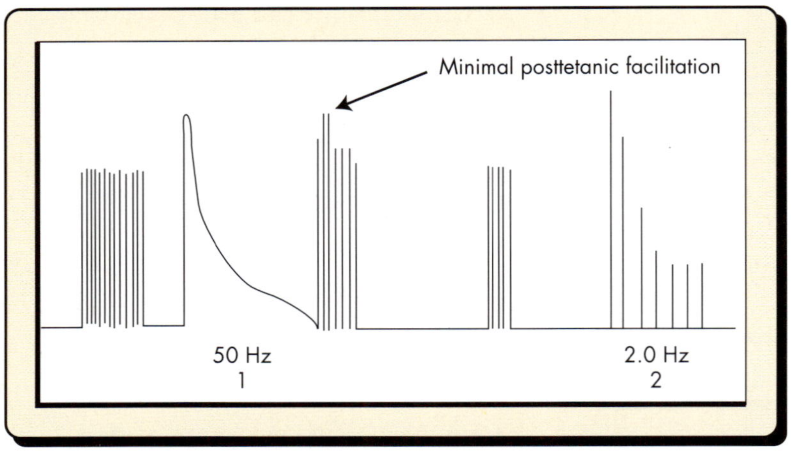

Figure 8-13. Features of block of presynaptic nicotinic receptors. If the presynaptic nicotinic receptors are blocked (by most nondepolarizing muscular blocking drugs, especially rocuronium) [15], then depression of the positive feed back mechanism occurs. This produces tetanic fade (50 Hz) (*1*) and train-of-four fade (2 Hz) (*2*) due to an inadequate rate of mobilization of reserve ACh to meet the increased demand.

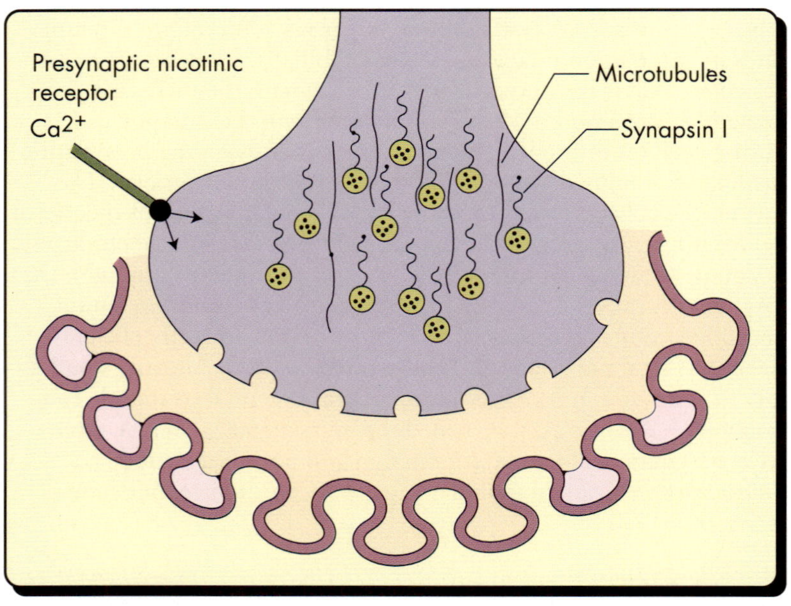

Figure 8-14. Mobilization of reserve vesicular ACh. Reserve ACh vesicles are tethered by a vesicular surface protein, synapsin 1, to formed microtubular elements in the axon. Calcium mobilizes the reserve vesicular ACh by stimulating a calmodulin-activated protein kinase. This induces a rupture of the terminal serine molecular bond, freeing the vesicle from the microtubule [16].

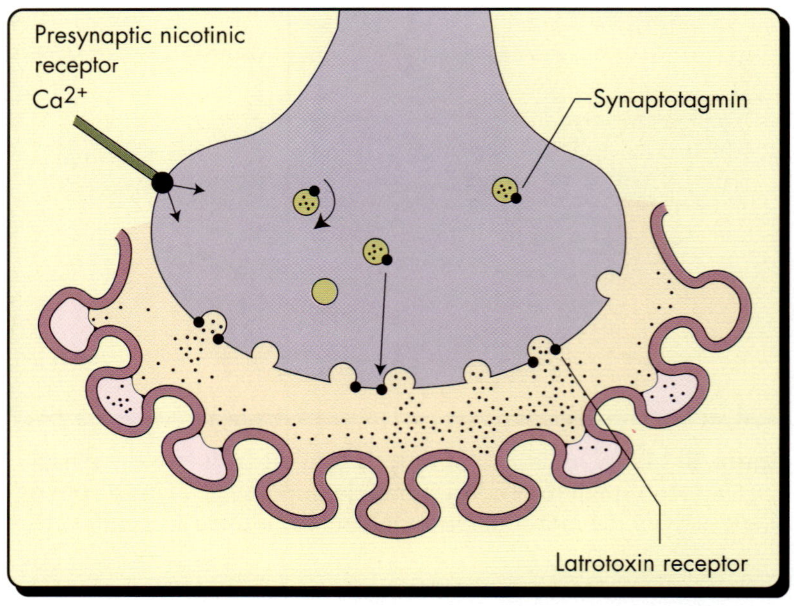

Figure 8-15. Activation of synaptotagmin-latrotoxin receptor by calcium. Calcium also speeds up the reaction of synaptotagmin on the vesicle surface with the latrotoxin receptor at the active zone of the presynaptic membrane, thus increasing the rate of release of ACh [17]. This process is blocked by botulinus toxin, which stabilizes the vesicle membrane by acting on a separate vesicular receptor [13].

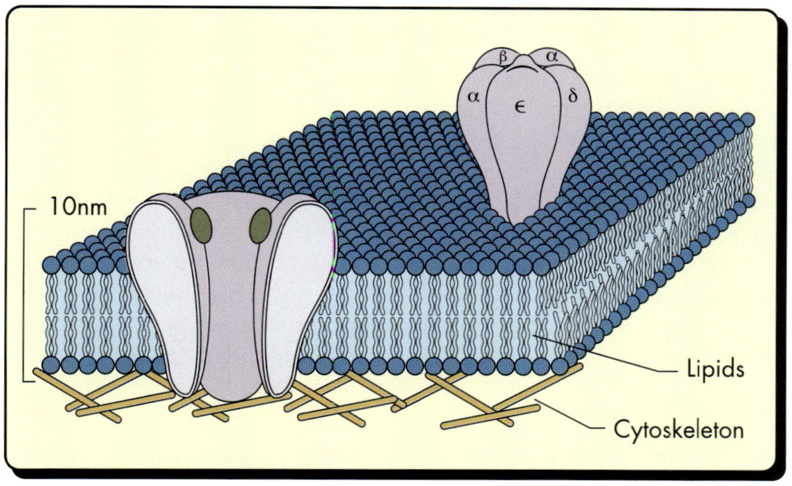

Figure 8-16. The postsynaptic ACh receptor (AChR). This receptor is a large structure about 10 nm long and 8.5 nm in diameter traversing the postsynaptic membrane. It protrudes from the surface of the postsynaptic membrane into the synaptic cleft. There is also a smaller intracellular projection. It is surrounded by an area of membrane rich in cholesterol and other steroids. (It has been suggested that volatile anesthetics alter the reactivity of this fatty pool.) The receptor is an asymmetric structure composed of five subunits (two alpha and one each of beta, delta and epsilon). In the newborn, and after denervation, the epsilon is represented by a gamma subunit. Each alpha unit has a beta subunit on one or the other of its sides and a delta or an epsilon on the other side.

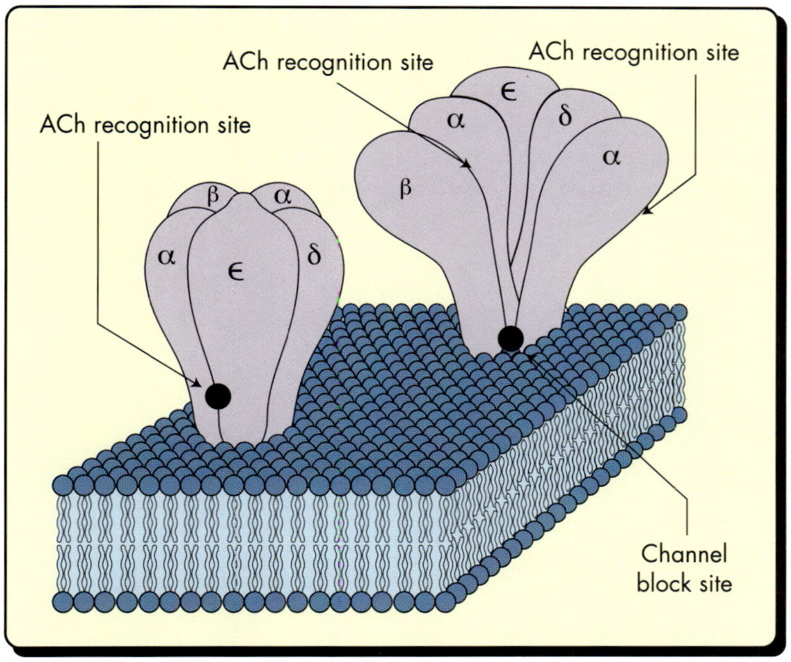

Figure 8-17. ACh recognition site. This small area (*left side of figure*) is situated on the alpha subunit at the junction with its intermembranous domain. Its characteristics are influenced by the chimera from the neighboring delta or epsilon subunit. Oocyte-expressed pentamers lacking delta and epsilon subunits do not respond to ACh although ganglionic nicotinic receptors composed of alpha and beta subunits do respond to ACh. Activation of both alpha subunits' receptor sites simultaneously causes an opening of the isthmus of the central ion channel of the pentamer (*right side of figure*). The isthmus lies beyond the extracellular vestibule, within the membranous part of the receptor. Drugs (local anesthetics, tricyclic antidepressants) may block this passage at the intracellular side of the vestibule producing channel block [18,19].

The opening of the ion channel is produced by the simultaneous activation of the ACh recognition sites on the two alpha subunits. Opening is believed to occur due to a twisting motion (likened to a Chinese puzzle in which shortening of the length increases the diameter of the structure) or to resemble the opening of petals in a bloom formation.

The ACh recognition site lies between 178 and 201 on the alpha helix and includes the important "sulfhydryl loop" between the cysteine molecules at 128 and 142. A sulfhydryl loop exists in all the subunits but it is only in the alpha receptors that it is capable of initiating the opening of the ion channel. Cysteine molecules at 192 and 193 and the tryptophan molecule at 187 appear to play an important part in binding antagonist drugs such as alpha bungarotoxin (these molecules are absent in some snakes and the mongoose, which are not poisoned by alpha bungarotoxin) [20,21]. The presence of the sulfhydryl loop is essential for ACh reactivity but because only the sites on the alpha subunits respond, a contribution from neighboring chimeras must be necessary. This must be at a site other than the 187 to 193 domain that binds alpha bungarotoxin, because the neuromuscular junction of the mongoose, in which different amino acids exist in these situations, readily reacts with ACh.

DEPOLARIZATION OF THE POSTSYNAPTIC MEMBRANE

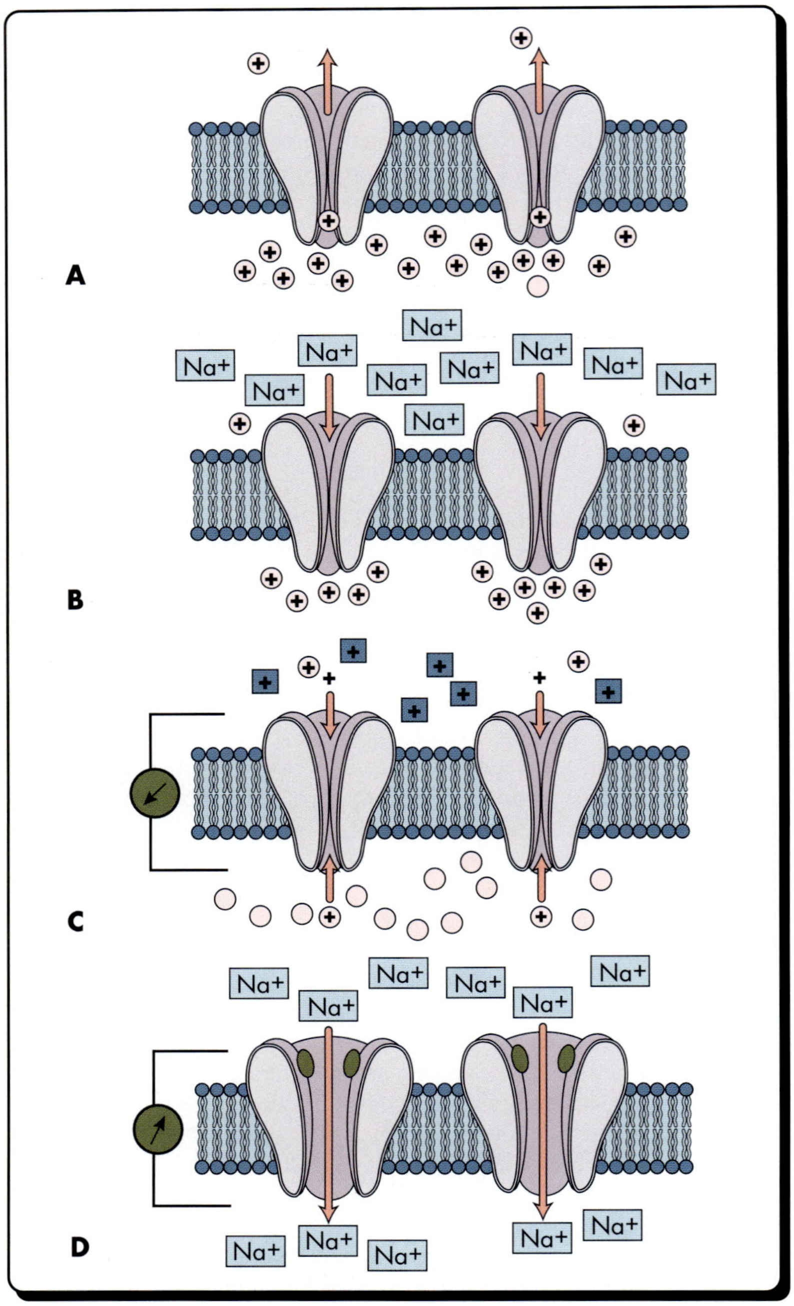

Figure 8-18. Ion movements associated with depolarization. The postsynaptic membrane has a resting potential of -90 mv. This results from the ion channel in the receptor allowing the free passage of the smaller hydrated K^+ ion but not the larger Na^+ in the closed state. Potassium ions are therefore free to pass along their concentration gradient from the intercellular fluid (ICF) (approximately 150 mmol/L) (**A**). In so doing, they increase the positive charge on the outside of the membrane, which is largely the result of the excess Na^+ ions in the extracellular fluid (ECF) (**B**). When the force of the increased positive charge outside the membrane is equal and opposite to the force produced by the concentration gradient for K^+, equilibrium will exist (**C**). At this point the resting membrane potential will be -90 mv. Once the ion channel dilates and allows Na^+ to pass into the cell, along its concentration gradient, the transmembrane potential falls toward zero (**D**).

The resting transmembrane potential is therefore the result of the unequal distribution of ions across a semipermeable membrane and can be described by the Nearest equation: (emf/F = RT/F x log e $[K_0]/[K_i]$), where R = universal gas constant, T = absolute temperature, F = Faraday constant, K_0 = concentration of K^+ in ECF, and Ki = concentration of K^+ in ICF.

(This ignores the small contribution of protein and other ions.) It follows that any disturbance of the ratio K_0/K_1 will alter the transmembrane potential. emf—electromotive force, in mV.

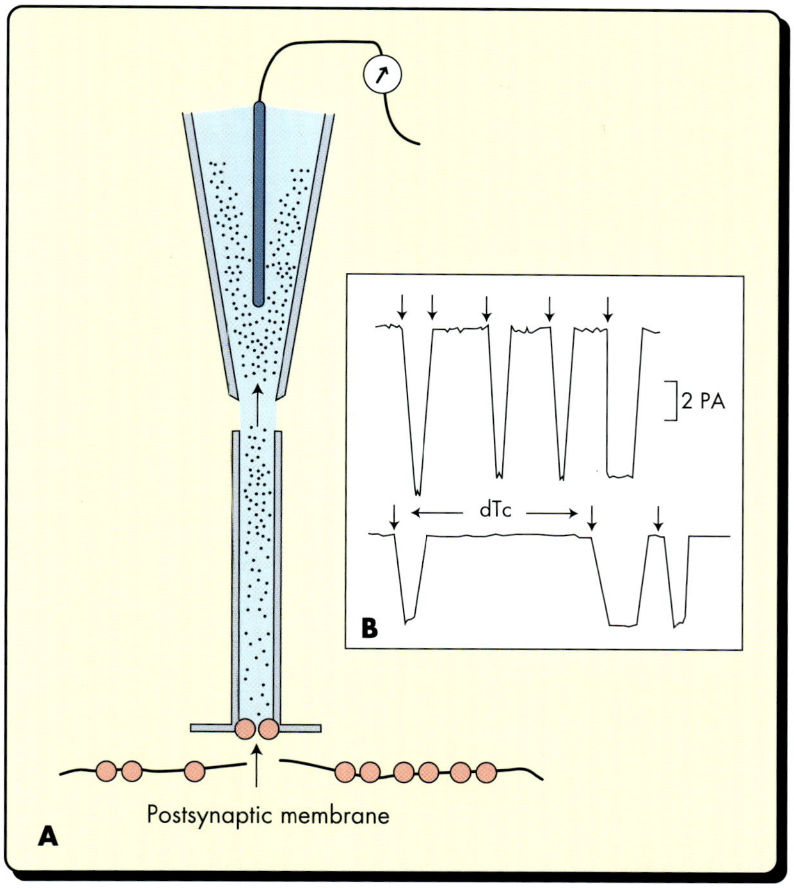

Figure 8-19. Studies of AChR response. The opening of one ion channel and the subsequent transient reversal of the membrane potential produces a picoamp (PA) current. This can be detected in patch clamp experiments. In these experiments a minute area of the postsynaptic membrane containing a single AChR is sucked onto the end of a micropipette [22] (**A**). ACh applied through the pipette produces a millisecond opening of the channel and a brief current flow [23]. If the channel opens repetitively, the channel open time is increased (**B**, *upper trace*). This effect is blocked by the application of D-tubocurare (dTc) through the pipette (*lower trace* in *panel B*) [24].

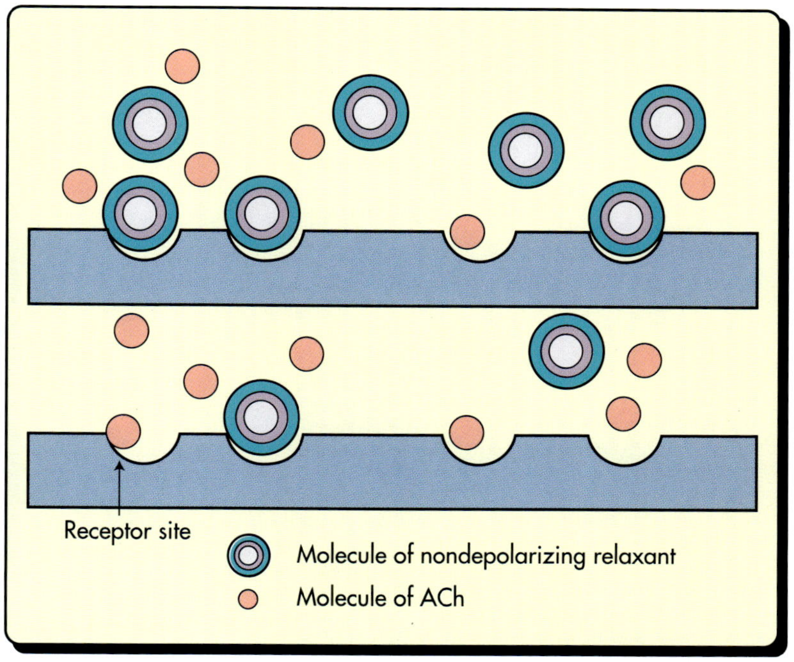

Figure 8-20. Recovery of action potential during washout of tubocurare. It requires many ion channels to open at the same time for the sum of the picoamp currents produced at each site to produce sufficient depolarization of the postsynaptic membrane to reach a threshold level and trigger off a propagated action potential.. It is envisaged that molecules of antagonist drugs (*eg*, D-tubocurare) produce their effect by competing with ACh for occupancy of the ACh recognition sites on the alpha subunits. If either ACh recognition site is occupied by an antagonist molecule, the receptor will not respond to ACh. The competition is not equal, however; antagonist drugs have a longer occupancy of the ACh recognition site than ACh itself, and this is reflected in their higher affinity (K_d). In the presence of a high ratio or concentration of drug molecules relative to ACh, most ACh recognition sites will be occupied and block will ensue (*top*). As the ratio is reduced, ACh molecules can react with the receptor, reversing the block (*bottom*). This effect is governed by the Law of Mass Action and depends upon the log of the relative concentrations of molecules.

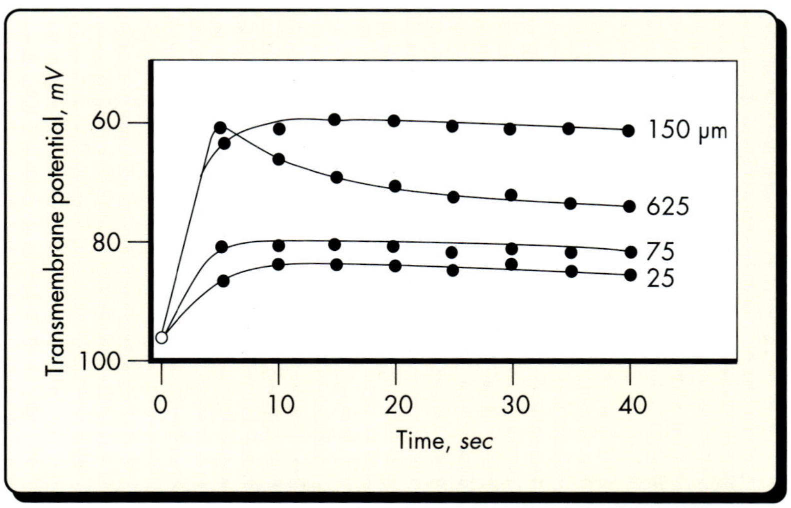

Figure 8-21. Action of agonist drugs. ACh transmission can also be blocked by reducing the transmembrane potential to a level at which further channel opening produces insufficient current to trigger off an action potential. This is analogous to cathodal block in a motor nerve produced by the prolonged application of a depolarizing current. A similar state at the postsynaptic membrane may be caused by the prolonged action of agonist drugs such as decamethonium or succinylcholine. The transmembrane potential falls as the concentration of the drug is increased up to a maximum, when repolarization starts to take place [25]. However, the fall in transmembrane potential that is recorded is seldom sufficiently great to produce a truly refractory membrane [26].

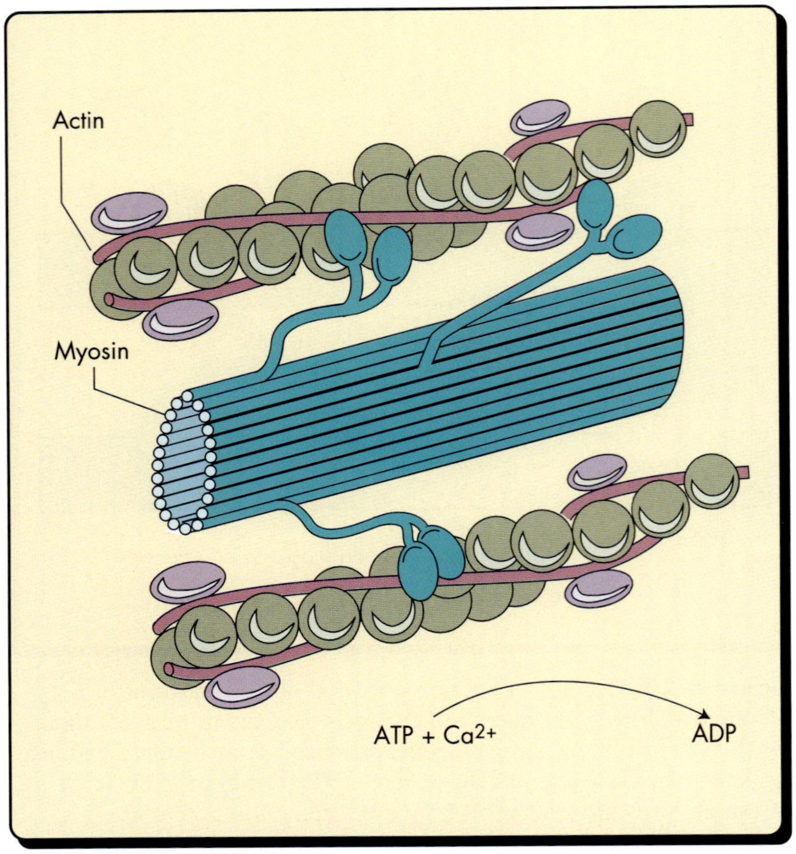

Figure 8-22. Muscle contraction. The propagated action potential necessary to cause depolarization of the postsynaptic endplate produces an influx of Ca^{2+} into sarcoplasmic reticulum of the adjoining muscle. This reacts with calmodulin-ATPase to produce the shortening of the cross-bridges between actin and myosin elements of striated muscle and hence leads to muscle contraction.

REFERENCES

1. Dale HH, Feldberg W: Chemical transmission at motor nerve endings in voluntary muscle. *J Physiol (Lond)* 1934, 81:39–42.
2. Dale HH, Feldberg W, Vogt M: Release of acetylcholine at voluntary nerve endings. *J Physiol (Lond)* 1936, 86:353–380.
3. Bacq AZ, Brown GL: Pharmacological experiments on mammalian voluntary muscle in relation to the theory of chemical transmission. *J Physiol (Lond)* 1937, 89:45–46.
4. Katz B, Miledi R: A re-examination of curare action at the motor endplate. *Proc R Soc Lond B Biol Sci* 1978, 203:119–133.
5. Narahashi T: Chemicals as tools in the study of excitable membranes. *Physiol Rev* 1974, 54:813–899.
6. Kirsch G, Narahashi T: 3-4 diaminopyridine: A potent potassium channel blocker. *Biophys J* 1978, 22:507–512.
7. Barrett JN, Makleby KL, Pallota BS: Properties of single calcium activated potassium channels in cultured muscle. *J Physiol* 1982, 332:211–230.
8. Birks RI, MacIntosh FC: Acetylcholine metabolism of a sympathetic ganglion. *Can J Biochem Physiol* 1961, 39:787–827.
9. Marshall IG, Prior C: Update on neuromuscular transmission. *Ballieres Clin Anaesthesiol* 1994, 294–315.
10. Parsons SM, Prior C, Marshall IG: Acetylcholine transport, storage and release. *Int Rev Neurobiol* 1993, 35:279–390.
11. Fatt P, Katz B: Spontaneous subthreshold activity at motor nerve endings. *J Physiol (Lond)* 1952, 117:109–128.
12. Bowman WC: Prejunctional and postjunctional cholinoceptors at the neuromuscular junction. *Anesth Analg* 1980, 59:935–943.
13. Glavinovic MI: Presynaptic action of curare. *J Physiol* 1979, 290:499–506.
14. Vizi ES, Somogyi GT, Nagashima H, *et al.*: D-tubocurarine and pancuronium inhibit the evoked release of acetylcholine from mouse hemidiaphragm preparations. *Br J Anaesth* 1987, 59:226–231.
15. Feldman SA, Khaw K: The effect of dose and rate of stimulation on the action of rocuronium. *Eur J Anaesthesiol* 1995, 12(suppl):15–19.
16. Bowman WC, Webb SN: Tetanic fade during partial transmission failure produced by non-depolarizing neuromuscular blocking drugs in the cat. *Clin Exp Pharmacol Physiol* 1976, 3:545–555.
17. Petrenko AG, Fried VA, Migoery GA, *et al.*: Phospholipid 19 binding by a synaptic vesicle protein homologous to the regulatory region of protein kinase C. *Nature* 1990, 345:260–263.
18. Forman SA, Miller KW: Molecular sites of anaesthetic action in postsynaptic nicotinic membranes. *Trends Pharmacol Sci* 1989, 10:447–452.
19. Dreyer F: Acetylcholine receptor. *Br J Anaesth* 1982, 54:115–130.
20. Barchan D, Kachalsky S, Neumann D, *et al.*: How the mongoose can fight the snake: the binding site of the mongoose acetylcholine receptor. *Proc Nat Acad Sci U S A* 1992, 89:7717–7721.
21. Fuchs S, Barchan D, Kachalsky S, *et al.*: Molecular evolution of the binding site of the acetylcholine receptor. *Ann NY Acad Sci* 1993, 681:126–139.
22. Neher E, Sackmann B: Single channel currents recorded from membrane of denervated frog muscle fibers. *Nature* 1976, 260:779–802.
23. Colquhoun D, Sackmann B: Fluctuations in the microsecond range of the current through single acetylcholine receptor channels. *Nature* 1981, 294:464–466.
24. Colquhoun D, Sheridan RE: The effects of tubocurarine competition on kinetics of agonist action on the nicotinic receptor. *Br J Pharmacol* 1982, 75:77–86.
25. Gissen AJ, Nastuk WL: Succinylcholine and decamethonium comparison of depolarization and desensitization. *Anesthesiology* 1970, 33:611–616.
26. Jenerick HP, Gerrard RW: Membrane potential and threshold of single muscle fiber. *J Cell Comp Physiol* 1953, 42:79–85.

9

Hemostasis and Thrombosis

Thomas F. Slaughter

In 1964, Macfarlane [1] and Davie and Ratnoff [2] independently proposed that a "cascade" or "waterfall" interaction between plasma coagulation proteins accounts for the explosive generation of clot occurring in response to a vascular injury. Over the intervening decades this scheme has remained the foundation for our understanding of the biochemical reactions associated with hemostasis. Plasma coagulation is characterized by an amplifying cascade of reactions during which inactive precursor molecules are proteolytically cleaved to generate hemostatically active enzymes. Rather than representing a series of independent pathways, as originally envisioned, recent insights gained from clinical and laboratory-based experiments clearly demonstrate the seamless integration of the intrinsic and extrinsic pathways, platelets, and vascular endothelium required to maintain normal hemostasis.

Although the plasma cascade is most often the focus in discussions of coagulation, the platelet plays an integral role in these reactions by providing a template on which plasma coagulation may occur [3]. Activation of the platelet results in structural and biochemical changes that allow the binding of coagulation factors into localized activation complexes. Only recently has the importance of these activation complexes to the propagation of plasma coagulation been recognized. Equally important are the roles of the platelet in providing structural stability and the delivery of hemostatically active proteins to the forming clot.

Many of the recent advances in our understanding of hemostasis and thrombosis have focused on interactions between the vascular endothelium and the cellular and plasma components of coagulation [4]. Although the contribution of the vascular endothelium to fibrinolytic degradation of the clot has long been recognized, only recently have additional mechanisms for the vascular endothelial–mediated regulation of hemostasis and thrombosis become apparent. Further investigations into the regulatory interactions among the vascular endothelium, plasma coagulation, and platelets will provide the foundation for new approaches to the management of bleeding and thrombosis in the surgical patient.

PLASMA COAGULATION

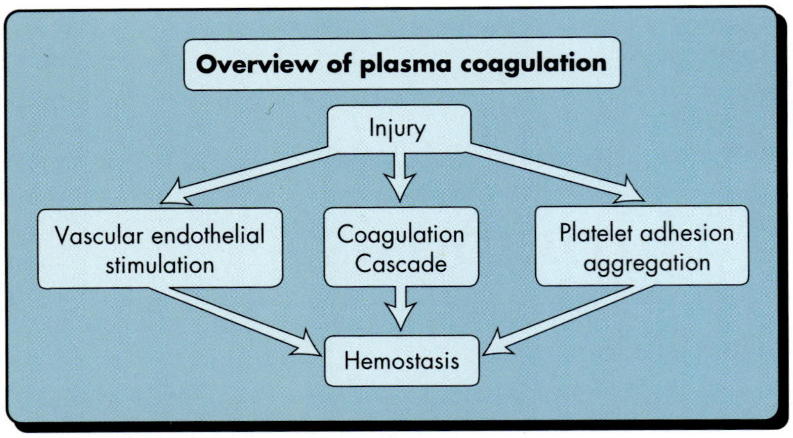

Figure 9-1. Overview of plasma coagulation. The normal hemostatic response to a vascular injury involves an integrated response among plasma coagulation proteins, platelets, and the vascular endothelium culminating in the formation of a stable hemostatic plug.

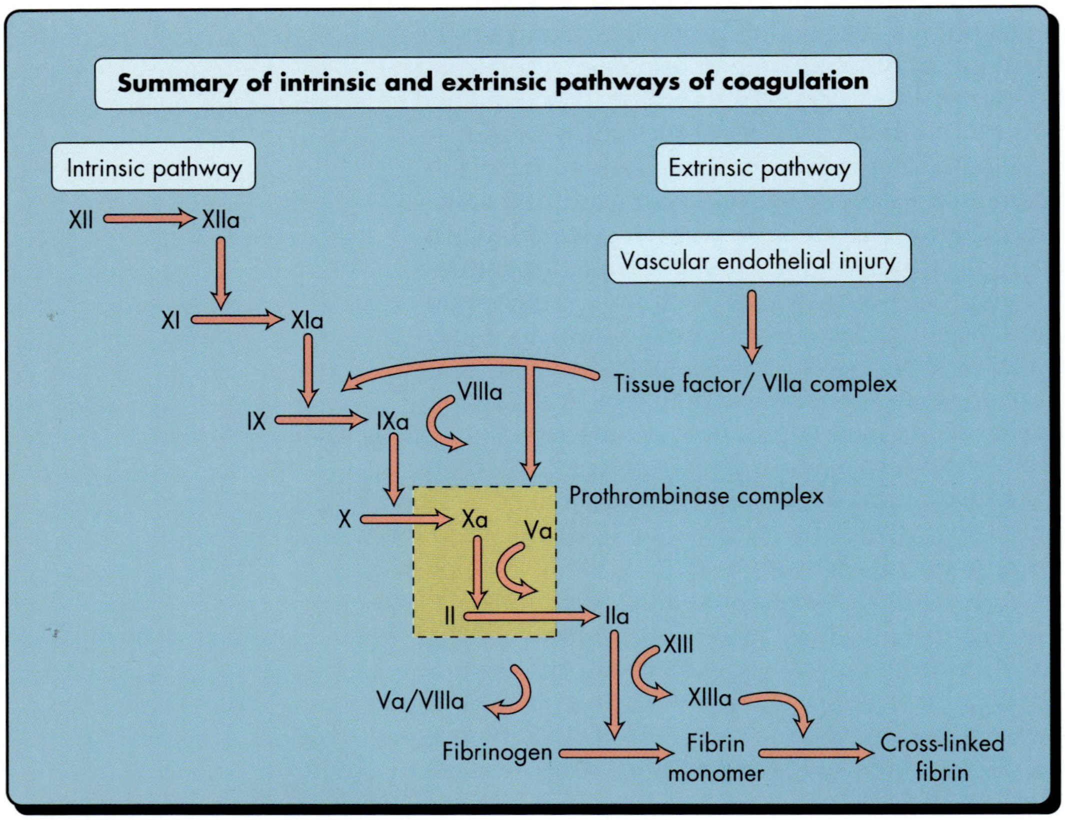

Figure 9-2. Summary of intrinsic and extrinsic pathways of coagulation. The coagulation pathway consists of intrinsic and extrinsic components, each of which is capable of activating the common pathway to generate fibrin clot [5]. Intrinsic and extrinsic pathways converge to activate factor X, thereby initiating the common pathway. Factor Xa converts prothrombin (factor II) to thrombin, and thrombin converts fibrinogen to fibrin clot. The cofactors Va and VIIIa are essential to formation of coagulation factor activation complexes that accelerate clot formation. The importance of these cofactors is, perhaps, best evidenced by an example of nature: deficiency of factor VIII results in the bleeding disorder hemophilia A. (*From* Slaughter [6]; with permission.)

CONCENTRATIONS OF COAGULATION PROTEINS IN PLASMA				
Protein	**Molecular Weight**	**μg/mL**	**Molarity**	**Relative Concentration/1000 Molecules of Fibrinogen**
Albumin	70,000	40,000	6×10^{-4}	60,000
α_1-Antitrypsin	54,000	2900	5×10^{-5}	5000
Fibrinogen	340,000	3500	1×10^{-5}	1000
Antithrombin III	65,000	250	4×10^{-6}	400
α_2-Macroglobulin	730,000	2600	4×10^{-6}	350
Plasminogen	90,000	150	1.7×10^{-6}	170
Prothrombin	72,000	100	1.4×10^{-6}	140
α_2-Antiplasmin	70,000	70	1×10^{-6}	100
Fibronectin	440,000	350	8×10^{-7}	80
Factor X	56,000	10	2×10^{-7}	20
Factor XIII	320,000	30	1×10^{-7}	10
Factor IX	56,000	5	9×10^{-8}	10
Factor V	330,000	10	3×10^{-8}	3
Thrombospondin	450,000	8	2×10^{-8}	2
Factor VII	50,000	0.5	1×10^{-8}	1
Factor VIII	330,000	0.1	3×10^{-10}	(0.03)

Figure 9-3. Plasma concentrations of coagulation proteins. (*Adapted from* Doolittle [7].)

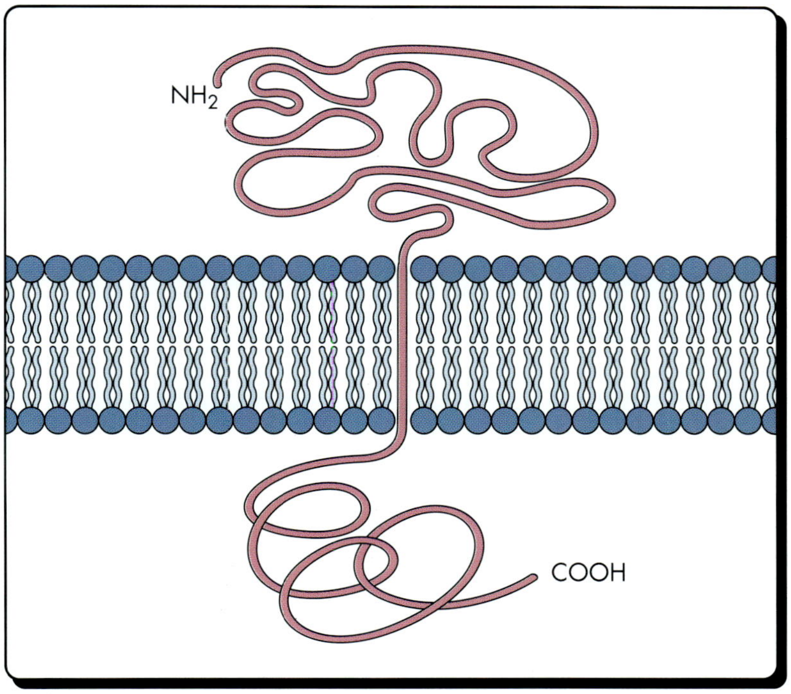

Figure 9-4. Structure of tissue factor. Tissue factor is an integral membrane lipoprotein with intracellular, transmembrane, and extracellular domains [10]. Under normal conditions, tissue factor is not expressed by tissues in contact with the plasma. However, vascular endothelial cells [11] and monocytes [12] may be induced to express tissue factor by inflammatory mediators such as thrombin and endotoxin. (*Adapted from* Nemerson [13].)

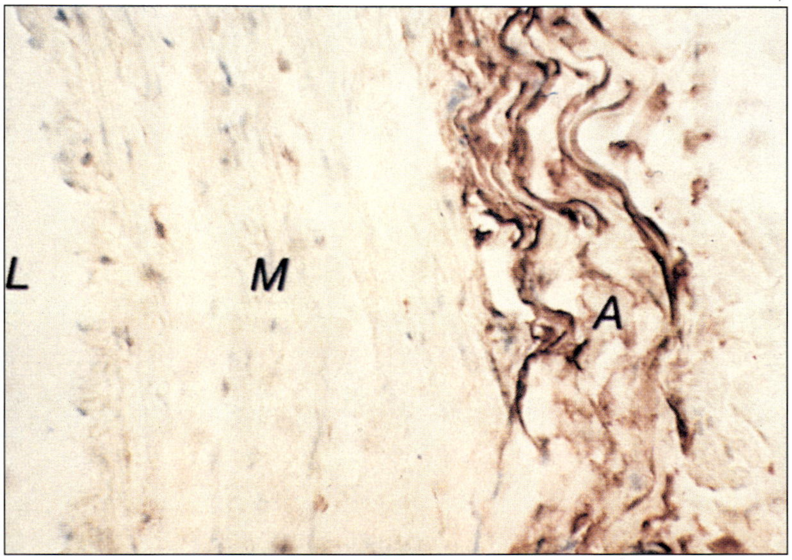

Figure 9-5. Localization of tissue factor within the vasculature. This photograph displays a cross section of the vessel wall consisting of the intima, media, and adventitia. The vessel lumen (L) is displayed at the left of the figure. The tissue has been incubated with an antibody-to-tissue factor and subseqently stained for identification. High concentrations of tissue factor are apparent within the adventitia. Injury to the vessel wall provides a mechanism for the interaction of plasma factor VIIa and tissue factor present in the adventitia, thereby initiating the extrinsic pathway of coagulation. (*Adapted from* Wilcox and coworkers [14].)

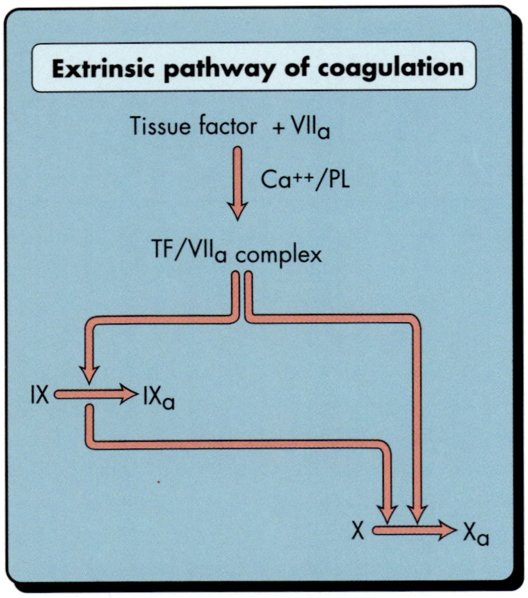

Figure 9-6. The extrinsic pathway of coagulation. On exposure to plasma, tissue factor (*TF*) binds calcium and factor VIIa to form an activation complex for factor X. The tissue factor–VIIa complex also activates factor IX, demonstrating one of the many interactions between the intrinsic and extrinsic pathways. Recent evidence suggests that the extrinsic pathway provides the primary mechanism for initiating the hemostatic response *in vivo* [9]. It would appear that the intrinsic pathway acts primarily as an amplification system to further propagate clot formation following activation of the extrinsic pathway. (*From* Schmaier [8]; with permission.)

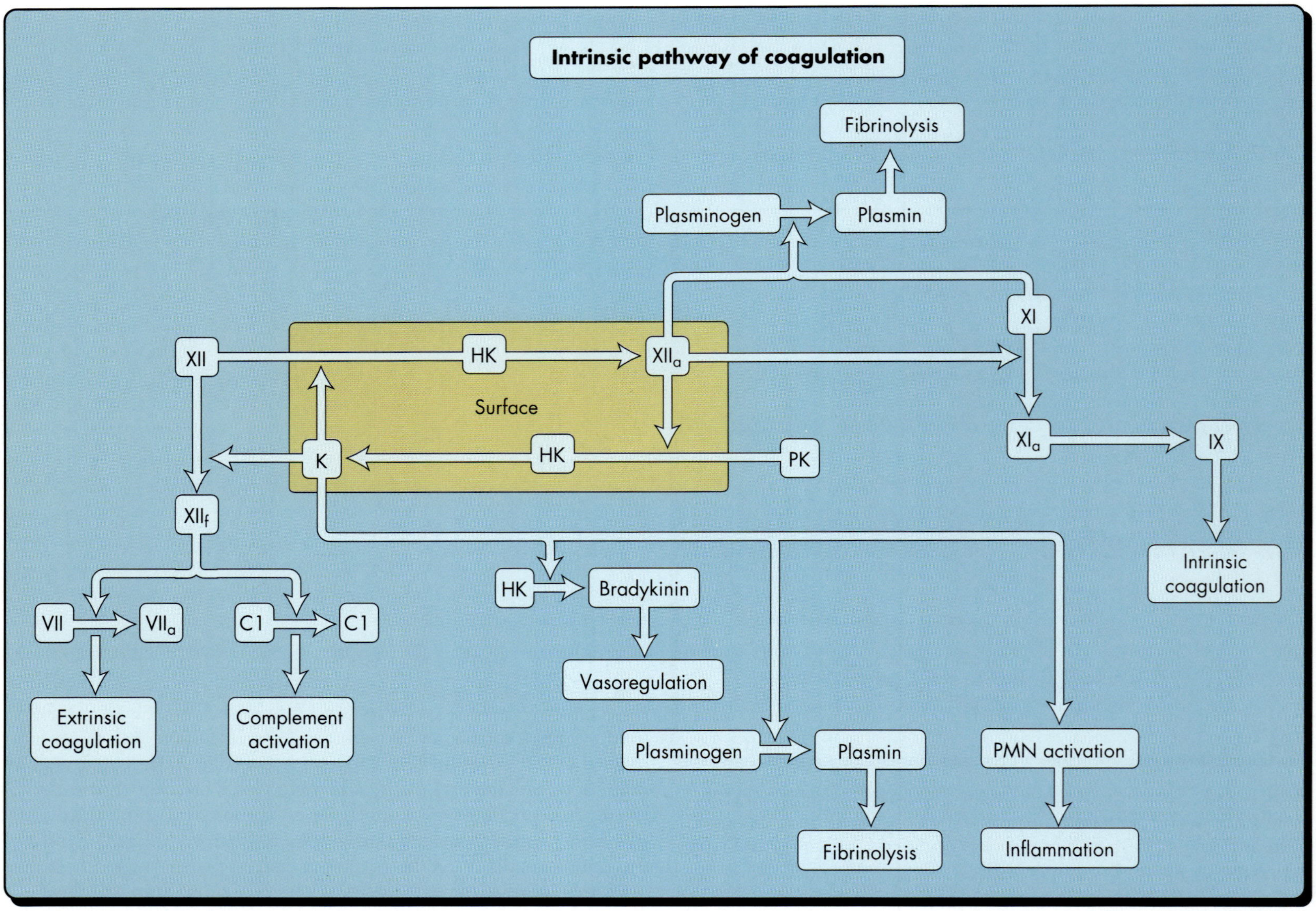

Figure 9-7. The intrinsic pathway of coagulation. The intrinsic pathway of coagulation provides an alternative mechanism to tissue factor for the activation of factor X. This pathway is typically initiated by the autoactivation of factor XII on a negatively charged surface. Factor XIIa subsequently catalyzes the formation of kallikrein (*K*) from prekallikrein (*PK*). High molecular weight kininogen (*HK*) acts as a cofactor in these surface-bound reactions and subsequently in the activation of factor XI. By-products generated from the intrinsic pathway affect a number of physiologic systems. For example, proteolytic cleavage of factor XII in plasma generates a Hageman factor fragment (XIIf) that activates both factor VII of the extrinsic pathway and the C1 component of the complement pathway. Proteolytic cleavage of high molecular weight kininogen by factor XIIa generates bradykinin, a vasoregulatory peptide. Furthermore, plasma kallikrein activates granulocytes and, with factors XIIa and XIa, contributes to fibrinolysis by the formation of plasmin. PMN—polymorphonuclear leukocyte. (*Adapted from* Schmaier [8]; with permission.)

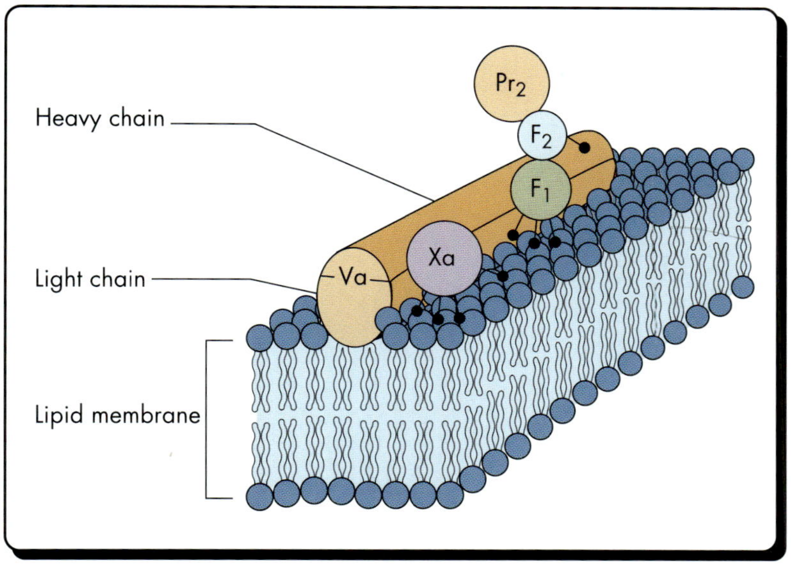

Figure 9-8. The role of activation complexes in coagulation. Contrary to popular belief, the propagation of coagulation does not occur in free plasma. Conversion of inactive coagulation precursors (zymogens) to active enzymes occurs at physiologically relevant rates only on phospholipid membrane surfaces [15]. Under most circumstances the platelet serves this role; however, activated monocytes and endothelial cells may also provide a suitable surface. Not only does the activation complex greatly amplify formation of the new enzyme product, but it also protects the components of the activation complex from inactivation by circulating protease inhibitors. This figure displays the prothrombinase activation complex consisting of the inactive zymogen prothrombin (F_1, F_2, Pr_2), the cofactor Va, and the active precursor enzyme factor Xa assembled on a phospholipid surface. Current models propose that propagation of the coagulation cascade occurs as the newly activated serine proteases are shuttled between adjacent activation complexes on the phospholipid surface. (*From* Rosenberg and Bauer [16]; with permission.)

EFFECT OF ACTIVATION COMPLEX ON RATE OF FORMATION OF BOVINE FACTOR Xa

Reaction Components	Relative Catalytic Efficiency
IXa	1
IXa, Ca^{2+}	8
IXa, Ca^{2+}, PL	58,000
IXa, Ca^{2+}, PL, VIIIa	1×10^9

Figure 9-9. The effect of the activation complex on rate of formation of bovine factor Xa. Note the increased catalytic efficiency afforded by the addition of phospholipid and the cofactor VIIIa to the reaction. PL—phospholipid. (*Adapted from* Bartha and coworkers [17].)

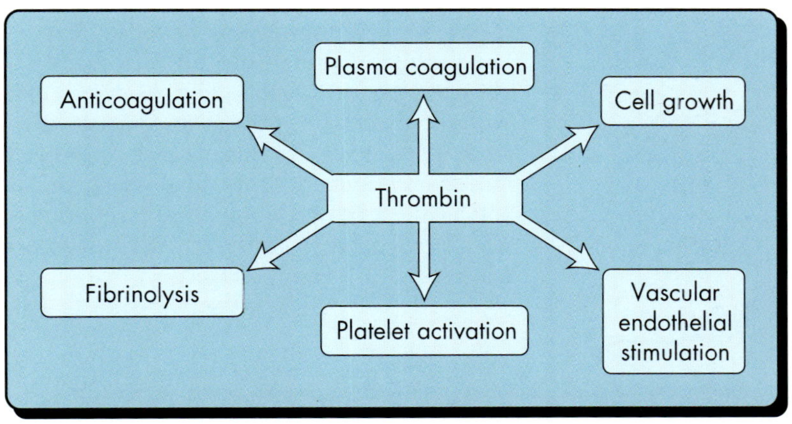

Figure 9-10. Physiologic roles of thrombin. Thrombin generation represents the key regulatory step in the hemostatic process. In addition to the recognized role of generating fibrin clot from fibrinogen, thrombin also activates platelets and provides a positive feedback mechanism to activate factor XI, factor XIII, and the cofactors V and VIII. Furthermore, thrombin interacts with vascular endothelial cells to express tissue factor [17] and to release von Willebrand factor and plasminogen activator inhibitor 1 (PAI-1). In addition to these procoagulant functions, thrombin simultaneously downregulates clot formation by inducing the release of tissue plasminogen activator (t-PA) [18], prostacyclin (PGI-2), and nitric oxide from vascular endothelial cells. Also, thrombin binds to thrombomodulin on the vascular endothelium, leading to activation of the anticoagulant protein C. Finally, thrombin is a potent mitogen, resulting in the migration and growth of vascular smooth muscle cells. These characteristics contribute not only to wound healing and tissue remodeling but also to the pathologic process of atherosclerosis.

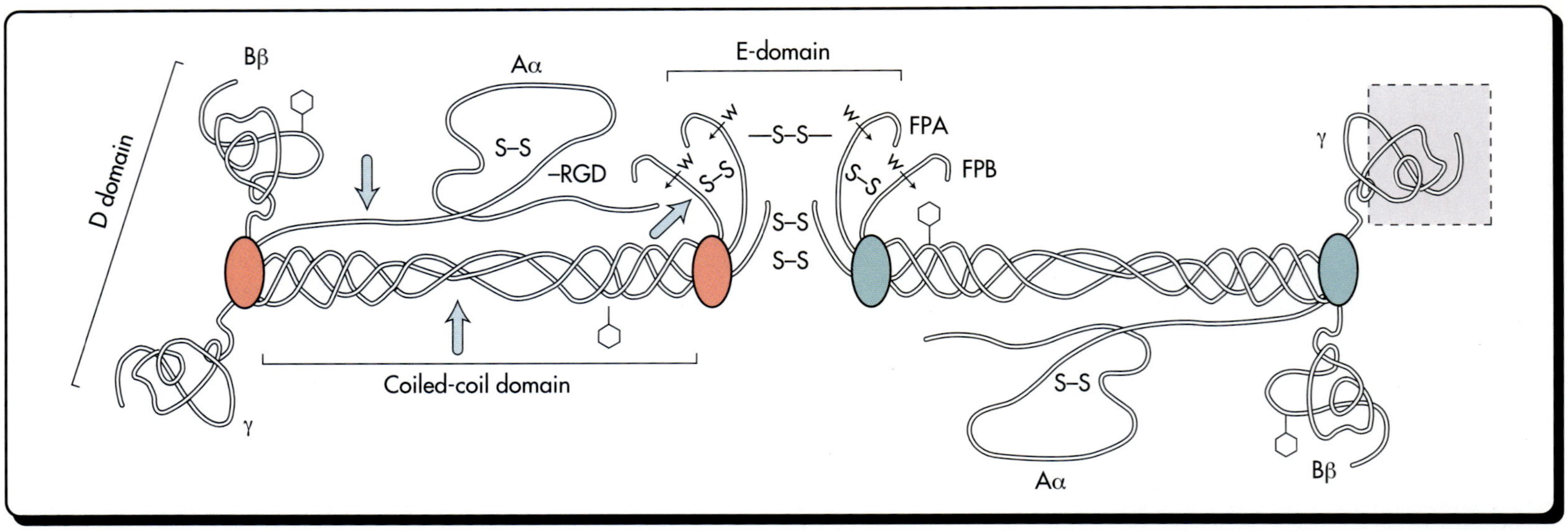

Figure 9-11. The structure of fibrinogen. The 340-kDa fibrinogen molecule is comprised of two identical halves, each of which contains three intertwined polypeptide chains termed Aα, Bβ, and γ [19]. The three chains are disulfide-bonded with a mirror image complex to form a trinodular structure consisting of two outer D domains and a central E domain. The amino terminals of the polypeptide chains, including the fibrinopeptides A and B (*FPA* and *FPB*), are located within the central E domain. The carboxy terminals of the polypeptide chains extend from the D domains and include cross-linking sites for factor XIII. The α chains also contain an RGD sequence, which provides a binding site for the platelet GPIIb-IIIa receptor. (*Adapted from* Mosesson [20]; with permission.)

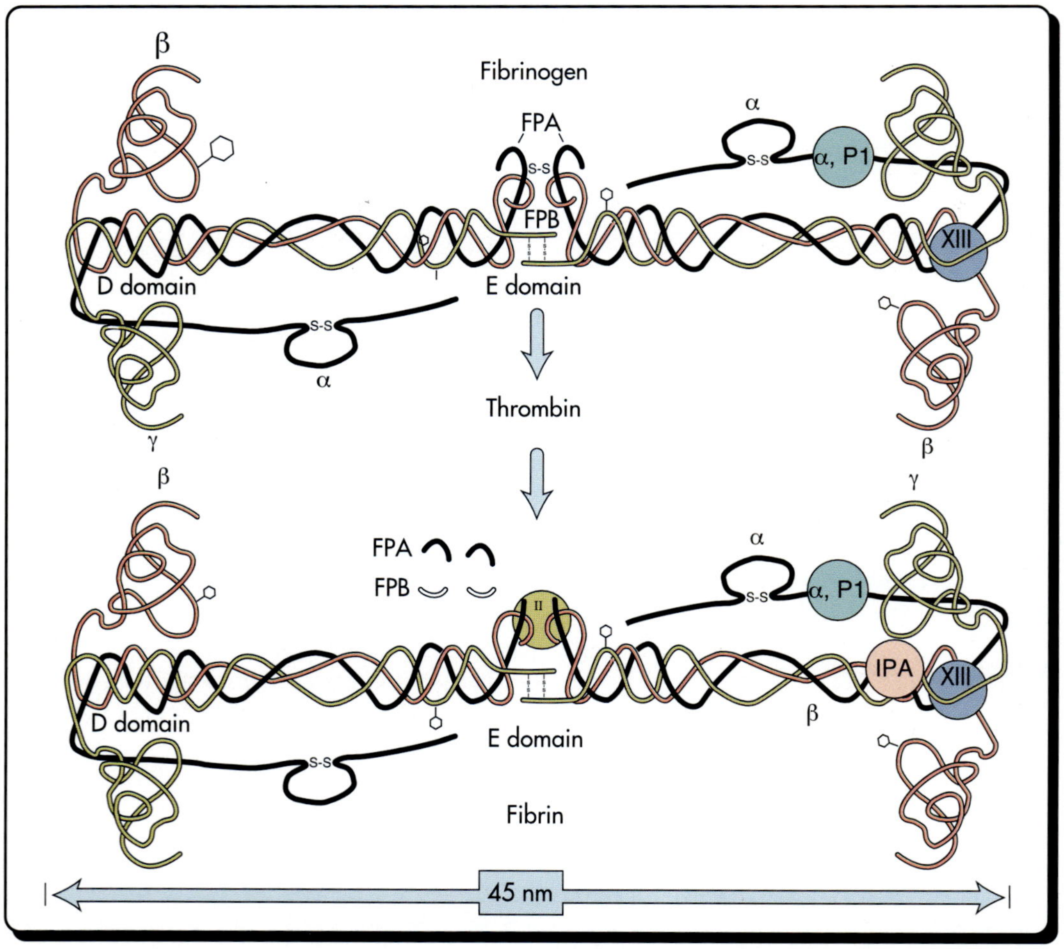

Figure 9-12. Interaction of thrombin and fibrinogen. The process by which fibrin is generated from fibrinogen begins as thrombin binds to and cleaves two specific arginine–glycine bonds located in the amino terminals of the Aα and Bβ chains of fibrinogen. This proteolytic activity of thrombin releases two activation peptides, fibrinopeptides A and B (*FPA* and *FPB*). The release of the fibrinopeptides exposes new binding sites within the central E domain, allowing the formation of noncovalent bonds with the D domains present in adjacent fibrinogen molecules. In this manner, fibrinogen molecules polymerize into a half-staggered arrangement of overlapping fibrin molecules which are called *protofibrils*. (*Adapted from* Mosesson [20]; with permission.)

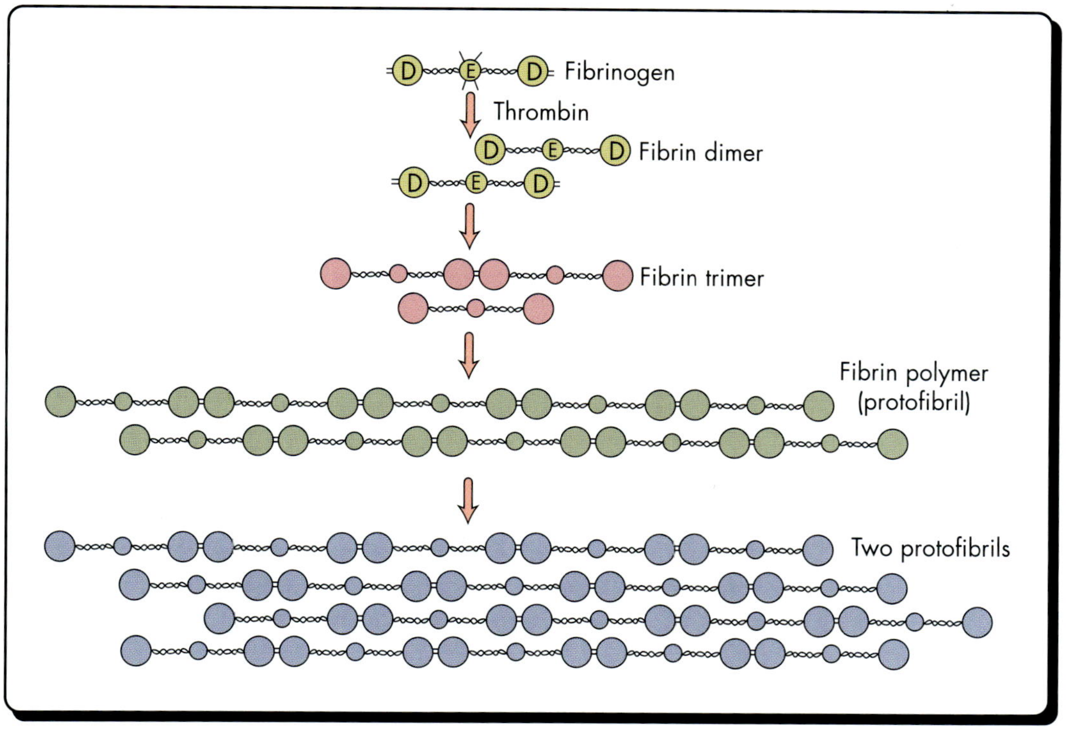

Figure 9-13. Fibrin polymerization and cross-linking. Protofibrils elongate and polymerize laterally to form a three-dimensional network of fibrin fibers. The process of fibrin polymerization is reversible, and the noncovalent bonds are easily disrupted. Only 20% of the volume of the fibrin gel consists of protein, with the remainder composed of solvent [21]. Factor XIII plays a crucial role in stabilization of the fibrin clot by covalently cross-linking adjacent Aα and γ polypeptide chains within the fibrin clot. In addition, factor XIII cross-links α_2-antiplasmin, the major physiologic inhibitor of plasmin, to the α chain of fibrinogen [22]. The cross-linking activities of factor XIII increase the ability of the clot to withstand mechanical and fibrinolytic degradation. D—terminal domain; E—central domain. (*From* Coleman and coworkers [23].)

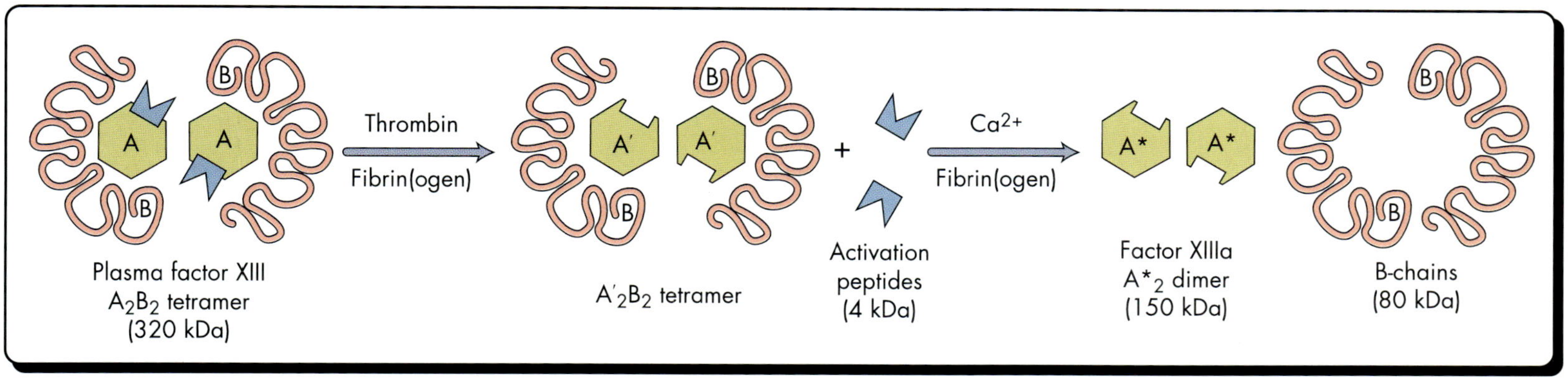

Figure 9-14. Activation of plasma factor XIII. Plasma factor XIII is a 320-kDa tetrameric molecule composed of two identical A chains and two identical B chains [24]. Thrombin initiates the activation of factor XIII by cleaving two activation peptides from the A chain to generate an inactive intermediate A′2B2. In the presence of calcium, the B chains dissociate from the A chains to expose the active site of the enzyme. Once the active site is exposed, factor XIII is capable of cross-linking fibrin and other substrates. *Asterisks* indicate activated enzyme. (*Adapted from* Greenberg [25]; with permission.)

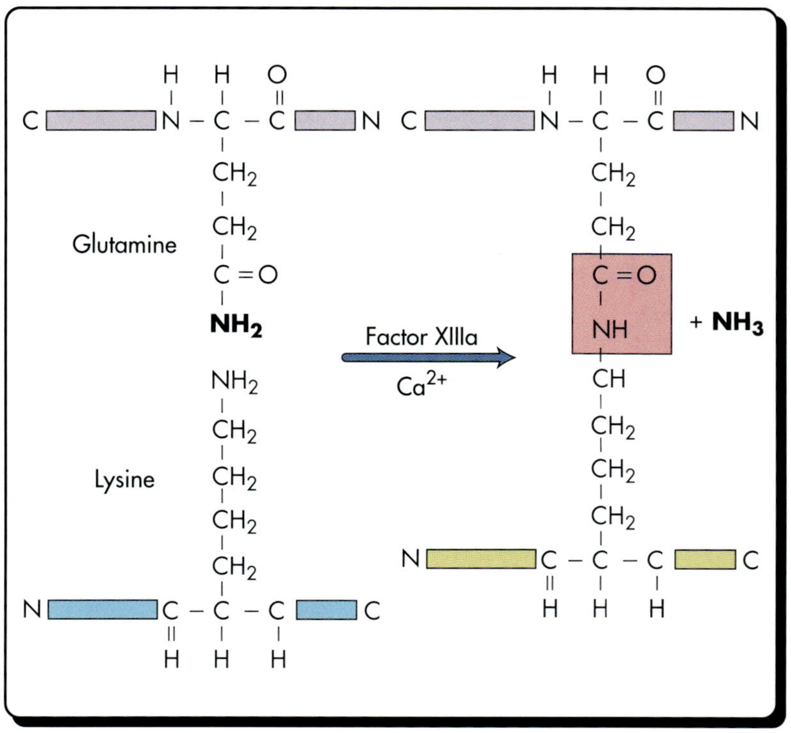

Figure 9-15. Isopeptide bond formation by factor XIII. The enzymatic activity of factor XIII is unique compared with other enzymes involved in coagulation. Rather than being a serine protease, factor XIII is a member of the transglutaminase gene superfamily [26]. The transglutaminases represent one of the earliest evolutionary forms of coagulation protein, with examples present in crustaceans and even bacteria. Once exposed, the active site cysteine of factor XIII generates highly stable isopeptide bonds between adjacent protein substrates. (*Adapted from* Greenberg [25]; with permission.)

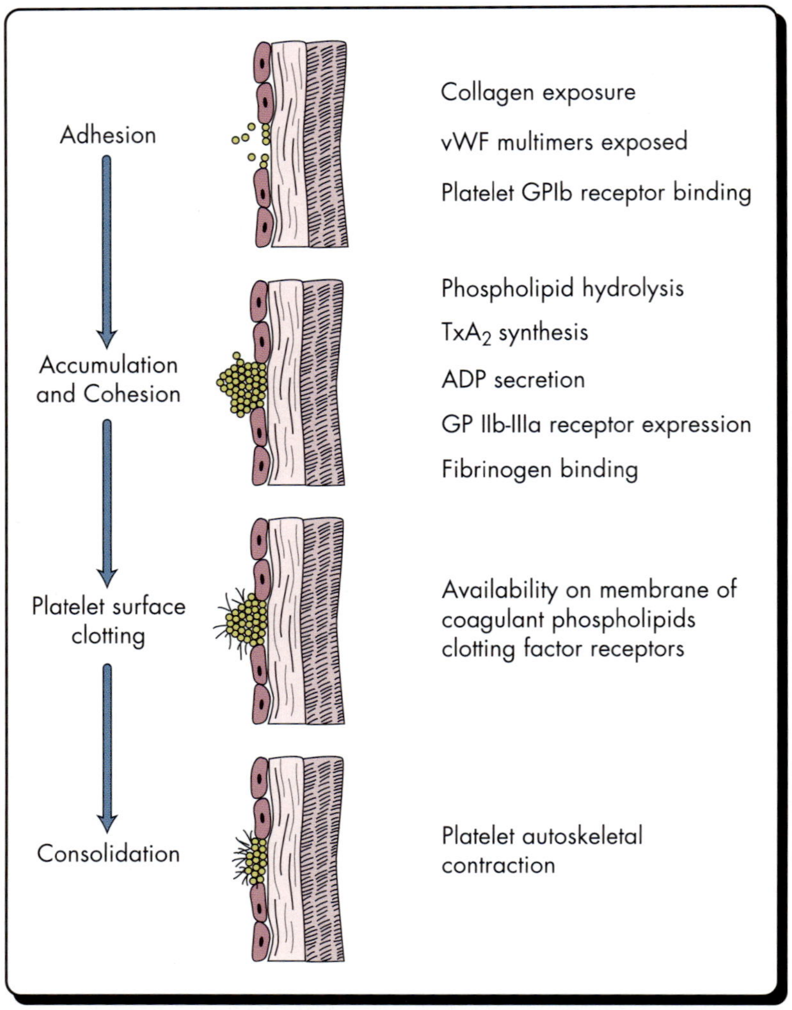

Figure 9-16. Overview of the platelet response in coagulation. The platelet plays a crucial role in clot formation by delivering hemostatically active proteins to the site of thrombosis, by adding to the structural integrity of the clot, and by providing a phospholipid surface on which plasma coagulation may occur. A typical response to vascular endothelial injury, with exposure of the extracellular matrix, would begin with platelet adhesion to exposed collagen. Interaction of the platelet with collagen results in platelet activation, with the biochemical formation and release of hemostatically active proteins. Thromboxane (TXA_2) and adenosine diphosphate (*ADP*) released from adhering platelets attract and activate additional platelets, leading to the accumulation of a platelet mass. Structural changes on the platelet surface provide a phospholipid template on which activation complexes assemble to generate fibrin and form an interconnected platelet–fibrin clot. Finally, contraction of the platelet cytoskeleton begins the process of consolidation and resolution of the clot [27]. GP—glycoprotein; vWF—von Willebrand factor. (*Adapted from* Rappaport [28]; with permission.)

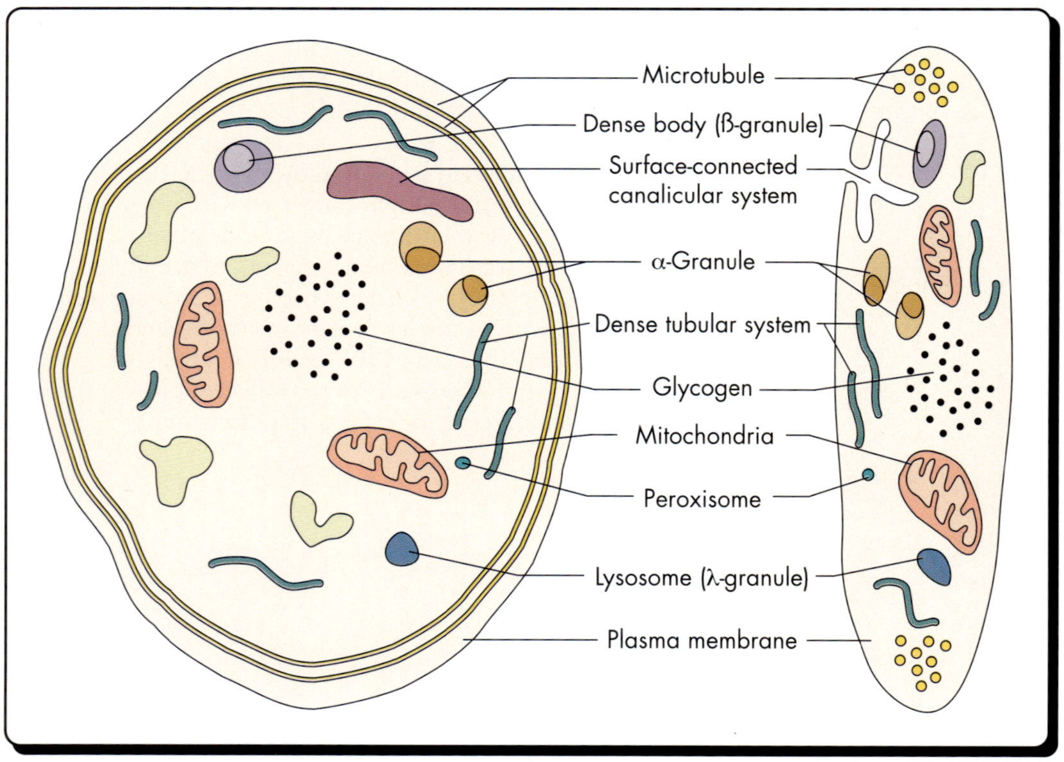

Figure 9-17. Structure of the human platelet. The interior of the platelet is characterized by three types of granules: α-granules, dense bodies, and lysosomes. These storage vesicles contain a variety of hemostatically active proteins, contributing to the regulation of clot formation and wound healing. One of the most distinctive features of the platelet is the surface-connected canalicular system. This extensive network of canals extending from the surface into the platelet provides a means for plasma proteins to rapidly interact with the interior of the platelet. Also, this network provides a conduit for release of platelet cytoplasmic contents into the extracellular space. An extensive cytoskeletal network of microtubules and actin supports the structural changes accompanying platelet activation. (*Adapted from* Lind [29].)

PLATELET CONTENTS

- Alpha granules
  - Adhesive proteins
    - Fibrinogen
    - Fibronectin
    - Thrombospondin
    - Vitronectin
    - von Willebrand factor
  - Albumin
  - Antifibrinolytics
    - α-2-antiplasmin
    - Plasminogen activator inhibitor-1
  - Coagulation factors
    - Factor V
    - Factor XI
    - Protein S
  - Immunoglobulins
  - Membrane proteins
    - P-selectin
    - GPIV
    - Osteonectin
  - Mitogens
    - Endothelial cell growth factor
    - Epidermal growth factor
    - Platelet-derived growth factor
    - Transforming growth factor-β
- Dense Bodies
  - ADP
  - ATP
  - Calcium
  - Pyrophosphate
  - Serotonin
- Other secreted proteins
  - α_2-Macroglobulin
  - α_1-Protease inhibitors
  - C1 inhibitor
  - Interleukin-1B
  - Factor XIII
  - High molecular weight kininogen
  - Peptidase
  - Protease nexin I and II
  - Tissue factor pathway inhibitor
  - Vascular permeability factor

Figure 9-18. Platelet granule and cytoplasmic contents. (*Adapted from* Ware and Coller [30].)

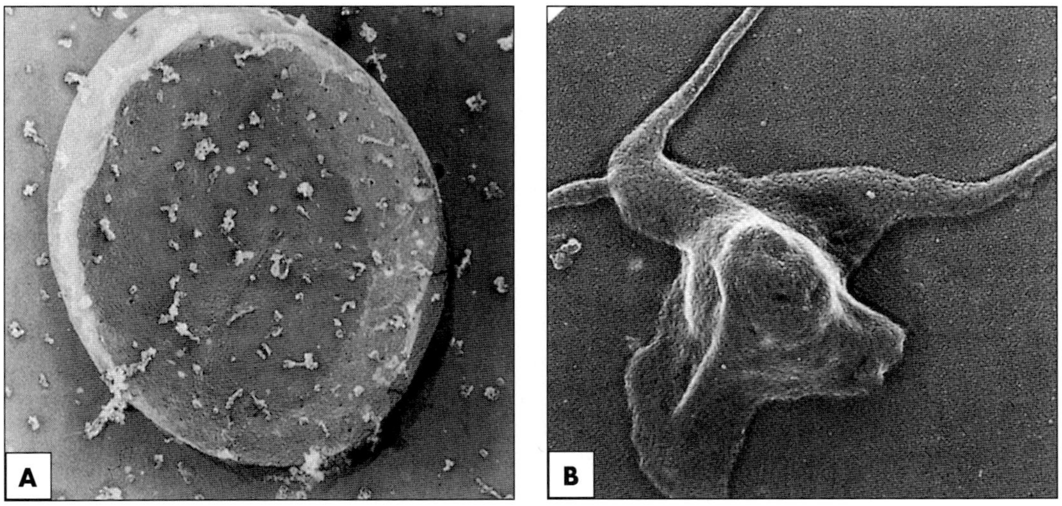

Figure 9-19. Morphology of resting and activated platelets. Electron micrographic images of resting (**A**) and activated (**B**) platelets. The resting platelet is an anuclear discoid cell less than 3 μm in size with a life span of approximately 10 days. Within minutes of activation the platelet undergoes dramatic alterations in shape and biochemical activity. Cyto-skeletal rearrangements generate pseudopod-like extensions from the cell membrane. Furthermore, the structural composition of the membrane changes to provide binding sites for plasma coagulation proteins. (*From* Lind [29]; courtesy of JH Hartwig.)

PLATELET SURFACE PROTEINS

Gene family	Common name	Platelet Chain Designation	Integrin Designation	Ligands	Platelet Specific	Function	Molecules on platelet surface (S) or internal (I)
Integrin	Fibrinogen receptor	GPIIb/IIIa	α_{IIb}/β_3	Fib, vWf,	+	Adhesion, aggregation, protein trafficking	(S) 40,000–80,000
				Fn, Vn, ?TSP	+		
	Collagen receptor	GPIa/IIa	$\alpha_2\beta_1$	Collagen	-	Adhesion	(S) ~ 1000
	Fibronectin receptor	GPIc*/IIa	$\alpha_5\beta_1$	Fn	-	Adhesion	(S) ~ 1000
	Laminin receptor	GPIc/IIa	$\alpha_6\beta_1$	Laminin	-	Adhesion	(S) ~ 1000
	Vitronectin receptor	α_v/GPIIIa	$\alpha_v\beta_3$	Vn, Fib, vWf, Fn, ?TSP	-	?Adhesion, ?protein trafficking	(S) ~ 100
Leucine-rich glycoproteins	von Willebrand factor receptor	GPIb/IX		vWf, Thrombin	?+	Adhesion (high shear)	(S) 25,000
					+	?Thrombin act	(S) 25,000
					+		(S) 25,000
		GPV			+		(S) 12,500
Immunoglobulin cell adhesion molecules	PECAM-I			Heparin	-	Platelets and endothelial cells	(S) 8,000
	Fcγ-RII			Immune complexes	-	Immune complex binding	(S) ~ 1000
	HLA-Class I				-	Histocompatibility	(S)
	ICAM-2			LFA-1	-	Platelet-leukocyte adhesion	(S) 2600
Selectins	P-Selectin (GMP 140; PADGEM)			Sialyl-Le	-	Platelet-leukocyte adhesion	(I) 20,000
Quadraspanin	p24			?	-	Activation	(S) 40,000
Miscellaneous	GPIV			Collagen, TSP	-	Adhesion	(S) 20,000
	Lamp 1			?	-	?	(I) 1200
	Lamp 2			?			
	Lamp 3 (granulophysin)						(I) 10,000
	67 kD Laminin receptor			Laminin	-	Adhesion	
	Leukosialin, sialophorin			ICAM-1	-	Adhesion	
Seven transmembrane domain (G protein-linked)	Thrombin receptor			Thrombin	-	Activation	~ 1800
	Thromboxane A_2 receptor			PGH_2/thromboxane A_2	-	Activation	~ 200
	α_2-Adrenergic receptor			Epinephrine	-	Activation	~ 250
	Vasopressin receptor			Vasopressin	-	Activation	~ 75

*Number of leucine-rich repeats.

Figure 9-20. Platelet surface proteins. CD—cluster of differentiation; Fib—fibrinogen; FN—fibronectin; GP—glycoproteins; PGH_2—prostaglandin H_2; TSP—thrombospondin; VLA—very late antigen; Vn—vitronectin; vWF—von Willebrand factor; +—yes; -—no. (*Adapted from* Ware and Coller [30]; with permission.)

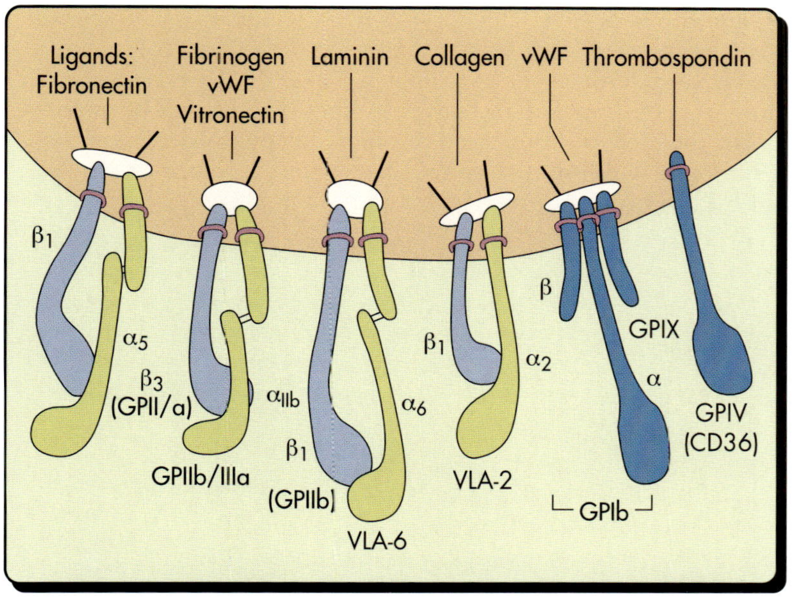

Figure 9-21. Platelet surface receptors. The platelet surface contains a variety of glycoprotein receptors, each of which binds a distinctive set of substrate ligands. Each receptor subtype varies in number from a few hundred to several hundred thousand receptor sites per platelet. These receptors are essential for normal platelet function. For example, Bernard-Soulier syndrome is an inherited bleeding disorder resulting from a deficiency of the glycoprotein (GP) Ib-IX receptor [31]. The GPIb-IX receptor allows the platelet to bind to subendothelial-associated von Willebrand factor, an essential step in platelet adhesion. CD—cluster of differentiation; VLA—very late antigen. (*From* Hawiger [32]; with permission.)

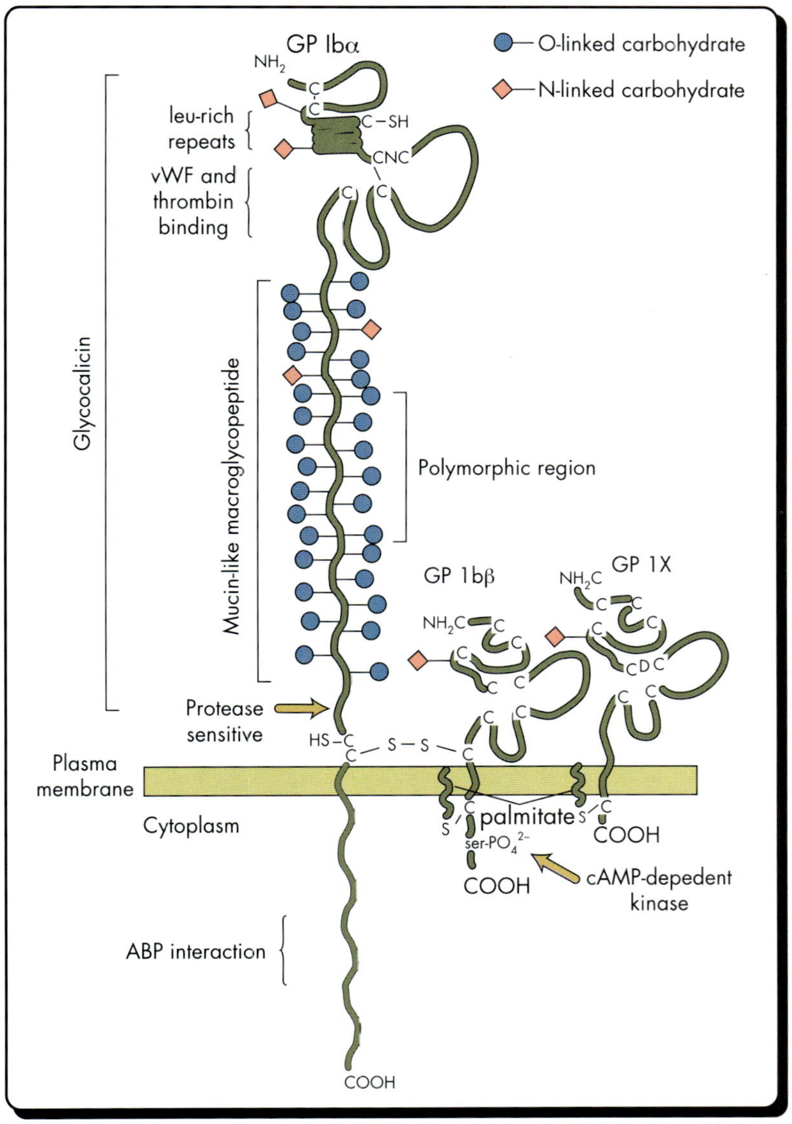

Figure 9-22. The glycoprotein (GP) Ib/IX receptor complex. This figure demonstrates the structural complexity associated with a single glycoprotein surface receptor. The GPIb-IX receptor participates in the binding of von Willebrand factor (vWF). Note the extensions of the receptor into the cytoplasm allowing for the initiation of intracellular signaling on binding of the vWF ligand. The presence of a protease-sensitive region near the transmembrane domain results in receptor degradation in the presence of fibrinolytic activity. This may serve as a means of down-regulating platelet activity following formation of the clot. ABP—actin binding protein; cAMP—cyclic adenosine monophosphate; GP—glycoprotein; leu-rich—leucine rich; vWF—vonWillebrand factor. (*Adapted from* Lopez [33]; with permission.)

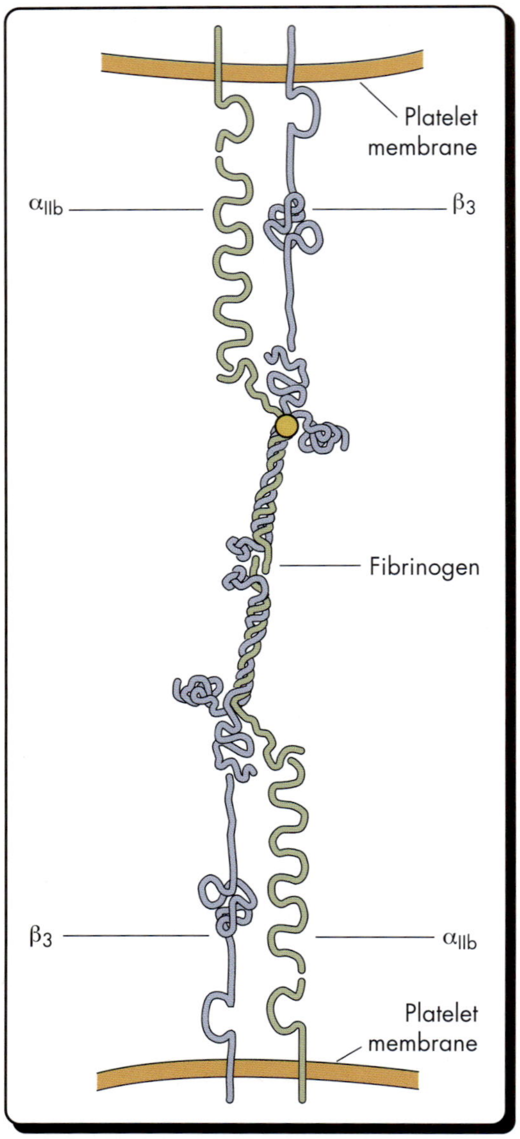

Figure 9-23. Fibrinogen–platelet interactions. The fibrinogen molecule plays an important role in platelet aggregation by bridging adjacent activated platelets through glycoprotein (GP) IIb-IIIa receptors [34]. Fibrinogen is incapable of binding the GPIIb-IIIa receptor until activation of the platelet produces conformational changes within the receptor. The importance of the fibrinogen–platelet interaction is evidenced by the bleeding disorder characterized by a congenital deficiency of the GPIIb-IIIa receptor, Glanzmann's thrombasthenia. α_{IIb}, β_3—components of the GPIIb-IIIa receptor. (*From* Harker and Mann [35].)

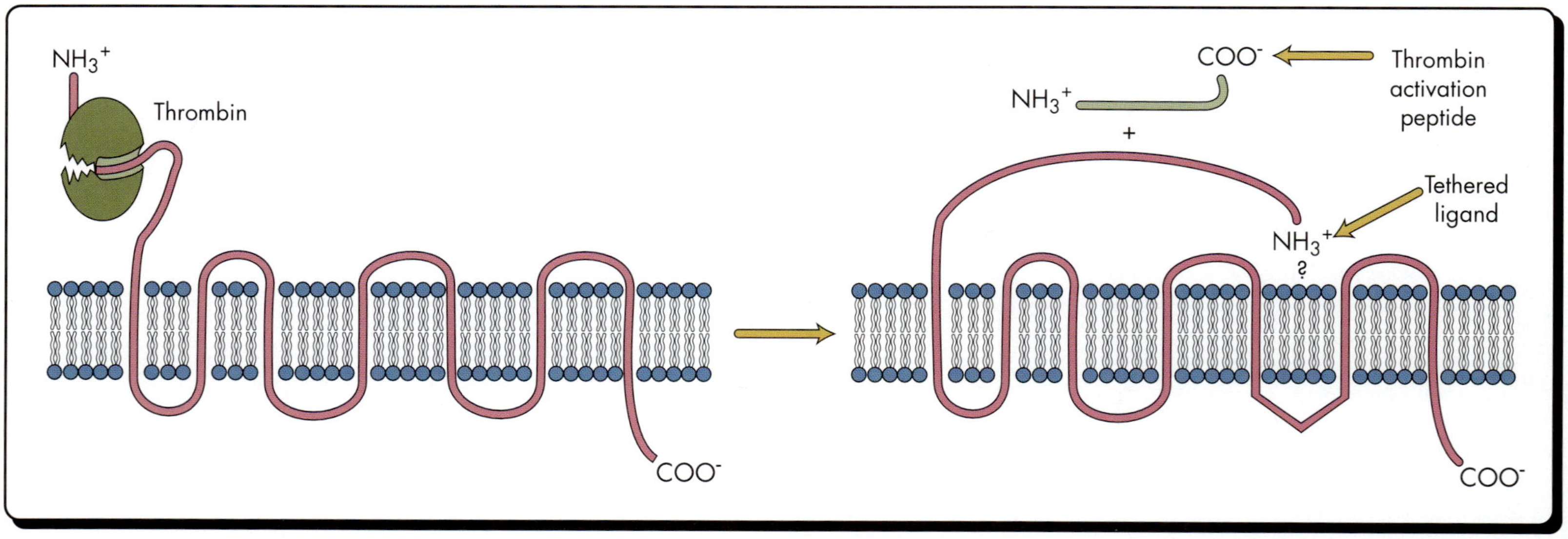

Figure 9-24. The platelet thrombin receptor. The thrombin receptor is a 425-amino-acid protein with seven membrane spanning domains. Thrombin binds to the extracellular portion of the receptor, cleaving an activation peptide from the amino terminal portion of the peptide [36]. Loss of the activation peptide exposes a new amino terminus, a tethered ligand, which binds to another portion of the receptor to activate the platelet. (*Adapted from* Vu and coworkers [37]; with permission.)

AGONISTS STIMULATING PLATELET ACTIVATION
Thrombin
Collagen
High shear stress
ADP
Epinephrine
Thromboxane A_2
Platelet-activating factor
Serotonin
Plasmin

Figure 9-25. Agonists stimulating platelet activation.

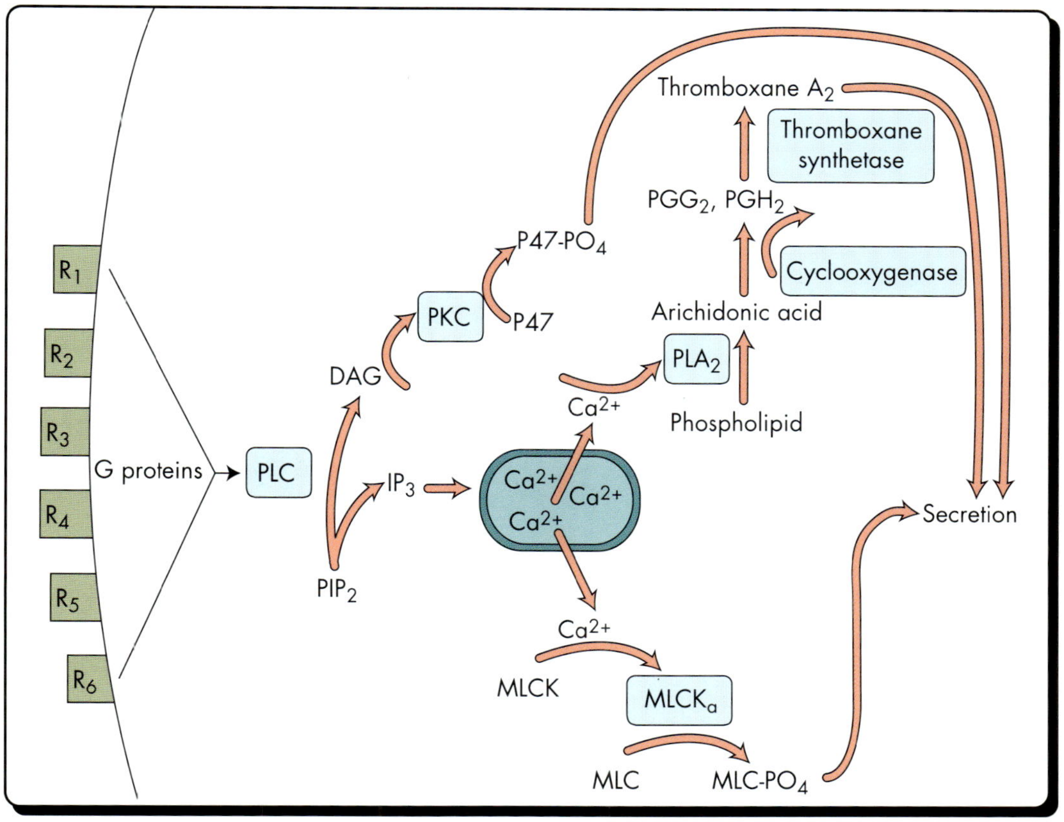

Figure 9-26. The biochemistry of platelet activation. Activation of the platelet generally occurs after an agonist binds to a specific surface receptor (R), triggering activation of membrane-bound GTP-binding proteins [38]. The G protein(s) activate phospholipase C (*PLC*), which subsequently hydrolyzes phosphatidyl inositol 4,5 -bisphosphate (PIP_2) to form diacylglycerol (*DAG*) and inositol 1,4,5-trisphosphate (*IP_3*). Diacylglycerol activates protein kinase C (*PKC*), providing a mechanism for protein phosphorylation (*ie*, phosphorylation of P47 contributes to the secretion of intracellular storage granule contents). IP_3 binds to receptors on the dense tubule system within the platelet to stimulate the release of intracellular calcium (*Ca^{2+}*). Intracellular calcium subsequently stimulates the activation of a variety of enzymes including certain forms of protein kinase C as well as phospholipase A_2 (*PLA_2*), the enzyme responsible for release of arachidonic acid from the phospholipid membrane during the initiation of prostanoid synthesis. MLC—myosin light chain; MLCK—myosin light chain kinase; MLC-PO_4—phosphorylated MLC. (*Adapted from* Colman and coworkers [23]; courtesy of Dr. A. Koneti Rao.)

BIOCHEMICAL AND STRUCTURAL CHANGES ASSOCIATED WITH PLATELET ACTIVATION
Storage granule secretion
Alpha granules
Dense granules
Lysosomes
Increased cytosolic calcium
Protein phosphorylation
Structural alterations in cytoskeleton
Surface receptor conformational changes (neoepitope expression)

Figure 9-27. Biochemical and structural changes associated with platelet activation.

MECHANISMS INHIBITING PLATELET ACTIVATION
Blood flow
Vascular endothelial anticoagulants
Nitric oxide
Prostacyclin
ADPases
Thrombin inhibitors
Antithrombin III
Thrombomodulin

Figure 9-28. Mechanisms inhibiting platelet activation.

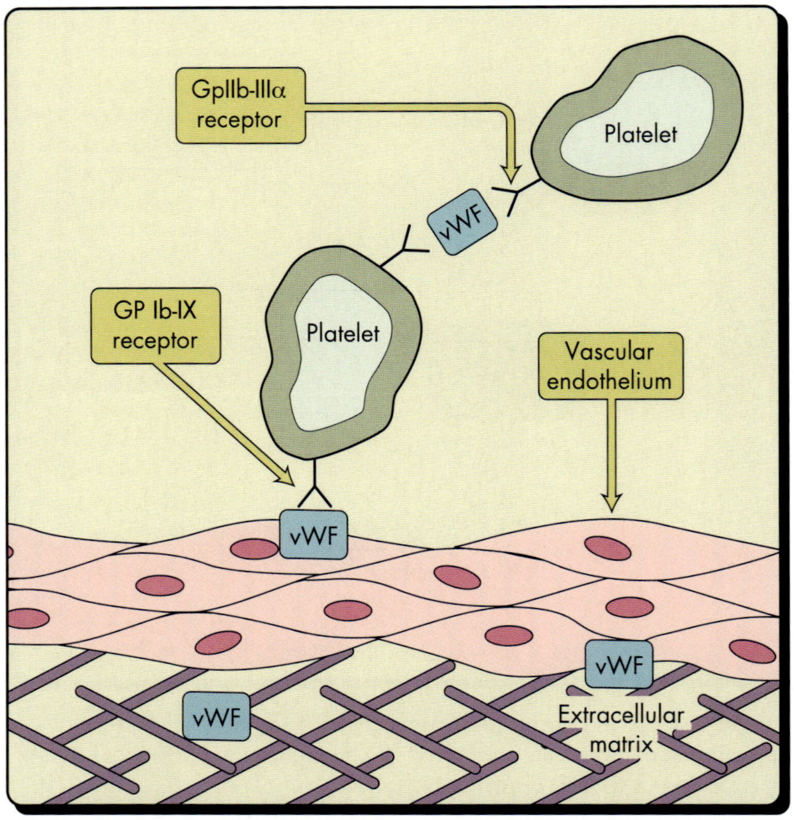

Figure 9-29. Hemostatic function of von Willebrand factor (vWF). vWF performs two major hemostatic functions. First, vWF acts as a bridge to facilitate binding of the platelet to the injured vessel wall by way of the glycoprotein (GP) Ib-IX receptor. Under conditions of high shear rate, as occur in the microcirculation, the presence of vWF is critical for normal platelet adhesion. Second, vWF acts as a carrier molecule for factor VIII. When bound to vWF, factor VIII is protected from proteolytic degradation. In fact, in the presence of a severe deficiency of vWF, factor VIII is often degraded to such an extent as to lead to an initial diagnosis of hemophilia A; however, when vWF is replaced in these patients, the factor VIII concentration spontaneously returns to normal [39].

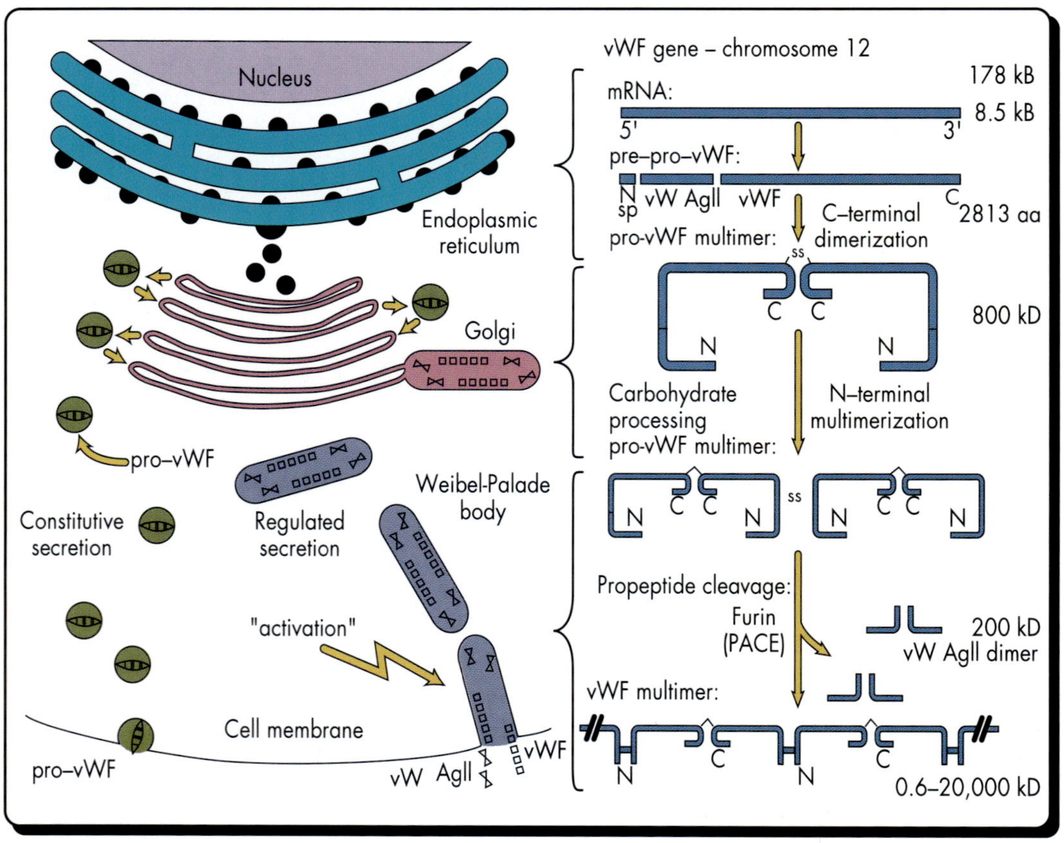

Figure 9-30. Cellular biosynthesis of von Willebrand factor (vWF). The gene for vWF, approximately 180 kb long, contains 52 exons and is located on the short arm of chromosome 12 [40]. The messenger RNA (*mRNA*) is initially translated into a pre-pro-vWF form, which subsequently undergoes cleavage of the signal peptide and disulfide bonding to generate a pro-vWF dimer. During passage through the Golgi, extensive post-translational processing occurs in concert with polymerization of the dimers into the final vWF multimer. The larger vWF multimers appear to be the most effective at facilitating platelet–endothelial binding. PACE—pulmonary angiotensin I converting enzyme. (*From* Montgomery and Coller [40]; with permission.)

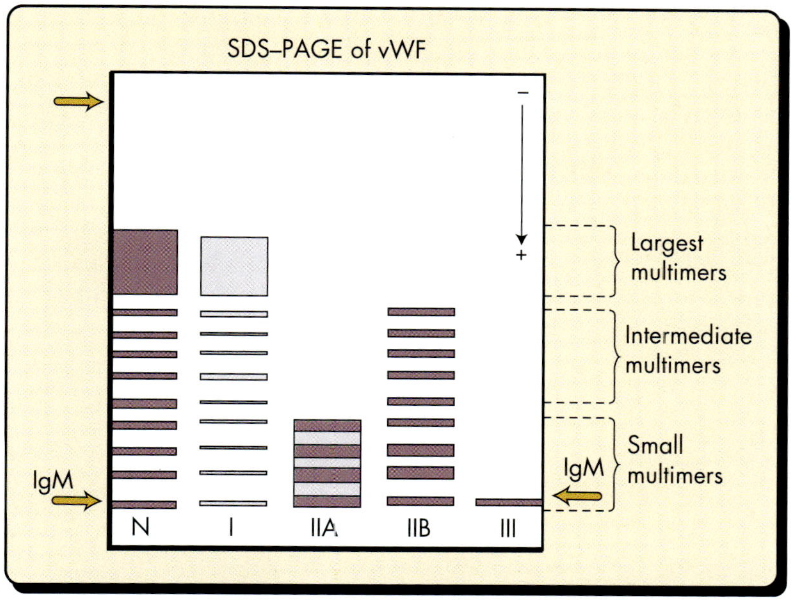

Figure 9-31. von Willebrand disease represents the most prevalent form of inheritable bleeding disorder, affecting nearly 1% of the population [41]. To date, at least 20 distinct subtypes of von Willebrand disease have been identified. For the sake of simplicity, subtypes of von Willebrand disease are described using three categories. Type I, a quantitative deficiency of von Willebrand factor (vWF), occurs in approximately 70% of patients. Type II von Willebrand disease represents a variety of qualitative disorders affecting the function of vWF. Type III may represent a homologous form of type I disease in that a severe deficiency of vWF occurs with little or no vWF measurable in plasma. Sodium dodecyl sulfate (*SDS*)–polyacrylamide gel electrophoresis (PAGE) of vWF multimers aids in the diagnosis of the specific subtype of von Willebrand disease. IgM—immunoglobulin M; N—normal plasma sample. (*Adapted from* Triplett [42].)

FIBRINOLYSIS

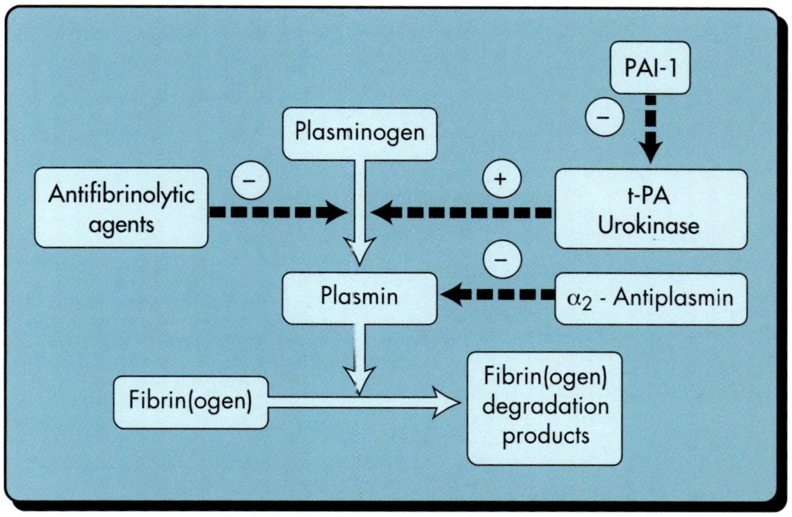

Figure 9-32. Overview of the fibrinolytic system. The fibrinolytic system characterizes the biochemical process by which the fibrin clot is degraded *in vivo*. The proteolytically active mediator of fibrinolysis is the enzyme plasmin. Under normal conditions, tissue plasminogen activator (*t-PA*) released from the vascular endothelium activates plasminogen to form plasmin [43]. A second plasminogen activator, urokinase, is generated by the urinary tract; however, this pathway accounts for only a small fraction of the fibrinolytic activity in plasma. Each step in the fibrinolytic pathway is regulated by specific inhibitory proteases. Plasminogen activator inhibitor-1 (*PAI-1*) inhibits the activity of both t-PA and urokinase. PAI-1, an acute phase reactant, is released from both the α-granules of platelets and the vascular endothelium. The major inhibitor of plasmin is the serine protease inhibitor (serpin) α_2-antiplasmin. Both t-PA and plasmin are relatively resistant to inhibition when bound to fibrin; this characteristic, as well as the presence of high plasma concentrations of protease inhibitors, limits the propagation of fibrinolytic activity beyond the clot. (*From* Slaughter [6]; with permission.)

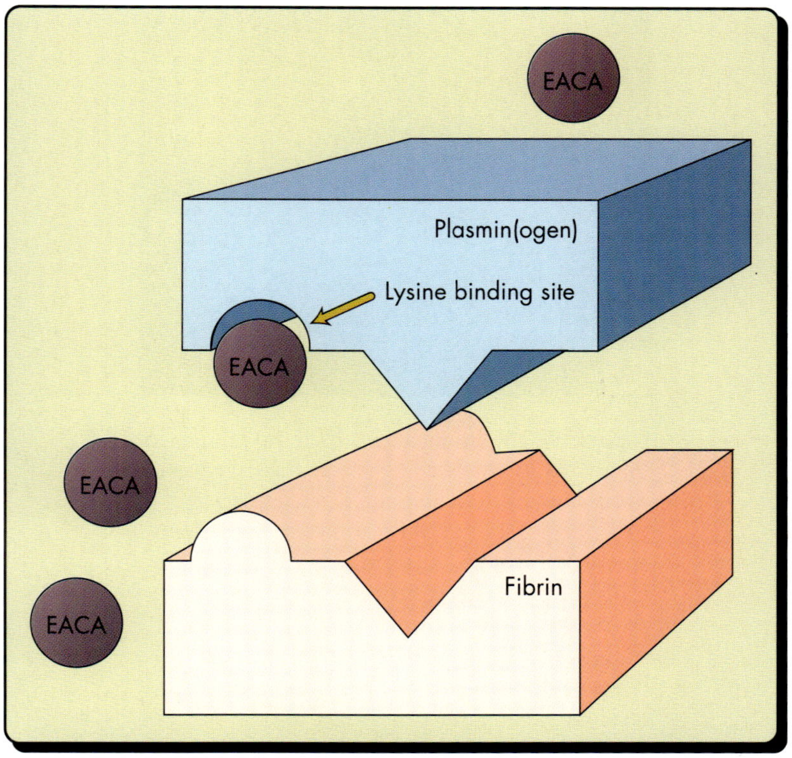

Figure 9-33. Pharmacologic inhibition of fibrinolysis. The binding of plasminogen to fibrin greatly accelerates the rate at which plasmin may be generated [44]. This regulatory mechanism acts to localize fibrinolytic activity to the region of a clot. Both plasminogen and plasmin bind to fibrin by way of lysine binding sites. Administration of lysine analogue drugs such as ε-aminocaproic acid (*EACA*) and tranexamic acid competitively inhibit the binding of both plasminogen and plasmin to the fibrin clot, thereby decreasing fibrinolysis [45]. (*From* Slaughter [6]; with permission.)

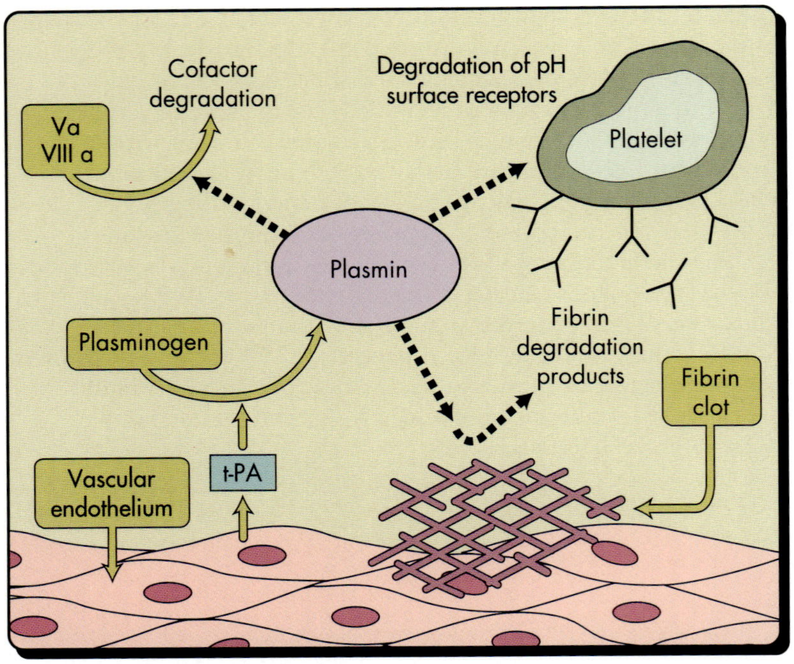

Figure 9-34. The effects of fibrinolysis on hemostasis. In addition to degradation of the fibrin clot, plasmin acts to suppress clot formation by a number of additional mechanisms. Fibrin degradation fragments act as anticoagulants by suppressing both fibrin polymerization and platelet aggregation [46]. Furthermore, the protease-sensitive domain of platelet glycoprotein receptors is susceptible to plasmin degradation resulting in loss of the receptor. Both of the cofactors Va and VIIIa are susceptible to proteolytic degradation by plasmin [47]. Loss of the cofactors limits the formation of membrane-bound activation complexes, thereby suppressing plasma coagulation. t-PA—tissue plasminogen activator.

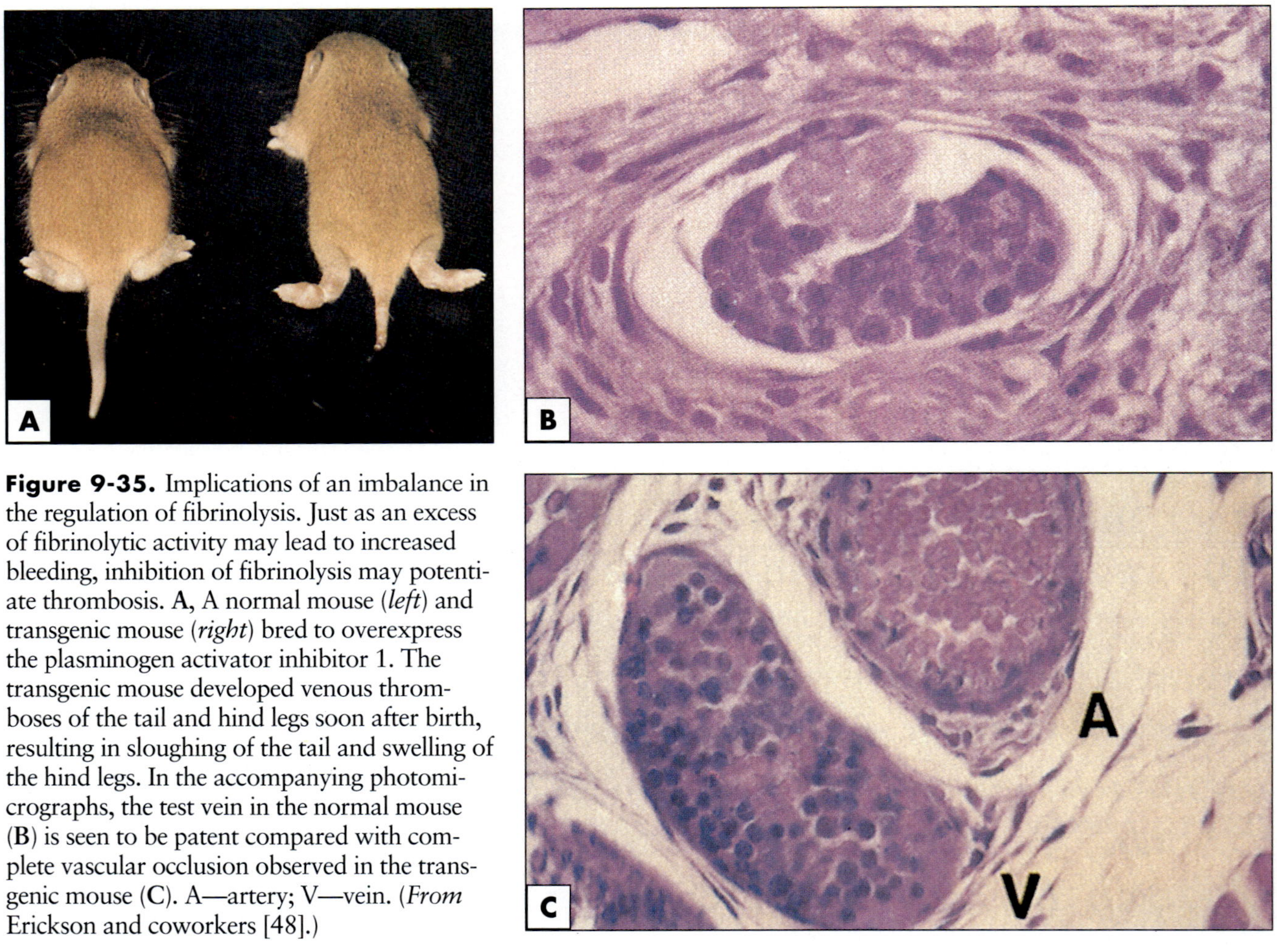

Figure 9-35. Implications of an imbalance in the regulation of fibrinolysis. Just as an excess of fibrinolytic activity may lead to increased bleeding, inhibition of fibrinolysis may potentiate thrombosis. **A**, A normal mouse (*left*) and transgenic mouse (*right*) bred to overexpress the plasminogen activator inhibitor 1. The transgenic mouse developed venous thromboses of the tail and hind legs soon after birth, resulting in sloughing of the tail and swelling of the hind legs. In the accompanying photomicrographs, the test vein in the normal mouse (**B**) is seen to be patent compared with complete vascular occlusion observed in the transgenic mouse (**C**). A—artery; V—vein. (*From* Erickson and coworkers [48].)

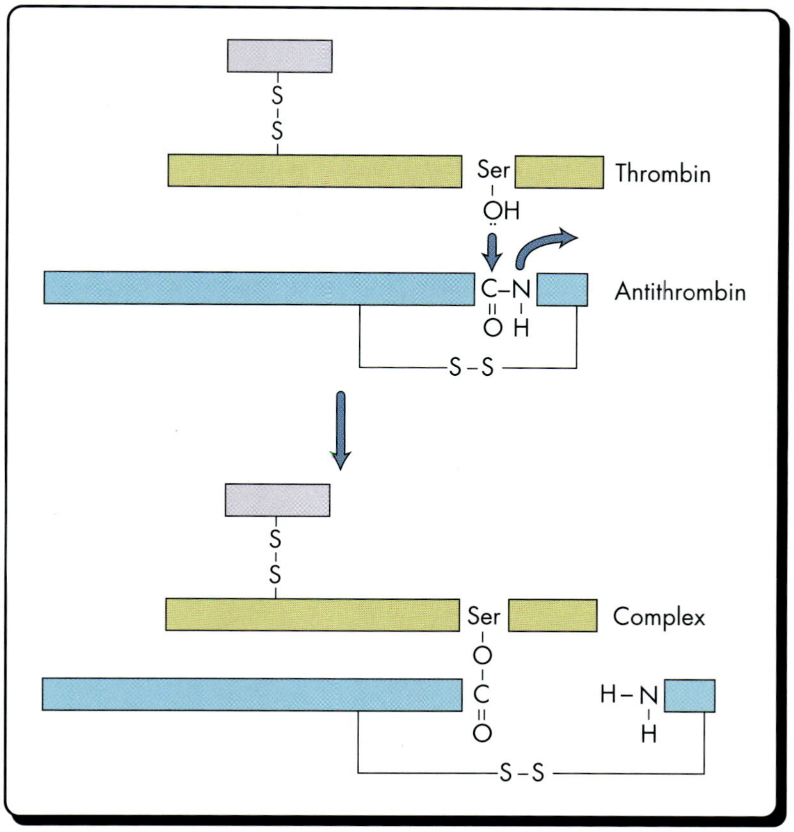

Figure 9-36. Mechanism of action of antithrombin III. In addition to the fibrinolytic pathway, a number of intrinsic anticoagulant mechanisms are present both in the plasma and on the vascular endothelial surface to limit the extent of clot propagation beyond the site of injury. Antithrombin III, a plasma serine protease inhibitor (serpin), provides a major mechanism for the elimination of thrombin and other activated coagulation factors from plasma [49]. Antithrombin III forms an irreversible covalent bond with the serine (*ser*) active site of target proteases (factors IIa, IXa, Xa, XIa, and XIIa). The inactive antithrombin III–protease complex is subsequently cleared from the circulation. Under normal conditions the interaction between antithrombin III and a target protease is relatively slow; however, in the presence of heparin or heparan sulfate (an intrinsic glycosaminoglycan present on vascular endothelial surfaces) this reaction is greatly accelerated [50]. (*From* Broze and Tollefsen [50]; with permission.)

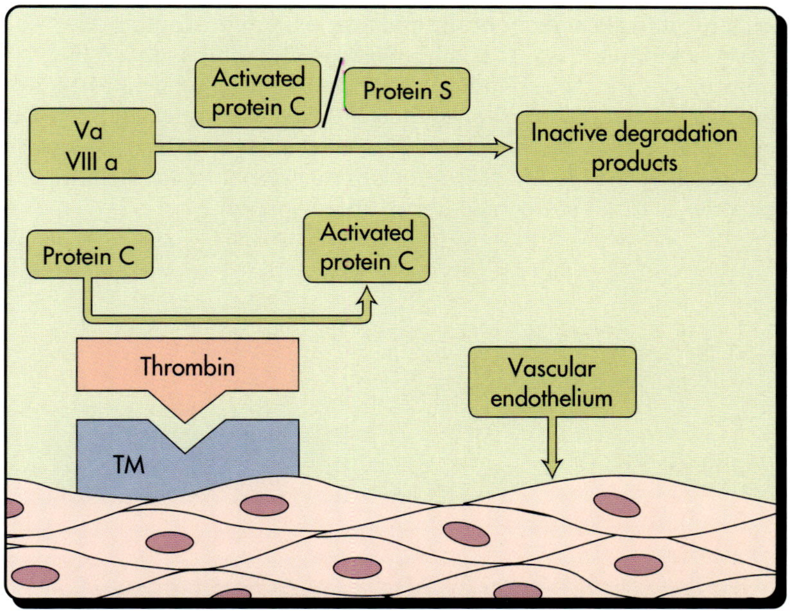

Figure 9-37. Mechanism of action of the thrombomodulin (TM)–protein C anticoagulant system. In addition to heparan sulfate, vascular endothelial cells are endowed with an additional mechanism for the inhibition of free thrombin. Each endothelial cell contains as many as 100,000 TM receptors, which are capable of binding and permanently inactivating thrombin [51]. In addition, the thrombomodulin–thrombin complex activates protein C, an anticoagulant protein with the ability to inactivate cofactors Va and VIIIa by proteolysis.

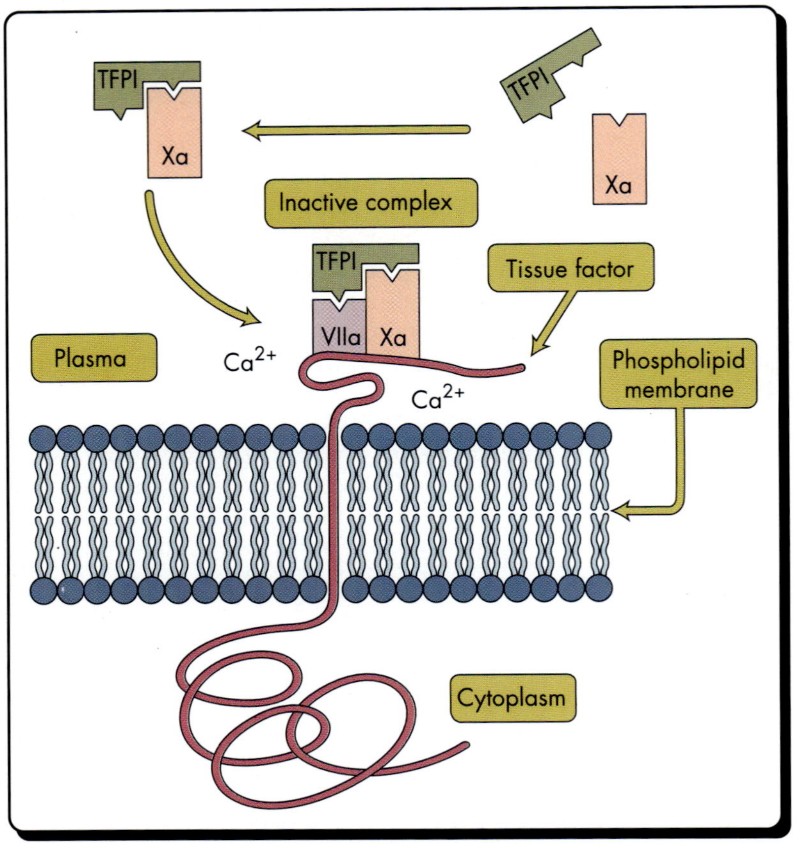

Figure 9-38. Mechanism of action of the tissue factor pathway inhibitor (*TFPI*). Recent identification of an inhibitor of the extrinsic pathway has led to new insights regarding the interdependency of the intrinsic and extrinsic pathways of coagulation. Shortly after release of tissue factor into the circulation, TFPI forms a quaternary complex with the tissue factor–VIIa complex and factor Xa, inhibiting the further activation of factor X by way of the extrinsic pathway. As the extrinsic pathway is downregulated, continuation of the hemostatic response becomes dependent on the intrinsic pathway to further amplify the initial thrombin formation. The recent identification of the TFPI explains the mystery of why patients with hemophilia A, a defect of the intrinsic pathway of coagulation, experience bleeding despite the presence of an intact extrinsic pathway [52]. Inhibition of TFPI may some day offer an additional approach to the management of hemostasis in the patient with hemophilia.

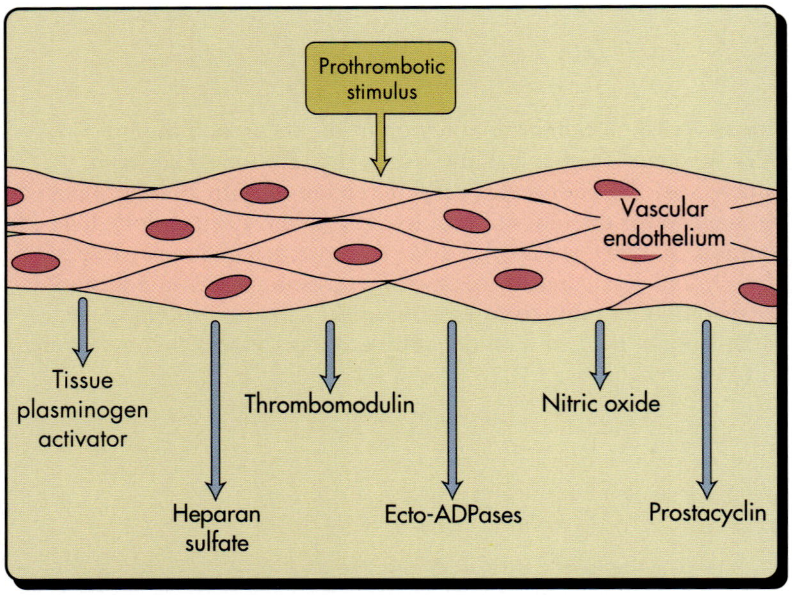

Figure 9-39. Intrinsic anticoagulant mechanisms of the vessel wall. The vascular endothelium provides a number of mechanisms to inhibit both plasma coagulation and platelet activation. Heparan sulfate, an endogenous glycosaminoglycan present on the endothelial surface, catalyzes activity of the anticoagulant antithrombin III. Thrombomodulin, as discussed in Figure 9-37, inhibits thrombin and provides for the activation of protein C. Nitric oxide, prostacyclin, and ecto-adenosine diphosphatases (ADPases) released from the endothelial cell inhibit platelet activation [53,54]. Finally, tissue plasminogen activator (t-PA) released from the vascular endothelium generates plasmin to degrade fibrin already present.

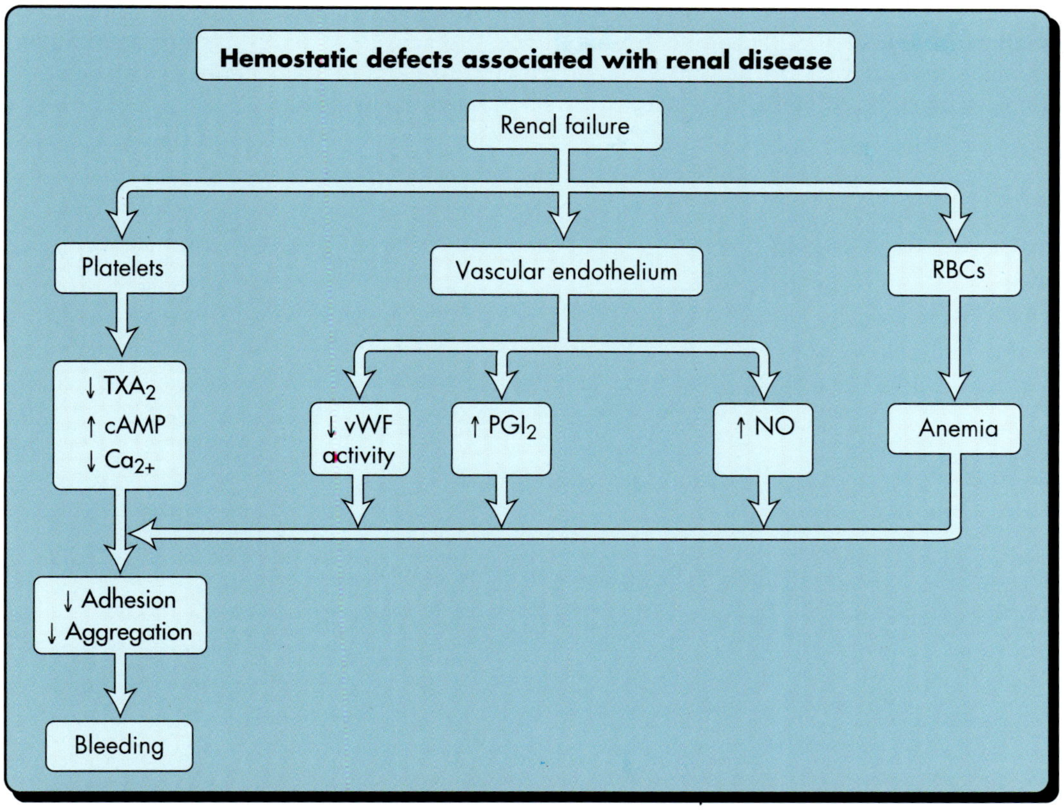

Figure 9-40. Hemostatic defects associated with renal disease. A variety of hemostatic abnormalities, primarily involving platelet adhesion and aggregation, have been described in patients with renal disease. The anemia associated with chronic renal insufficiency alters platelet interactions with the vessel wall. In fact, the bleeding time in patients with renal failure correlates inversely with hematocrit [55]. Defects in platelet glycoprotein receptors and decreased thromboxane production further contribute to platelet dysfunction. Also, increased generation of prostacyclin and nitric oxide (*NO*) by the vascular endothelium may increase the bleeding propensity by inhibiting platelet activation [56,57]. PGI_2—prostacyclin; RBC—red blood cells; TXA_2—thromboxane A_2; cAMP—cyclic adenosine monophosphate; vWF—von Willebrand factor.

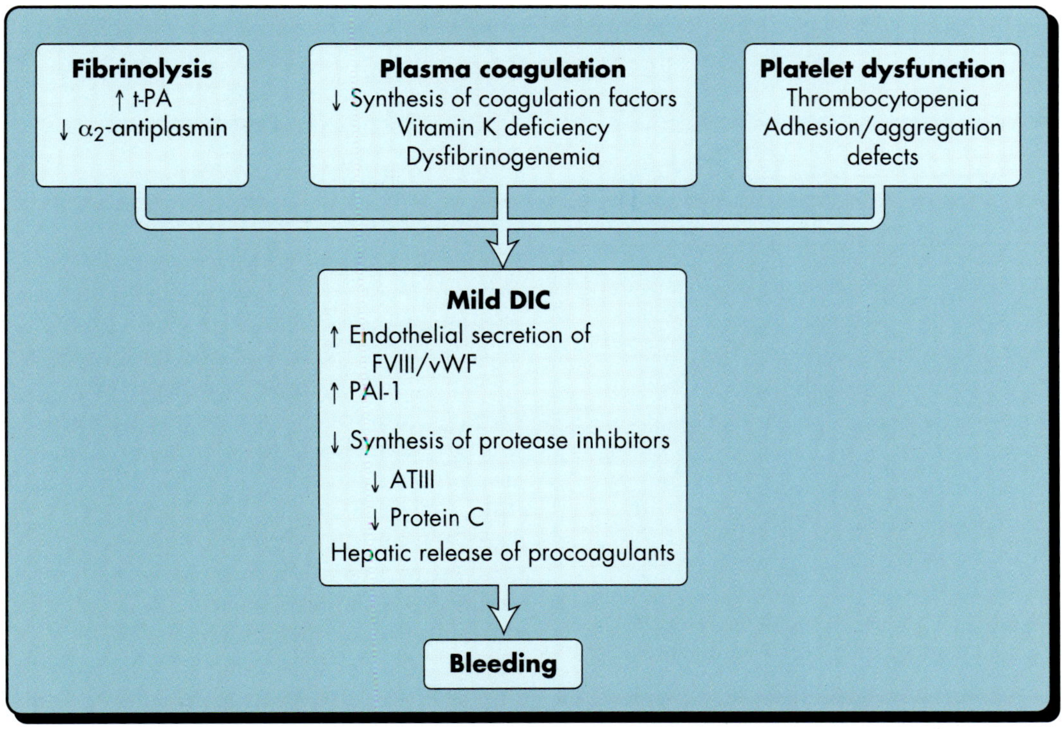

Figure 9-41. Hemostatic defects associated with liver disease. Severe hepatic dysfunction results in significant alterations in plasma coagulation, platelet function, and fibrinolytic activity [58]. Declining synthetic function of the liver results in decreased production of the plasma coagulation factors. Furthermore, malabsorption leads to vitamin K deficiency and the synthesis of aberrant forms of the vitamin K–dependent clotting factors. In addition to thrombocytopenia related to splenic sequestration, defects in platelet adhesion and aggregation are observed in some patients. Increased fibrinolytic activity is a common finding in these patients related primarily to decreased synthesis of the plasmin inhibitor $alpha_2$-antiplasmin and to the decreased ability of the liver to clear fibrinolytic enzymes from the circulation. In some patients, procoagulants released from damaged liver cells initiate chronic disseminated intravascular coagulation (*DIC*) further contributing to the hemostatic defects of liver disease. ATIII—antithrombin III; PAI-1—plasminogen activator inhibitor 1; t-PA—tissue plasminogen activator.

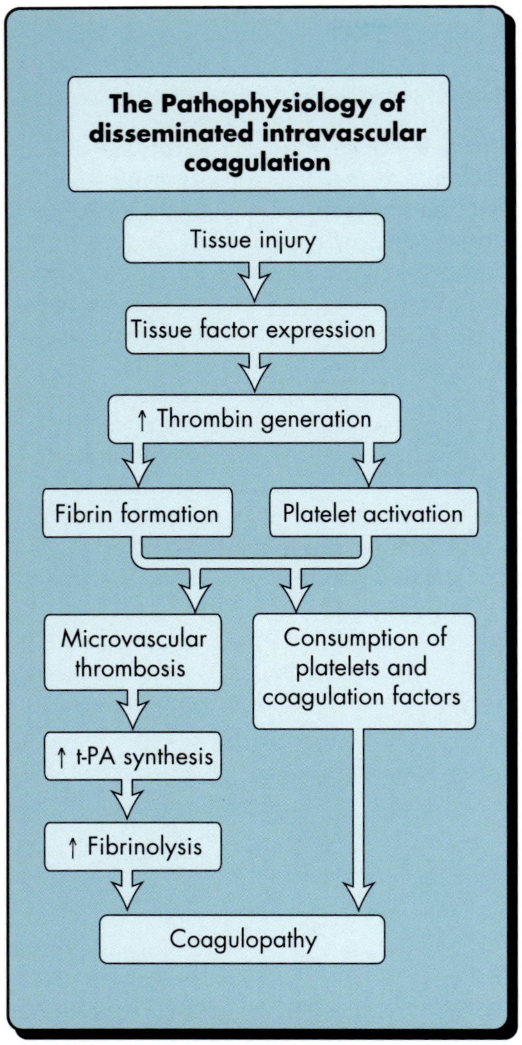

Figure 9-42. Disseminated intravascular coagulation (DIC). DIC is characterized by extensive microvascular thrombosis accompanied by fibrinolytic activity [59]. Although a wide variety of stimuli may trigger DIC, vascular injury resulting in the exposure or expression of tissue factor is most often involved. Fibrinolysis occurs as tissue plasminogen activator (t-PA) is released by the vascular endothelium in response to thrombin, endotoxin, and other inflammatory mediators. Thrombin formation leads to activation and consumption of both plasma coagulation factors and platelets. Increased fibrinolytic activity coupled with depletion of hemostatic components generally results in impaired hemostasis.

DRUG-INDUCED DEFECTS IN COAGULATION

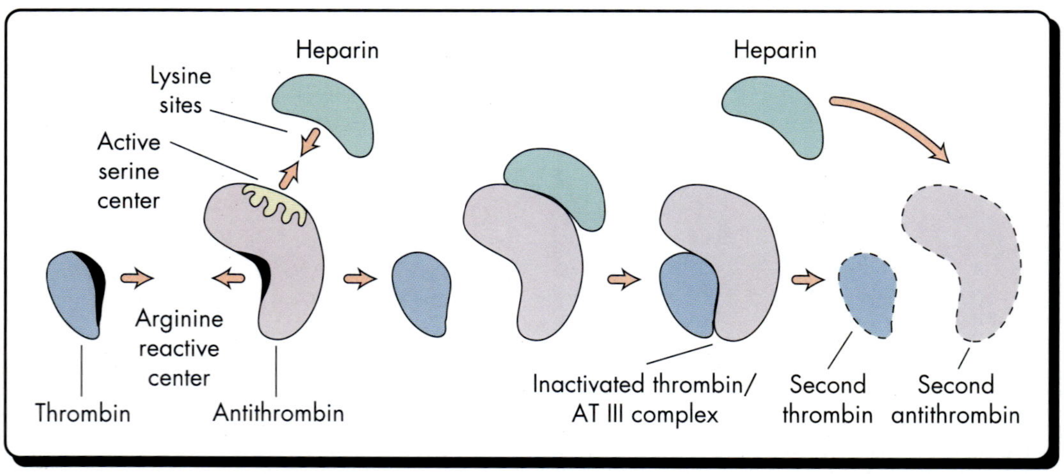

Figure 9-43. Mechanism of action of heparin. Heparin is a heterogeneous glycosaminoglycan synthesized within mast cells and commercially purified from porcine intestinal mucosa and bovine lung [60]. Heparin catalyzes the interaction between antithrombin III and the activated coagulation proteins thrombin, IXa, Xa, XIa, and XIIa. Once the covalent bond between antithrombin III and a target protease is established, heparin is released to catalyze additional reactions. Heparin also catalyzes the inhibition of thrombin by way of heparin cofactor II, although the *in vivo* importance of this reaction remains unclear.

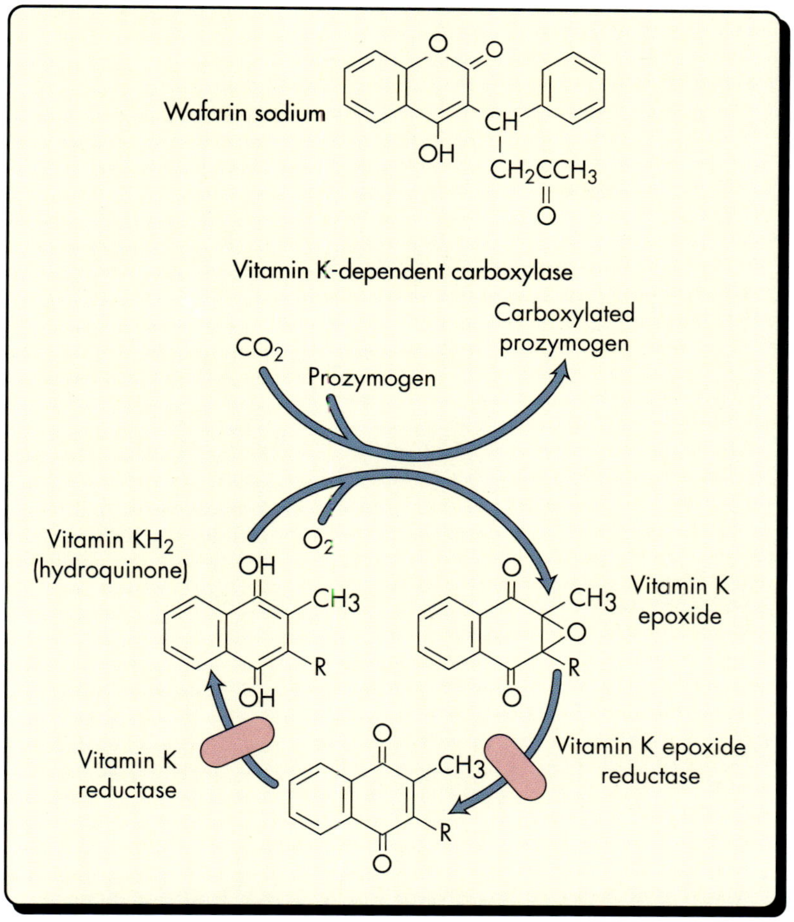

Figure 9-44. Mechanism of action of the vitamin K antagonists. Vitamin K antagonists, such as warfarin sodium, prevent the generation of reduced vitamin K by inhibition of the enzyme vitamin K epoxide reductase [61]. In the absence of reduced vitamin K, the procoagulant factors II, VII, IX, and X are unable to synthesize the carboxylated calcium binding sites necessary for formation of phospholipid-bound activation complexes. Vitamin K antagonists inhibit the activity of the anticoagulant proteins C and S by a similar mechanism. (*From* Furie and coworkers [62].)

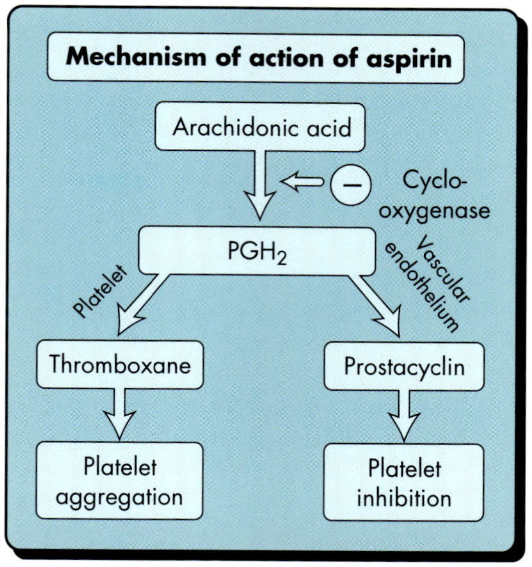

Figure 9-45. Mechanism of action of aspirin. Aspirin and nonsteroidal anti-inflammatory drugs inhibit the enzyme cyclooxygenase, thereby preventing the formation of the prostanoid intermediate PGH_2 from arachidonic acid. Inhibition of cyclooxygenase disrupts the generation of both thromboxane and prostacyclin. Although platelet synthesis of thromboxane is inhibited for the life of the platelet, vascular endothelial synthesis of prostacyclin resumes as cyclooxygenase activity returns [63].

REFERENCES

1. Macfarlane RG: An enzyme cascade in the blood clotting mechanism and its function as a biochemical amplifier. *Nature* 1964, 202:498–499.
2. Davie EW, Ratnoff OD: Waterfall sequence of intrinsic blood coagulation. *Science* 1964, 145:1310–1312.
3. Kalafatis M, Swords NA, Rand MD, Mann KG: Membrane-dependent reactions in blood coagulation: role of the vitamin K-dependent enzyme complexes. *Biochimica et Biophysica Acta* 1994, 1227:113–129.
4. Marcus AJ, Safier LB: Thromboregulation: multicellular modulation of platelet reactivity in hemostasis and thrombosis. *FASEB* 1993,7:516–522.
5. Furie B, Furie BC: Molecular and cellular biology of blood coagulation. *N Engl J Med* 1992, 326:800–806.
6. Slaughter TF: The coagulation system and cardiac surgery. In *Cardiac Anesthesia: Principles and Clinical Practice*. Edited by Estafanous FG, Barash PG, Reves JG, *et al.* Philadelphia: JB Lippincott; 1994:622, 623, 628.
7. Doolittle RF: The Molecular Biology of Fibrin. In *The Molecular Basis of Blood Diseases*, edn 2. Edited by Stamatoyannopoulos G, Nienhuis AW, Majerus PW, Varmus H. Philadelphia: WB Saunders; 1994:701—723.
8. Schmaier AH: Contact Activation. In *Thrombosis and Hemorrhage*. Edited by Loscalzo J, Schafer AI. Boston: Blackwell Publications; 1994:87–105.
9. Gailani D, Broze GJ: Factor XI activation in a revised model of blood coagulation. *Science* 1991, 253:909–912 .
10. Bach RR: Initiation of coagulation by tissue factor. *Crit Rev Biochem* 1988, 23:339–368.
11. Colucci M, Balconi G, Lorenzet R, *et al.*: Cultured human endothelial cells generate tissue factor in response to endotoxin. *J Clin Invest* 1983, 71:1893–1896.
12. Rivers RPA, Hathaway WE, Weston WL: The endotoxin-induced coagulant activity of human monocytes. *Br J Haematol* 1975, 30:311–316.
13. Nemerson Y: The tissue factor pathway of blood coagulation. In *Hemostasis and Thrombosis: Basic Principles and Clinical Practice*, edn 3. Edited by Colman RW, Hirsh J, Marder VJ, Salzman EW. Philadelphia: JB Lippincott; 1994:81–93.
14. Wilcox JN, Smith KM, Schwartz SM, Gordon D: Localization of tissue factor in the normal vessel wall and in the atherosclerotic plaque. *Proc Natl Acad Sci USA* 1989, 86:2839–2843.

15. Mann KG, Nesheim ME, Church WR, *et al.*: Surface-dependent reactions of the vitamin K dependent enzyme complexes. Blood *1990,* 76:1–16.
16. Rosenberg RD, Bauer KA: Prothrombinase generation and the regulation of coagulation. In *Thrombosis and Hemorrhage.* Edited by Loscalzo J, Schafer AI. Boston: Blackwell Scientific Publications; 1994:13–25.
17. Van Dieijen G, Tans G, Rosing J, Hember HC: The role of phospholipid and factor VIIIa in activation of bovine factor X. *J Biol Chem* 1981, 256:3433–3442.
17a. Bartha K, Brisson C, Archipoff G, *et al.*: Thrombin regulates tissue factor and thrombomodulin mRNA levels and activities in human saphenous vein endothelial cells by distinct mechanisms. *J Biol Chem* 1993, 268:421–429.
18. Levin EG, Marzec U, Anderson J, Harker LA: Thrombin stimulates tissue plasminogen activator release from cultured human endothelial cells. *J Clin Invest* 1984, 74:1988–1995.
19. Mossesson MW: The roles of fibrinogen and fibrin in hemostasis and thrombosis. *Sem Hematol* 1992, 29:177–88.
20. Mosesson MW: Fibrin polymerization and its regulatory role in hemostasis. *J Lab Clin Med* 1990, 116:8–17.
21. Carr ME, Hermans J: Size and density of fibrin fibers from turbidity. Macromolecules *1978, 11:46–158.*
22 Sakata Y, Aoki N: Significance of cross-linking of alpha 2 plasmin inhibitor to fibrin inhibition of fibrinolysis and in hemostasis. *J Clin Invest* 1982, 69:536–542.
23. Coleman RW, Marder VJ, Salzman EW, Hirsh J: Overview of Hemostasis. In *Hemostasis and Thrombosis: Basic Principles and Clinical Practice*, edn. 3. Edited by Colman RW, Hirsh J, Marder VJ, Salzman EW. Philadelphia: JB Lippincott;1994:7, 3–18.
24. Lorand L, Losowsky MS, Miloszewski KJ: Human factor XIII: fibrin-stabilizing factor. *Prog Hemost Thromb* 1980, 5:245–290.
25. Greenberg CS: Fibrin formation and stabilization. In *Thrombosis and Hemorrhage.* Edited by Loscalzo J, Schafer AI. Boston: Blackwell Scientific Publications; 1994:107–126.
26. Greenberg CS, Birckbichler PJ, Rice RH: Transglutaminases: multifunctional cross-linking enzymes that stabilize tissues. *FASEB* 1991, 5:3071–3077.
27. Cohen I: The contractile system of blood platelets and its function. *Methods Achieve Exp Pathol* 1979, 9:40–86.
28. Rappaport SI: *Introduction to Hematology*, edn 2. Philadelphia: JB Lippincott; 1987: 439.
29. Lind SE: Platelet morphology. In *Thrombosis and Hemorrhage.* Edited by J Loscalzo, AI Schafer. Boston: Blackwell Scientific Publications; 1994:201–218.
30. Ware JA, Coller BS: Platelet morphology, biochemistry, and function. In *William's Hematology*, edn 5. Edited by Beutler E, Lichtman MA, Coller BS, Kipps TJ. New York: McGraw-Hill; 1995:1164, 1170–1171.
31. George JN, Shattil SJ: The clinical importance of acquired abnormalities of platelet function. *N Engl J Med* 1991, 324:27–39.
32. Hawiger J: Adhesive interactions of blood cells and the vascular wall. In *Hemostasis and Thrombosis. Basic Principles and Clinical Practice*, edn 3. Edited by Colman W, Hirsh J, MarderVJ, Salzman EW. Philadelphia: JB Lippincott; 1994:762–796.
33. Lopez JA: The platelet glycoprotein Ib-IX complex. *Blood Coag Fibrinolysis* 1994, 5:97–119.
34. Phillips DR, Charo IF, Parise LV, Fitzgerald LA: The platelet membrane glycoprotein IIb-IIIa complex. *Blood* 1988, 71:831–843.
35. Harker LA, Mann KG: Thrombosis and fibrinolysis. In *Thrombosis in Cardiovascular Disorders.* Edited by Fuster V, Verstraete M. Philadelphia: WB Saunders; 1992, 1–16.
36. Vu T-KH, Wheaton VI, Hung DT, Coughlin SR: Molecular cloning of a functional thrombin receptor reveals a novel proteolytic mechanism of receptor activation. *Cell* 1991, 64:1057–1068.
37. Vu T-KH, Wheaton VI, Hung DT, *et al.*: Domains specifying thrombin-receptor interaction. *Nature* 1991, 353:674–677.
38. Kroll MH, Schafer AI: Biochemical mechanisms of platelet activation. *Blood* 1989, 74:1181–1195.
39. Sadler JE: Von Willebrand factor. *J Biol Chem* 1991, 266:22777–22780.
40. Montgomery RR, Coller BS: von Willebrand Disease. In *Hemostasis and Thrombosis: Basic Principles and Clinical Practice*, edn 3. Edited by Colman RW, Hirsh J, Marder VJ, Salzman EW. Philadelphia: JB Lippincott; 1994:134–168.
41. Rodeghiero F, Castaman G, Dini E: Epidemiological investigation of the prevalence of von Willebrand's disease. *Blood* 1987, 69:454–459.
42. Triplett DA: Laboratory diagnosis of von Willebrand's disease. *Mayo Clin Proc* 1991, 66:832–840.
43. Collen D: On the regulation and control of fibrinolysis. *Thromb Haemost* 1980, 43:77–89.
44. Hoylaerts M, Rijken DC, Lijnen HR, Collen D: Kinetics of the activation of plasminogen by human tissue plasminogen activator. Role of fibrin. *J Biol Chem* 1982, 257:2912–2919.
45. Hoylaerts M, Lijnen HR, Collen D: Studies on the mechanism of antifibrinolytic action of tranexamic acid. *Biochim Biophys Acta* 1981,673:75–85.
46. Haverkale F, Timan G, Nieuwenhuizen W: Anticlotting properties of fragments D from human fibrinogen and fibrin. *Eur J Clin Invest* 1979, 9:253–255.
47. Omar MN, Mann KG: Inactivation of factor Va by plasmin. *J Biol Chem* 1987, 262:9750–9755.
48. Erickson LA, Fici GJ, Lund JE, *et al.*: Development of venous occlusions in mice transgenic for the plasminogen activator inhibitor-1 gene. *Nature* 1990, 346:74–76.
49. Pratt CW, Church FC: Antithrombin: structure and function. *Semin Hematol* 1991, 28:3–9.
50. Broze GJ, Jr, Tollefsen DM: Regulation of blood coagulation by protease inhibitors. In *The Molecular Basis of Blood Diseases*, edn 2. Edited by Stamatoyannopoulos G, Nienhuis AW, Majerus PW, Varmus H. Philadelphia: WB Saunders; 1994:629–656.
51. Esmon CT: The roles of protein C and thrombomodulin in the regulation of blood coagulation. *J Biol Chem* 1989, 264:4743–4746.
52. Broze GJ: Why do hemophiliacs bleed? *Hosp Pract* 1992, 27:71–87.
53. Marcus AJ, Brockman MJ, Drosopoulos JHF, *et al.*: The endothelial cell ecto- ADPase responsible for inhibition of platelet function is CD39. *J Clin Invest* 1997, 99:1351–1360.
54. Radomski MW, Palmer RMJ, Moncada S: Comparative pharmacology of endothelium-derived relaxing factor, nitric oxide and prostacyclin in platelets. *Br J Pharmacol* 1987, 92:181–187.
55. Vignano G, Benigni A, Bool, SD,*et al.*: Recombinant human erythropoietin to correct uremic bleeding. *Am J Kidney Dis* 1991, 18:44–49.
56. Kyrle PA, Stockenhuber F, Brenner B, *et al.*: Evidence for an increased generation of prostacyclin in the micovasculature and an impairment of the platelet α-granule release in chronic renal failure. *Thromb Haemost* 1988, 60:205–208.
57. Remuzzi G, Perico N, Zoja C, *et al.*: Role of endothelium-derived nitric oxide in the bleeding tendency of uremia. *J Clin Invest* 1990, 86:1768–1771.
58. Carr JM: Disseminated intravascular coagulation in cirrhosis. *Hepatology* 1989, 10:103–110.
59. Bick RL: Disseminated intravascular coagulation and related syndromes: a clinical review. *Semin Thromb Hemost* 1988, 14:299–338.
60. Hirsh J: Heparin. *N Engl J Med* 1991, 324:1565–1574.
61. Hirsh J: Oral anticoagulant drugs. *N Engl J Med* 1991, 324:1865–1875.
62. Furie B, Liebman HA, Blanchard RA, *et al.*: Comparison of the native prothrombin antigen and the prothrombin time for monitoring oral anticoagulant therapy. *Blood* 1984, 64:445–451.
63. Weksler BB, Pett SB, Alonso D, *et al.*: Differential inhibition by aspirin of vascular and platelet prostaglandin synthesis in atherosclerotic patients. *N Engl J Med* 1983, 308:800–805.

10

Injury and Inflammation

Teiji Sawa, Jeanine P. Wiener-Kronish, and Michael A. Gropper

Inflammation consists of a panoply of responses by which the host defends itself against various injurious agents, including pathogens, and tissue trauma. Inflammatory responses include the responses that initiate structural and functional repair of injured tissue.

The earliest stages of inflammation include the release of vasoactive mediators from tissue mast cells (histamine, leukotrienes), platelets, and plasma components (bradykinin). This release results in vasodilation and edema formation and contributes to the rubor and calor associated with inflammatory processes. These local inflammatory response are followed by systemic responses known as the acute-phase reaction, in which the systemic production of the acute-phase reaction proteins is enhanced in the liver and in other organs to help host defense and promote tissue repair. Many chemical mediators that belong to the different cascades, such as the kinin system, the complement system, the lipid mediators, and the cytokines, play important roles not only in inducing these local inflammatory responses but also in mediating local responses to the systemic inflammatory reaction.

Activation of the kinin system, which includes kallikrein and bradykinin, leads to vasodilation and edema at a site of local inflammation. The kinin system can also activate the blood coagulation cascade, the fibrinolytic cascade, and the complement system. Through the activation of the complement cascade, C3a and C5a increase neurtrophil chemotaxis, C3b opsonizes foreign bodies, and the membrane attack complex enhances cytotoxicity of pathogens. Lipid mediators (prostaglandins, leukotrienes, platelet-activating factor or PAF) also contribute to these early responses. These mediators also cause vasodilation and lead to neutrophil chemotaxis to the inflammatory site.

Recent studies have shown that many cytokines play important roles in regulating the inflammatory response. The local release of cytokines—interleukin-1 (IL-1), interleukin-8 (IL-8), and tumor necrosis factor (TNF)—coordinates the inflammatory response in the local sites and promotes neutrophil chemotaxis to sites of inflammation. Some cytokines released from local inflammatory sites, such as IL-1, IL-6, and TNF, mediate the systemic response by inducing fever, the acute-phase reaction, and neutrophil mobilization from the bone marrow and promote lymphocyte proliferation. Some biologic functions are mediated by more than one cytokine, and each cytokine has many different functions; these features of the cytokines are called *functional redundancy* and *pleiotrophy*. The molecular mechanism of these characteristics of the cytokines has been elucidated through investigation of the structure of the cytokine receptors and investigation of the mechanisms of receptor signaling. These new insights have improved our understanding of the complexity of the cytokine network.

A complex interplay of these diverse systems usually leads to tissue repair and to the return of normal structure and function. Under unclear conditions, chronic inflammation occurs instead, leading to the persistence of pathogens and granuloma formation. For unknown reasons irreversible injury of tissue occurs, apparently when the host response is inadequate or too exuberant or when the insult is overwhelming and has disabled normal host defenses.

The cells and plasma systems involved in the inflammatory response are reviewed in this chapter, and the complement, cytokine, and cyclooxygenase systems are explored for their importance and their complex interactions in this fundamental lifesaving response.

ACUTE PHASE OF INFLAMMATION

Response / Cascades	Acute phase: Early stage (minutes to hours) Vasodilation →	Edema →	Chemotaxis (Adhesion)	(Chemotactic factors)
Mast cells Platelets	Histamine Serotonin	Histamine Serotonin	Histamine	
Plasma components	Bradykinin			
Complement		C5a/3a	C5a/3a	C5a/3a
Cytokine			IL-1 IL-8 TNF	IL-8
Lipid mediators	LTC_4/D_4 PGE_2/I_2 PAF	LTC_4/B_4 PAF	PAF	LTB_4

Figure 10-1. The acute phase of inflammation. The major acute responses such as vasodilation, edema formation, and chemotaxis are mediated by several chemical mediators from several different cascades. Vasodilation and edema formation are mediated by histamine, serotonin, bradykinin, fragments of the complement system (C5a, C3a), leukotrienes (LTC_4, D_4), prostaglandins (PGE_2, I_2), and PAF. Neutrophil chemotaxis is mediated by histamine, fragments of the complement system (C5a, C3a), cytokines (IL-1, IL-8, TNF), PAF, and leukotriene B_4 (LTB_4).

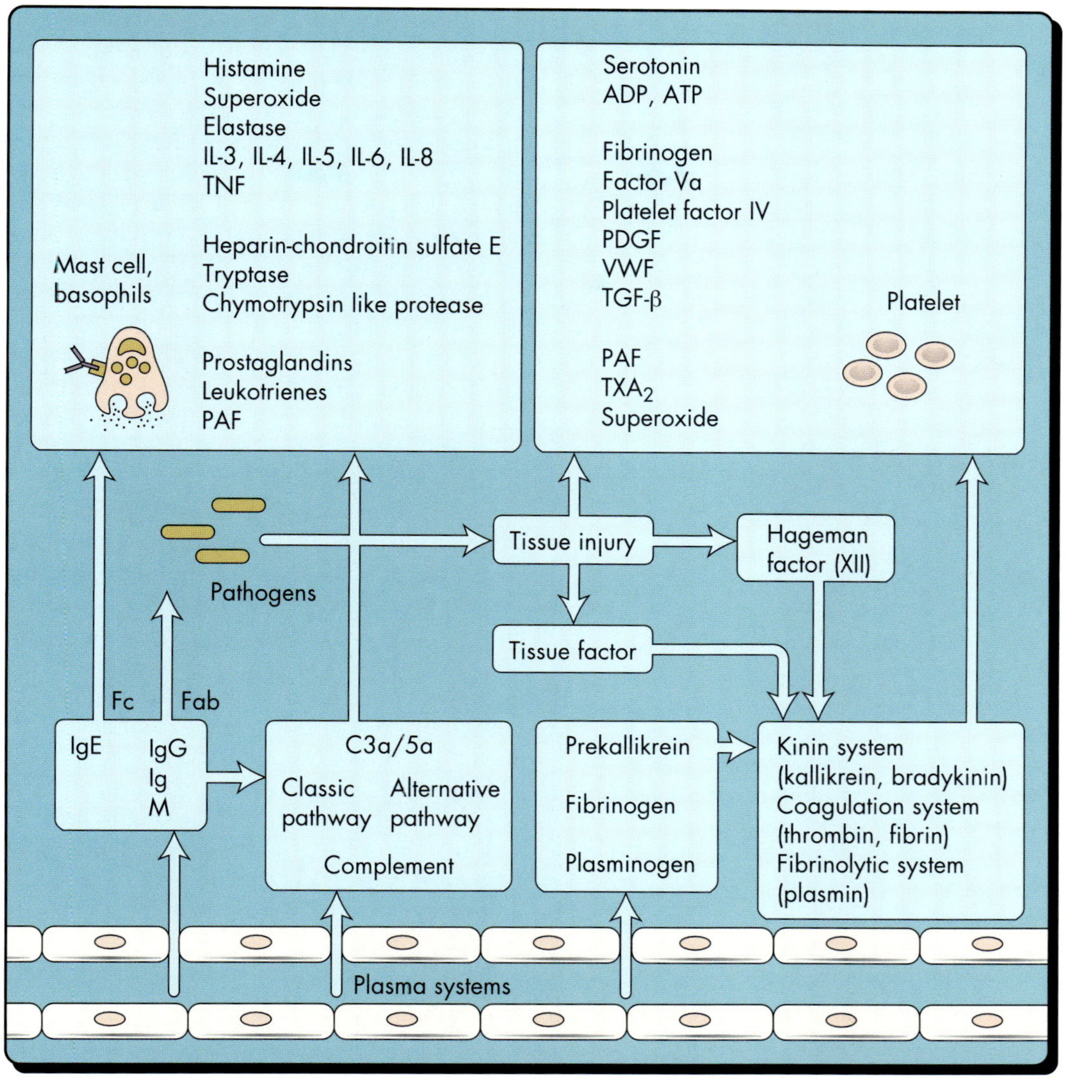

Figure 10-2. Products from cells and plasma systems that mediate inflammation. Mast cells, basophils and platelets are important sources of histamine and serotonin (5-hydroxytryptamine), which produce vasodilatation, increase vascular permeability, and lead to edema formation. The immune system can interact with these cells and cause the release of these mediators; mast cells and basophils have high affinity receptors for IgE, which allow the antigen-specific triggering of granule release from the cells. Mast cell mediators include the preformed and eluted (histamine, superoxide, elastase, cytokines such as IL-3, IL-4, IL-5, IL-6, IL-8, and TNF), the preformed and granule-associated (heparin-chondroitin sulfate E, tryptase, chymotrypsin), and the newly generated (leukotrienes C_4, D_4, E_4, PAF, prostaglandin D_2). Platelets produce serotonin, ADP, ATP, fibrinogen, factor Va, platelet factor 4, platelet-derived growth factor (PDGF), von Willebrand factor (VWF), transforming growth factor-β (TGF-β), PAF, thromboxane A_2 (TXA_2), superoxide, and so forth.

Several plasma systems have a role in inflammation, including the kinin system, the coagulation system, the fibrinolytic system, immunoglobulins, and the complement system. The Fab portion of the immunoglobulins can bind to epitopes on target antigens whereas the Fc portion can bind to inflammatory cells, which leads to complement activation.

Activation of the coagulation can be initiated in inflammation if factor XII occurs or procoagulants are formed, such as tissue factor. When thrombin forms at inflammatory sites, platelet aggregation occurs and platelets and endothelial cells secrete more inflammatory mediators.

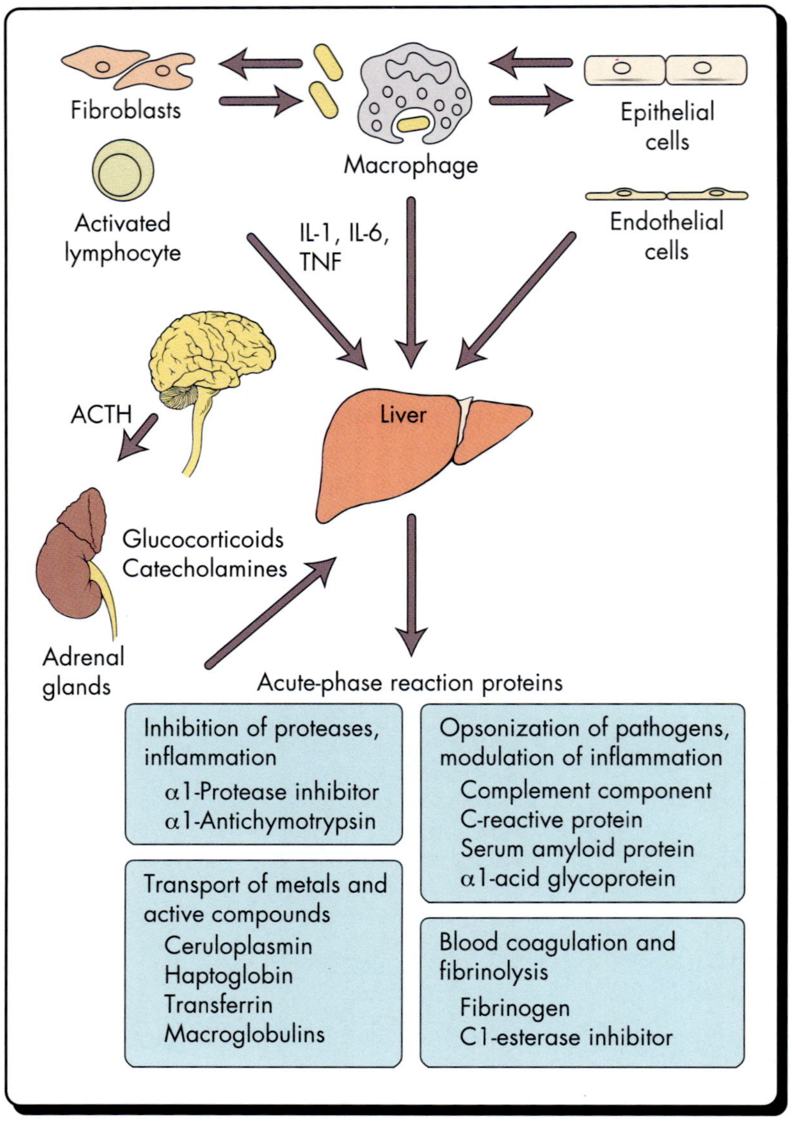

Figure 10-3. The acute phase reaction. Once inflammation has occurred, a rapid change in the pattern of hepatic protein synthesis occurs. Multiple cytokines produce this change; supernatants from stimulated macrophages cause liver cells *in vitro* to produce proteins typical of the acute-phase reaction. Hormones also influence this pattern of hepatic protein production; sex steroid hormones particularly influence the synthesis of pregnacy zone protein, a member of the α_2-macroglobulin family. Glucocorticoids decrease the acute-phase reaction; IL-1 and IL-6 both induce the production of corticotrophin (ACTH) in the pituitary, which stimulates the production of glucocorticoids in the adrenal cortex.

The acute-phase reaction proteins are also made outside the liver. Monocytes and neutrophils produce α1-protease inhibitor and monocytes produce C3, C4, factor B, and other complement components. The choroid plexus also produces transthyretin and transferrin.

The proteins produced by the liver during the acute-phase reaction are all helpful to the patient for host defense against infection as well as for tissue repair. Serum amyloid A is a protein that increases 100- to 1000-fold in the serum after an inflammatory stimulus. This protein is found in association with high-density lipoprotein 3, suggesting that serum amyloid A may be useful in the elimination of the lipids or toxins derived from pathogens that associate with lipoproteins. The other acute-phase proteins include C-reactive protien, which is produced in great quantities during an acute-phase reaction. This protein binds to a large number of microorganisms (including the C polysaccharide of *Streptococcus pneumoniae*), as well as to polysaccharides, phospholipids, and polycations.

Acid glycoprotein (orosomucoid) has an extremely high carbohydrate content. The polysaccharide chains of this protein appear to be important for the ability of the protein to interact with parasites, including those causing malaria.

Haptoglobin binds to hemoglobin and helps dispose of hemoglobin at sites of inflammation. Haptoglobin may have antiprotease activity and may be able to modify prostaglandin production. Haptoglobin also appears to affect the immune system; *in vitro* the addition of haptoglobin suppresses lymphocyte blastogenesis and monocyte chemotaxis.

Fibrinogen is very important in coagulation but is also an opsonin for staphylococci and streptococci. Fibrinogen also affects the immune system by blocking T-cell mitogen reactions and macrophage chemotaxis.

α1-Proteinase inhibitor is the major protease inhibitor in plasma; this inhibitor stops serine proteases in the coagulation, fibrinolytic, kinin, and complement systems. Patients deficient in this proteinase inhibitor can develop emphysema at a young age from the unopposed lung tissue destruction that occurs if they smoke.

Ceruloplasmin is the major transporter of copper. This protein may also be able to scavenge oxygen radicals and may be important for the removal of iron from hemoglobin. Finally, complement proteins B, C, and C4 are important in host defense against pathogens.

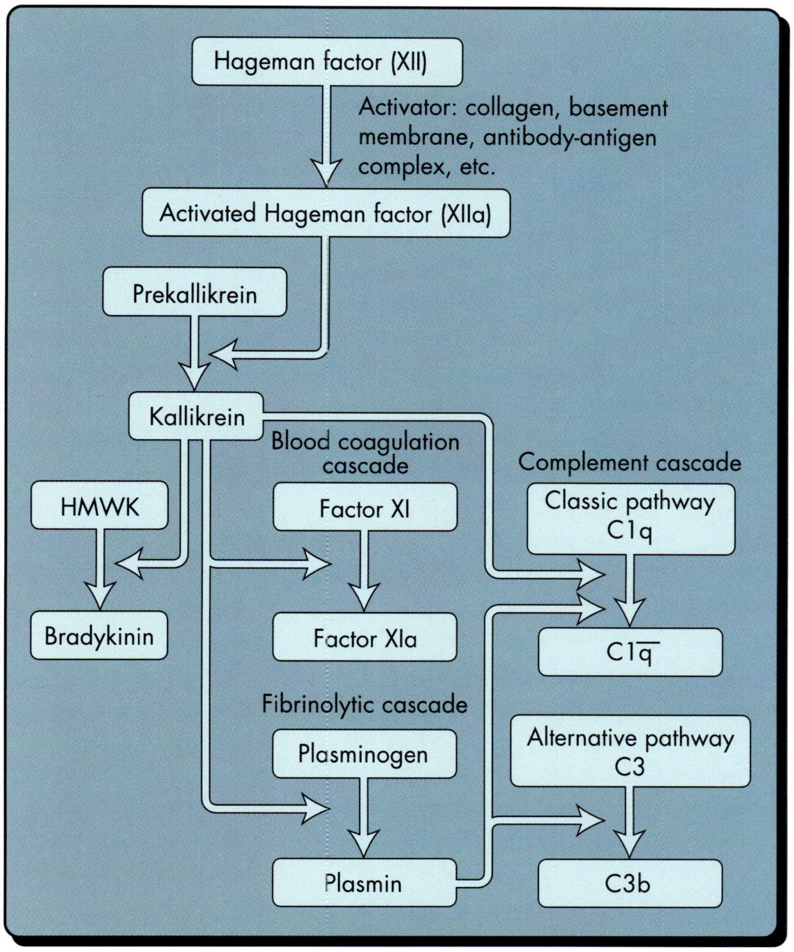

Figure 10-4. Activation of the kinin system. The immediate response to injurious agents includes the fast-acting mediators, including products of the kinin system and products from mast cells, basophils, and platlets. Activated Hageman factor (XIIa) acts on prekallikrein to generate kallikrein, which releases bradykinin. Kallikrein also activates complement via C1q and activates both the coagulation and fibrinolytic cascades by activating both factor XI and plasminogen.

Bradykinin is a potent vasoactive peptide that causes smooth muscle contraction, increased vascular permeability, venular dilatation, electrolye secretion, activation of phospholipase A_2, ion transport, and cellular proliferation. Activation of the kallikrein-kinin system is thought to occur in septic shock; activation of factor XII might be due to endotoxin or to TNF. Other disease states that have been associated with activation of the kinin system include carcinoid syndrome, allergic rhinitis, postgastrectomy dumping syndrome, hereditary angioedema (due to a deficiency of C1 inhibitor), nephrotic syndrome, rheumatoid arthritis, and the adult respiratory distress syndrome. HMWK—high-molecular-weight kininogen.

ARACHIDONIC ACID METABOLITES IN INFLAMMATION

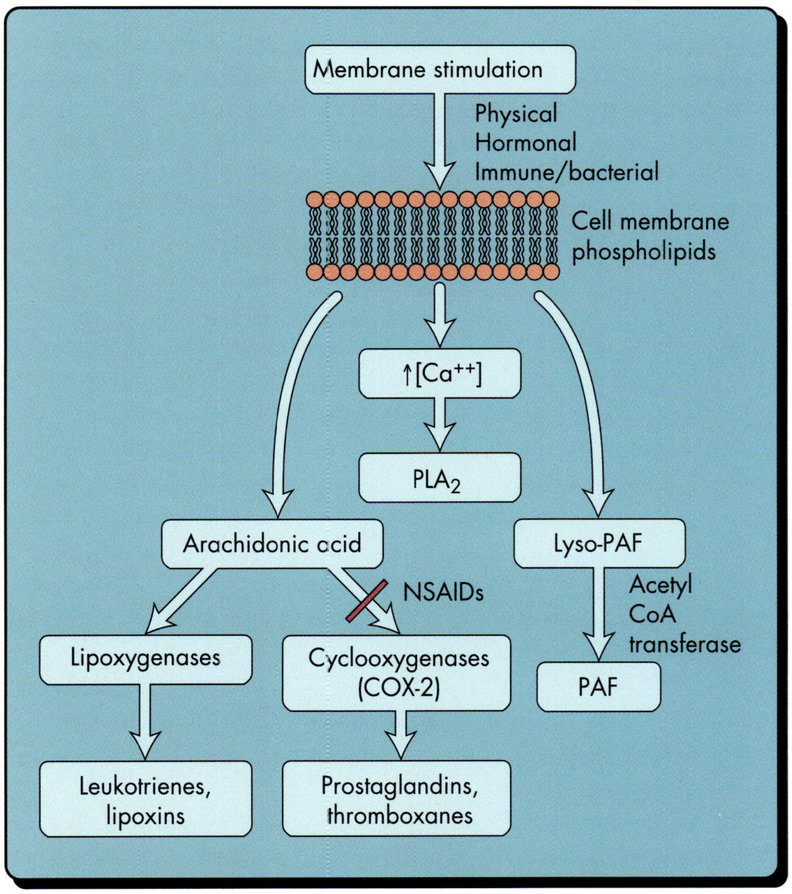

Figure 10-5. Overview of arachidonic acid metabolism. An essential component of the inflammatory response is the generation of lipid mediators. These mediators are not stored intracellularly but are formed through the breakdown of membrane phospholipids by the action of specific phospholipases. For example, phospholipase A_2 (PLA_2) is activated by an increase in intracellular calcium concentration, resulting in the liberation of arachidonic acid from phosphatidylcholine, phosphatidylethanolamine, or phosphatidylinositol. Free arachidonic acid can then be acted upon by cyclooxygenases or lipoxygenases resulting in the formation of prostaglandins (PGs), thromboxanes, leukotrienes, and lipoxins. PAF is formed through the action of PLA_2 on membrane-bound phosphatidylcholine, resulting in the liberation of lyso-PAF and free fatty acid. Lyso-PAF is acetylated by acetyl CoA transferase, yielding PAF. The initial step in the production of these lipid mediators is the activation of PLA_2. A number of different stimuli can result in an increase in intracellular calcium, including cell injury, hormones, and other mediators including cytokines, chemokines, and lipids. This mechanism allows the cell to respond to a number of different stimuli with generation of lipid mediators. The biologic actions of the PGs and PAF are many. NSAIDs—nonsteroidal anti-inflammatory drugs.

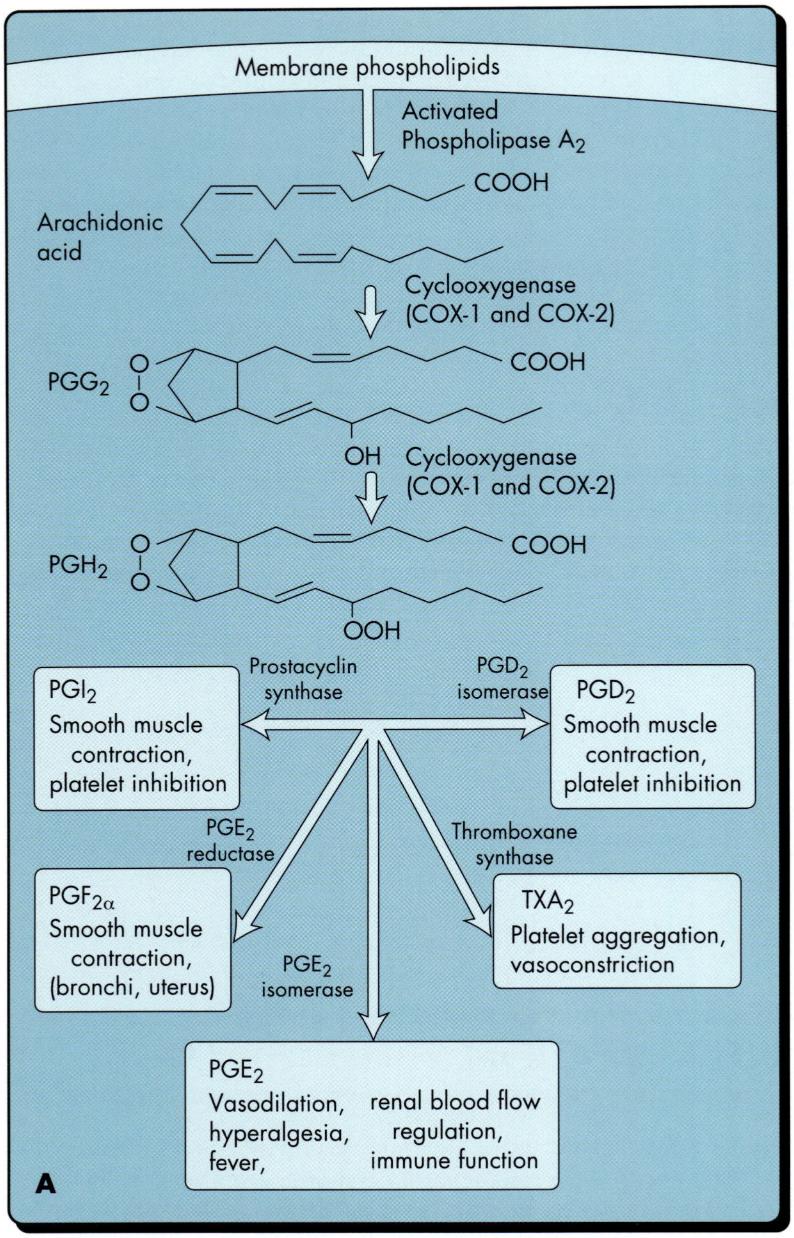

Figure 10-6. Formation of prostaglandins. Prostaglandins (PGs) (**A** and **B**) are the major product of arachidonic acid metabolism in mammalian cells. The basic structure of PG is a 20-carbon carboxylic acid containing a cyclopentane ring. Oxygen substitution at different positions of the cyclopentane ring results in formation of the different species of PGs (PGD, PGE, PGF, PGG, and PGH). Cyclooxygenase (also known as PG endoperoxide G/H synthase) has two catalytic activities; cyclization of arachidonic acid to form PGG_2 and hydroperoxidation of PGG_2 to form PGH_2. PGH_2 is acted upon by specific synthases to result in formation of specific PGs and thromboxanes. Cell-specific expression of the various synthase enzymes determines the PG profile in different cell types. For example, renal endothelial cells produce primarily prostacyclin, whereas platelets produce mostly thromboxanes. Recent experiments have demonstrated the existence of two isoforms of cyclooxygenase, termed COX-1 and COX-2. COX-1 is thought to be the constitutive form of the enzyme, responsible for cellular "housekeeping" functions including gastric protection, epithelial differentiation, and regulation of renal blood flow. Regular use of aspirin has been shown to decrease the incidence of colon cancer, which is mediated through COX-1 inhibition. COX-2, which is not normally present in unstimulated cells, is induced with various inflammatory stimuli. Both isoforms of cyclooxygenase are inhibited by aspirin and glucocorticoids. Specific inhibitors of the COX-2 isoform are currently under development.

B. BIOLOGIC ACTIVITY OF PROSTAGLANDINS AND PAF

Agent	Biologic Activity
PGD_2	Smooth muscle contraction
	Inhibition of platelet aggregation
PGE_2	Increase in vascular permeability
	Pain
	Vasodilation
	Immunomodulation
	Fever
	Regulation of renal blood flow/natriuresis
	Gastric protection
$PGF_{2\alpha}$	Smooth muscle contraction, bronchoconstriction, uterine contraction
PGI_2	Vasodilation
	Inhibition of platelet aggregation
TXA_2	Platelet aggregation
	Vasoconstriction
PAF	Neurophil and platelet activation
	Anaphylactoid reaction
	Vasoconstriction
	Increased vascular permeability
	Bronchoconstriction
	Stimulation of eicosanoid production

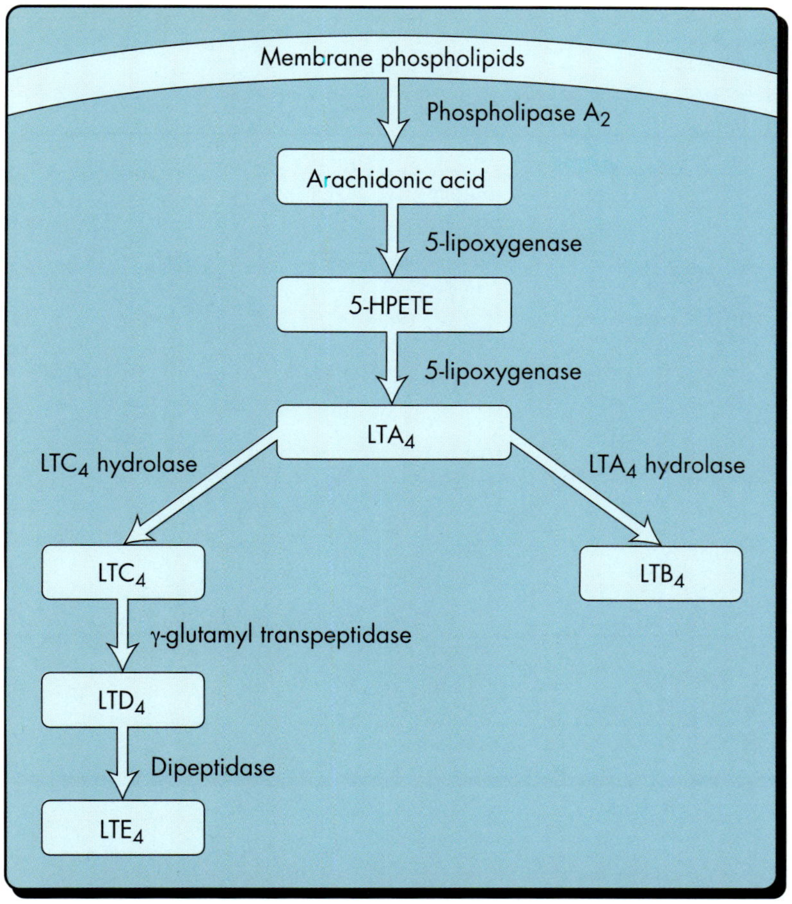

Figure 10-7. Formation of leukotrienes. Leukotrienes (LTs) are formed through the action of the lipoxygenase family of enzymes on arachidonic acid. The enzyme 5-lipoxygenase catalyzes the insertion of an oxygen at C-5 of arachidonic acid and the subsequent formation of a hydroperoxide (hydroperoxy eicosatetranoic acid [HPETE]) and then a peroxide LTA_4. LTA_4 is then hydrated or conjugated to form other members of the LT family. The combination of LTC_4, LTD_4, and LTE_4 when released by mast cells was previously referred to as slow-reacting substance of anaphylaxis. Not all cells contain the 5-lipoxygenase enzyme. These cells may participate in "transcellular metabolism" by taking up LTA_4 produced by other cells and then performing subsequent conversion into other LTs. LTB_4 is a very potent stimulator of neutrophil activity, resulting in margination at endothelial cells, degranulation, diapedesis, and generation of the respiratory burst with superoxide generation and activation of eicosanoid synthesis. This stimulation improves the ability of neutrophils to both phagocytose and kill bacteria. LTB_4 acts synergistically with PGE_2 to increase vascular permeability and has been identified as an important mediator of arthritis, cystic fibrosis, and psoriasis. LTC_4, LTD_4, and LTE_4 are referred to as the "peptido"-LTs and act to cause smooth muscle constriction in the lung and blood vessels in addition to increasing vascular permeability. These compounds have been implicated in hypersensitivity reactions and asthma. All the LTs have been demonstrated to have both cellular and humoral immunomodulatory effects.

Lipoxins are formed by the interaction of lipoxygenase with arachidonic acid, particularly the oxygenation of LTA_4 in platelets. These compounds have been demonstrated to cause neutrophil chemotaxis but not adhesion or diapedesis (unlike LTB_4). These compounds appear to have an anti-inflammatory role in inhibiting the activity of natural killer cells and blocking the activity of LTC_4 and LTD_4. High levels of lipoxins have been found in the lavage fluid of patients with pneumonia, the significance of which is unclear.

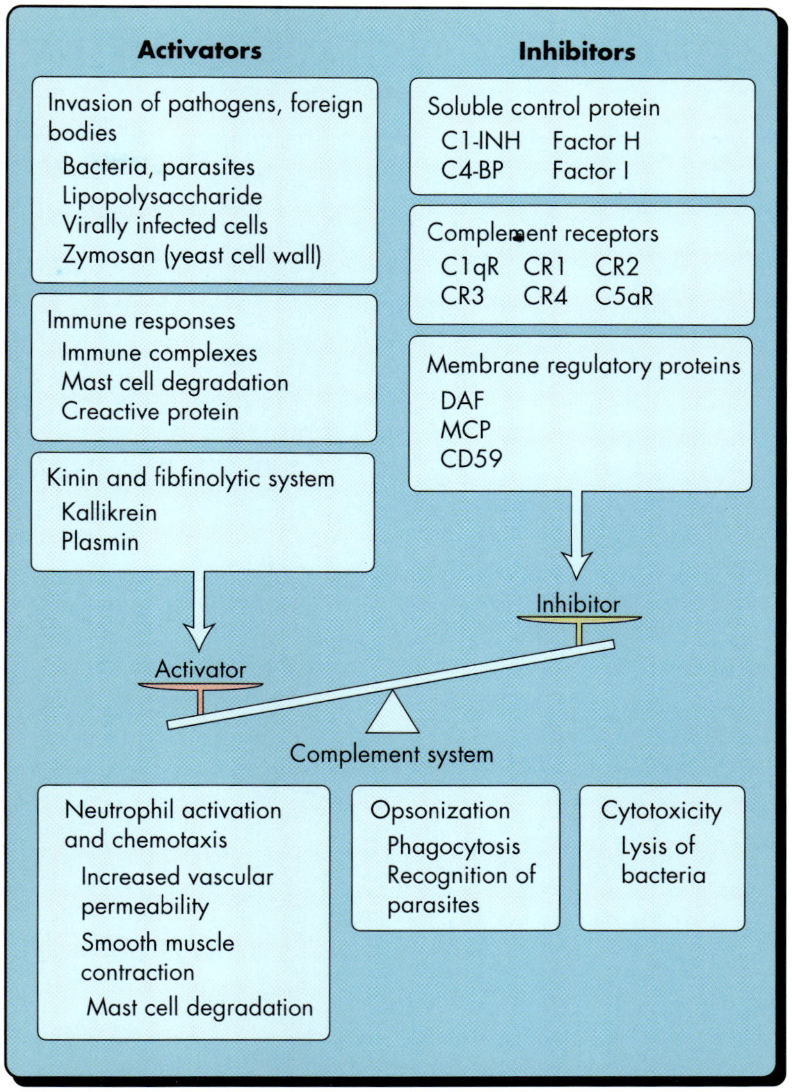

Figure 10-8. The complement system. The complement system is composed of distinct proteins, including regulatory and inhibitory proteins. The complement components are inactive in the circulation and become sequentially activated after some inciting event. Complement activation occurs after many events, including mast cell degranulation; bacterial invasion (secondary to contact with microbial polysaccharides, endotoxin, or immunoglobulin bound to the pathogen); the aggregation of antibodies; or the exposure to proteases, urate crystals, yeast cells, x-ray contrast material, or dialysis membranes. Kallikrein activates C1q (as well as plasminogen). Complement activation leads to cytotoxicity and lysis as well as chemotaxis and smooth muscle contraction. DAF—decay-accelerating factor; MCP—membrane cofactor protein.

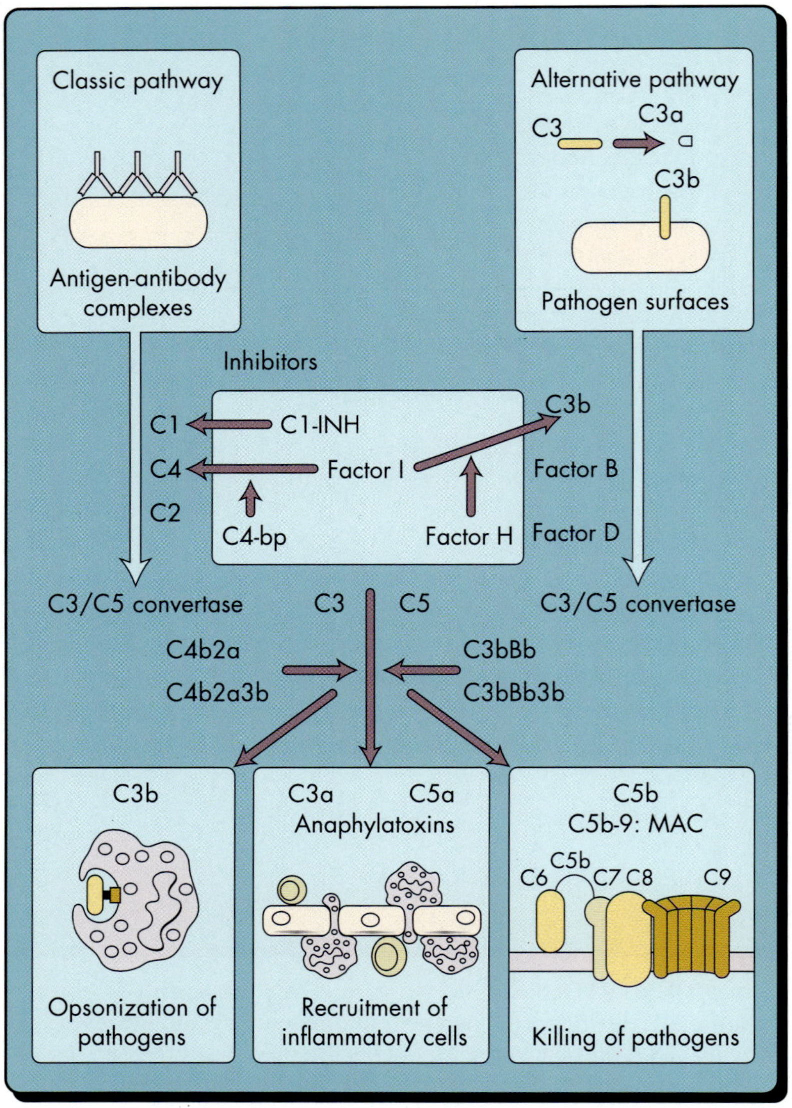

Figure 10-9. Overview of the complement cascade. There are two pathways of complement activation. The reactions that are activated by antibody binding to antigen as part of the adaptive humoral immunity are called the classic pathway, because this pathway was discovered first. The other pathway is called the alternative pathway; these reactions are triggered without antibody. The complement pathways are part of humans' "innate immunity" and probably arose early in evolution. Both pathways generate a protease called a C3/C5 convertase, which generates the main effector molecules. Three main consequences of complement activation are recruitment of inflammatory cells and opsonization and direct killing of pathogens.

The major components are numbered as they were discovered. Activated complement is symbolized by a *line* over the component. The cleavage products of complement proteins are designated by added lowercase letters (a, b, etc.). Note that, in the center of this cascade, there is an inhibitory system that regulates the activation of the both pathways. C1 inhibitor inhibits C1s, factor I inactivates C4b and C3b, factor H accelerates inactivation of C3b by factor I, and C4-binding protein accelerates cleavage of C4b by factor I. MAC—membrane attack complex.

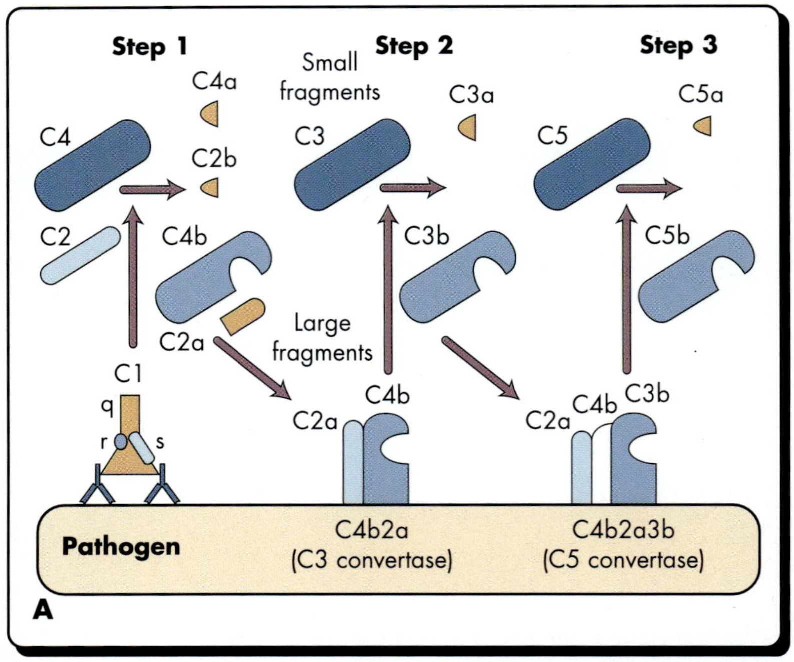

B. FUNCTIONS OF THE COMPONENTS OF THE CLASSICAL PATHWAY

Component	Fragment	Function
C1	C1q	Binds to IgM and IgG that has bound to antigen and activates C1r
	C1r	Cleaves C1s to yield the active serine protease
	C1s	Cleaves C4 into C4a and C4b, and C4a-bound C2 into C2a and C2b
C4	C4a	Weak mediator of inflammation
	C4b	Opsonizes the pathogen; binds C2 for cleavage by C1s
C2	C2b	Unknown
	C2a	Makes C3 convertase with C4b to cleave C3
C3	C3a	Mediator of inflammation
	C3b	Opsonizes the pathogen; Makes C5-convertase with C4b2a; amplifies the alternative pathway

Figure 10-10. The classic pathway. **A**, This pathway is initiated when C1 binds to either IgG or IgM antibodies that are fixed to antigens. C1 is composed of three subcomponents, C1q, C1r, and C1s. Binding of C1q to antibody activates C1r, which activates the serine protease C1s. Activated C1s cleaves C4 and C2 to form C4b2a, which is termed *C3 convertase*. This enzyme has the ability to cleave C3 to form two biologically important fragments, C3a and C3b. The bound C3b to the surface of the pathogen is the major opsonin of the complement system. In addition, C3b binds to C4b2a to form C4b2a3b, which is termed *C5 convertase*. Cleavage of C5 by this enzyme yields C5a and C5b. C5b leads to the membrane attack complex composed of C5b-9, which can lyse the pathogens.The small fragments, C3a and C5a, that are also formed are called anaphylatoxins. **B**, Functions of the components of the classical pathway. (Part B *adapted from* Janeway and Ravers [2]; with permission.)

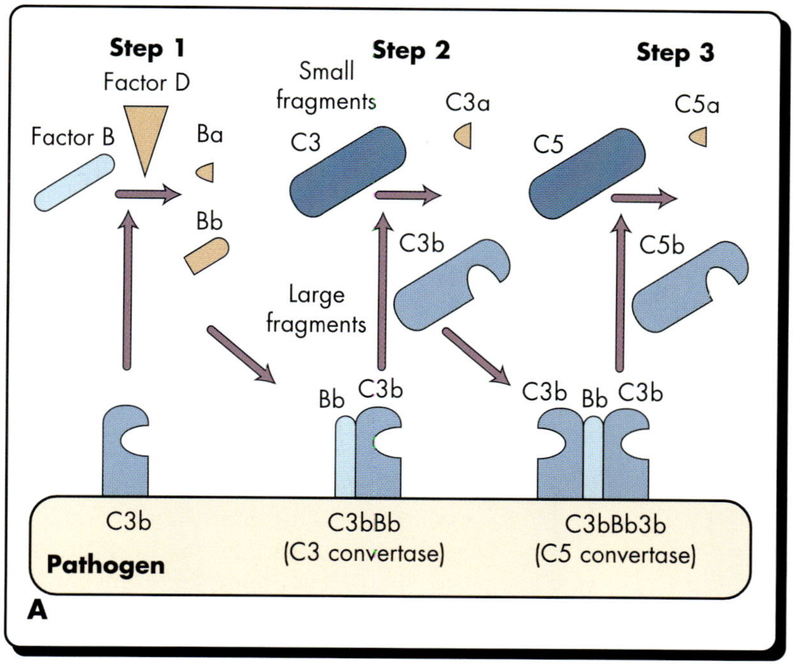

Figure 10-11. The alternative pathway. **A**, This pathway can be initiated directly by the surface of the pathogens, which facilitates the initial binding of a few molecules of naturally formed C3b to factor B. Bound factor B is then cleaved by plasma protease factor D into Ba and Bb to form C3bBb and C3bBb3b, which are termed *C3 convertase* and *C5 convertase*, respectively. These enzymes can cleave C3 to C3b and C5 to C5b to create a positive feedback cycle of this reaction, leading to the formation of the membrane attack complex. Note that the formation of the membrane attack complex occurs as a terminal event in both complement pathways. **B**, Functions of the components of the alternative pathway. (Part B *adapted from* Janeway and Ravers [2]; with permission.)

B. FUNCTIONS OF THE COMPONENTS OF THE ALTERNATIVE PATHWAY

Component	Fragment	Function
C3	C3a	Mediator of inflammation
	C3b	Opsonizes the pathogen; binds to factor B for cleavage by factor D and makes C3 convertase with Bb and C5 convertase with C3bBb; amplifies the alternative pathway
Factor B	Ba	Unknown
	Bb	Makes C3/C5 convertase with C3b
Factor D		Cleaves C3b-bound factor B into Ba and Bb

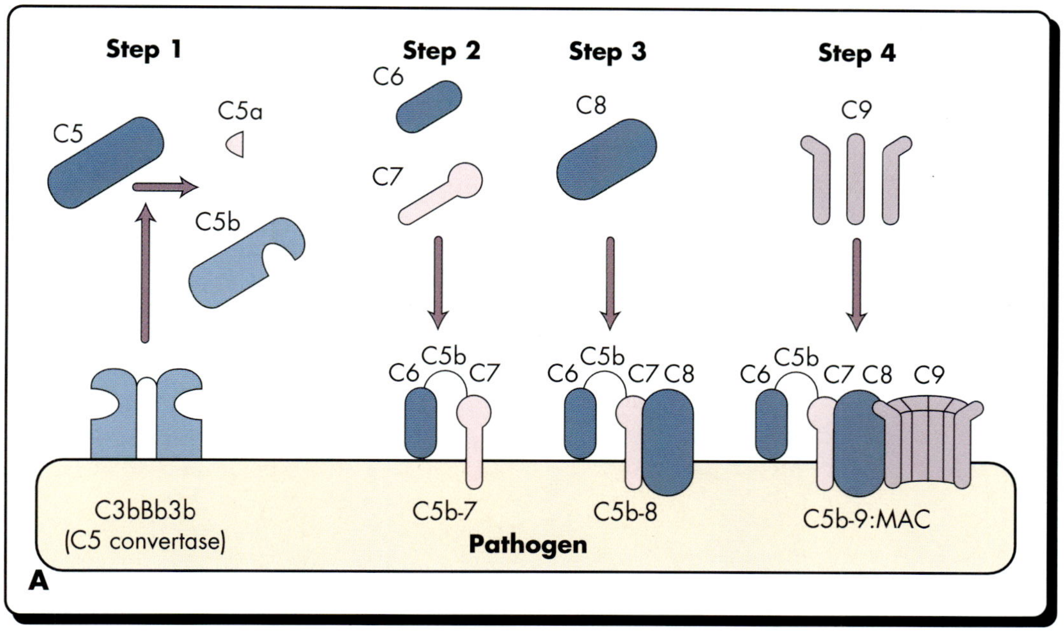

Figure 10-12. The membrane attack complex (MAC). **A**, This complex is formed when C5b67 inserts into the lipid bilayer and C8 and multiple molecules of C9 polymerize to form a cylindrical structure. The outer portion of this complex is lipophilic. The inner hydrophilic channel allows passage of water and small ions, so that the cell swells and cell lysis occurs. The membrane adjacent to the C5b-C9 complex may leak as well, as the complex disrupts the membrane lipids and phospholipids. Cells that can be disrupted by this complex include lymphocytes, erythrocytes, platelets, bacteria, viruses, virus-infected cells, tumor cells, spirochetes, and protozoa. **B**, Functions of the various fragments of the MAC. (Part B *adapted from* Janeway and Ravers [2]; with permission.)

B. FUNCTIONS OF THE COMPONENTS OF THE MAC

Component	Fragment	Function
C5	C5a	Strong mediator of inflammation
	C5b	Initiates making the MAC
C6		Bind C5b
C7		Binds C5b-6 and inserts in membrane
C8		Binds C5b-7 and initiates C9 polymerization
C9		Binds C5b-8 and forms membrane-spanning channel to lyse the pathogen

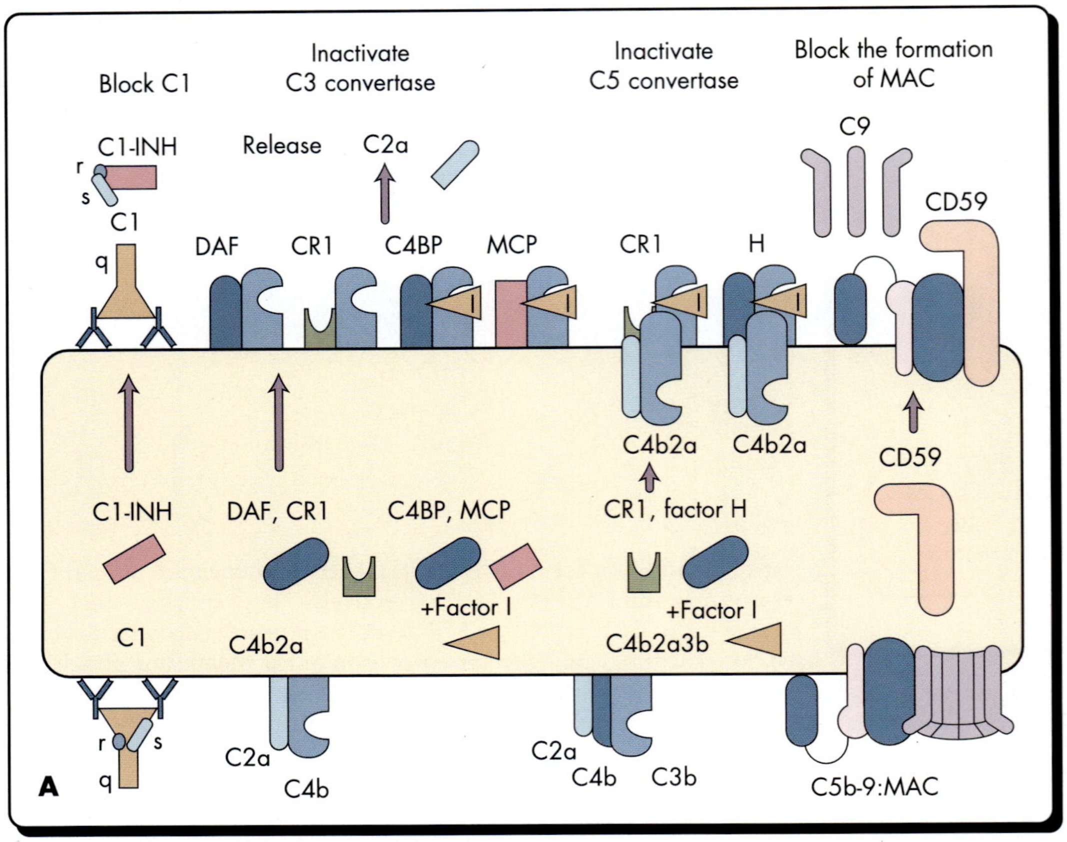

B. FUNCTIONS OF THE PROTEIN FRAGMENTS IN THE COMPLEMENT CASCADE

Protein	Component	Function
Soluble control protein	C1-INH	Binds to C1 and inactivates it
	C4-BP	Binds to C4b to inactivate C3 convertase with factor I
	Factor H	Binds C3b with C4-bp, factor H, MCP, or CR1
	Factor I	Cleaves C3b with C4-bp, factor H, MCP or Cr1
Receptor	CR1	Binds C4b or C3b to inactivate C3/C5 convertase with factor I
Membrane regulatory proteins	DAF	Membrane protein that binds C4b or C3b to inactivate C3/C5 convertase
	MCP	Membrane protein that binds C4b or C3b to inactivate C3/C5 convertase
	CD59	Prevents formation of MAC

Figure 10-13. The inhibitory system. **A**, The complement cascade is tightly regulated by proteins that are both in the fluid phase and membrane bound. The classic pathway is regulated by soluble and membrane-bound proteins. Three soluble control proteins are the C1 inhibitor (C1-INH), factor I, and C4 binding protein (C4 BP) . C1 inhibitor is a serine proteinase inhibitor that binds and inactivates C1r and C1s. Factor I breaks down C4b, blocking the formation of C4b2a. C4 binding protein also breaks down C4b and increases the dissociation of C2a from C4b2a. The membrane-bound proteins that regulate the classic pathway activation include the decay-accelerating factor (DAF), CR1, and membrane cofactor protein (MCP). DAF or CR1 inhibits the binding of C2 to C4b and either of these control proteins increases the dissociation of C2a from C4b2a. MCP or CR1 also increases the catabolism of C4b by factor I. The complement control proteins share a domain of about 60 amino acids. This family of proteins are encoded in a gene cluster on chromosome 1 and include factor H, C4-BP, DAF, MCP, and CR1 and CR2.

The alternative pathway is regulated by a protein in the soluble phase, factor H, of the complement control proteins. Factor H increases the dissociation of Bb from C3i and from C3b. Factor H also increases the catabolism of C3i and C3b by associating with factor I. The membrane-bound proteins that regulate the alternative pathway are DAF and CR1, again complement control proteins (and the membrane-bound proteins that regulated the classic pathway). DAF and CR1 increase the dissociation of the C3bBb C3 convertase enzyme, so that there is an increase in the release of C3b from the complex. CR1 and MCP are cofactors for factor I and increase the cleavage of C3b. CD59 is a protein that is anchored into the cell membrane via a glycophospholipid foot. This protein is found in many cell membranes and inhibits the insertion of C9 or its polymerization onto complexes of C5b-8, and therefore blocks the formation of the membrane attack complex (MAC). Homologous restriction factor (HRF) is another glycophospholipid-linked membrane protein that similarly blocks C9 insertion and therefore blocks MAC formation. **B**, Functions of the protein fragments involved in the complement cascade. (Part B *adapted from* Janeway and Ravers [2].)

SIMILARITIES BETWEEN FACTORS OF THE CLASSIC AND ALTERNATIVE PATHWAYS

Function		Class	Alternative	Structural Features
Binding to antigen-antibody complexes		C1q	—	
Activating enzymes	Initiating the pathway; serine protease	C1r, C1s	D	Serine esterase domain
	C3/C5 convertase	C2b	Bb	Serine esterase domain, short consensus repeats
Covalent binding to cell surface	Opsonins	C4b	C3b	Internal thioester bond
Control of activation	Complement receptors, complement inhibitors	CR1, C4-bp	H	Short consensus repeat
Main effector molecules	Opsonins	C3b		
	Local inflammation	C3a, C5a		
	Membrane attack protein	C5b, C5b-C6		Pore-forming molecules

Figure 10-14. Similarities between the factors of the classic and alternative pathways. The proteins of the two pathways are the products of genes that have duplicated and then diverged in sequence or are, in fact, the product of identical genes. The proteins C4 and C3, for example, are homologous and contain an unstable thioester bond that is required for membrane binding. The regulatory proteins, factor H, CR1, and C4-bp, share a repeat sequence that is common to complement regulatory proteins.

The initiation of the two complement pathways is different. C1 is composed of three components; one of these components, C1q, binds to the Fc region of antibody. In contrast, the initiation of the alternative pathway does not require the presence of antibody and requires the presence of factor D, which is not similar to C1.

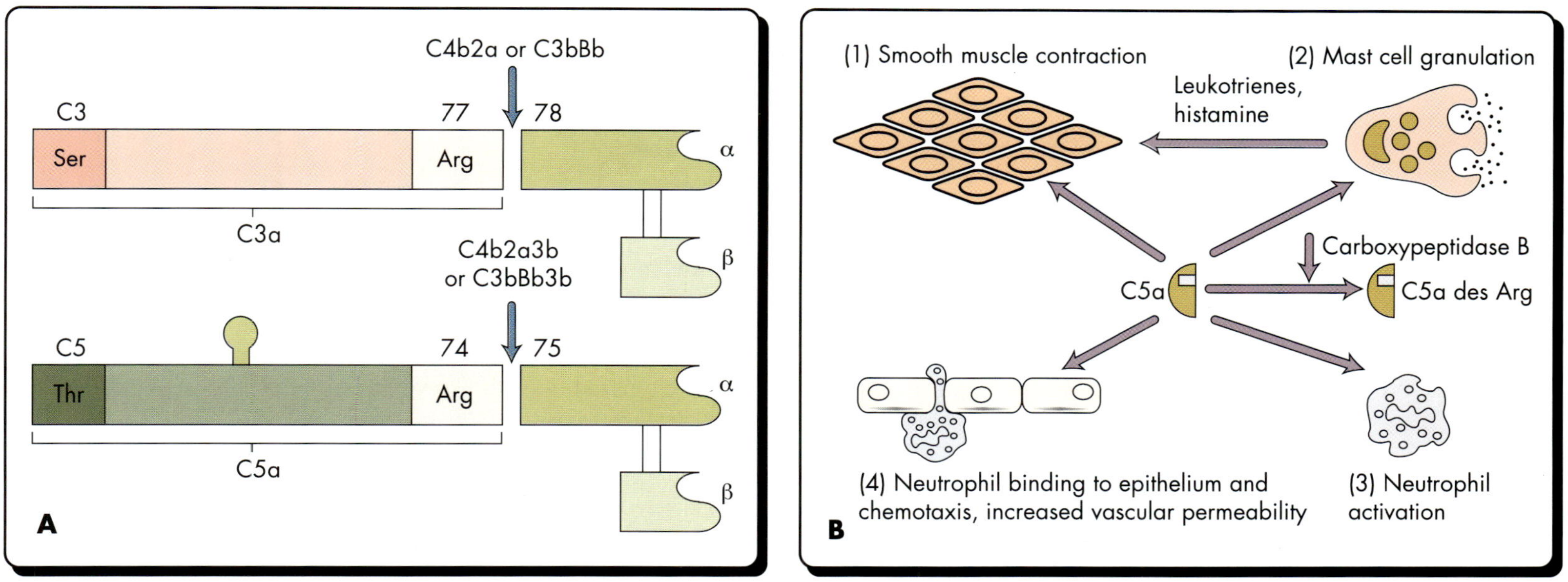

Figure 10-15. Anaphylatoxins. **A**, Anaphylotoxin formation. The generation of two fragments of complement, C3a and C5a, induces chemotaxis for neutrophils and can trigger the degranulation of mast cells and basophils. The degranulation of these cells leads to the release of substances associated with anaphylaxis. C5a causes smooth muscle contraction, which is further affected by the histamine and leukotriene release that occurs secondary to C5a-induced mast cell degranulation. C5a may also induce the release of IL-1 and TNF, which are proinflammatory cytokines. The effects of C3a and C5a are mediated by the binding of these fragments to specific receptors. The receptor for C5a is located on neutrophils and belongs to the rhodopsin superfamily of receptors; these receptors produce a signal via intracellular GTP-binding proteins. Once C5a is bound, C5a is internalized and degraded to inactive fragments. Activation of other enzyme systems can cleave C3, C4, and C5, including the activation of plasmin, kallikrein, tissue and leukocyte lysosomal enzymes, and bacterial proteases. **B**, Biologic effects of C5a and C5a-des-Arg. (Part B *adapted from* Walport [3].)

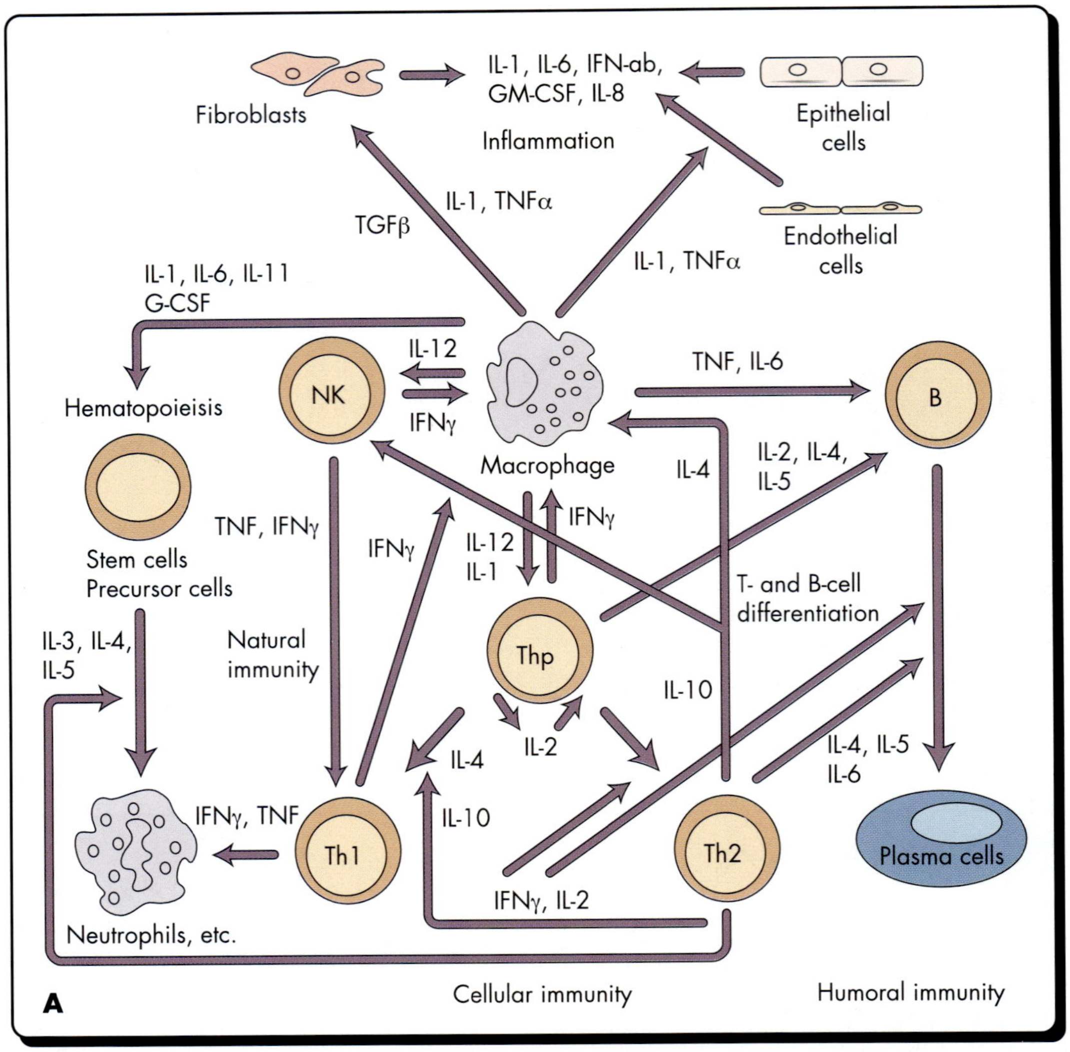

Figure 10-16. Overview of cytokines. Communication between cells in both the immune system and the hematopoietic systems is accomplished by cytokines (**A**). Most of the cytokines behave in a redundant manner, *ie*, each cytokine has multiple biologic effects and different cytokines act on the same cell type and even mediate similar effects (**B**, *opposite page*). Cytokines produce responses associated with inflammation, including fever, the production of acute-phase proteins, and chemotaxis; other effects include tumor regression and hematopoiesis. Cytokine production is tightly regulated. This is accomplished by limited receptor expression, such that one cytokine may limit the secretion of another by the production of specific inhibitory proteins that compete at the receptor or by the shedding of the extracellular domain of the cytokine receptor, which then binds to the cytokine in the fluid phase so that the cytokine can no longer interact with its receptors on the cell membrane. BCGF—B-cell growth factor; GM-CSF—granulocyte-macrophage colony-stimulating factor; GRO/MGSA—growth-regulated oncogene/melanoma growth-stimulatory activity; IFN—interferon; IL—interleukin; MCP—membrane cofactor protein; MIP—macrophage inflammatory protein; NK—natural killer (cell); TCGF—T-cell growth factor; TGFβ—transforming growth factor β; Th1—T-helper 1 (cell); TNF—tumor necrosis factor.

B. CYTOKINES

Family	Member	Main Source	Main Biologic Activities	Receptor type
β-Trefoil	IL-1α IL-1β	Macrophages, endothelial cells, T and B cells, fibroblasts, epithelial cells, etc.	Induce acute-phase reaction of inflammation; endogenous pyrogen	Type IV
Hematopoietins	IL-2	T cells	Stimulates T-cell proliferation; TCGF	Type I
	IL-3	T cells, mast cells	Stimulates hemotopoiesis; multi-CSF	
	IL-4	T cells, mast cells, stroma cells	Stimulates B-cell proliferation; BCGF-1	
	IL-5	T cells	Induces BCGF-2; promotes eosinophil growth	
	IL-6	Macrophages, T cells, fibroblasts, endothelial cells, etc.	Stimulates acute-phase protein production	
	IL-7	Stroma cells	Stimulates B and T cells	
	IL-9	T cells	Stimulates T-cell proliferation	
	IL-11	Stroma cells	Stimulates megakaryocyte colony formation	
	IL-12	Macrophages, T and B cells	Enhances differentiation of T cells into Th1 cells	
	IL-13	T cells	Stimulates B-cell growth	
	Epo	Kidney cells, liver cells	Stimulates the formation of erythrocytes	
	GM-CSF	T cells, endothelial cells, fibroblasts, macrophages, stroma cells	Stimulates the formation of granulocytes and macrophages	
	G-CSF	Macrophages, fibroblasts, endothelial cells, stroma cells	Stimulates the formation of granulocytes	
	IL-10	T cells, macrophages	Inhibits cytokine production by Th1 cells	Type II
	IFNα	Leukocytes	Induces antiviral state; induces class I HLA on cell surfaces	
	IFNβ	Fibroblasts, epithelial cells		
	IFNγ	T cells, NK cells	Activates macrophages; increases class II HLA expression	
	M-CSF	Lymphocytes, monocytes, fibroblasts, endothelial cells, epithelial cells	Stimultes the formation of macrophages	Tyrosine kinase Type III
TNF	TNFα	Macrophages, T cells, NK cells, keratinocytes	Cytolytic and cytostatic for transformed and virus-infected cells; activates granulocytes and macrophages; stimulates acute-phase protein release	
	LT (TNFβ)	T cells, B cells		
Cysteine knot	TNFβ	Macrophages, megakaryocytes, chondrocytes	Inhibits the growth of a variety of normal and transformed cells; promotes extracellular matrix formation	Serine/threonine kinase
Chemokine	IL-8	Macrophages, fibroblasts, endothelial cells, epithelial cells	Chemoattractive for neutrophils	Rhodopsin superfamily
	MIP-2α, β	Monocytes, macrophages	Chemoattractive for neutrophils	
	GRO/MGSA	Macrophages, fibroblasts, platelets	Chemoattractive for neutrophils	
	MIP-1α, β	T cells, B cells, macrophages	Chemoattractive for macrophages	
	MCP-1	Monocytes, T cells, fibroblasts, endothelial cells	Chemoattractive for macrophages	

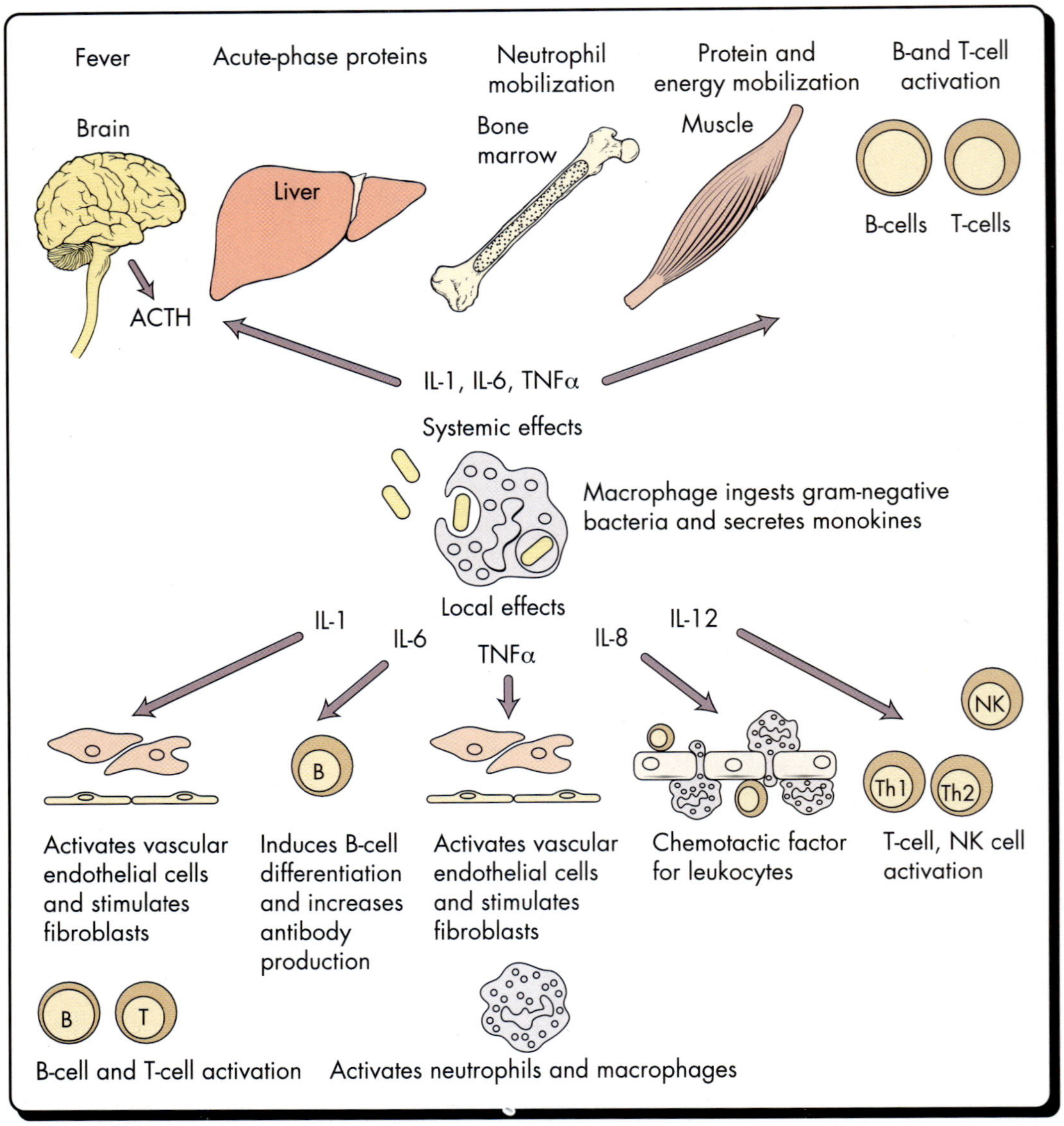

Figure 10-17. Production by macrophages of cytokines that are helpful in host defense. The macrophage ingests bacteria, and in particular, produces cytokines when gram-negative bacteria are ingested. Macrophages produce tumor necrosis factor α (TNFα) after exposure to lipopolysaccharide, a component of gram negative bacterial cell walls; TNFα has been shown to be important in the killing of microorganisms. Transgenic mice produced to lack the TNF1 receptor die of overwelming *Listeria monocytogenes* infections, whereas their genetic littermates that have the receptor survive the same infection [3]. Similarly, the intratracheal administration of recombinant TNFα helped mice eliminate *Legionella pneumophila* from their lungs and increased their survival [4,5].

Macrophages produce interleukins IL-1, IL-6, and IL-12 when exposed to gram-negative bacteria. All of these cytokines have local as well as systemic effects. In particular, IL-6 has effects on hepatocytes, which cause the synthesis of acute-phase proteins (*see* Fig. 10-3). The acute-phase proteins act as opsonins and their activity is enhanced by the recruitment of neutrophils that occurs, in part, due to the production of IL-8.

Interleukin-1 and IL-6 act on the hypothalamus, leading to changes in temperature regulation. These two cytokines also alter energy mobilization by their actions on fat and muscle cells. The alteration in energy mobilization also leads to elevations in body temperature. At elevated body temperatures, both bacteria and viruses have more difficulty in replicating. Both IL-1 and IL-6 also activate B and T cells and enhance antigen processing. ACTH—corticotropin; NK—natural killer (cell).

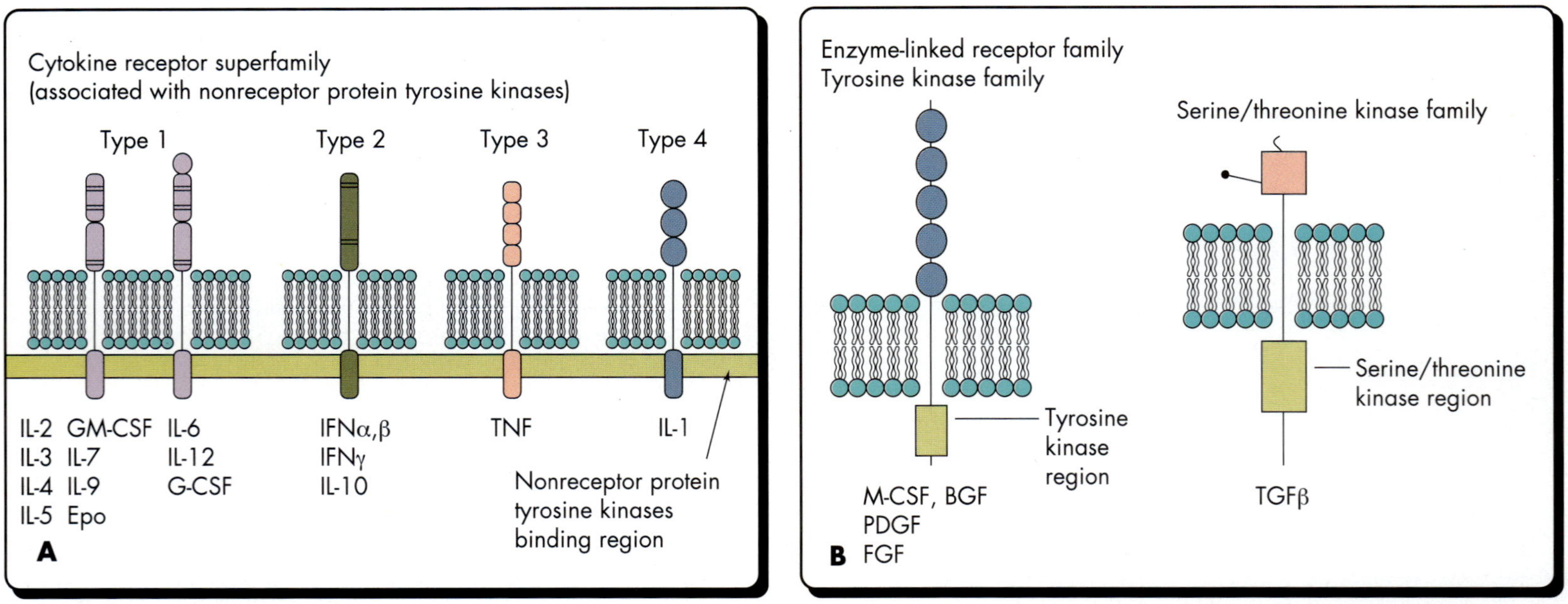

Figure 10-18. Cytokine receptors. There are four types of receptors used by cytokines. Most of the cytokine receptors are type 1 membrane glycoproteins; these receptors have been named the cytokine receptor superfamily (**A**). This family includes four subtypes based on a characteristic structural motif found in their extracellular ligand-binding domains. The cytoplasmic regions of these receptors have no intrinsic protein kinase domains, but nonreceptor types of tyrosine kinase can bind the cytoplasmic region and invoke intracellular signalling. Some of these receptors function as monomers, but most consist of more than two subunits. An example is IL-2R, which consists of three subunits, the α, β, and γ chains.

(*Continued on next page*)

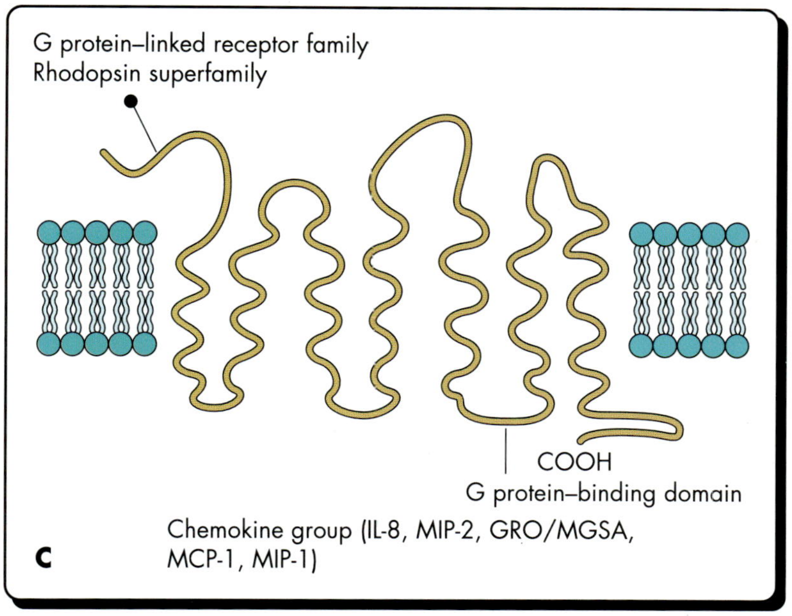

Figure 10-18. (*Continued*) The receptor for macrophage colony-stimulating factor (M-CSF) and the receptors for many of the cytokine growth factors are tyrosine kinase–linked receptors (**B**). Similarly, the receptor for transforming growth factor β (TGFβ) is a serine/threonine kinase–linked receptor. Therefore, these receptors form a group of enzyme-linked receptors. The chemokines form a group of cytokines that bind to a very different receptor; these cytokines bind to G protein–linked receptors (the rhodopsin superfamily) (**C**). EGF—epidermal growth factor; FGF—fibroblast growth factor; GM-CSF—granulocyte-macrophage colony-stimulating factor; GRO/MGSA—growth-regulated oncogene/melanoma growth-stimulatory activity; IFN—interferon; MCP-1—membrane cofactor protein; MIP-1—macrophage inflammatory protein; PDGF—platelet-derived growth factor. (Part A *modified from* Taniguchi [6]; parts B and C *modified from Callard and Gearing* [7].)

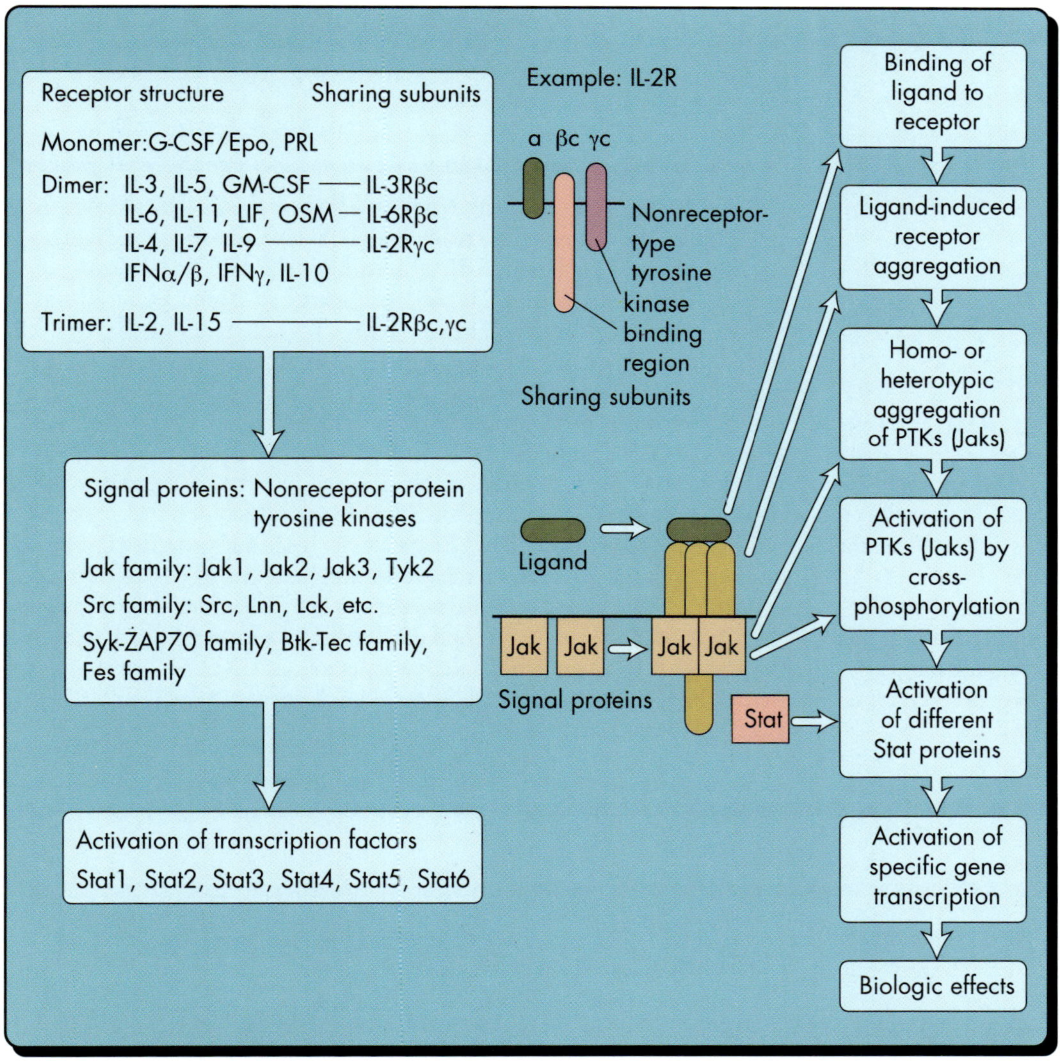

Figure 10-19. Cytokine receptor signaling. The remarkable features of cytokines are their functional redundancy and pleiotropy (*see* Fig. 10-23). This family of cytokine receptors has been found to have three general characteristics: (1) they share receptor subunits among different cytokines; (2) they utilize distinct signal proteins (nonreceptor type tyrosine kinases) to transmit the cytokine signal to the cell interior; and (3) they activate distinct transcription factors.

First, one receptor subunit is often shared among different cytokine receptors. For example, IL-2Rβc is also a subunit of IL-15R; IL-2Rγc is also a subunit of IL-4R, IL-7R, and IL-9R. IL-3Rβc is also a subunit of IL-5R and the receptor for granulocyte-macrophage colony-stimulating factor (GM-CSF). Finally, IL-6Rβc is also a subunit of IL-11R, the leukemia inhibitory factor receptor (LIFR), and the oncostatin M receptor (OSMR).

Second, several families of signal proteins (nonreceptor type tyrosine kinases, *eg*, Jak, Src), which can bind to the cytoplasmic region of the receptor subunit, transmit the cytokine signal to the cell interior. These proteins aggregate after there is ligand binding to the cytokine receptor; the aggregation leads to receptor hetero- or homodimerization. The aggregation of one or more signal proteins leads to phosphorylation of the other or the phosphorylation of nearby structures.

For example, the Janus kinase (Jak) family of signal proteins has been investigated. This family consists of Jak1, Jak2, Jak3 and Tyk2. When there is aggregation of the cytokine receptor, there is aggregation of Jak2, which leads to increasing catalytic activity and to Jak2 phosphorylating itself as well as the cytokine receptor and other substrates near the receptor complex.

The second pattern of association occurs in the cytokine receptors that have two interleukin chains (IL-3R, IL-6R). Jak2 associates with the β common subunit of these cytokine receptors. When the receptor β subunit aggregates, signal transduction occurs. In the third pattern of association, two subunits in the receptor are required for the cell signaling. IL-2 and interferon (IFN) have such receptors.

The cytokine receptors can also activate other signaling pathways through other signaling proteins, including Src, and the Syk-ZAP family. The great number of effects seen after cytokine release is probably due to the large number of signaling proteins that are activated by a cytokine attaching to its own receptor and to other common cytokine receptor subunits.

Cytokine receptors also activate transcription factors called signal transducers and activators of transcription (STAT). The Stat family of transcription factors regulates the expression of many genes, including the genes responsible for acute-phase responses, immunoglobulin class switching, cell surface proteins, and immunoglobin receptors. PRL—prolactin receptor; PTK—protein kinase. (*Adapted from* Ihle [8].)

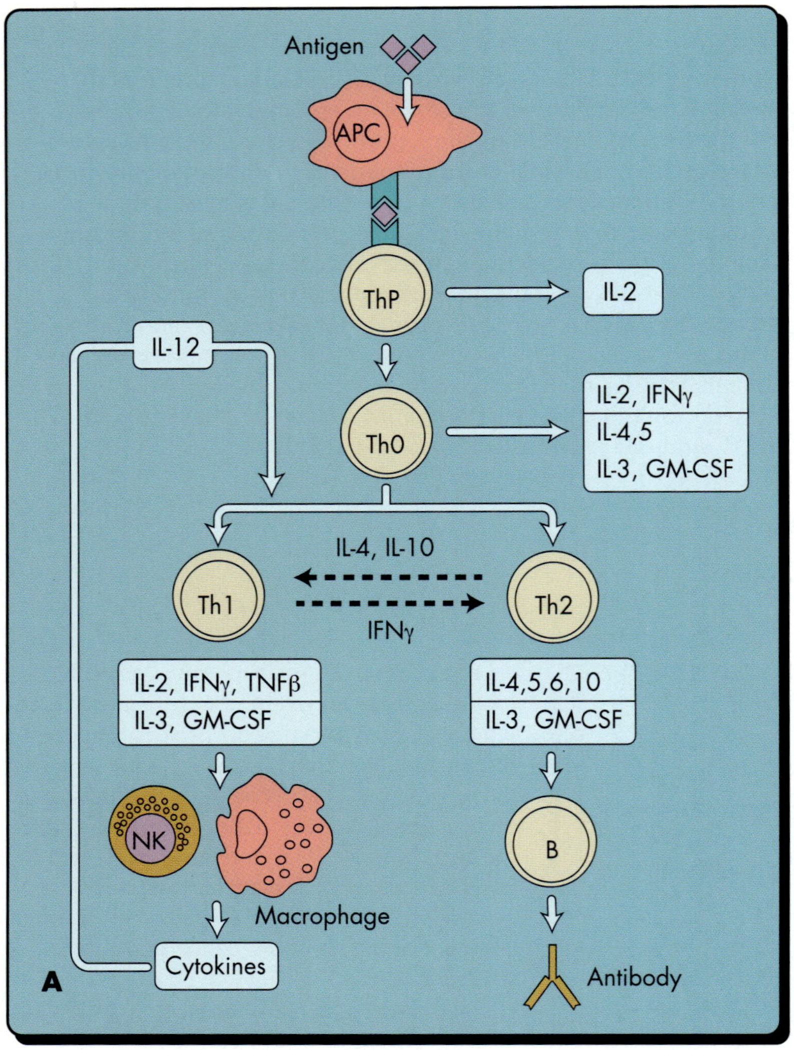

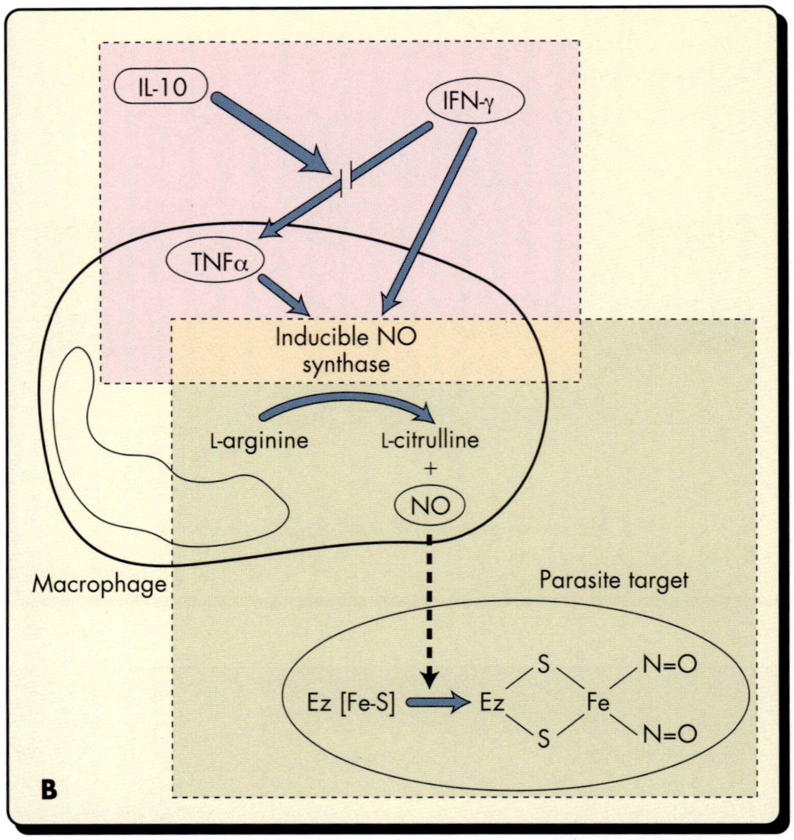

Figure 10-20. Regulation of the immune system by cytokines. How the host reacts to a particular pathogen is a complex interaction of events involving cytokines at multiple levels. **A,** The cell-mediated immune response alone is influenced at several levels by cytokines. In the cell-mediated immune response, the antigen-presenting cells (APCs) bear the particular processed antigen of th einfecting agent to the T-helper (Th) cells. The Th cells recognize particular epitopes and based on that selection activate appropriate effectors cells. The Th cell stimulates the B cells to make antibody or the Th cell makes cytokines to stimulate natural killer cells, macrophages, granulocytes, or antibody-dependent killer cells. Recently, it has become clear that there are two types of Th cells, defined primarily by the different patterns of lymphokines (cytokines) they synthesize. Short-term stimulation of Th cells leads to cells that can be distinguished as Th1 or Th2 cells. The Th1 cells release IL-2 (interleukin-2) and interferon γ (IFNγ), and the Th2 cells release IL-4, IL-5, and IL-10. Th1 cells would then activate macrophages and Th2 cells would increase the production of eosinophils, mast cells, and IgE. **B,** Each pattern of response tends to regulate the other; IL-10 produced by the Th2 cells inhibits IFNγ produced by the Th1 cells. Examples of this regulation have been shown to occur in infections; macrophages stimulated by IFNγ induce the endogenous sythesis of TNFα, which is a required costimulant for activation of nitric oxide (NO) production by the macrophage. Exposing the macrophage to IL-10 prior to or along with IFNγ will block the production of TNFα as well as the production of NO and will decrease parasitic killing. Therefore, IL-10 regulates the action of IFNγ but also secondarily blocks the production of TNFα; in this respect IL-10 is an anti-inflammatory cytokine. GM-CSF—granulocyte-macrophage colony-stimulating factor. (Part A *adapted from* Rook [9]; part B *adapted from* Sher *et al.* [10].)

REFERENCES

1. Eichenfield LF, Johnston RB Jr: The complement system. In *Immunology and Inflammation.* Edited by Sigal LH, Ron Y. New York: McGraw-Hill; 1994:251–252.
2. Janeway CA Jr, Ravers P: The complement system in humoral immunity. *Immunobiology.* 1994, 8:35–54.
3. Walport M: Complement. In *Immunology*, edn 3. Edited by Roitt I, Brostoff J, Male D. St. Louis: Mosby; 1993:12:12–13.
4. Rothe J, Lessiauer W, Lotscher H, *et al.*: Mice lacking the tumor necrosis factor receptor 1 are resistant to TNF-mediated toxicity but highly susceptible to infection by *Listeria monocytogenes*. *Nature* 1993, 364:798–802.
5. Blanchard DK, Djeu JY, Klein TW, *et al.*: Protective effects of tumor necrosis factor in experimental *Legionella pneumophila* infections of mice via activation of PMN function. *J LeukocBiol* 1988,43:429–435.
6. Taniguchi T: Cytokine signaling through nonreceptor protein tyrosine kinases. *Science* 1995, 268:251–255.
7. Callard R, Gearing A: *Cytokine Facts Book*. London: Academic Press; 1994.
8. Ihle JN: Cytokine receptor signalling. *Nature* 1995, 377:591–594.
9. Rook G: Cell-mediated immune reactions. In *Immunology*, edn 3. Edited by Roitt I, Brostoff J, Male D. Mosby; St. Louis: 1993:8:1–16.
10. Sher A, Gazzinelli RT, Oswald IP, *et al.*: Role of T-cell derived cytokines in the downregulation of immune responses in parasitic and retroviral infection. *Immunol Rev* 1992, 127:183–204.

11

Pain Processing

Tony L. Yaksh and Linda S. Sorkin

Certain unconditioned thermal or mechanical stimuli of sufficient intensity will induce escape behavior and verbal reports describing the experience as painful or noxious. This information has long been appreciated as being carried by spinal projections to the brain.

Increasing the stimulus intensity will lead to increased pain reports, whereas removing the stimulus will abolish the sensation. If the stimuli are of sufficient intensity, tissue will be injured and the injury will become an adequate stimulus to sustain the pain behavior and report. Electrophysiologic studies correlating activity in the sensory afferent fibers reveal that traffic in small myelinated and unmyelinated afferents appears to encode noxious stimuli by modality and frequency, *eg*, certain afferents (Aδ) may be selectively activated by high-intensity thermal and mechanical stimuli, whereas others (C fibers) with free nerve endings may be activated by high-intensity thermal or mechanical causes, and/or importantly, by chemicals released secondary to injury of the tissue or vasculature. In each case, the frequency of the activity appears to covary with the intensity of the stimulus.

This information, with intensity encoded as frequency, traveling over different populations of primary afferents, enters through the dorsal root entry zone (DREZ) to terminate largely within the segment of entry in the spinal dorsal horn. Small afferents terminate shallow in the substantia gelatinosa and larger afferents terminate in deeper laminae. These afferents serve to excite a variety of second-order neurons that project rostrally. Of these cells, several functionally distinct families of neurons can be observed: nociceptive selective neurons and those called wide-dynamic-range (WDR) neurons, which respond over a broad range of stimulus intensities with an increasing frequency of discharge. Many of these WDR cells receive convergent afferent input from a variety of organs and sensory modalities. These cells are believed to account for the phenomenon of referred pain.

Many of these spinal neurons project in both crossed and uncrossed pathways in the ventrolateral quadrant of the spinal cord. The contralateral pain deficit produced by a unilateral cordotomy emphasizes the crossed nature of the pain pathway. Tracing the rostral projections of these ascending systems emphasizes that such projections may terminate at virtually all levels from the pons up into the mesencephalon and as far rostrally as several thalamic nuclei. From here, ascending projections into a variety of cortical areas have been described. Recent studies using positron emission tomography (PET) to define neuronal activation have identified a number of specific regions, notably the anterior cingulate cortex, that may play a surprisingly selective role in pain perception.

Afferent transmission can be characterized by its connectivity, by the nature of the transmitters released and the receptors on which they act. Best identified in this regard is the primary afferent, for which it is appreciated that small afferents may contain and release several peptides or excitatory amino acids.

This connectivity just described suggests a hardwired connection in which a given stimulus input will yield a given output. It is now appreciated that this input-output relationship can be modified to either decrease or increase the gain and that these manipulations can accordingly enhance or diminish the pain states induced by a given stimulus. Several pharmacologic systems exist whereby the input-output relationship may be reduced. Of particular interest are those receptors for opiates and amines that may act by blocking the release of transmitters from small primary afferents. Importantly, these receptors are postsynaptic to a powerful endogenous modulatory system that projects from the brain stem to the spinal cord to release, *eg*, noradrenalin, which by acting upon the α_2-adrenergic receptor can regulate spinal nociceptive processing.

In addition to the downregulation of the gain, persistent small afferent input can serve to augment the gain of the output system. This suggests that after tissue injury, when a persistent afferent barrage is induced, there may be a routine state of hyperalgesia in animals and in humans. Recent studies have emphasized that this facilitated state may be induced in part by the spinal release of glutamate and the initiation of a cascade that includes the release of prostanoids from the spinal cord. Such studies suggest that the modulatory pharmacology of the spinal dorsal horn is quite complex.

It has long been appreciated that after nerve injury a variety of anomalous pain states can be observed, including pain induced by light touch (allodynia) or exaggerated pain in the presence of a given noxious stimulus (hyperalgesia). Current thinking has emphasized that nerve injury may lead to a variety of changes in activity and connectivity that may account in part for the anomalous pain. Importantly, this post–nerve injury pain state has been shown to have a distinct pharmacology as compared with pain induced by tissue injury.

Our growing appreciation of the complexity of the nociceptive systems increases the likelihood that considerable progress will occur in managing various pain states. The two most widely used classes of agents are the opioids and the nonsteroidal anti-inflammatory agents (NSAIDs). Work in this area has shown, using the focal delivery of drugs to specific sites, that opiates may interact at a number of supraspinal and spinal sites to reduce the excitatory drive induced by small afferent input. Recently, it has been shown that in the case of peripheral inflammation, opiates may exert an antihyperalgesic effect through local opiate receptors at the site of injury. Work with the NSAIDs has also shown considerable complexity, but it seems that a portion of their action may be mediated by these agents' ability to inhibit the formation of prostanoids by inhibiting cyclooxygenase. Prostanoids can be released at the site of injury to sensitize the afferent terminal and can be released from the spinal cord, where they act to enhance afferent transmitter release.

PAIN PATHWAYS

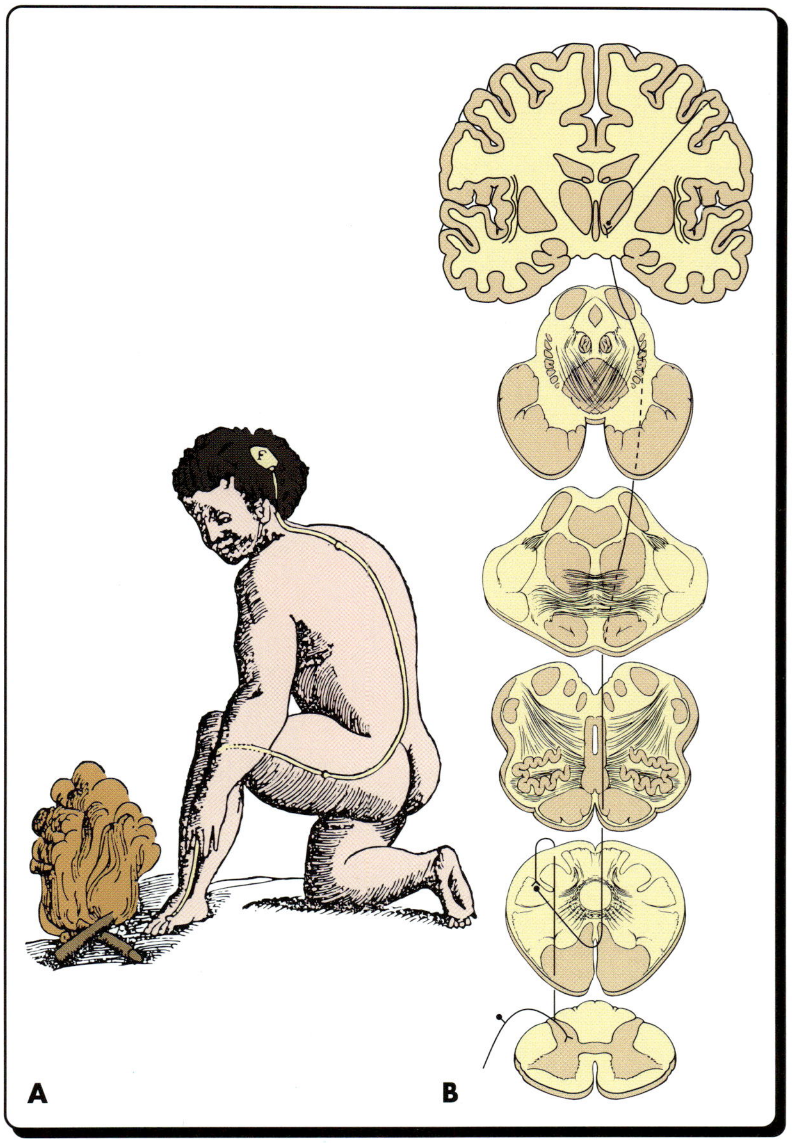

Figure 11-1. The ascending pain pathway. A, This cartoon, published by Descartes in his 1606 work entitled *L'Homme*, is considered to be one of the earliest systematic representations of the organization whereby a noxious stimulus (the fire) activates systems that travel through the nerves to the spinal cord and thence to the brain. A contemporary view of the neuraxis [1]. Though differing in detail, B, this representation shares with the Cartesian organization the concept that afferent input excited by an adequate, potentially tissue-damaging, stimulus enters the spinal cord through the nerve roots and ascends from the spinal cord to the brain. (Part B *from* Kandel and Schwartz [1].)

PERIPHERAL TRANSDUCTION AND TRANSMISSION

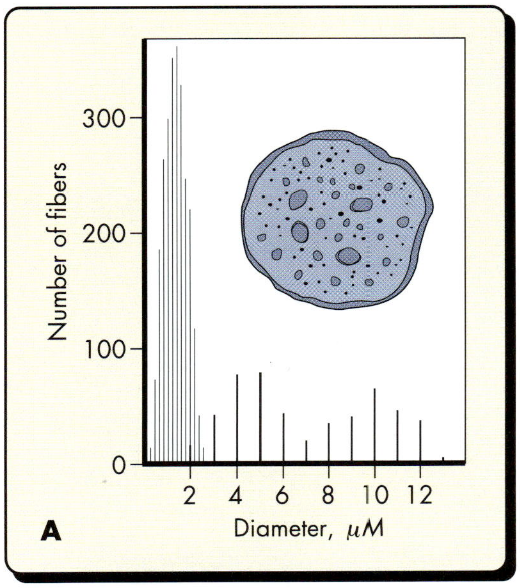

Figure 11-2. The peripheral sensory nerve. A, A typical histogram presenting the number of fibers in a mixed (sensorimotor) nerve as a function of axon diameter, emphasizing the large number of small unmyelinated profiles.

(*Continued on next page*)

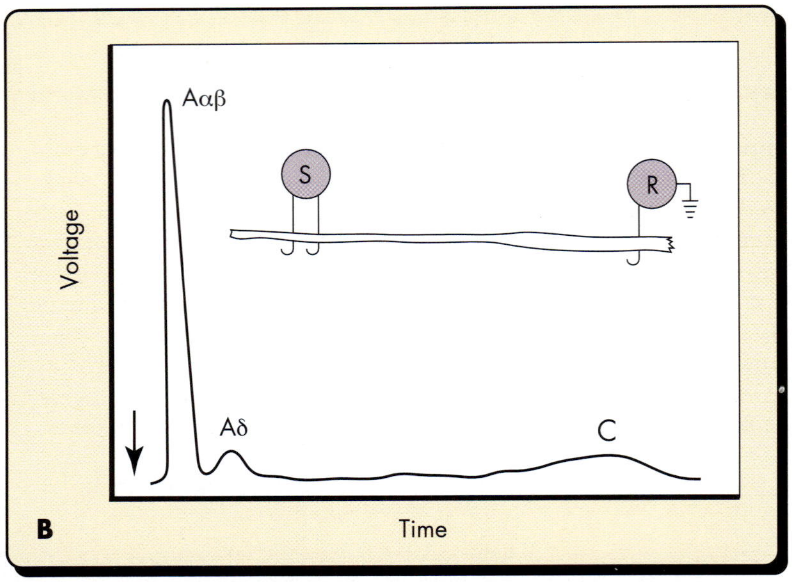

Figure 11-2. (*Continued*) B, The results of applying a brief electrical stimulus to a nerve and recording from the nerve monopolarly at a short distance. Stimulation at the time indicated by the *arrow* results in three separate waves of depolarization recorded (R) at a point distant from the stimulation (S) site. The evoked potential resulting from C-fiber activation has the longest latency because of the slow conduction velocity of these fibers; it has the lowest voltage because the individual C fibers emit smaller electrical potentials than the larger A fibers. C, The three classes of sensory axons. Note that Aδ axons may be subdivided on the basis of their sensitivity to specific stimuli. In contrast, a C fiber may respond to several classes of high-intensity stimuli and is referred to as a "C-polymodal nociceptor" [2]. Aβ/Aδ/C classes are from the Erlanger-Gasser classification and refer to anatomic characteristics. II/III/IV is the Lloyd-Hunt classification defined on the basis of conduction velocity in muscle afferents.

C. CLASSES OF SENSORY AXONS

Fiber Class	Conduction Velocity	Receptor Type
Aβ (large myelinated) Group II (12–20 µm diameter)	> 25–28 m/s	Low-threshold mechanoreceptors Specialized nerve endings (Pacinian corpuscles)
Aδ (small myelinated) Group III (1–4 µm diameter)	2 < x < 25 m/s	Low-threshold mechano- or thermoreceptors High-threshold mechano- or thermoreceptors Specialized nerve endings
C (small unmyelinated) Group IV (0.5–1.5 µm diameter)	< 2 m/s	High-threshold thermo-, mechano-, or chemoreceptors Free nerve endings

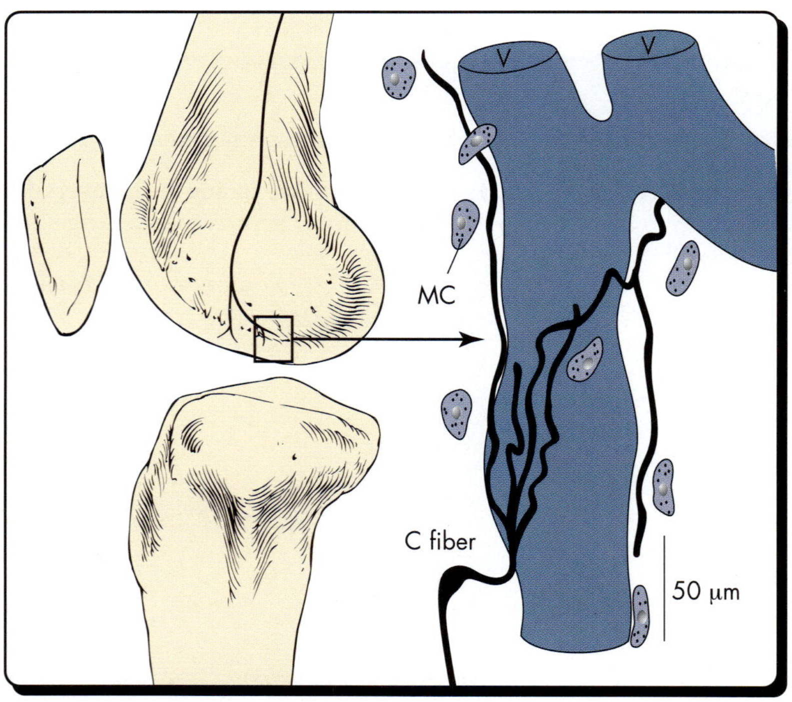

Figure 11-3. Structure of the peripheral terminal environment of the free nerve ending. Free nerve endings of nociceptive primary afferent fibers are unencapsulated, without a perineurium, for up to 400 µm from their distal ends. Frequently they are in close contact with distal arterioles, venules (V), and mast cells (MC). This common triad suggests an important functional relationship between nociceptive terminals, MCs, and small blood vessels. (*Adapted from* Heppelmann and coworkers [3].)

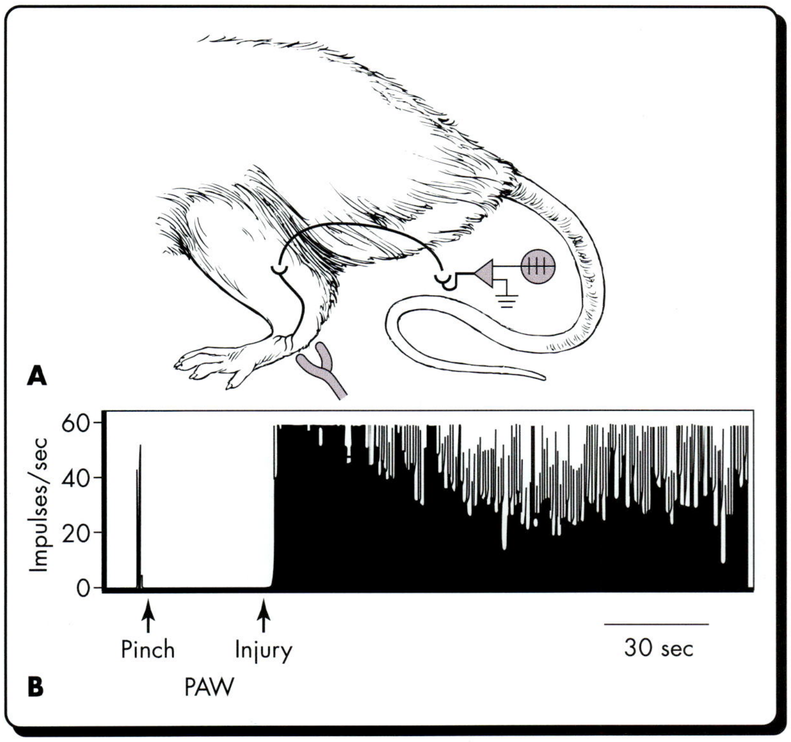

Figure 11-4. Temporal response evoked by an intense mechanical stimulus inducing a local injury. The firing rate of a single small afferent in response to pinch and to a tissue crush is shown. The peripheral nerve of the anesthetized rat (**A**) is dissected and a few filaments are teased free and mounted on a small electrode. **B**, In the absence of stimulation, there is no spontaneous activity in this small afferent axon. A brief pinch evokes a transient stimulus-linked discharge. The induction of local injury by a crush resulting in local tissue injury leads to a prolonged ongoing discharge. (*Adapted from* Fitzgerald and Gibson [4].)

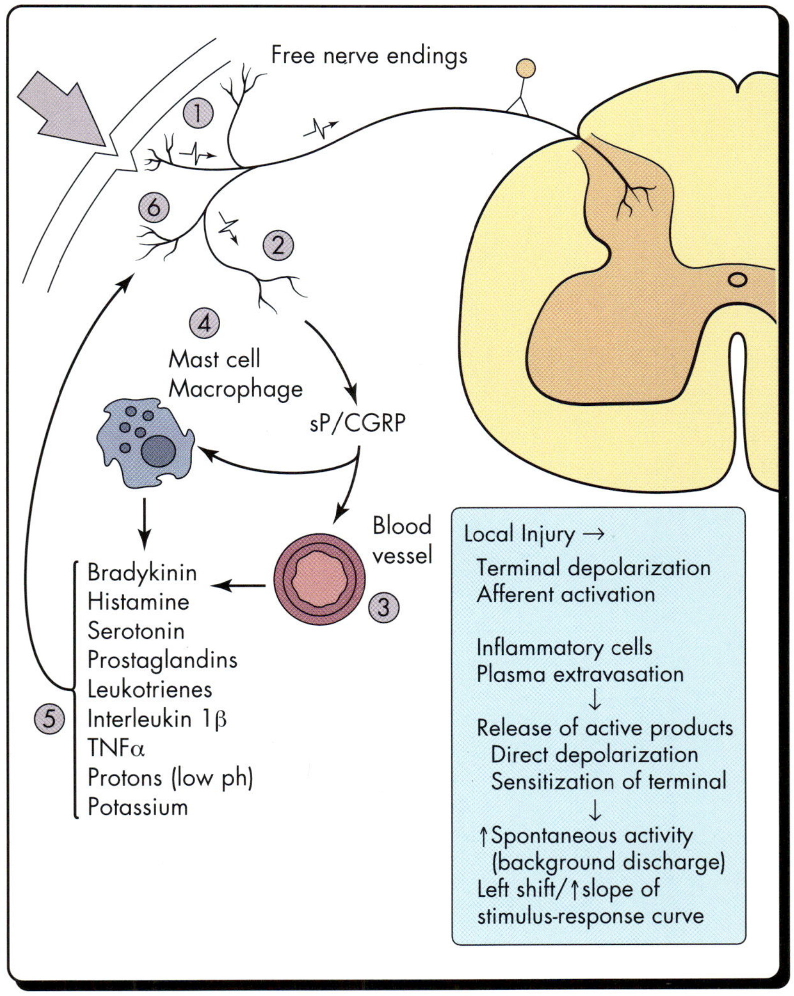

Figure 11-5. Periterminal milieu after local injury. Local damaging stimulus leads to firing of the fine afferents and local activation of inflammatory cells (*1*). Afferent fibers display antidromic release of neuropeptides such as substance P and calcitonin gene–related peptide (sP/CGRP) (*2*). Hormones, such as bradykinin, prostaglandins, and cytokines, or K+/H+ released from injured tissue, inflammatory cells, and plasma extravasation (*3, 4, 5*), result in stimulation and sensitization of free nerve endings (*6*) [5]. TNFα—tumor necrosis factor α.

SPINAL ORGANIZATION

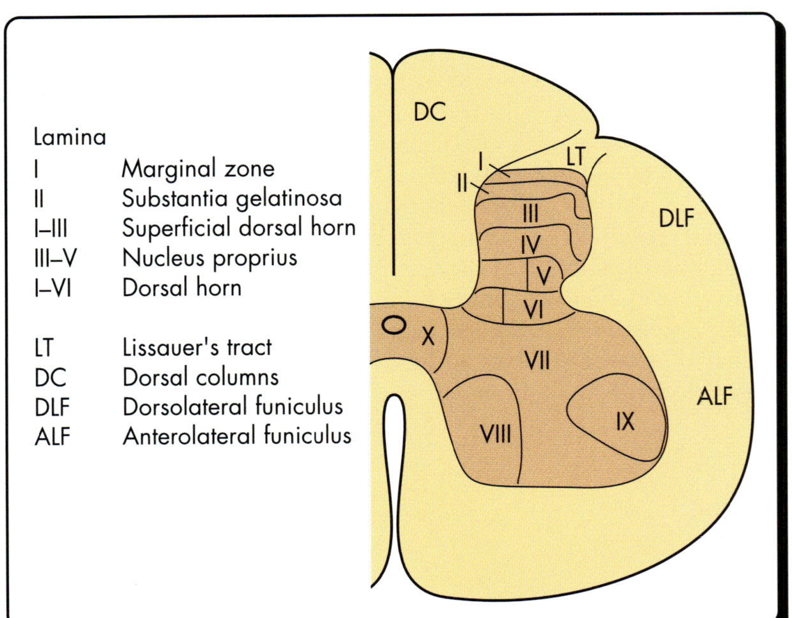

Figure 11-6. 7. Rexed lamination showing organization of the spinal gray matter. The principal anatomic subdivisions correspond to the more detailed lamination patterns defined by Rexed [6]. The majority of descending bulbospinal modulatory pathways travel in the dorsolateral funiculus (DLF) whereas axons of the more prominent ascending projection systems are in the anterolateral funiculus.

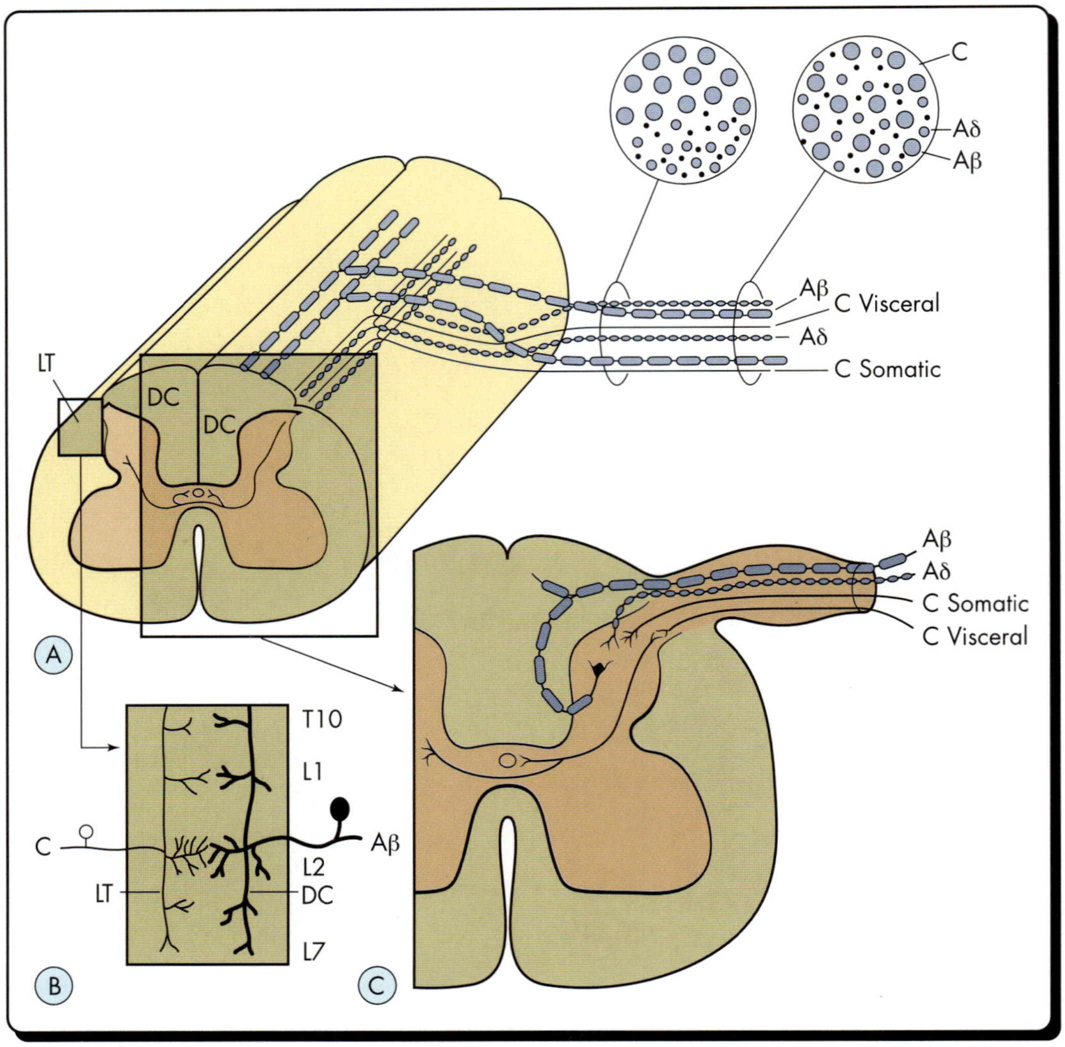

Figure 11-7. Organization of primary afferent terminal distribution within the spinal dorsal horn. All afferents, upon entry, may trifurcate, sending projections directly into the dorsal horn at the segment of entry as well as both rostrally and caudally. The collaterals of the large afferent travel in the dorsal columns (DC) whereas those of the small afferent travel in Lissauer's tract (LT).

Inset A, Sections through the root reveal that large and small axon profiles are randomly distributed in fascicles through the cross-section. Upon approach into the DREZ, there is a tendency for the large myelinated fibers to move medially in the root and for the smaller axons to move laterally. Although the majority of afferents enter through the DREZ, a small fraction may also enter through the ventral root [7,8].

Inset B, The horizontal plane of the rostrocaudal ramification of Aβ (*right*) and C fibers (*left*) in the dorsal horn. Cutaneous C fibers have only an ascending branch, which travels in the LT. Visceral C fibers have both ascending and descending branches. Their rostral spread is greater than that of cutaneous C fibers but less than that of Aβ fibers. Some visceral C fibers send branches to the contralateral cord. Each axon has its densest projections at the segments of entry; however, periodically axon collaterals emerge and terminate in the underlying laminae. At sites distal to the level of entry, the projections and synaptic contacts become less dense and the input presumably exerts less excitatory influence.

Inset C, In the coronal plane, Aβ fibers curve around the medial edge of the dorsal horn to enter the gray matter. Terminations are throughout laminae III and IV. Aδ and C fibers both enter from the lateral aspect. High-threshold Aδ terminate in laminae I, II(outer), and V. C fibers end primarily in lamina II. Lamina X is the area around the central canal and receives some direct input from visceral C fibers [9].

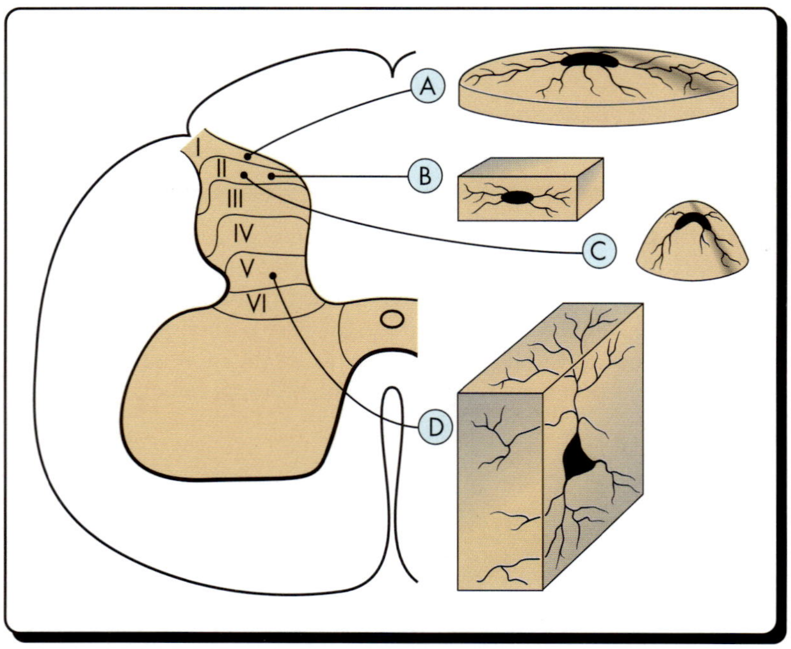

Figure 11-8. Distribution of cell types known to receive nociceptive information. A cross-section of the lumbar spinal cord shows the approximate laminar distribution of cells types known to receive nociceptive input. **Insets A, B, C, D**, The dendritic distribution and morphology of four cell types, showing their relative sizes [10]. **Inset A**, Marginal cell of lamina I. These are oriented horizontally and their dendrites can encompass the entire lamina. Their distribution allows them to integrate input from small afferents that terminate along the mediolateral aspect of the segment. Many of these cells project rostrally out of the spinal cord and belong to the spinothalamic or spinomesencephalic tracts. **Insets B and C**, Stalked/Islet cells of lamina II. These small interneurons of lamina II have restricted dendritic trees and may play a local role: (1) in exciting the dendrites of more deeply lying neurons, perhaps through the release of glutamate (*see* Fig. 11-34) or (2) in exerting inhibitory influences by presynaptic modulation of the terminals of large and small afferents by the release of, *eg*, inhibitory modulators such as γ aminbutyric acid/glycine or enkephalin (see Fig. 11-37). **Inset D**, Pyramidal cell of lamina IV and V. Dendrites of these large cells radiate in all directions. Frequently their axons project to supraspinal structures.

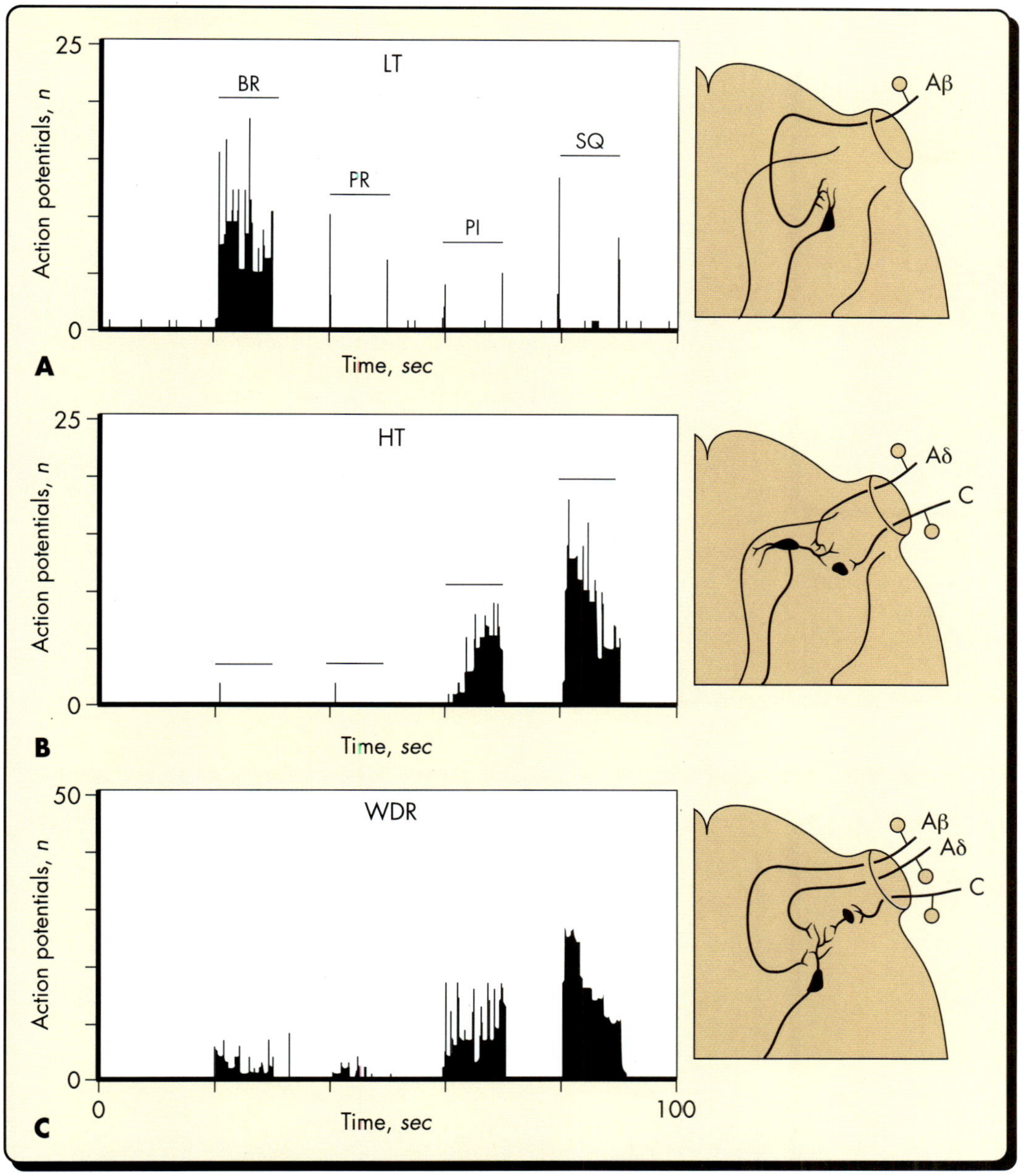

Figure 11-9. Electrophysiologic properties of neurons activated by somatosensory stimuli. Three simple types of dorsal horn cells may be identified based on their pattern of responses to mechanical stimuli applied to their receptive fields (*left*) over a range of intensities from light touch, firm pressure, to hard pinch. The intervals of stimulus application are indicated by the *horizontal bars*.These response profiles suggest the organization indicated in the dorsal horn (*right*) [11]. **A**, Low-threshold (LT) cells respond to a repetitive brush stimulus (BR) but not to a maintained mechanical pressure (PR) or to a frankly noxious pinch (PI) or tissue-damaging squeeze (SQ). This cell receives input selectively from low-threshold mechanoreceptors (in this case hair follicle afferents).

B, High-threshold cells (HT) respond exclusively to the more noxious stimuli and receive excitatory input directly or indirectly from Aδ or C fibers. **C**, WDR cells respond over the range from innocuous to noxious, but their peak response is to noxious stimulation. They receive input from Aβ fibers, Aδ fibers, and/or C fibers. Accordingly, the WDR cell is able to map in a frequency-dependent fashion the input over a wide range of stimulus intensities. Note that this example indicates the importance of afferent convergence on a single cell. No population of sensory afferent fibers possesses this "dynamic range" of responding, and the encoding of stimulus intensity by frequency would not be possible without such convergence.

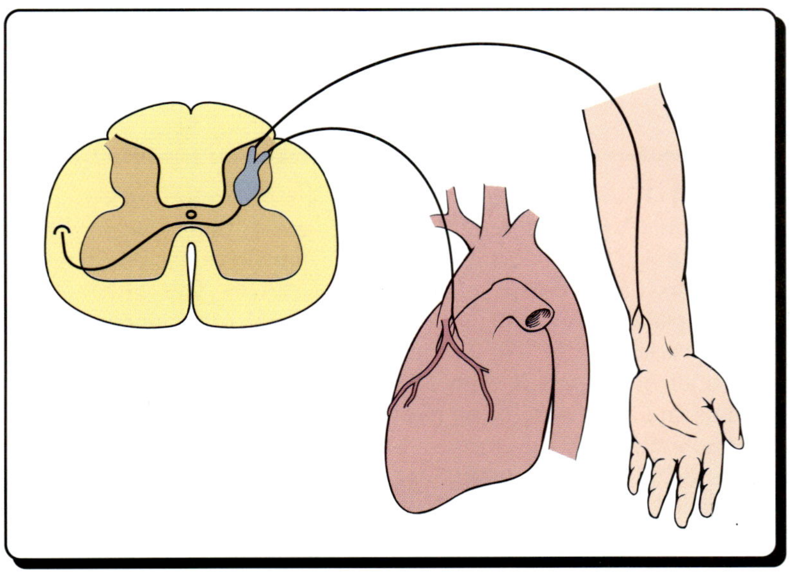

Figure 11-10. Referred pain: role of modality convergence of afferent input onto dorsal horn neurons. Dorsal horn cells that receive convergent input from deep structures and skin are referred to as somatovisceral cells. Somatic nociceptive afferents from visceral (*eg*, heart, esophagus, bowel) and somatic structures (skin and muscle) may thus both drive the same dorsal horn neurons. Cells in the left thoracic dorsal horn (approximately T4) may be excited by input from the skin of the upper arm and shoulder and from noxious stimuli applied to the coronary afferent. This organization is believed to underlie the phenomenon of referred pain. Such dermatomal coprojections with other visceral organ systems, such as the esophagus (midsternal pain), appendix (lower right quadrant), and pancreas (upper left quadrant), correspond with the skin dermatomes with which the respective referred pain states are associated.

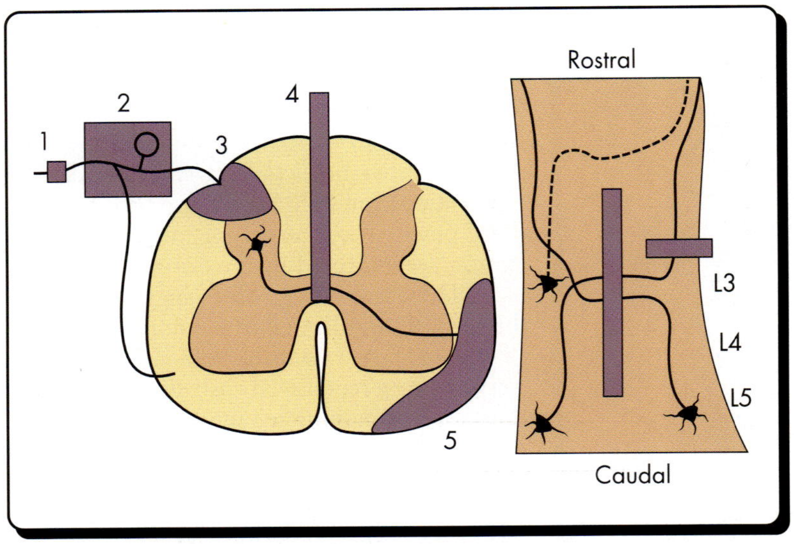

Figure 11-11. Spinal lesions and pain perception. The schematic displays the principal projections in the coronal (*left*) and horizontal (*right*) plane, which are impacted upon by lesions that produce sensory anesthesia or analgesia. Neurosurgical interventions provide insight into the nature of the pathways that are involved in the transmission of nociceptive information. Such interventions include (*1*) neurectomy, in which sectioning of a nerve leads to a reduction in sensibility in the distribution of the sensory nerve; (*2*) dorsal root ganglionectomy, which removes the cell bodies of origin of all afferents; (*3*) lesions of the DREZ were initially targeted at the turn of the century to selectively destroy small afferents that moved laterally upon entry into the spinal parenchyma, sparing the large afferents; this lesion evolved into destruction of the entry zone and frequently encompasses portions of the marginal layer and underlying parenchyma—it is occasionally used for deafferentation syndromes; (*4*) midline myelotomy, which constitutes a longitudinal section though the midline of the spinal cord and serves to section crossing fibers, resulting in a bilateral analgesia—the growing appreciation of the distribution of axons arising in lamina X and axons in the postsynaptic dorsal column tract raises the possibility that such lesions may involve systems other than those that are crossing; and (*5*) ventrolateral cordotomy, first suggested by Gowers in 1888 [12] and practiced by Martin and by Beer in 1912 for pain of sacral metastasis, resulting in a thermal analgesia in contralateral dermatomes that are one to two segments below section.

SPINAL PROJECTIONS

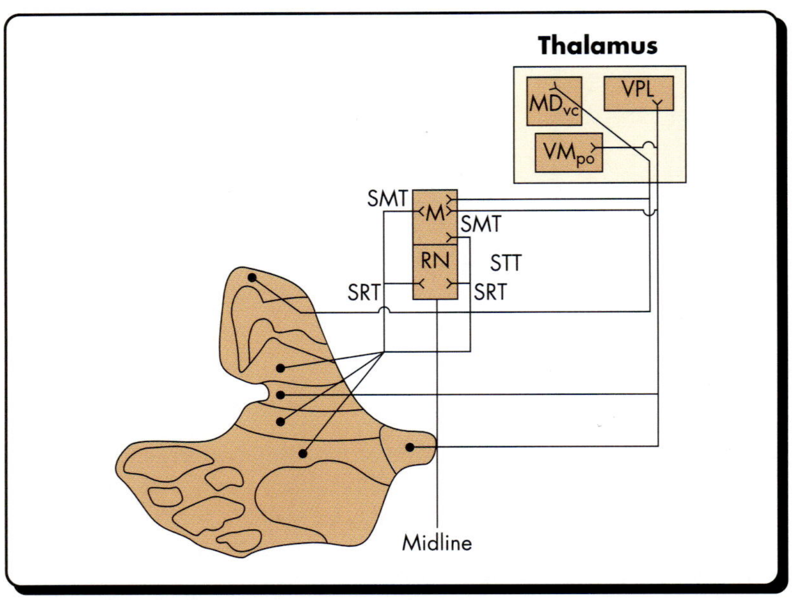

Figure 11-12. Ascending pain pathways. The three classic tracts implicated in pain transmission with axons in the ventrolateral quadrant of the spinal cord show their primary cells of origin and their supra-spinal projection sites [9]. The spinothalamic tract (STT) projection originates from laminae I/II and III-VI, and these projections are predominantly contralateral from lumbar cord (90%) but are bilateral from the upper cervical spinal cord. At the thalamic levels the STT has strong projections into a number of nuclear groups, notably the ventroposterior lateral (VPL) nuclear groups (also known as the ventrobasal complex). The mediodorsal ventral component (MD_{vc}) may receive projections originating exclusively in high-threshold lamina I neurons in the contralateral dorsal horn.

The spinomesencephalic (SMT) tract originates in a fashion similar to the STT cells but has a stronger bilateral projection into the medial mesencephalon, notably the mesencephalic reticular formation and the periaqueductal gray matter. The spinoreticular tract (SRT) originates widely throughout the nucleus proprius and upper motor horn (laminae V through VIII). Its projections are bilateral throughout its extent. M—midbrain; RN—reticular nuclei; VM_{po}—posterior portion of the ventral medial nucleus.

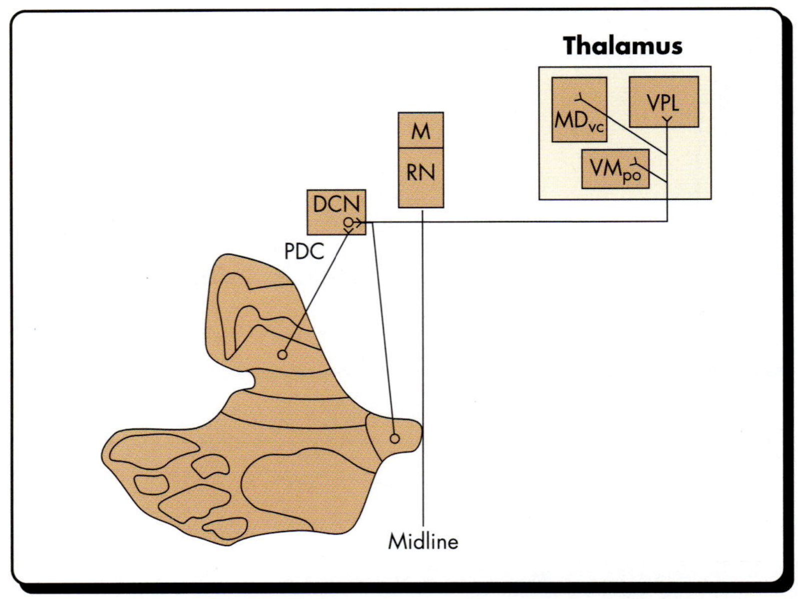

Figure 11-13. Ascending pain pathways. Cells in the nucleus proprius (lamina V) are known to give rise to axons that travel in the ventral portion of the dorsal columns. This projection is referred to as the postsynaptic dorsal column (PDC) pathway. This pathway projects ipsilaterally through the dorsal columns to the dorsal column nuclei (DCN). The component of the pathway originating primarily from lamina X of the sacral cord travels in the deep dorsal columns and appears to be an important visceral pain pathway. M—midbrain; MD_{vc}—ventral caudal portion of the medial dorsal nucleus; RN—reticular nuclei; VM_{po}—posterior portion of the ventral medial nucleus; VPL—ventral posterior lateral nucleus.

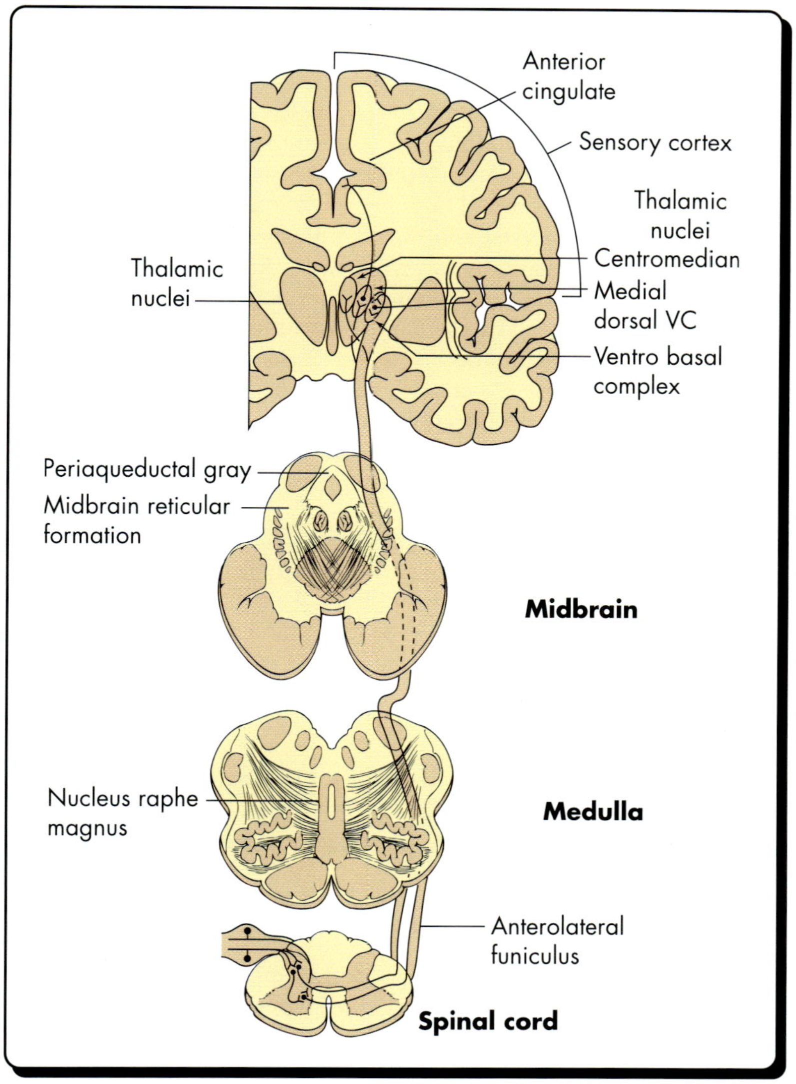

Figure 11-14. Projections of ascending anterolateral projections. The general organization is shown of the important rostral projection of the pathway by which information passes through crossed pathways and up the ventrolateral tract to send collaterals into the medulla and mesencephalon to terminate in the thalamus. VC—ventral component.

SUPRASPINAL ORGANIZATION

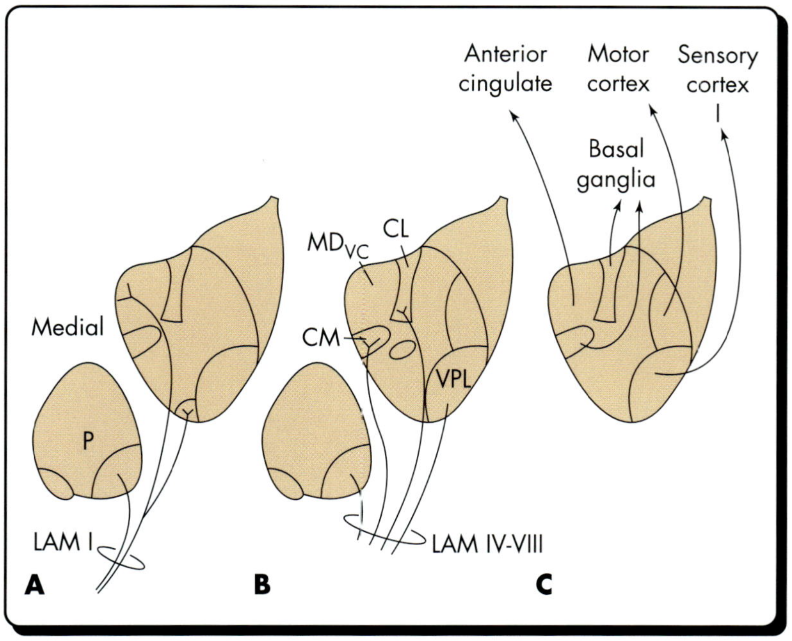

Figure 11-15. Organization of spinothalamic and thalamocortical projections presenting sections through the right thalamus. Only the more prominent nuclei are included. **A** and **B**, Distribution of input from spinothalamic projections. **C**, Several primary outputs from the thalamus, summarized in the accompanying table (**D**). The ventrobasal complex maintains a somatotopic mapping of the body surface and possesses neurons that frequently respond to low-threshold input and cells that respond as WDR neurons (see Fig. 11-11). The mediodorsalis ventral component (MD_{vc}) receives input almost exclusively from high-threshold marginal cells and provides strong projections to the anterior cingulate gyrus. CL—central nucleus; CM—centromedian; P—posterior nucleus; VM_{po}—posterior portion of the ventral medical nucleus; VPL—ventral posterior lateral nucleus.

D. INPUT/OUTPUT FROM SPINOTHALAMIC PROJECTIONS

Thalamic Nuclei	Input	Output
Posterior nuclei	Laminae I and V	Retroinsular cortex
Centromedian	Laminae V, VII, VIII	Basal ganglia frontal cortex (?)
Mediodorsal$_{vc}$	Lamina I	Anterior cingulate
Ventrobasal		
VPL/VPM	Laminae I, IV–VI	Somatosensory cortex I
VPI	Laminae IV–VII	Somatosensory cortex II
VM_{po}	Lamina I	Frontal

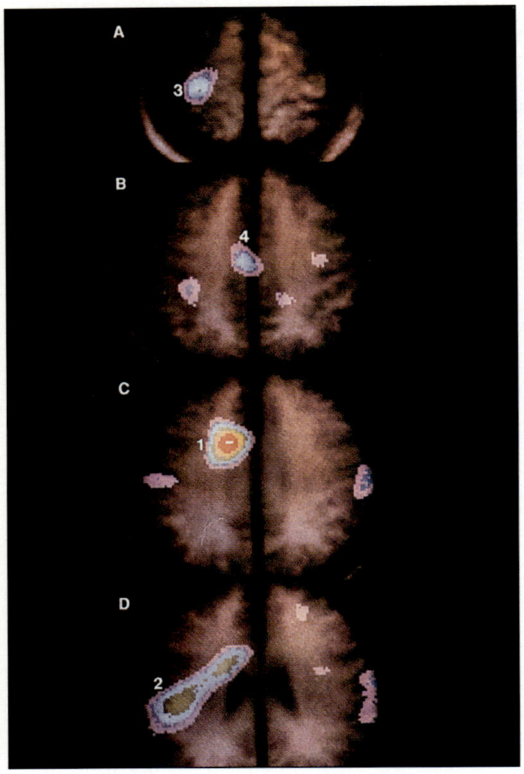

Figure 11-16. Cortical PET scans of pain sites representing horozontal planes (most superior, **A**, to most most inferior, **D**) obtained from human subjects by magnetic resonance imaging and PET scans. The PET scan indicates increased regions of local blood flow (indicating neuronal activation). Subjects were examined with magnetic resonance imaging and PET scanning after application of a warm (non-noxious) stimulus to the right forearm and, after some delay, application of a hot (noxious) stimulus to the same site. The scans represent the subtracted difference between the local blood flow in the various regions measured during the nonnoxious and noxious stimuli. *Intense coloration* indicates regions that show a higher flow during the noxious than during the nonnoxious stimulus. As indicated, a mild increase in blood flow was noted in the contralateral somatosensory cortices (*plane A, site 3; plane D, site 2*), corresponding to the primary and secondary somatosensory projection mapping of the body surface. Intense increases in blood flow were also noted in the contralateral anterior cingulate cortex (*plane B, site 4; plane D, site1*). This contrasts with the limited activation of the somatosensory cortex produced by non-noxious vibrotactile stimuli. These results suggest that certain cortical regions, such as the anterior cingulate in the forebrain (a region thought to regulate emotions), may contain an unexpected, specific representation of pain (*From* Talbot and coworkers [13].)

TRANSMITTER PHARMACOLOGY OF SENSORY AFFERENTS

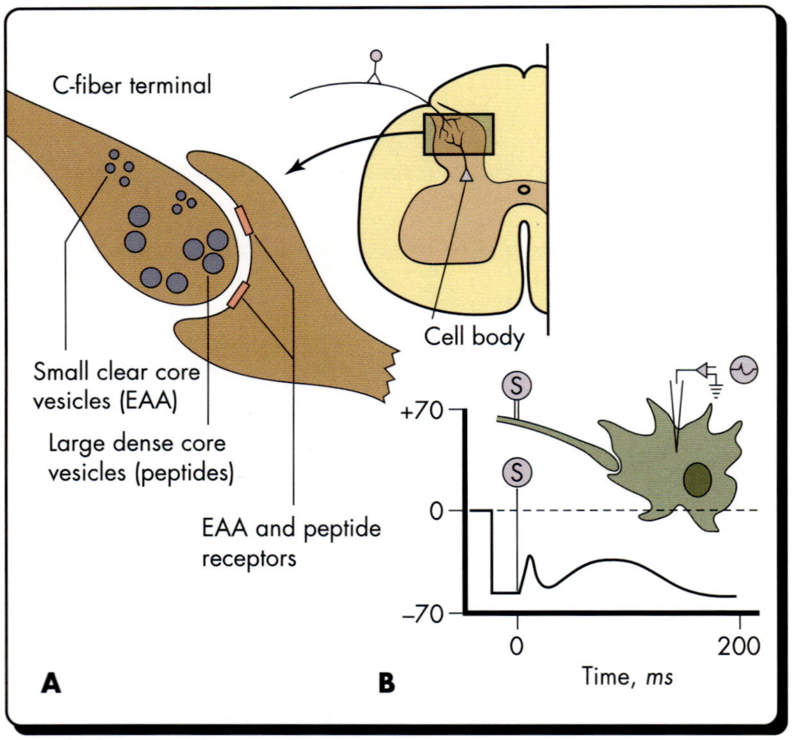

Figure 11-17. Primary afferent neurotransmitter function. Characteristics of the primary afferent transmitters released from small, capsaicin-sensitive, primary afferents: C primary afferents [18]. **A**, Peptides and excitatory amino acids (EAA) are co-contained in dorsal root ganglion cells (type B) and in vesicles in their central terminals. **B**, The intracellular response to a stimulus (S) applied to a single filament innervating a neuron *in vitro*. After stimulation, a rapid, early depolarization is seen that is believed to be mediated by release of an excitatory amino acid (glutamate), followed by a delayed and long-lasting depolarization believed to be mediated by a peptide (*eg*, substance P).

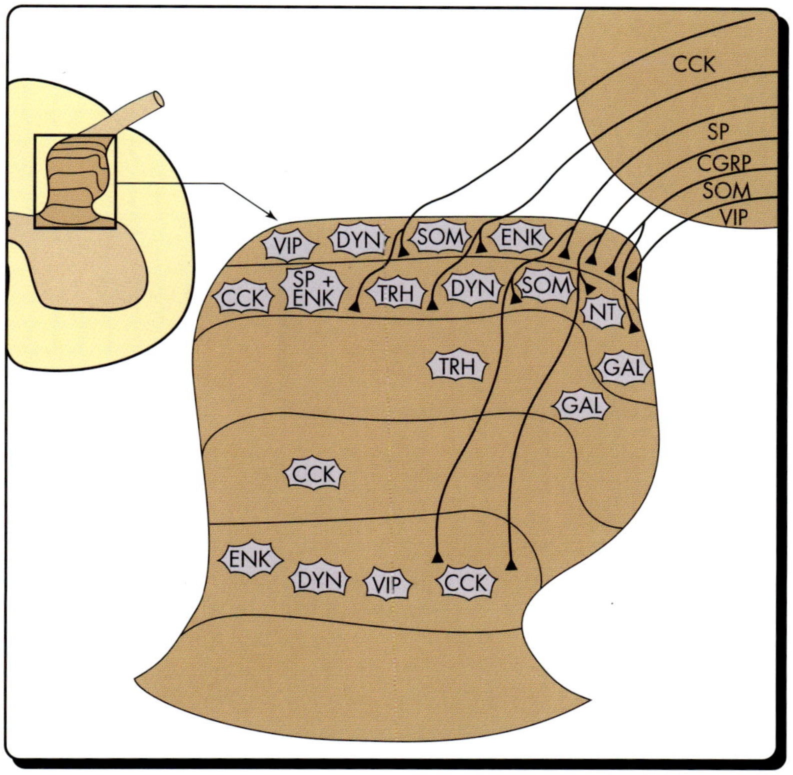

Figure 11-18. Distribution of small afferent terminals containing peptides and intrinsic dorsal horn neurons. Peptides in the dorsal horn may arise from intrinsic neurons, primary afferents, or bulbospinal projections. The first two possibilities are shown here. Several details are emphasized. (1) Cell bodies containing peptides are concentrated in laminae I and II. (2) Laminae 1 and 2 are also the sites of the most dense primary afferent projections for the majority of primary afferent peptides. (3) The endogenous opiates dynorphin (DYN) and enkephalin (ENK) are located only in cell bodies and not in primary afferent fibers. This also appears to be true for thyrotropin-releasing hormone (TRH) and neurotensin (NT). (4) Conversely, dorsal horn calcitonin gene–related peptide (CGRP) is exclusively from primary afferent sources. (5) Intrinsic substance P (SP) is always colocalized with enkephalin, but enkephalin is also found in some spinothalamic tract and other spinofugal projection cells. CCK—cholecystokinin; GAL—galanin; SOM—somatostatin; VIP—vasoactive intestinal peptide [15].

MODULATION OF THE AFFERENT MESSAGE

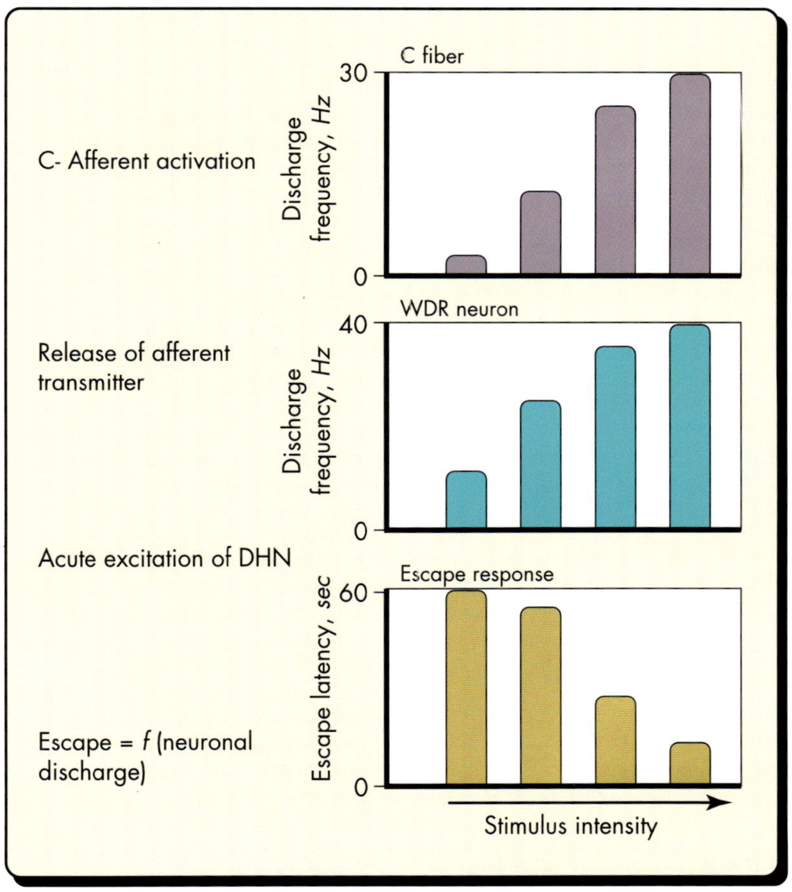

Figure 11-19. Summary of the parallel relationship between stimulus intensity and activity in sensory C fiber (*top*), activity in spinal dorsal horn neurons (DHN) (WDR neurons) (*middle*), neurons, and the latency to escape (*bottom*) in the unanesthetized organism. Physiologic and behavioral studies have suggested that there is typically a monotonic covariance between these measured endpoints for an *acutely* presented stimulus. There are several instances in which this relationship between stimulus intensity and pain behavior can be substantially altered.

A. COMMON PROPERTIES OF SPINAL RECEPTORS

Characteristics	Receptors: $\mu/\delta/\alpha_2$/NPY	GABA-B
Electrophysiologic changes		
↓ C-fiber excitation of WDR	x	o
Binding		
Dorsal > ventral	x	x
Rhizotomy or capsaicin	x	o/?
Physiology		
Reduce sP/CGRP rel (↓ ICa)	x	x
Hyperpolarize WDR (↑ IK; Gi)	x	x

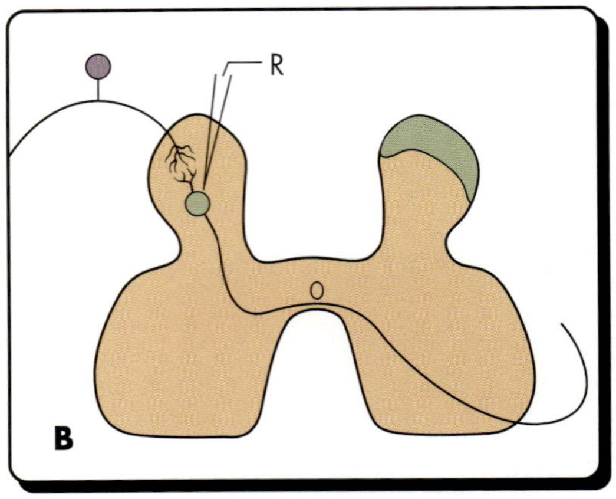

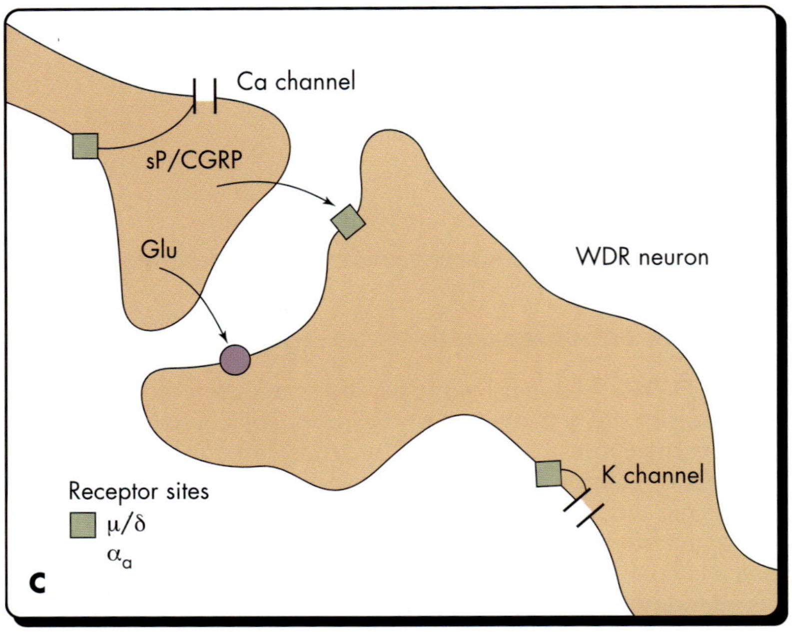

Figure 11-20. Inhibitory pharmacology of spinal excitation induced by small afferent input: common properties of several families of spinal receptor systems that regulate acute pain processing by regulating C-fiber input [15]. The common characteristics of these receptor systems are presented in **A**. Recording (R) from wide dynamic range (WDR) neurons in the dorsal (**B**) have shown them to receive convergent input from large (AB) and small (C) fibers. A variety of agents such as μ, δ, α_2 agonists have been shown to selectively reduce the activity evoked by C fiber input and produce a powerful analgesia after spinal delivery. Several points are relevant. First, the majority of active agents bind predominantly in the superficial dorsal horn of the spinal cord. As indicated for several families of receptors, a large fraction of receptor binding is located on primary afferents in view of the reduction induced by rhizotomy or by treatment with C-primary afferent fiber neurotoxin (capsaicin).

This presynapatic localization (**C**) serves to reduce depolarization-evoked release of peptides. This has been demonstrated for μ and δ opioids and for α_2-adrenergic receptors. Some agents, such as baclofen, have presynaptic binding but fail to significantly reduce release of peptides such as substance P (sP). This suggests that binding of γ aminobutyric acid may be on terminals that do not contain the relevant peptide. Presynaptic inhibition is mediated by the blocking of the normal opening of voltage-sensitive Ca^{2+} channels responsible for transmitter release. In addition, all compounds listed have potent effects upon the postsynaptic excitation evoked by the local application of depolarizing agents, such as glutamate. The mechanism of postsynaptic inhibition (**C**) has not been defined for all agents. However, for μ, δ, and α_2 receptors, studies have emphasized that they may hyperpolarize the membrane by a G protein–coupled increase in K^+ conductance. These joint pre- and postsynaptic effects are believed to account for the potent antinociceptive actions of μ, δ, α_2 agonists. CGRP—calcitonin gene-related peptide; GABA—gamma aminobutyric acid; Glu—glutamate; NPY—neuropeptide Y; SP—substance P.

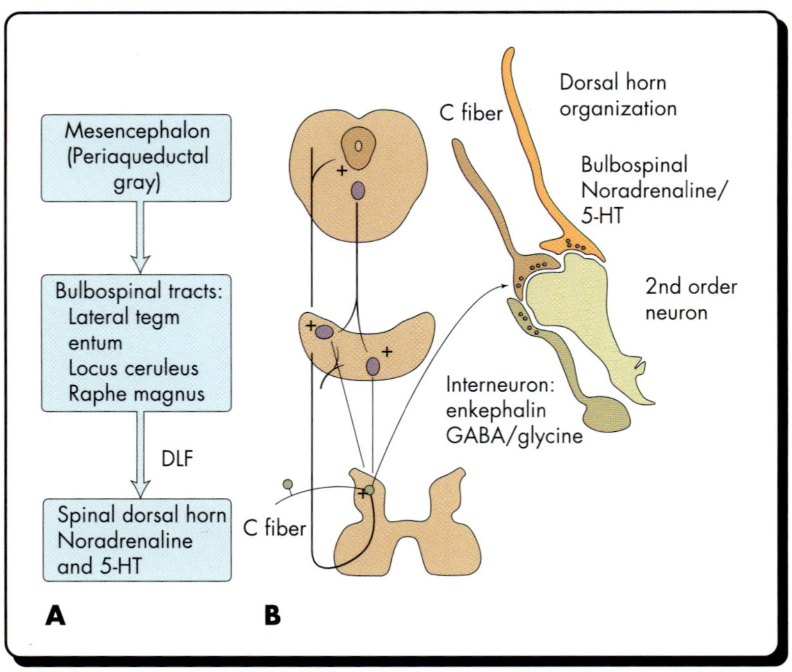

Figure 11-21. Bulbospinal systems that regulate spinal excitation. **A**, The bulbospinal projection through the dorsolateral funiculus (DLF) of noradrenergic and serotonergic (5-HT) tracts into the dorsal horn, originate from the locus ceruleus/lateral tegmentum and raphe magnus, respectively. **B**, At the level of the dorsal horn, these bulbospinal pathways are believed to exert actions pre- and postsynaptic to the primary afferent. At this level, there are also several families of local interneurons that contain peptides such as enkephalin and amino acids such as γ aminobutyric acid (GABA) and glycine. These interneurons exert a similar inhibitory action pre- and postsynaptic to the primary afferent. Both sets of systems serve to modulate the excitability of the synapse by altering the release of primary afferent neurotransmitters and the postsynaptic excitability of the second-order neuron [16].

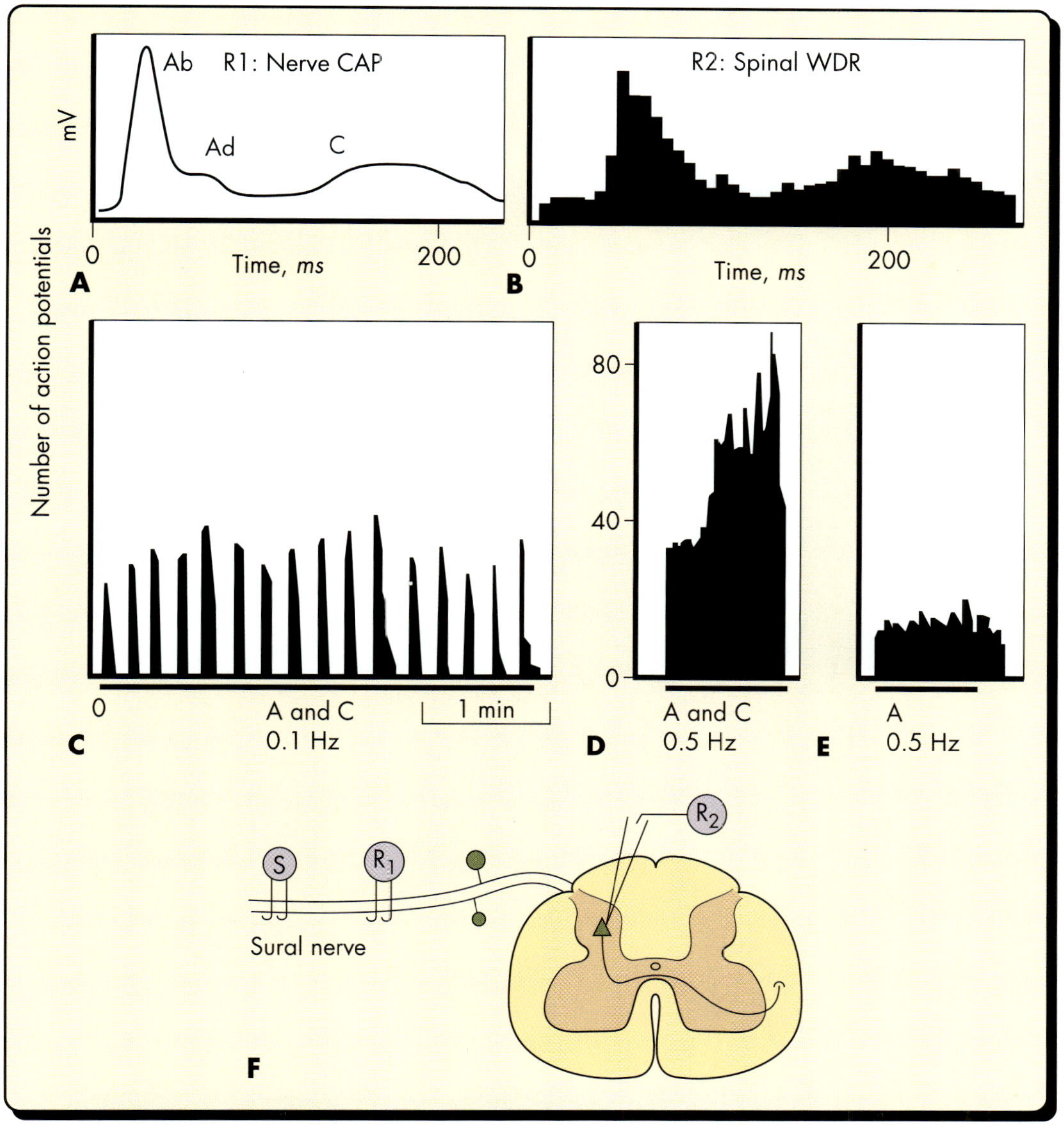

Figure 11-22. Role of persistent small afferent–evoked excitation and central facilitation. **A,** Compound action potential (CAP) recorded from sural nerve (from site R1 in the cord) evoked by a single, brief, high-intensity electrical stimulus to the nerve. Note the rapidly conducting Aβ/Aδ and the slowly conducting C component.

B, Post–stimulus-time histogram, plotting the frequency of firing over time of a single WDR neuron, as recorded with an electrode (R2) inserted into the dorsal horn. Note that the activity evoked by the same single stimulus as that in the CAP and measured over an interval of approximately 200 ms shows an initial component reflecting the activity evoked by the rapidly conducting Aβ afferents, whereas the later discharge reflects the excitation produced by the more slowly conducting Aδ and the most slowly conducting C fibers. This emphasizes that this cell received convergent input from these several types of afferents.

C, Post–stimulus-time histogram displaying response over an interval of approximately 2–3 min showing the response of the single WDR neuron shown in *panel B* to sequential electrical stimuli at an intensity that activates large (A) and small (C) afferents delivered at 0.1 Hz. As indicated, a reliable, stimulus-linked response is evoked at this frequency. In contrast, when the stimulation rate is increased to 0.5 Hz, there is a progressive increase in the magnitude of the response generated by the stimulation. This is called "wind-up" (**D**). This facilitation is not observed when the stimulus intensity is lowered to evoke only an Aβ CAP (**E**). **F,** Location of electrical stimulus on sural nerve. (Parts C, D, and E *adapted from* Dickenson and Sullivan [17].)

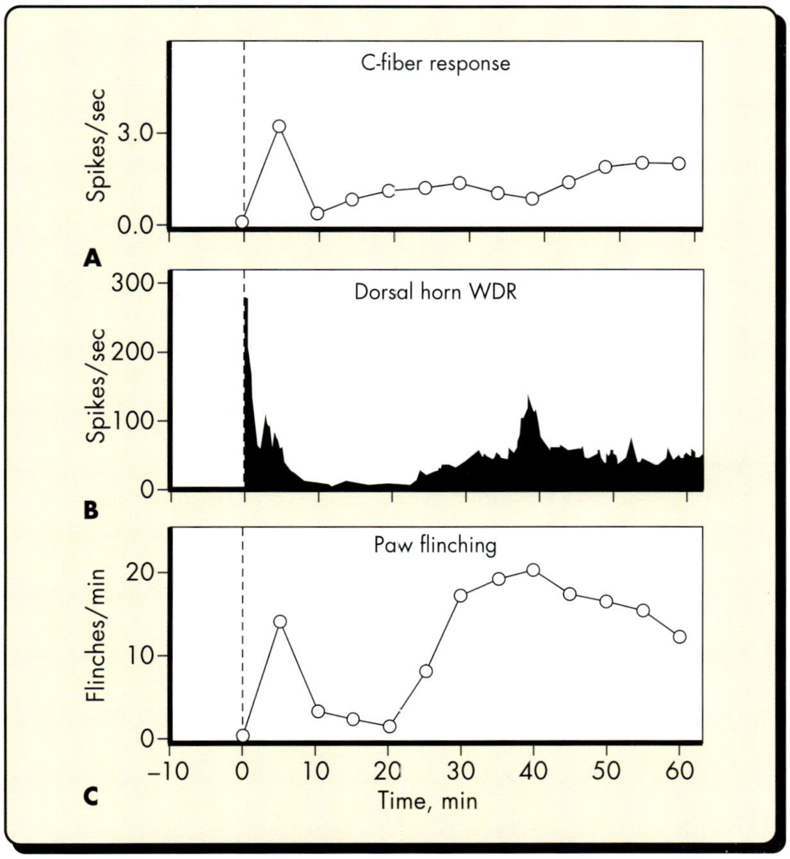

Figure 11-23. Effect of persistent afferent input evoked by paw formalin on neural activity and behavior in the rat. The three panels display the small afferent activity measured in the sural nerve of the anesthetized rat (**A**); activity recorded in a dorsal horn WDR neuron in the halothane-anesthetized rat (**B**); and the number of flinches per minute in the unanesthetized rat (**C**) measured before and after the ipsilateral subcutaneous injection of formalin into the hind paw at the time indicated by the *vertical dashed line*. Note the low level of afferent input during the second phase, when dorsal horn activity and behavior suggestive of pain (flinching) are high. (Part A *adapted from* Puig and Sorkin [17a]; part B *adapted from* Dickenson and Sullivan [18]; part C *adapted from* Malmberg and Yaksh [19].)

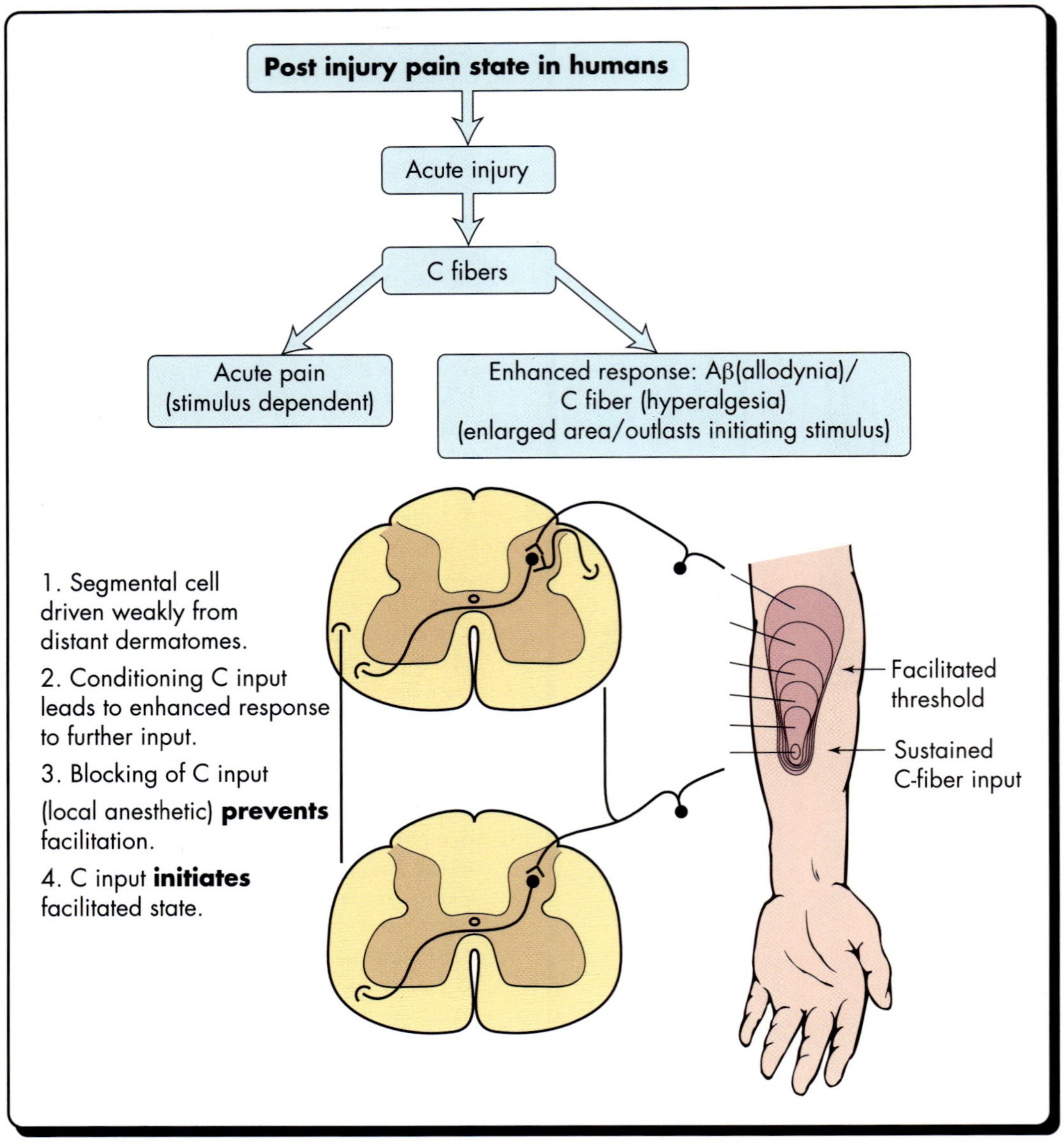

Figure 11-24. Induction of local hyperalgesia by local activation of C fibers in humans: the effects of injecting the C-fiber stimulant capsaicin under the skin. **Top,** Injection generates an intense local pain sensation that persists for 20 to 30 minutes. This sensation diminishes and the patient or observer reports a large area of secondary hyperalgesia that persists for hours. Importantly, if the area of the injection is anesthetized with local anesthetic prior to capsaicin delivery, then when the initial capsaicin effect is gone and the local anesthesia reverses, the observer reports no secondary hyperalgesia. [20,21]. **Bottom,** A component of the effect may be mediated by the spread of excitation to dorsal horn neurons that lie in adjacent segments (see Fig. 11-7).

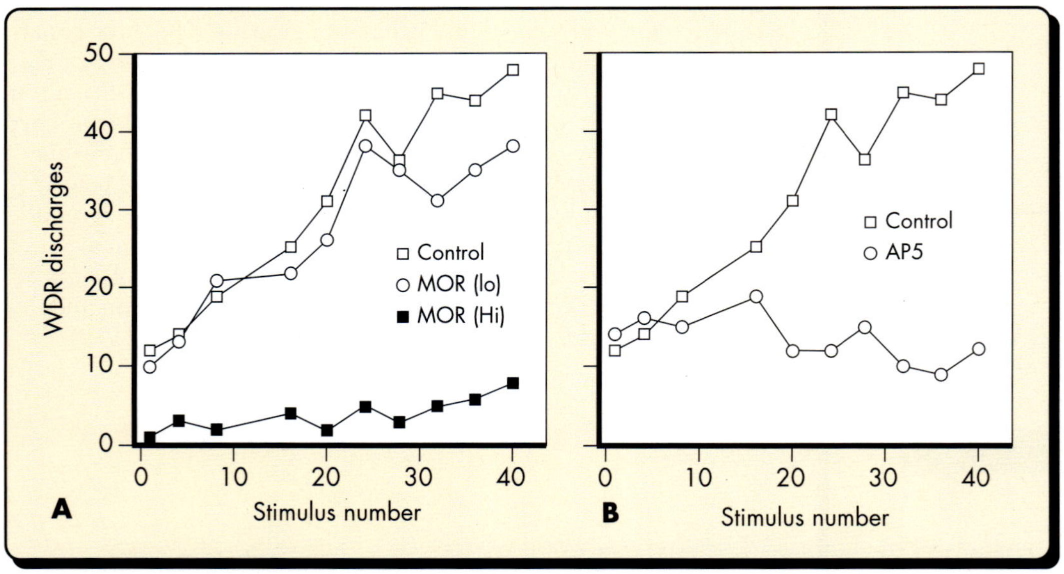

Figure 11-25. Pharmacology of wind-up. In rats under halothane anesthesia, electrical stimuli of the peripheral nerve will evoke discharge. WDR neurons fire in response to sequential electrical stimuli applied to the peripheral nerve. *N*-methyl-D-aspartate (NMDA) receptors are believed to mediate the facilitated response evoked by repetitive (postinjury) C-fiber input. With each sequential stimulus, the number of spikes displayed by the cell increases. This is wind-up. The spinal delivery of an analgesic (Hi) dose of morphine (MOR) results in a suppression of the initial discharge and wind-up does not occur; a low dose (Lo) has no initial effect and does not prevent wind-up (**A**). In contrast, the NMDA antagonist 2-amino-5 phosphonovalorate (AP5) does not block initial input but prevents wind-up (**B**). The NMDA receptor is a calcium ionophore that is activated by glutamate. Note that morphine blocks wind-up but also blocks the initial input (*panel A*). The NMDA receptor is believed *not* to be postsynaptic to the primary afferent, and thus NMDA antagonists do not block the initial evoked discharge. Nevertheless, the interneuron that releases glutamate exerts its facilitative effects at the NMDA site (see Fig. 11-29) [22,23]. (Part B *from* Dickenson and Sullivan [22].)

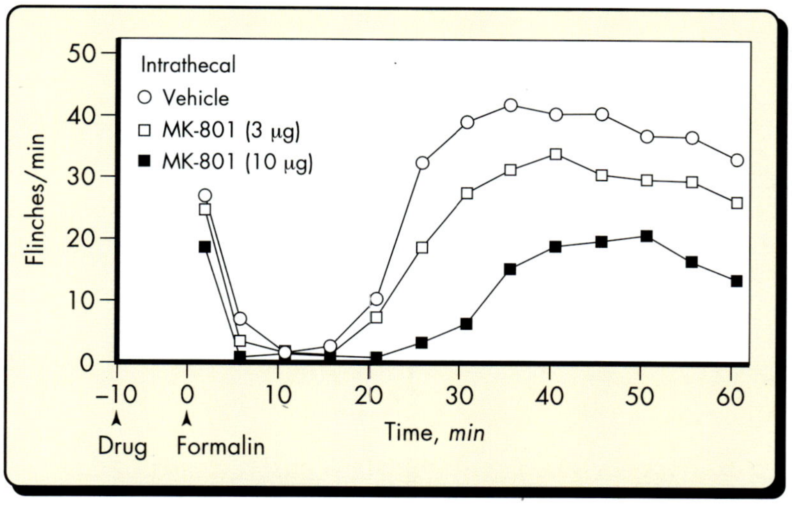

Figure 11-26. Effect of administering a spinal *N*-methyl-D-aspartate (NMDA) antagonist (MK-801) on formalin response. In rats prepared with an intrathecal catheter, the injection of formalin into a single hind paw will induce a biphasic licking and flinching of the injected paw over the ensuing hour. The graphs show the number of flinches per minute after the injectin of formalin at time = 0. The intrathecal injection of MK-801 results in a dose-dependent reduction in the second phase of the formalin test. The second phase of the postformalin state is believed to reflect a state of facilitated processing (see Fig. 11-25) [23].

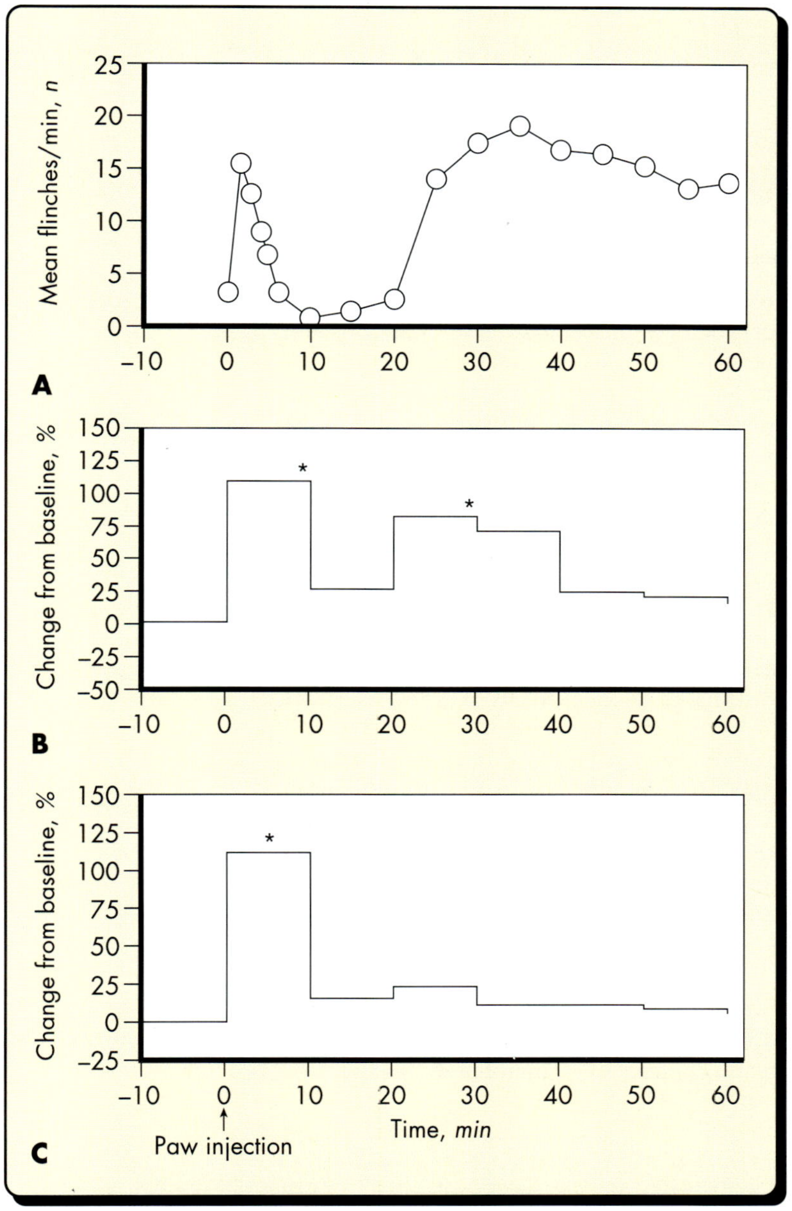

Figure 11-27. Spinal release of glutamate and prostaglandin E_2 (PGE_2) from the spinal cord by paw formalin. In unanesthetized rats prepared with a spinal loop dialysis catheter, the injection of formalin into the hind paw results in a biphasic flinching behavior (**A**). Concurrent measurement of the concentration of PGE_2 (**B**) and glutamate (**C**) into the spinal cord dialysate reveals an increase in glutamate release concurrent with phase 1 and a release of PGE_2 concurrent with phase 1 and phase 2. These results show that the initial release of glutamate initiates a cascade that leads to a facilitated state of processing, which is mediated in part by the spinal release of cyclooxygenase products [24]. *Asterisk* indicates $p < 0.05$ compared with baseline. (*From* Malmberg and Yaksh [24].)

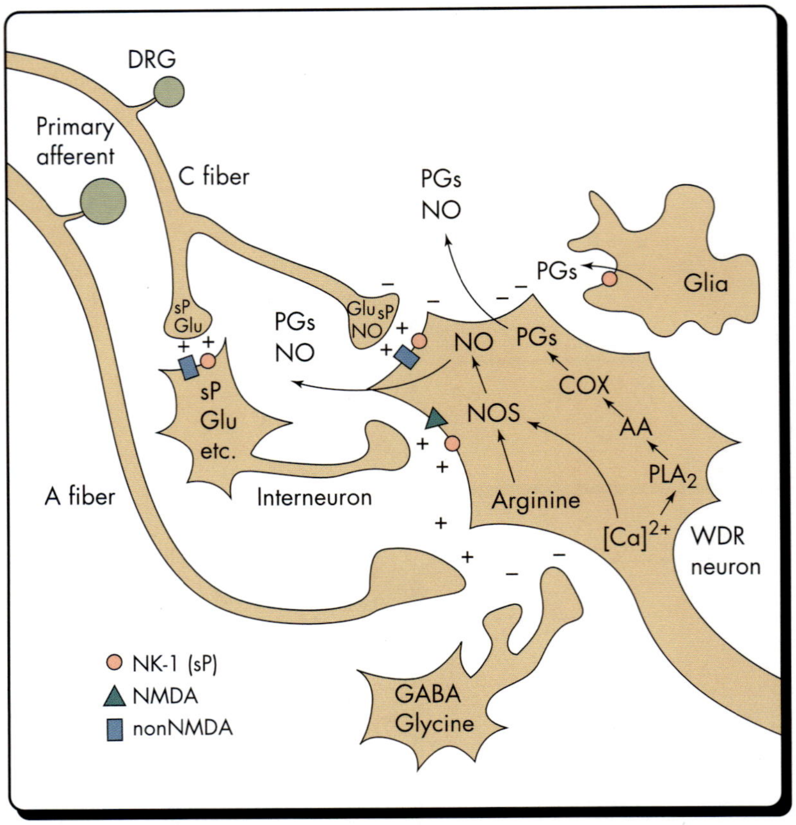

Figure 11-28. Dorsal horn afferent transmitter organization: functional organization of elements in the dorsal horn that impact on the processing of afferent input. This organization reflects the response to acute stimulation, development of the hyperalgesic state induced by repetitive small afferent stimulation, and the development of anomalous pain states secondary to large afferent stimulation. Elements of this organization include the following:

(1) Sensory C fibers release both peptides such as substance P (sP) and calcitonin gene–related peptide and excitatory amino acids such as glutamate (Glu). Small dorsal root ganglion (DRG) cells as well as postsynaptic cells contain nitric oxide synthase (NOS) and are thus able, upon depolarization, to synthesize and release nitric oxide (NO).

(2) Peptides and excitatory amino acids, acting transsynaptically, can evoke excitation in second-order neurons (see Fig. 11-18). For glutamate, it is believed that the excitation is mediated by non-*N*-methyl-D-aspartate (NMDA) receptors. Antagonists for the NMDA or the neurokinin (NK-1) receptor for sP will not block C–fiber evoked excitation, (*ie*, the monosynaptic primary afferent excitation of WDR neurons is not mediated by the NMDA or NK-1 receptor) but will prevent the development of wind-up.

(3) Interneurons excited by the small afferent barrage evoke excitation in subsequent neuronal populations by an action mediated via an NMDA receptor, leading to an increase in intracellular Ca^{2+} and activation of a number of kinases and phosphorylating enzymes. Based on the effects of various enzyme inhibitors, it has been determined that cyclooxygenase (COX) products (prostaglandins or PGs) and NO are formed and released. These agents move extracellularly to facilitate transmitter release from primary and nonprimary afferent terminals.

(4) Intervening products, such as the prostanoids, may arise from nonneuronal structures such as glia by the action of sP.

(5) In certain instances, second-order neurons receive convergent excitatory input from large afferents. Based on the effects of various inhibitory amino acid antagonists, it appears that the excitatory effects of large afferents is under the modulatory control of γ aminobutyric acid (GABA)/glycine, removal of which results in an allodynia (see Fig. 11-29).

(6) Interneurons containing peptides such as enkephalin, or bulbospinal pathways containing monoamines (norepinephrine, serotonin) and peptides (enkephalin, neuropeptide Y), may be activated by afferent input and "reflexly" exert a modulatory influence on the release of C-fiber peptides and postsynaptically hyperpolarize projection neurons (see Fig.11-23). AA—arachidonic acid; PLA_2—phospholipase A_2. (*Adapted from* Yaksh and Malmberg [15].)

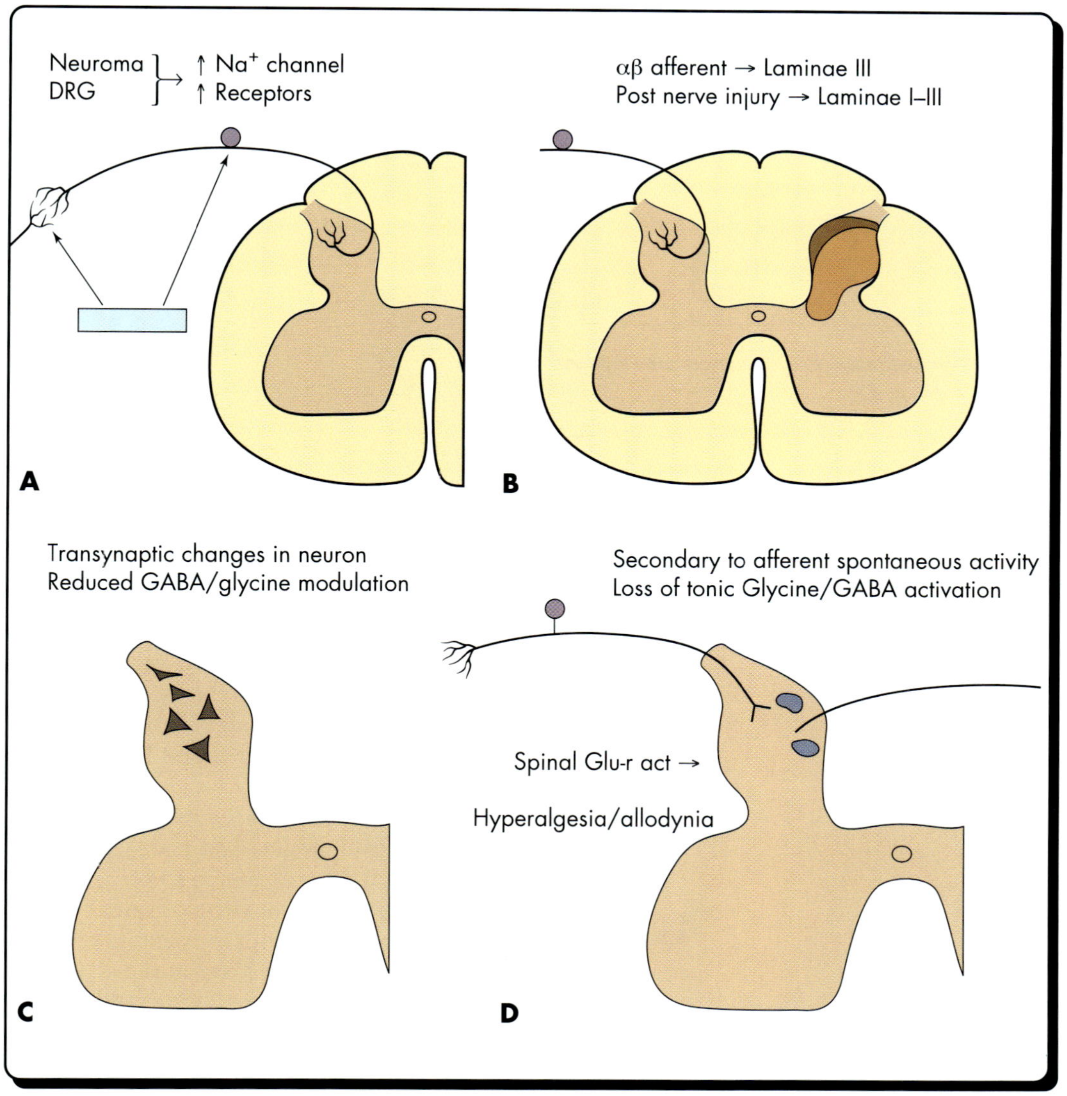

Figure 11-29. Post–nerve injury alteration in spinal and nerve function: Four major events that transpire in the spinal dorsal horn after peripheral nerve injury [25]. **A**, Spontaneous activity develops in the injured terminal (neuroma) *and* in the dorsal root ganglion (DRG) cell of the injured axon. Sprouted terminals also display significant mechanical sensitivity and develop a responsiveness to a number of humoral factors, such as prostaglandins, catecholamines, and cytokines. In addition, it is known that these regenerating terminals display significant increases in the densities of various ion channels, notably those for sodium (Na) [26]. **B**, After peripheral injury, there is a prominent sprouting of large afferents up from lamina III into laminae I and II. Thus, large afferents, normally encoding low-threshold information, will now gain access to spinal termination regions that originally received input only from high-threshold (pain) afferents (see Fig. 11-7) [27]. **C**, Morphologic changes have been identified in the spinal dorsal horn ipsilateral to nerve injury, including appearance of dark-staining neurons that are believed to presage cell death. The region is high in cells that contain γ-aminobutyric acid (GABA) and glycine (inhibitory transmitters). Loss of such GABAergic and glycinergic tone by acute spinal inhibition of these receptors has been shown to induce an allodynic state [28]. **D**, There is an increase in the spinal release of glutamate. Activation of spinal glutamatergic receptors (Glu-r) will induce a spinal hyperalgesia and tactile allodynia. The origins of this increased release are not known, but it is believed to be secondary to the loss of local inhibition and increased spontaneous afferent activity.

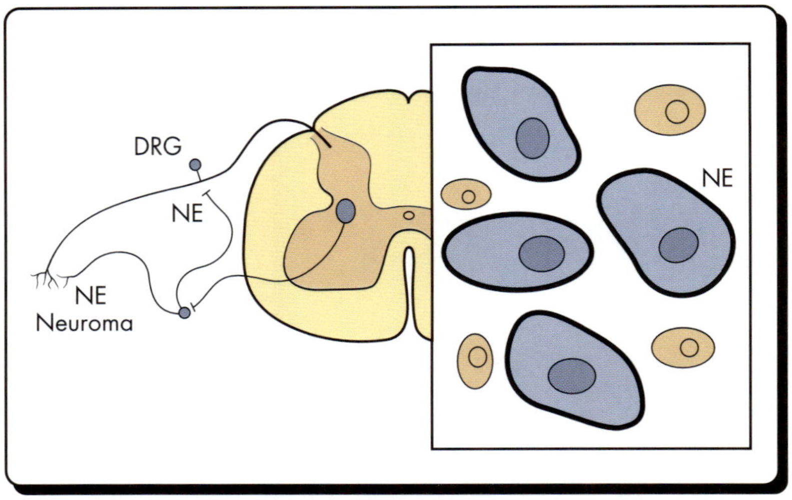

Figure 11-30. Nerve injury and sympathetic innervation of neuroma and dorsal root ganglion (DRG) cells. After peripheral injury, the injured tissue displays a significant increase in sympathetic innervation that occurs concurrently with the revascularization and healing. This increased innervation is particularly prominent in the neuroma of the resprouting afferent nerve. In addition, prominent changes in the DRG of the injured nerve have also been seen. Thus, postganglionic sympathetic terminals proliferate and form basketlike projections around DRG cells, particularly the large type A ganglion cells [29]. Importantly, this sympathetic innervation has been shown to exert an excitatory drive on both the neuroma *and* independently on the respective DRG cell; NE—norepinephine. (*From* McLachlan and coworkers [30].)

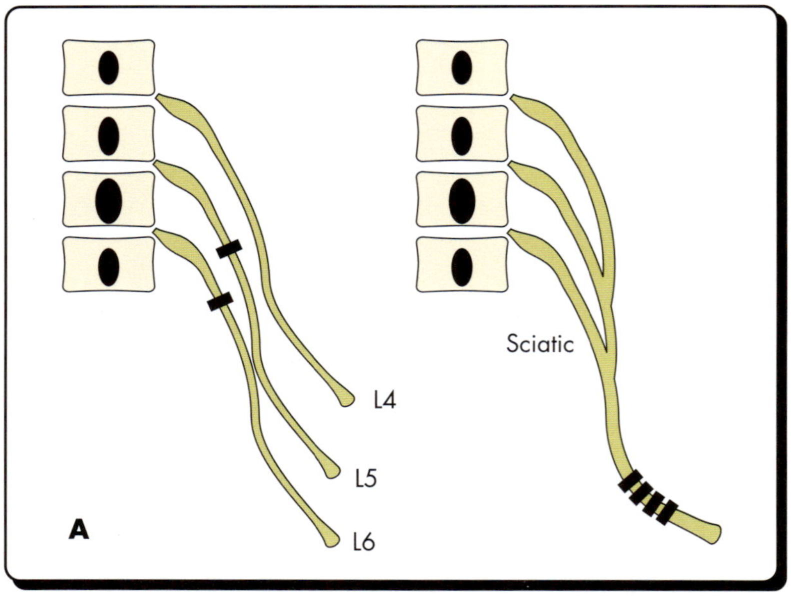

Figure 11-31. Pharmacology of neuropathic pain states. **A**, Models of post–nerve injury or neuropathic pain. Two animal models are the Chung model of neuropathic pain created by the tight ligation of the Lδ and Lβ dorsal roots. This induces a sympathetically dependent tactile allodynia [37] (*left*). A second model is that induced by the placement of loose ligatures on the sciatic nerve. This induces a thermal hyperalgesia [29] (*right*). **B**, Components of the pharmacology for intrathecally delivered agents in the rat on acute nociceptive processing (as defined by the escape latency on a 52°C hot plate test) and on the tactile allodynia of the Chung model and the thermal hyperalgesia of the Bennett and Xie [31] model. Several points may be emphasized [25].

The modest effects of *opiates* in models of allodynia as compared with acute pain models (hot plate) correspond with the relatively poor effect of these agents in some neuropathic conditions in humans. The marginal effect of spinal opiates in the neuropathic pain model as compared with the acute thermal response is consistent with the probable role of C fibers in the acute pain models and of A fibers in the neuropathic model. Importantly, some neuropathic states, such as that generated in the Bennett and Xie [31] model, are opiate sensitive. α_2 *agonists* such as clonidine have been reported to be effective in neuropathic states in humans as well as animals. This effect may be mediated by the sympatholytic action of spinal α_2 agonists. Current observations indicate that there is increased spinal *glutamate* release after a peripheral nerve injury is sustained, and the time course of this increase corresponds with the hyperalgesia and allodynia that appear after injury. Spinally delivered agents that block the receptor/channel will produce a dose-dependent reduction in the allodynic state. *Intravenous local anesthetics* such as parenteral lidocaine attenuates allodynia and hyperalgesia in the post–nerve injury states (see Fig. 35). CCI—chronic constriction injury; EAA—excitatory amino acid; GABA—γ aminobutyric acid; HP—hot plate; IT strych—spinal strychnine; IV—intravenous; M—motor effects are limiting; NMDA—*N*-methyl-D-aspartate; NK-1—neurokinin-1.

B. SPINAL PHARMACOLOGY OF HYPERESTHETIC STATES

Drug Class	Pain State			
	Acute	Hyperesthesia		
Agonists	HP	CCI Thermal	IT Strych Tactile	ChungTactile
Opioid				
μ/δ	++	++	0	0
K	+	+	0	0
α_2	++	++	0	++
Aden (A1)	+(M)	+	++	++
GABA				
A	+(M)	+(M)	+	+
B	+(M)	+(M)	+	+
Antagonists				
EAA				
NMDA	0	++	++	++
Glycine site	0	++	++	++
Non-NMDA	0	++	++	++
NK-1	0	0	0	0
Calcium channel				
N-type	0	?	++	++
P-type	0	?	?	0
IV blockers				
Lidocaine	0	0	+	++

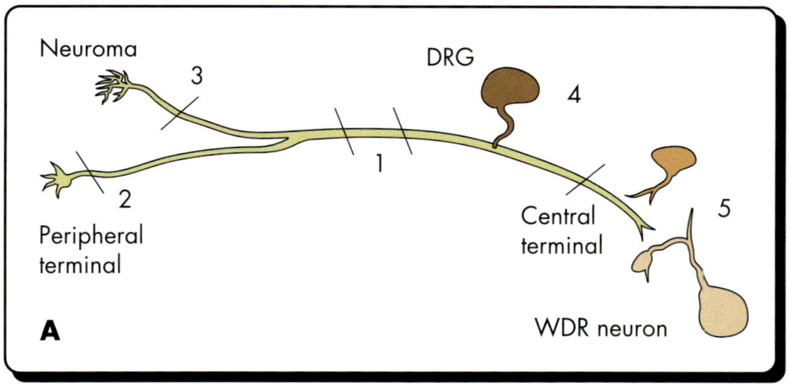

B. LIDOCAINE AND POST–NERVE INJURY PAIN

Site	Blockade	Estimated plasma concentration, *µg/mL*
(1)	Axon conduction	10–15
(2)	SA in injured fiber (rabbit cornea) [33]	5–10
(3)	Neuroma-SA (rat sciatic nerve) [34]	3–5
(4)	DRG-SA (rat sciatic nerve) [34]	1–3
(5)	Glutamate-evoked excitation (intrathecal glutamate) [32]	1–3

Figure 11-32. Action of systemic sodium channel blocker (lidocaine) in altering the post–nerve injury pain production. **A**, Five sites of generation of spontaneous activity. **B**, Approximate estimated plasma concentrations that will reduce that spontaneous activity in the rat. Note that the spontaneous generators are blocked by lower lidocaine concentrations than those required to produce frank conduction block of an intact nerve [32]. DRG—dorsal root ganglion; SA—spontaneous activity.

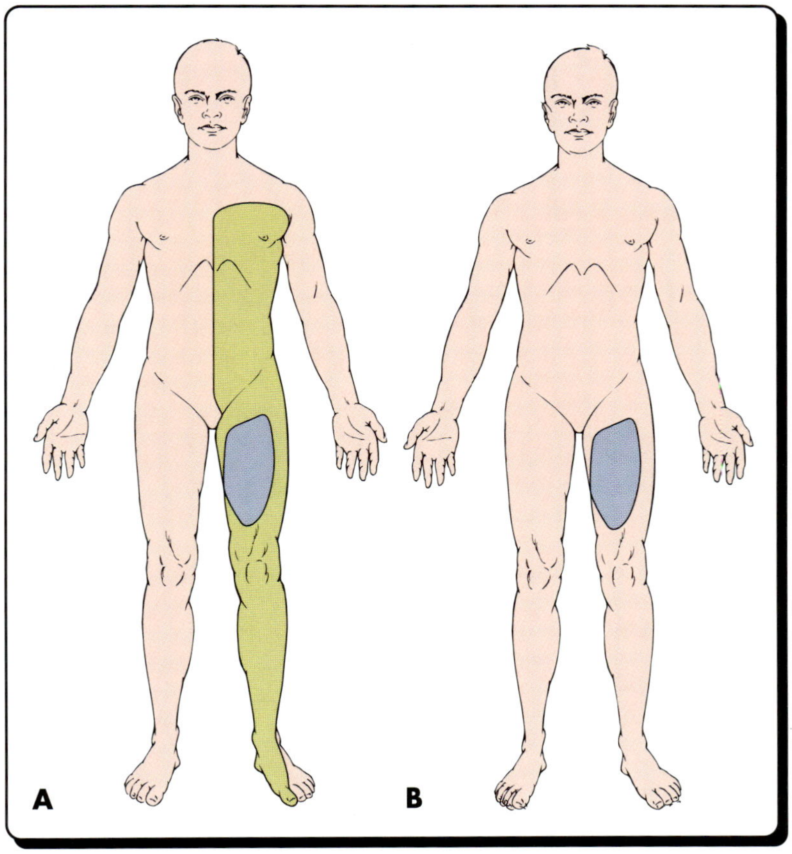

Figure 11-33. Intrathecal *N*-methyl-D-aspartate (NMDA) antagonist in the human neuropathic pain state. A patient presented with severe and intractable neuralgia mediolaterally in the left thigh, probably due to injury of the anterior cutaneous branches of the femoral nerve. **A**, Mapping with low-threshold stimuli indicated that the area of pain sensation (*yellow area*) extended far beyond the territory of the femoral nerve (*purple area*). **B**, Following intrathecal administration of an NMDA antagonist, pain evoked by light touch was limited to the territory of the injured nerve. The remaining pain was not influenced by spinal lidocaine block, strongly implying that it was due to neuropathologic changes at the supraspinal level. Thus, the spinal NMDA antagonist may have reversed all of the plastic changes in pain transmission at the spinal level. (*From* Kristensen and coworkers [35].)

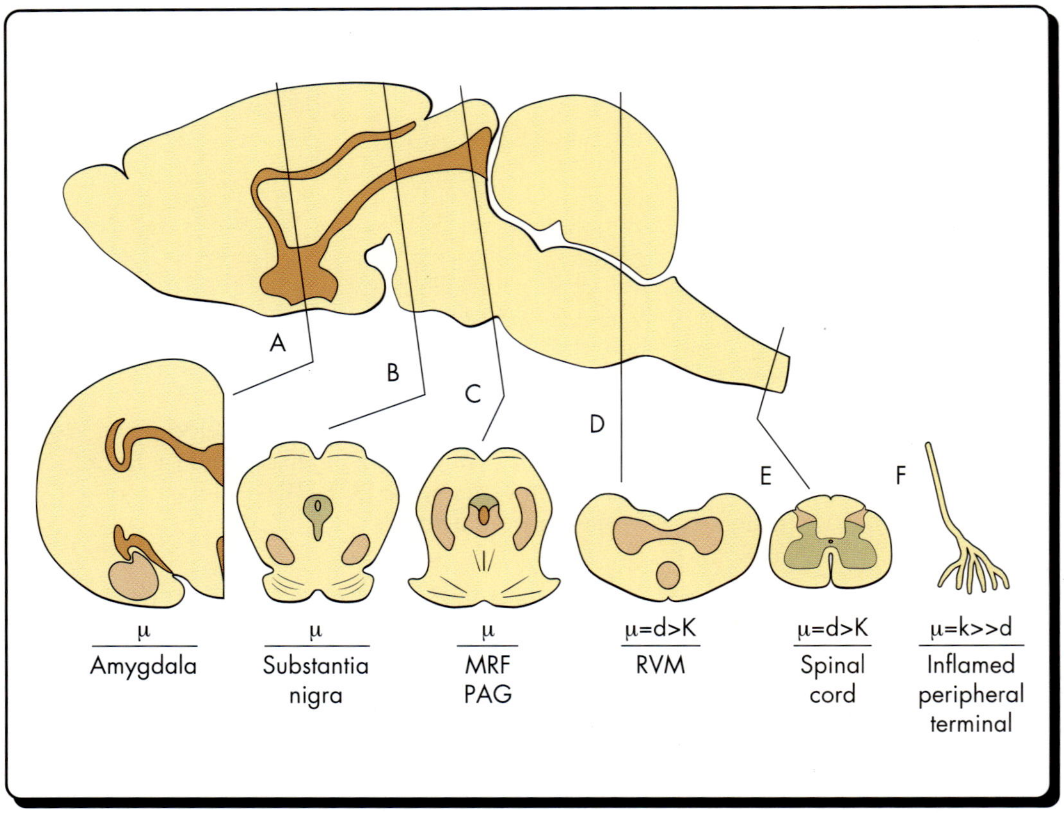

Figure 11-34. Sites of action where opiates exert an antinociceptive action. At these sites within the neuraxis, opiate injections result in a prominent increase in the nociceptive threshold. The approximate planes of section at which the coronal sections are taken are indicated. The *orange area* indicates the cerebral aqueductal location. The *lighter orange area* indicates the active regions. **A**, Diencephalic: active regions within the basolateral amygdala. **B**, Mesencephalic: active sites within the substantia nigra. **C**, Mesencephalic: lateral regions are the mesencephalic reticular formation (MRF); medial region is the periaqueductal gray (PAG) matter. **D**, Medulla: site indicates the rostral ventral medulla (RVM) with the midline structure corresponding to the raphe magnus. **E**, Spinomedullary: active regions refer to the substantia gelatinosa in the spinal and medullary dorsal horn. **F**, Peripheral sensory terminal in an inflamed state. The pharmacology as defined by agonist and antagonist studies is presented under each respective site [44].

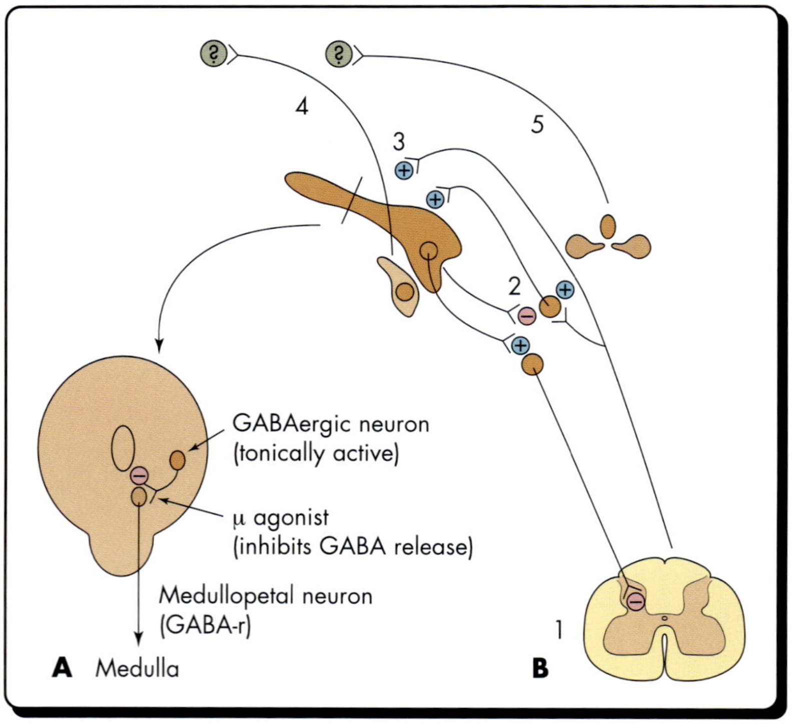

Figure 11-35. Systems underlying antinociceptive effects of periaqueductal gray (PAG) morphine. **A**, Organization of opiate action within the periaqueductal gray matter. μ-Opiate actions block the release of gamma aminobutyric acid (GABA) from tonically active systems that otherwise regulate the projections to the medulla, leading to an activation of PAG outflow. **B**, Overall organization of several mechanisms whereby PAG μ-opiate agonists can alter nociceptive processing. The following mechanisms are hypothesized: PAG projections to the medulla, which serve to activate bulbospinal projections releasing serotonin or noradrenaline at the spinal level (*1*); PAG outflow to the medulla, where local inhibitory interactions result in an inhibition of ascending medullary projections to higher centers (*2*); opiate binding within the PAG may be preterminal on the ascending spinofugal projection; this preterminal action would inhibit input into the medullary core and the mesencephalic core (*3*); outflow from the PAG can act to modulate excitability of dorsal raphe (*4*) and locus ceruleus (*5*), from which ascending serotonergic and noradrenergic projections originate to project to the limbic system and forebrain. (*From* Yaksh [36].)

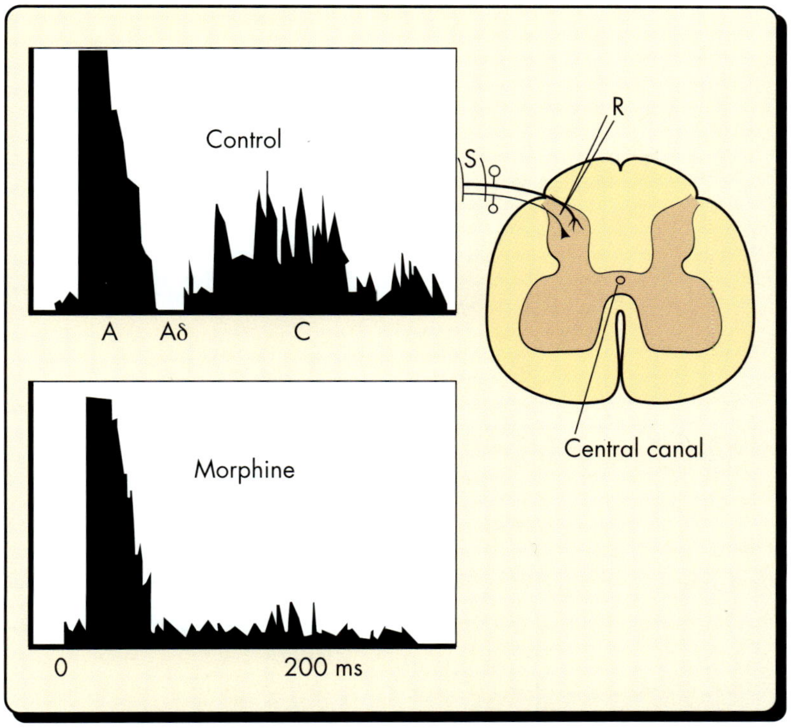

Figure 11-36. Effects of systemic morphine on the discharge of a WDR neuron. In an unanesthetized decerebrate spinal cat, the electrical stimulation (S) of the sciatic nerve will induce a potent activation of a dorsal horn WDR neuron as measured with a single unit electrode (R). The early phase is consistent with the activation generated by the rapidly conducting Aβ afferents, whereas the delayed discharge is believed to be evoked by the more slowly conducting C fibers. As indicated, the late-phase activation is preferentially sensitive to morphine (5 mg/kg, intravenously) as compared with the early component. These effects are readily reversed by naloxone. (*Adapted from* Yaksh [37]).

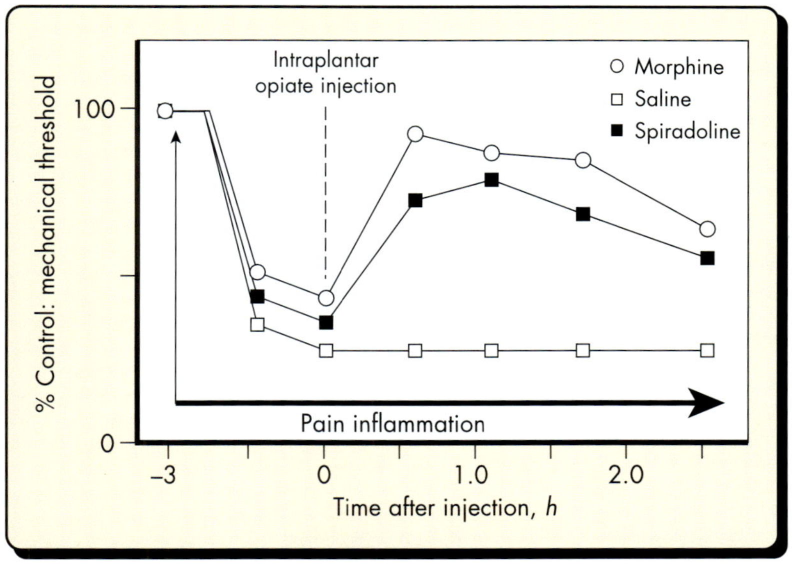

Figure 11-37. Effects of intradermal opiates on inflammation-evoked hyperalgesia. In rats with inflamed paws, the mechanical pain threshold is significantly lowered. The injection of μ (morphine) or K (Spiradoline) agonists will reverse the hyperalgesic components. The effects are naloxone reversible, and similar doses given parenterally do not exert this action. In the uninflamed paw, this local action does not occur. This action is believed to reflect a local effect on the hyperalgesic inflamed state.

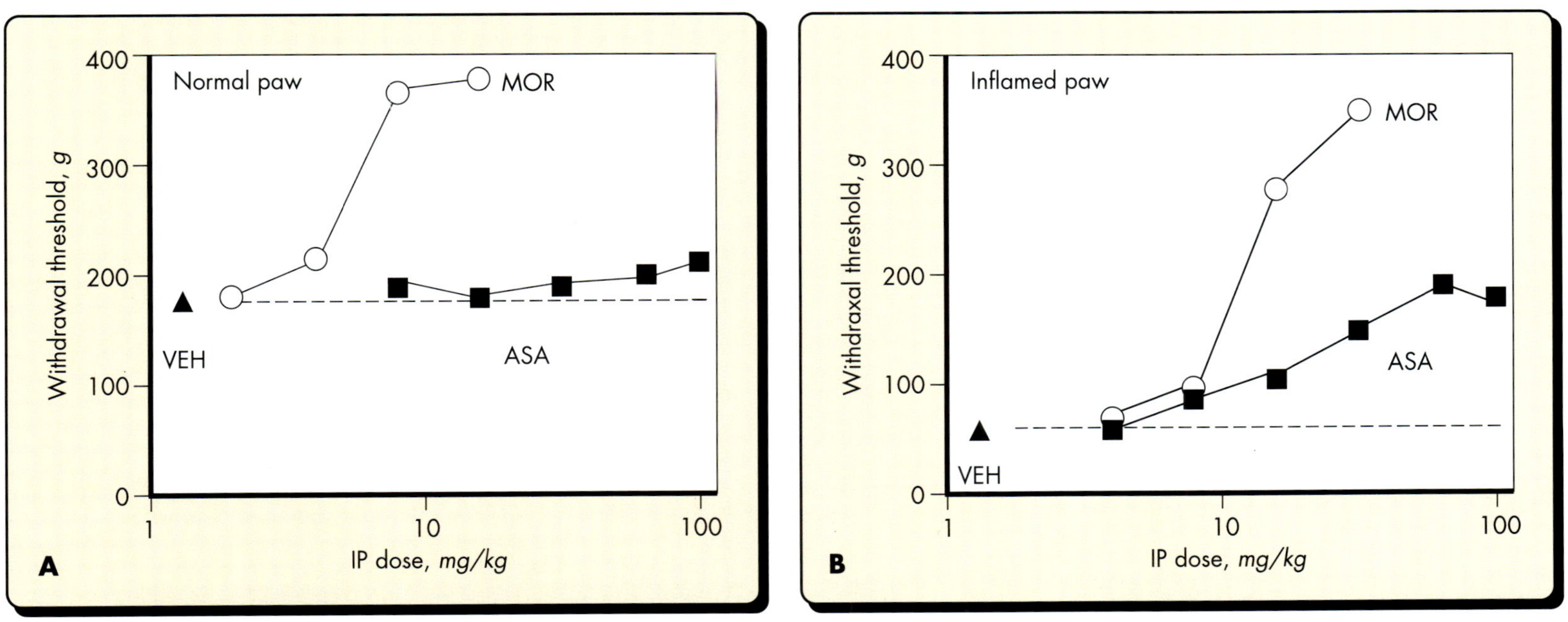

Figure 11-38. Comparison of the effects of morphine (MOR) and acetylsalicylic acid (ASA) on mechanical threshold in normal versus inflamed rat paws. Dose-response curves for systemic morphine and ASA in rats show the effects of these agents in the threshold pressure in grams required to produce a withdrawal of the hindpaw in a normal paw (**A**) and in a paw inflamed previously by the local injection of carrageenan (**B**). As indicated, the carrageenan-injected paw shows a lower threshold than the normal paw injected with vehicle (VEH) or a hyperalgesia. Morphine elevates the threshold to maximum (400 g) in both paws (though it takes higher doses for the inflamed paw) whereas ASA elevates threshold only of the inflamed paw (but not the normal paw). The effect of ASA is limited to reversing the hyperalgesic component. (*From* Yaksh [38].)

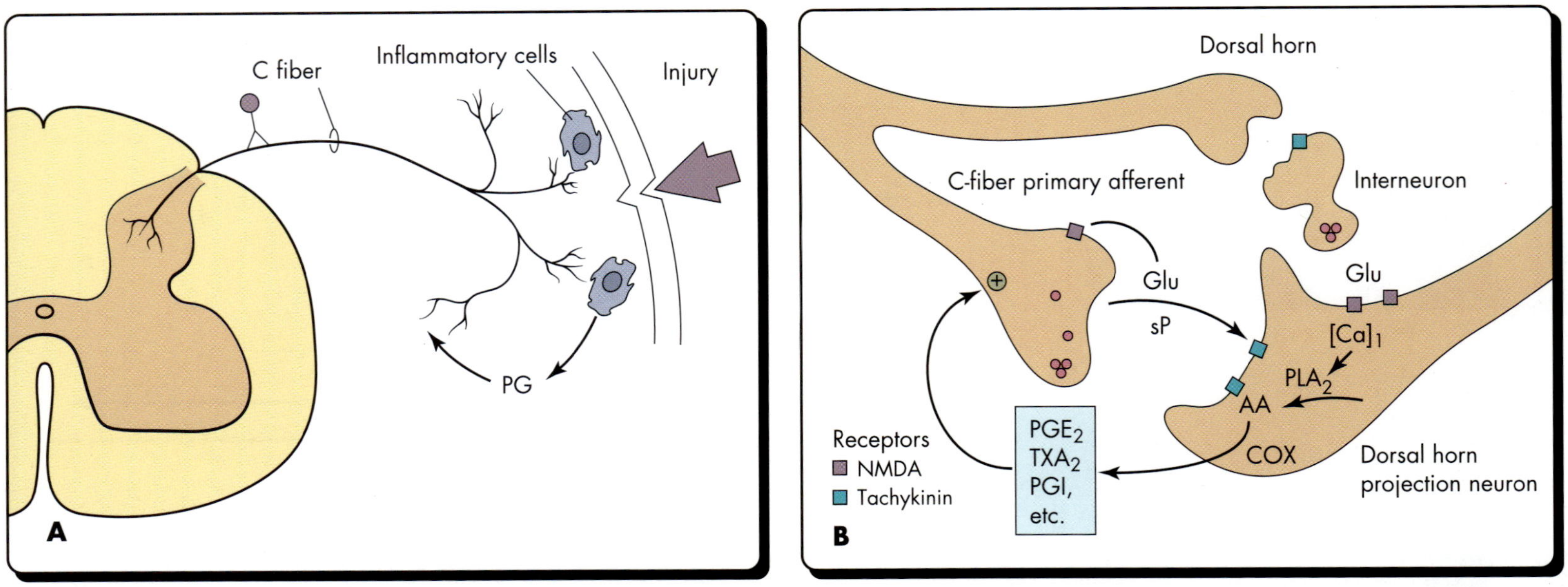

Figure 11-39. Peripheral and central actions of NSAIDs: Potential mechanisms whereby cyclooxygenase (COX) inhibitors can alter the hyperalgesic component of the post–injury pain state [39]. **A**, Peripheral effects. Tissue injury yields local secretion of prostanoids, which when applied locally yield pain reports and an increase in discharge of sensory nerves. Agents classified as NSAIDs are potent inhibitors of cyclooxygenase and prevent the synthesis and release of prostaglandins (PGs). Assays employing somatomotor nociceptive reflexes evoked by acute high-intensity stimuli are opiate- but not NSAID-sensitive. In contrast, pain models employing local irritants or inflammation are sensitive to both opiates and cyclooxygenase inhibitors. **B**, Central effects. It has been shown that repetitive C-fiber activation yields a release of a variety of excitatory neurotransmitters, including substance P (sP) and glutamate (Glu). This results in an increased intracellular calcium, which in turn results in the activation of a number of intracellular enzymes, including phospholipase A_2 (PLA_2). This results in an increase in free arachidonic acid (AA), which then enters the cyclooxygenase cascade leading to the formation of a variety of PGs that gain access to the extracellular space. Several of these prostanoids have been shown to increase intracellular calcium in sensory afferents and thus would serve to facilitate afferent transmitter release. NMDA—*N*-methyl-D-aspartate; TXA_2—thromboxane A_2.

REFERENCES

1. Kandel ER, Schwartz JH: *Principles of Neural Science*. New York:Elsevier:1981.
2. Raja SN, Meyer RA, Campbell JN: Peripheral mechanisms of somatic pain. *Anesthesiology* 1988, 68:571–590.
3. Heppelmann B, Messlinger K, Neiss W, *et al.*: Fine sensory innervation of the knee joint capsule by group II and group IV nerve fibers in the cat. *J Comp Neruol* 1995, 351:415–432.
4. Fitzgerald M, Gibson S: The postnatal physiological and neurochemical development of peripheral sensory C fibers. *Neuroscience* 1984, 13:933–944.
5. Handwerker HO, Reeh PW: Pain and inflammation. *Pain Res Clin Manage* 1991, 4:59–70.
6. Rexed B: A cytoarchitectonic atlas of the spinal cord of the cat. *J Comp Neurol* 1954, 100:297–380.
7. Kerr FWL: Neuroanatomical substrates of nociception in the spinal cord. *Pain* 1975, 1:325–356.
8. Coggeshall RE, Applebaum ML, Fazen M, *et al.*: Unmyelinated axons in human ventral roots: a possible explanation for the failure of dorsal rhizotomy to relieve pain. *Brain* 1975, 98:157–166.
9. Willis WD, Coggeshall RE: *Sensory Mechanisms of the Spinal Cord*. New York: Plenum Press; 1993.
10. Brown AG: Organization in the Spinal Cord: The Anatomy and Physiology of Identified Neurons. Berlin: Springer Verlag; 1981.
11. Sorkin LS, Ferrington DG, Willis WD Jr: Somatotopic organization and response characteristics of dorsal horn neurons in the cervical spinal cord of the cat. *Somatosens Res* 1986, 3:323–338.
12. Gowers WR: *Manual of Diseases of the Nervous System*. Philadelphia: 1888.
13. Talbot JD, Marrett S, Evans AC, *et al.*: Multiple representations of pain in human cerebral cortex. *Science* 1991, 251:1355–1358.
14. Levine JD, Fields HL, Basbaum AI: Peptides and the primary afferent nociceptor. *J Neurosci* 1993, 13:2273–2286.
15. Yaksh TL, Malmberg AB: Central pharmacology of nociceptive transmission. In *Textbook of Pain*. Edited by Wall PD, Melzack R. New York: Churchill Livingstone; 1994:165–200.
16. Fields HL, Heinricher MM, Mason P: Neurotransmitters in nociceptive modulatory circuits. *Annu Rev Neurosci* 1991, 14:219–245.
17. Dickenson AH, Sullivan AF: Evidence for a role of the NMDA receptor in the frequency dependent potentiation of the deep rat dorsal horn nociceptive neurons following C fiber stimulation. *Neuropharmacology* 1987, 26:1235–1238.

17a. Puig S, Sorkin L: Formalin-evoked activity in identified primary afferent fibers: Systemic Lidocaine suppresses phase-2 activity. *Pain* 1995, 64:345–355.

18. Dickenson AH, Sullivan AF: Subcutaneous formalin-induced activity of dorsal horn neurones in the rat: differential response to an intrathecal opiate administered pre or post formalin. *Pain* 1987, 30:349–360.
19. Malmberg AB, Yaksh TL: Antinociceptive actions of spinal nonsteroidal anti-inflammatory agents on the formalin test in the rat. *J Pharmacol Exp Ther* 1992, 263:136–146.
20. LaMotte RH, Lundberg LE, Torebjõrk HE: Pain, hyperalgesia and activity in nociceptive C units in humans after intradermal injection of capsaicin. *J Physiol* 1992, 448:749–764.
21. Torebjõrk HE, Lundberg LE, LaMotte RH: Central changes in processing of mechanoreceptive input in capsaicin-induced secondary hyperalgesia in humans. *J Physiol* 1992, 448:765–780.
22. Dickenson AH, Sullivan AF: A cure for wind up: NMDA receptor antagonists as potential analgesics. *Trends Pharmacol Sci* 1990, 11:307–309.

23. Yaksh TL, Chaplan SR, Malmberg AB: Future directionsin the pharmacological management of hyperalgesic and allogynic pain states: The NMDA receptor. In *Medications Development for the Treatment of Pregnant Addicts and Their Infants*. NIDA Research Monograph Series #149. Edited by Chiang CN, Finnegan LP. Rockville, MD: US Dept. of Health and Human Services; 1995:84–103.
24. Malmberg AB, Yaksh TL: Cyclooxgenase inhibition and the spinal release of prostaglandin E2 and amino acids evoked by paw formalin injection: A microdialysis study in unanesthetized rats. *J Neurosci* 1995, 15:2768–2776.
25. Yaksh TL: Neurologic mechanisms of pain. In *Clinical Anesthesia and Management of Pain*, edn 2. Edited by Cousins MJ, Bridenbaugh PO. Philadelphia: Lippincott-Raven; 1997: in press.
26. Devor M: Neuropathic pain and injured nerve: Peripheral mechanisms. *Br Med Bull* 1991, 47:619–630.
27. Woolf CJ, Shortland P, Coggeshall RE: Peripheral nerve injury triggers central sprouting of myelinated afferents. *Nature* 1992, 355:75–78.
28. Sugimoto T, Bennett GJ, Kajander KC: Transsynaptic degeneration in the superficial dorsal horn after sciatic nerve injury: Effects of a chronic constriction injury, transection, and strychnine. *Pain* 1990, 42:205–213.
29. Kim SH, Chung JM: An experimental model for peripheral neuropathy produced by segmental spinal nerve ligation in the rat. *Pain* 1992, 50:355–363.
30. McLachlan EM, Janig W, Devor M, Michaelis M: Peripheral nerve injury triggers noradrenergic sprouting within the dorsal root ganglia. *Nature* 1993, 363:543–546.
31. Bennett GJ, Xie YK: A peripheral mononeuropathy in rat that produces disorders of pain sensation like those seen in man. *Pain* 1988, 33:87–107.
32. Chaplan SR, Bach FW, Shafer SL, Yaksh TL: Prolonged alleviation of tactile allodynia by intravenous lidocaine in neuropathic rats. *Anesthesiology* 1995, 83:775–785.
33. Tanelian DL, MacIver MB: Analgesic concentrations of lidocaine suppress tonic A-δ and C fiber discharges produced by acute injury. *Anesthesiology* 1991, 74:934–936.
34. Devor M, Wall PD, Catalan N: Systemic lidocaine silences ectopic neuroma and DRG discharge without blocking nerve conduction. *Pain* 1992, 48:261–268.
35. Kristensen JD, Svensson B, Gordh T Jr: The NMDA-receptor antagonist CPP abolishes neurogenic "wind-up pain" after intrathecal administration in humans. *Pain* 51:249–253.
36. Yaksh TL: Pharmacology and mechanisms of opioid analgesic acitivity. *Acta Physiol Scan* 1997, 41:94–111.
37. Yaksh TL: Inhibition by etorphine of the discharge of dorsal horn neurons: Effects upon the neuronal response to both high- and low-threshold sensory input in the decerebrate spinal cat. *Exp Neurol* 1978, 60:23–40.
38. Yaksh TL: Central and peripheral mechanisms for the antialgesic action of acetylsalicylic acid. In *Acetylsalicyclic Acid: New Uses for an Old Drug*. Edited by Barnet JM, Hirsh J, Mustard JF. New York: Raven Press; 1982:137–152.
39. Malmberg AM, Yaksh TL: Spinal actions of non-steroidal anti-inflammatory drugs: Evidence for a central role of prostanoids in nociceptive processing. In *Progress in Pharmacology and Clinical Pharmacology* vol 10. New York: Gustav Fischer Verlag; 1993:91–110.

12

Principles of Molecular Biology

Marcel E. Durieux

It has become virtually impossible for the clinical anesthesiologist to ignore the explosive entry of molecular biology in the clinical sciences [1]. The number of laboratory tests based on molecular techniques is increasing at an ever more rapid pace, and there are no signs that this trend will slow in the years to come. There is hope that at some point in the future we may have access to rapid, precise blood tests for such important diseases as the hemophilias and malignant hyperthermia. At the same time, research is in full progress on a more daunting task: the cure of genetically determined diseases. Although the prognosis for gene therapy is still guarded, initial experiments have at least shown the feasibility of replacing a lacking gene in humans [2]. In the future more remote concepts may be considered, such as recombinant drug delivery targeted to only those cells that need the therapy.

To those uninitiated in molecular biology, many of these advances may seem almost magical. Yet they are all logically based on conceptually simple building blocks. This chapter provides a concise overview of the techniques of molecular biology, focusing on concepts rather than practicalities. After a brief review of the necessary background of gene expression, basic techniques are discussed. Then it is shown how these basic techniques are used in succession to generate clinically useful procedures. Diagnosis *of* nucleic acids and *with* nucleic acids is discussed, as well as the technique of DNA sequencing. The basics of cloning are illustrated in sections covering vectors and nucleic acid preparation. Techniques for localizing, amplifying, and expressing DNA are discussed, after which a series of examples of actual gene cloning procedures illustrate the manner in which these techniques are applied together. Finally, the area of mutagenesis requires attention. Examples from applications relevant to anesthesiologists are provided to clarify complex issues, and the figures are cross-referenced to indicate the way in which advanced applications depend on simpler building blocks, as well as to help the reader in returning to a previous explanation for a quick refresher. Important terms are *italicized*.

Molecular biology is a very elegant discipline, and the concepts of the techniques can be understood easily, without the need for detailed procedural information. An understanding of these basics will hopefully enable the clinician to approach advances in molecular biology not only with less trepidation but also with an appreciation for the investigators who, over the past decades, have developed these remarkable techniques. For readers who desire additional information, several excellent textbooks on the subject are available [3,4]. In addition, a recent series of review articles gives a good introduction to the subject [5–8].

GENE EXPRESSION

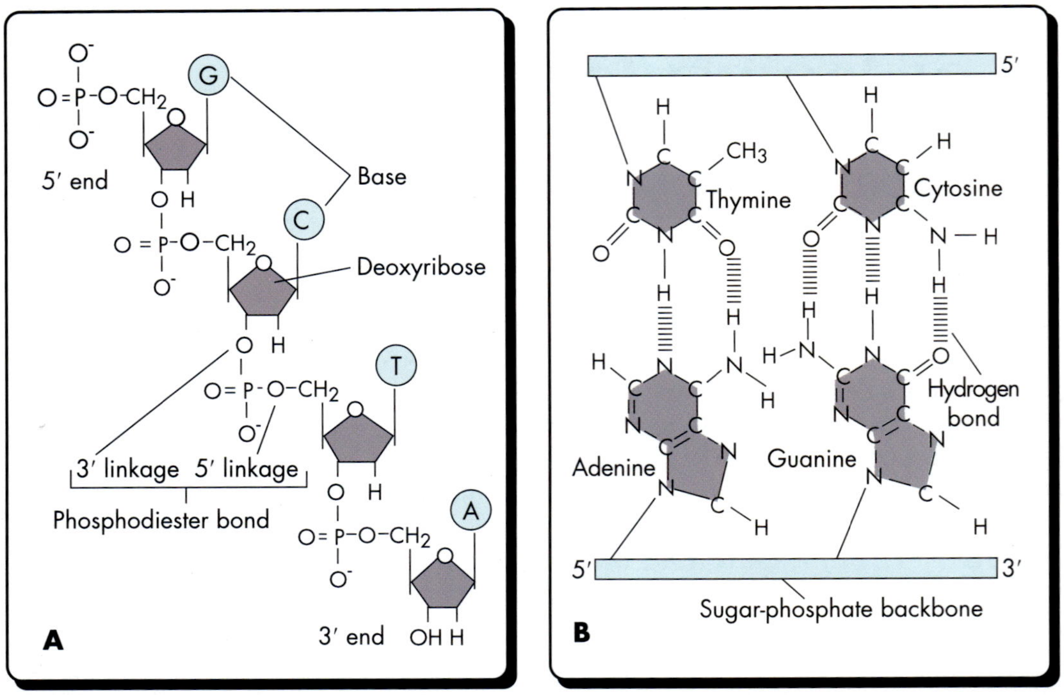

Figure 12-1. DNA structure. Deoxyribonucleic acid (DNA) is a linear polymer of nucleotides. The backbone of the polymer (**A**) consists of deoxyribose (note the colored H) groups connected by phosphodiester bonds between 5′ and 3′ carbon of the sugar moieties. One end of this backbone has a free phosphate group (the 5′ end), whereas the other end has a free hydroxyl group (the 3s′ end). Attached to the sugar moieties are bases (**B**): the pyrimidines thymine (T) and cytosine (C), and the purines adenine (A) and guanine (G). A base with attached sugar is calleda *nucleoside*. A nucleotide with attached phosphate group is called a *nucleotide*.The order of these bases constitutes the information encoded in DNA. In contrast to RNA (see Fig. 12-4), DNA consists of double-stranded molecules, with complementary bases from opposite strands pairing through specific hydrogen bonding. Hence, thymine always pairs with adenine, and cytosine always pairs with guanine (see Fig. 12-2). Therefore, both strands of the DNA molecule contain the same information, and a complementary strand can be constructed based on the information in a single one. This is the basis for the replication (see Fig. 12-3) and repair mechanisms of DNA, as well as the principle for RNA transcription (see Fig. 12-5). (*From* Alberts and coworkers [4].)

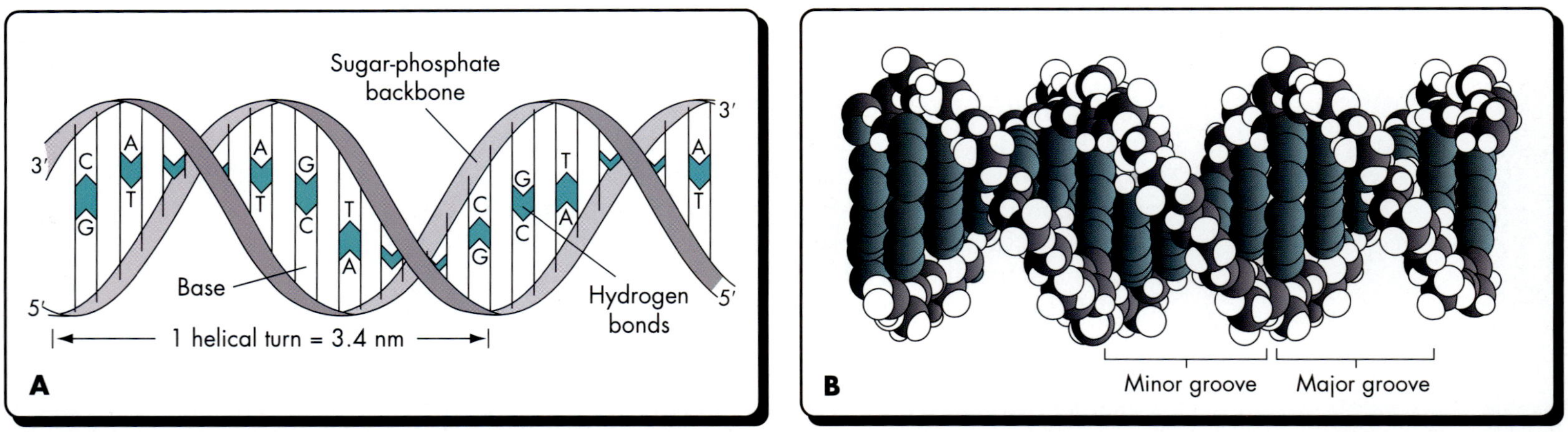

Figure 12-2. The double helix. The essential feature of DNA allowing it to serve as a replicatable, repairable, and transcribable carrier of genetic information is the double encoding of information in two complementary strands (**A** and **B**). These two strands of DNA are twisted around each other in antiparallel fashion (*ie*, one strand runs 5′ to 3′, the other 3′ to 5′) in a right-handed double helix. The bases, paired by hydrogen bonding (see Fig. 12-1) lay within the helix, and the sugar-phosphate backbone occupies the outside. This conformation leads to two grooves in the outer surface of the helix, the major and minor grooves, which allow access for enzymes and regulatory proteins. One turn of the helix is 3.4 nm in length, and contains approximately 10 nucleotides. (*From* Alberts and coworkers [4].)

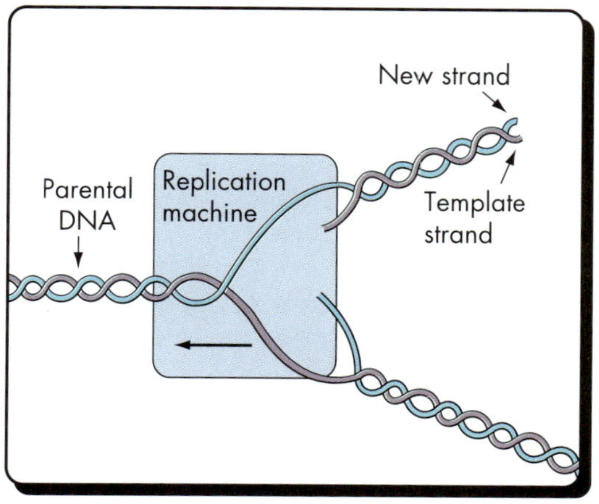

Figure 12-3. DNA replication. Replication of DNA allows the two daughter cells that result from cell division each to have its own full complement of genetic material. Replication is accomplished by opening up the double helix (see Fig. 12-2) as a zipper and using each strand as a template for the construction of a complementary strand. The result is two separate, identical, double-stranded DNA molecules. The process, dubbed *semiconservative replication*, is accomplished by a complex array of enzymes, including *DNA polymerases* (which create a DNA strand based on a template), primases (which lay down short primers needed by the polymerases), helicases (which unwind the double helix), and helix-destabilizing proteins (which help keep the helix unwound). A number of proofreading mechanisms built into the enzymes, as well as separate mechanisms that repair mismatches, ensure very high fidelity in the copying process. The total assembly of enzymes is at times called the *"replication machine."* The figure obviously gives a schematized view of this highly complex process.

The requirement for a primer to begin DNA synthesis is used in several techniques employing DNA synthesis *in vitro*, such as reverse transcription (see Fig. 12-25), polymerase chain reaction (PCR) (see Fig. 12-30), DNA sequencing (see Fig. 12-17), and site-directed mutagenesis (see Fig. 12-43).

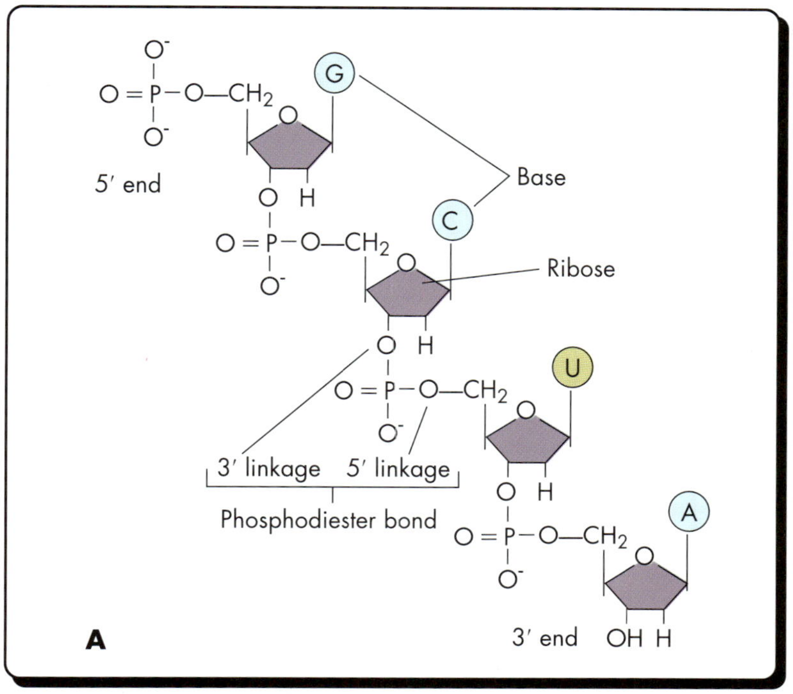

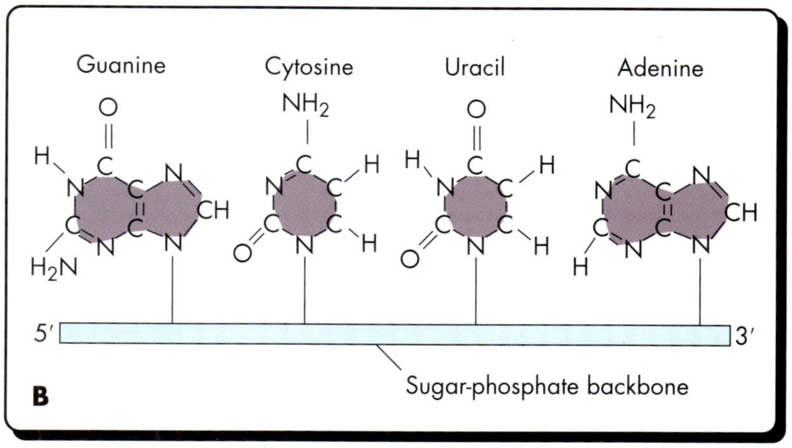

Figure 12-4. RNA structure. There are three differences between the structures of ribonucleic acid (RNA) and DNA (see Fig. 12-1): (1) the sugar-phosphate backbone of RNA (**A**) contains ribose rather than deoxyribose (note the colored OH groups); (2) RNA contains the base uracil instead of thymine; and (3) RNA generally exists as a single-stranded molecule rather than as a double-stranded helix. However, an RNA molecule can fold back on itself, and sections within the same RNA molecule can basepair as in DNA. This allows RNA to assume complex conformational states not unlike those of proteins. Indeed, RNA molecules can act as enzymes, and current thinking on molecular evolution postulates the existence of an RNA-world before the appearance of either DNA or proteins. Some remnants of this are still seen in the presence of structural and catalytic RNA in ribosomes (see Fig. 12-8) and spliceosomes (see Fig. 12-6). However, DNA has a stabler structure, and the variety of amino acids provides proteins with much more structural flexibility than the four bases of RNA (**B**) can accomplish. As a result, DNA evolved to become the prime carrier of genetic information, proteins evolved to become the main structural and catalytic components of the cell, and RNA retained a place only in the conversion of information between the two (see Figs. 12-5 through 12-9). (*From* Alberts and coworkers [4].)

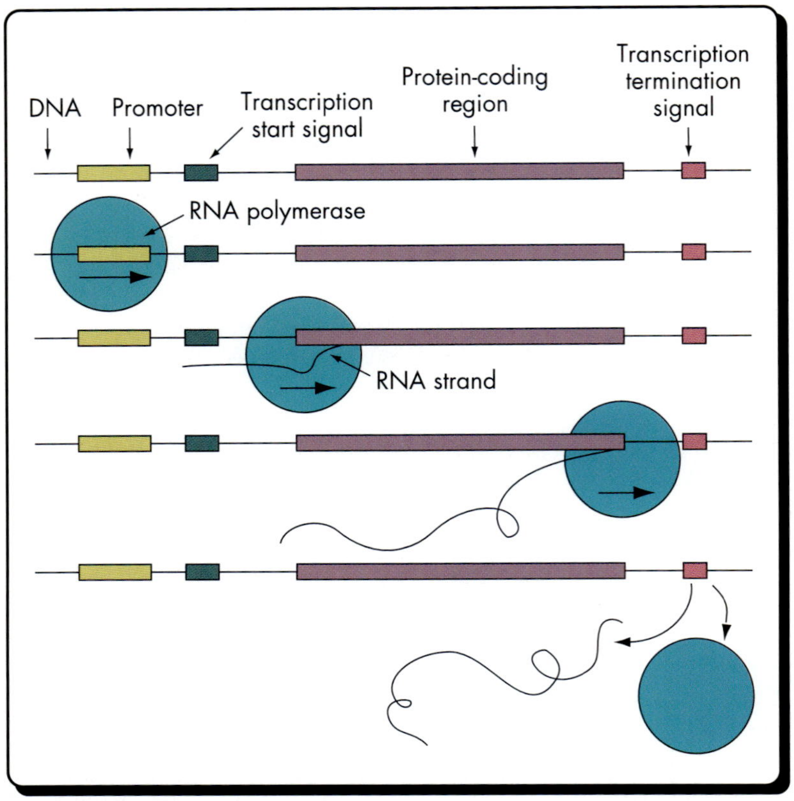

Figure 12-5. RNA transcription. In order for a segment of DNA encoding a protein (a gene) to be translated into protein, it first needs to be copied into RNA, a process called *transcription*. The regulation of this process is shown in Figure 12-10, and the mechanics are discussed here. Transcription is accomplished by a large enzyme, *RNA polymerase*. This enzyme binds to a region on the DNA just in front of the area to be transcribed (*the promoter*). It then moves along the DNA, partially unwinding the helix in the process, until it encounters a *transcription start signal*. At this point, the polymerase begins creating an RNA copy complementary to one strand of the DNA helix (the promoter determines in which direction the polymerase moves along the DNA, and this direction in turn determines which strand is transcribed). The RNA elongates in a 5′ to 3′ direction at a rate of approximately 30 nucleotides per second. Finally, when a *transcription termination signal* is reached, the RNA chain is released and the polymerase dissociates from the DNA template. The RNA can now be processed (see Fig. 12-6) and translated (see Fig. 12-7).

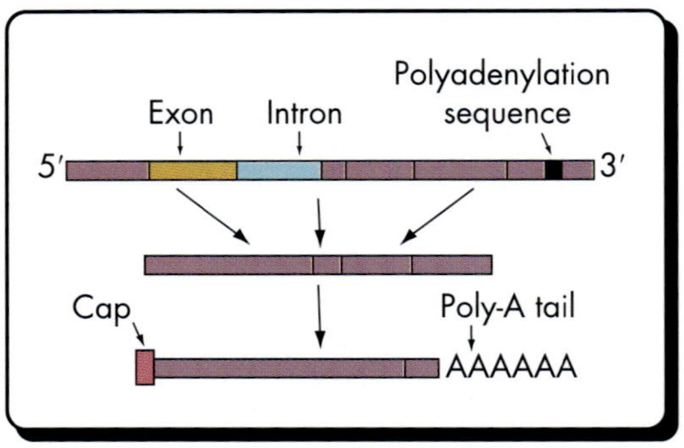

Figure 12-6. RNA processing. Before the RNA can be translated into protein (see Fig. 12-8), several modifications are made. At the 5′ end a methylated guanine nucleotide is added (*capping*); this helps efficient initiation of protein translation. The 3′ end is cleaved 10 to 30 nucleotides upstream (*ie*, 5′) from a *polyadenylation sequence*, and a string of 100 to 200 adenine nucleotides is added. This *poly-A tail* probably prevents degradation of the RNA and forms the basis for a technique of mRNA selection (see Fig. 12-22). Within the area that encodes the protein, eukaryotic DNA often contains sequences of noncoding DNA, called *introns*. Areas actually coding for amino acids are called exons. Introns are removed from the RNA in a process called splicing, by mixed RNA-protein enzymes called *spliceosomes* (a remnant of the RNA-world; see Fig. 12-4). Alternative splicing (see Fig. 12-7) can produce multiple proteins from a single RNA transcript. After processing, the resulting *messenger RNA* (mRNA) is packaged with small protein and ribonucleoprotein particles and transported to the cytoplasm for translation into protein (see Fig. 12-8).

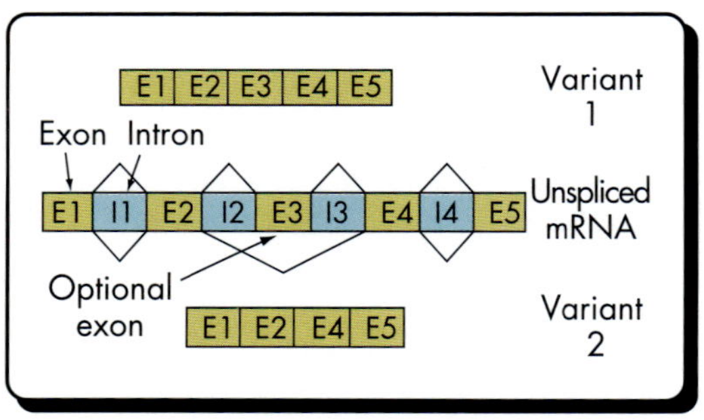

Figure 12-7. Alternative splicing. Although the function of introns (see Fig. 12-6) is poorly understood, they do offer the cell's information handling systems an opportunity to generate different proteins out of a single RNA transcript. In the process of alternative splicing, regulatory molecules direct the splicing machinery to selectively cut out or retain specific exons and introns. An example of an "optional exon" is shown. Other forms of *alternative splicing* include optional introns, mutually exclusive exons, and internal splice sites, where the alternatively spliced variant employs a splice site inside an intron.

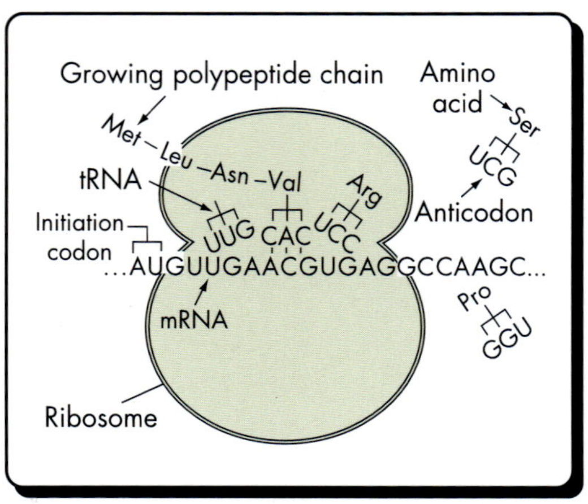

Figure 12-8. Protein synthesis. After transcription (see Fig. 12-5) and processing (see Figs. 12-6 and 12-7), the mRNA is transferred to the cytoplasm, where it is translated into protein. Protein synthesis takes place on ribosomes, complex multisubunit molecules comprised of proteins and ribosomal RNA (rRNA, a remnant of the RNA-world; see Fig. 12-4). In order for translation of an RNA message into protein to occur, the four nucleotide types of RNA must be able to encode the 20 amino acids used to construct proteins. This is done using the genetic code (see Fig. 12-9), where a group of three nucleotides (a *codon*) represents a single amino acid. The genetic code is virtually the same for all organisms, indicating that it evolved early in evolution. Translation starts at an *initiation codon* (AUG, encoding methionine) and proceeds in a 5′ to 3′ direction. Transfer RNA (tRNA) performs the actual translation. Each tRNA molecule displays a triplet of nucleotides (termed an *anticodon*) on one side, which can pair with a complementary codon on the mRNA. On the other side the tRNA carries a single amino acid that is attached by the ribosome to the growing polypeptide chain. Translation ends at a stop codon (see Fig. 12-9).

First Position	Second Position: U	C	A	G	Third Position
U	Phe	Ser	Tyr	Cys	U
	Phe	Ser	Tyr	Cys	C
	Leu	Ser	Stop	Stop	A
	Leu	Ser	Stop	Trp	G
C	Leu	Pro	His	Arg	U
	Leu	Pro	His	Arg	C
	Leu	Pro	Gln	Arg	A
	Leu	Pro	Gln	Arg	G
A	Ile	Thr	Asn	Ser	U
	Ile	Thr	Asn	Ser	C
	Ile	Thr	Lys	Arg	A
	Met	Thr	Lys	Arg	G
G	Val	Ala	Asp	Gly	U
	Val	Ala	Asp	Gly	C
	Val	Ala	Glu	Gly	A
	Val	Ala	Glu	Gly	G

THE GENETIC CODE

Figure 12-9. The genetic code. The *genetic code* indicates how each triplet of bases in mRNA (a *codon*) is translated in an amino acid. It will be obvious that most amino acids can be encoded by several codons, *ie*, the genetic code is *degenerate*. Usually, the degeneracy of the code is in the third base of the codon. Translation always begins with the *initiation codon* AUG, encoding methionine. Hence, all newly synthesized proteins start with methionine, although this amino acid can later be removed. Three stop codons signal termination of translation, resulting in release of the polypeptide chain from the ribosome. Examples of an initiation codon (ATG in the DNA sequence), a stop codon (TAA), and codon usage to encode amino acids is found in Figure 12-18.

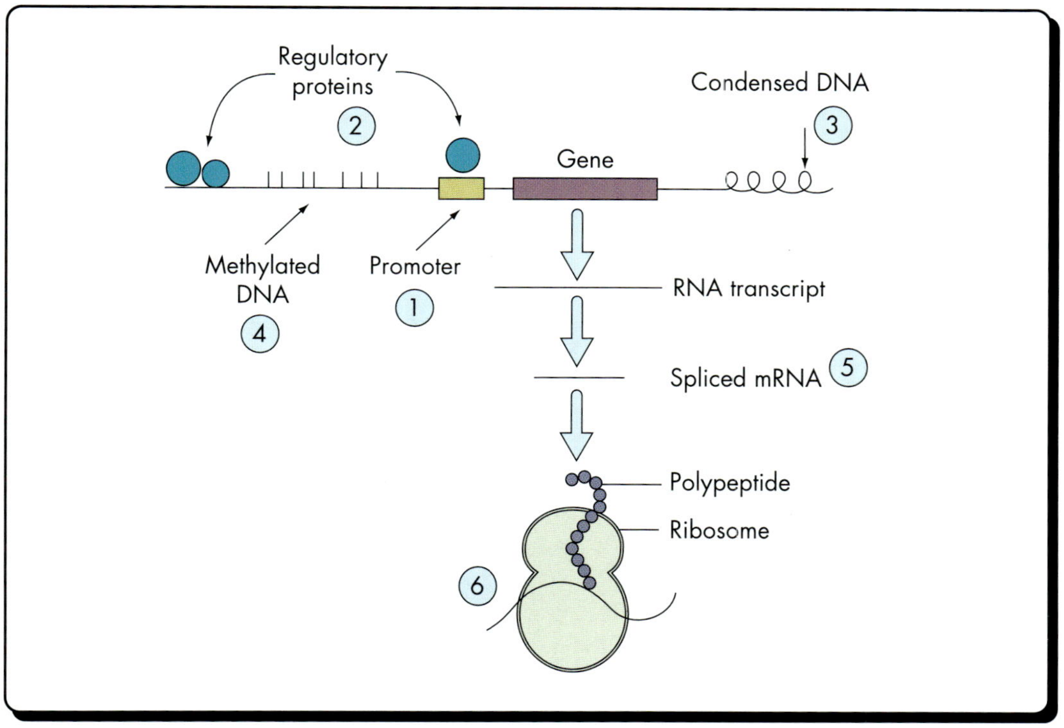

Figure 12-10. Regulation. Although the machinery that transcribes RNA and translates it into protein can create a protein out of every message contained in the DNA, this would be of little use if the expression of these genes was not regulated tightly. All somatic cells within an organism have the same complement of DNA; it is selective expression of proteins that causes the remarkable variability between cell types. Protein expression also must be carefully regulated in order to respond to changes in the environment. Because this issue is so critical, a variety of mechanisms have evolved to regulate the expression of genes. These should be divided into *transcriptional* and *posttranscriptional* regulation. Transcriptional control is most efficient, as no metabolic energy is wasted on the creation of intermediaries that are later discarded.

(1) Promoter strength, or the ability of the promoter (see Fig. 12-5) to initiate transcription, can vary significantly between genes and is a major regulator of gene expression. *(2) Regulatory proteins* bind to DNA and either repress or enhance transcription. *Operons* are a well-studied example in prokaryotes. *Steroid hormone receptors* are a eukaryotic example. *(3)* Eukaryotic DNA can be condensed into a form called *heterochromatin*, which is inaccessible for transcription. An extreme example is the condensation of a whole X chromosome in women into a Barr body. *(4) DNA methylation* is an additional form of regulation and has the advantage that it can be passed on during DNA replication (see Fig. 12-3). *(5) Alternative splicing* (see Fig. 12-7) is a form of posttranscriptional regulation. *(6) mRNA stability* can also regulate the amount of protein produced. Eukaryotic mRNA has a half-life of several hours, but this can differ significantly between messages. Stability is built into the 3s′ untranslated region (see Fig. 12-6). Other regulatory strategies undoubtedly await discovery.

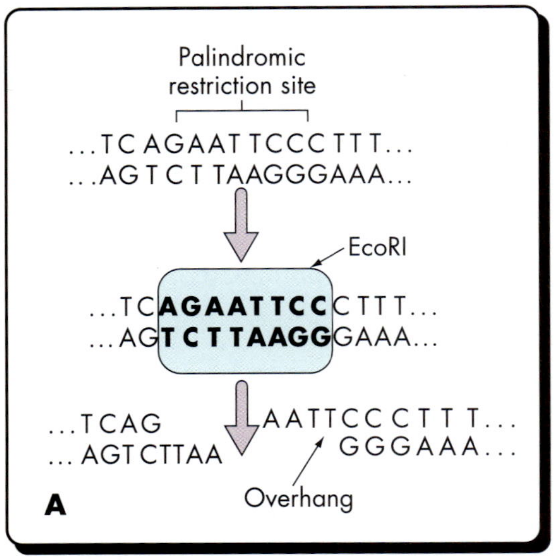

Figure 12-11. Restriction digestion. The essential invention of molecular biology is to use enzymes from living organisms to perform complex operations on DNA and RNA, rather than to manipulate these macromolecules in standard chemical ways. In a way, progress in molecular biology has been commensurate with the number of enzymes known, isolated, and induced to perform their functions *in vitro*. The first step on this path, and still one of those most often used, is restriction digestion of DNA.

B. RESTRICTION SEQUENCES OF SOME RESTRICTION ENZYMES

Enzyme	Sequence	Notes
Taq I	5′ . . . T↓CG A. . . 3′ 3′. . . A GC↑T. . . 5′	4 base pair recognition sequence creates 5′ overhang
Dde I	5′ . . . C↓TNA G. . . 3′ 3′. . . G ANT↑C. . . 5′	4 base pair recognition sequence allows any base in center
*Eco*RI	5′ . . . G↓AATT C. . . 3′ 3′. . . C TTAA↑G. . . 5′	6 base pair recognition sequence creates 5′ overhang
Pst I	5′ . . . CT GCA↓G. . . 3′ 3′. . . GA↑CGT C. . . 5′	6 base pair recognition sequence creates 3′ overhang
*Eco*RV	5′ . . . GAT↓ATC. . . 3′ 3′. . . CTA↑TAG. . . 5′	6 base pair recognition sequence creates blunt ends
Not I	5′ . . . GC↓GGC CGC. . . 3′ 3′. . . CG CCG↑CGC. . . 5′	8 base pair recognition sequence creates 5′ overhang

Restriction enzymes are present in bacteria, where they have the function of destroying foreign DNA (such as from bacteriophages) by cutting it at specific sites that in the bacterial DNA are protected by methylation. Restriction enzymes cut DNA at specific restriction sites, which are short (four to eight nucleotides) palindromic sequences (*ie*, showing the same sequence on both DNA strands) of DNA (**A**). The figure shows how the enzyme *Eco*RI (*ie*, first restriction enzyme obtained from *Escherichia coli* strain R) cuts DNA. The table (**B**) shows restriction sites for representative other restriction enzymes. Note that many enzymes do not cut in the center of the restriction sequence but instead create 5′ and 3′ overhangs ("sticky ends"). These are extremely useful for linking together pieces of DNA (see Fig. 12-12).

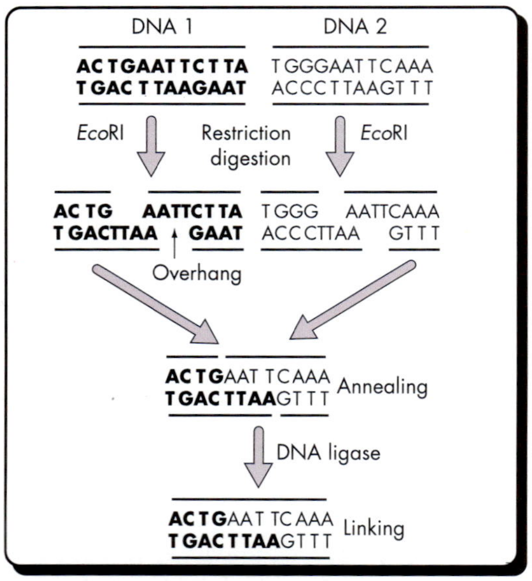

Figure 12-12. Linking. DNA cut by restriction enzymes usually has overhangs or "sticky ends" (see Fig. 12-14). These overhangs can be used to link fragments of DNA from various sources together. If the DNA from both sources is cut with the same restriction enzyme (or a different enzyme yielding the same overhangs), mixing the resulting fragments will result in the basepairing (annealing) of complementary single-stranded ends. Treatment with the enzyme DNA ligase will reconnect the sugar-phosphate backbone, creating a new covalently linked DNA molecule. Thus, restriction enzymes and ligases are powerful tools for removing, moving, and replacing fragments of DNA. For example, they are used to clone segments of DNA into vectors (see Fig. 12-20).

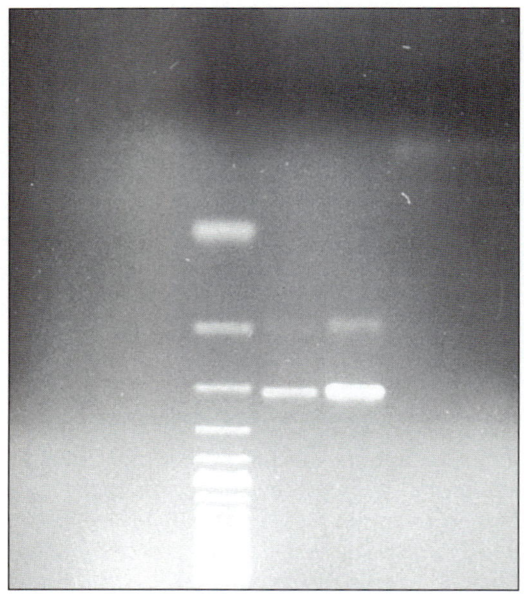

Figure 12-13. Gel electrophoresis. To analyze the fragments of DNA produced by a restriction enzyme (see Fig. 12-11), these fragments must be separated by size. This is done by gel electrophoresis. Agarose is used most commonly, and an example of an agarose gel is shown here. When an electrical field is applied to the gel, the negatively charged DNA molecules move toward the positive pole with a velocity proportional to their molecular weight, which, conveniently, is proportional to their length. The DNA can be stained using the intercalating dye ethidium bromide, and bands can be cut out of the gel to continue processing the separated DNA. RNA can be separated using similar techniques (see Fig. 12-28). (Courtesy of C.K. Chan, MS.)

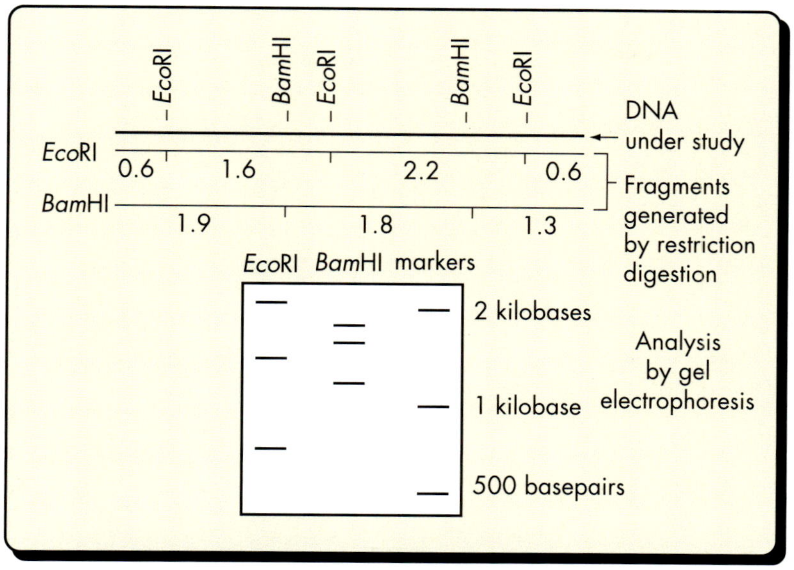

Figure 12-14. Restriction mapping. The particular complement of restriction sites (see Fig. 12-11) in a fragment of DNA forms a marker for the particular piece of DNA. In order to produce such a restriction map the DNA is cut with several enzymes, and the products are separated by gel electrophoresis (see Fig. 12-13). The number and sizes of the resulting fragments form a signature for the particular piece of DNA. This technique forms the basis for diagnosis by restriction fragment length polymorphisms (see Fig. 12-15). In the example, cutting with *Eco*RI results in fragments of 0.6, 1.6, 2.2, and 0.6 kb, whereas cutting with *Bam*HI results in fragments of 1.9, 1.8, and 1.3 kb. Separated on an agarose gel, the resulting bands provide a signature of the DNA from which they were obtained.

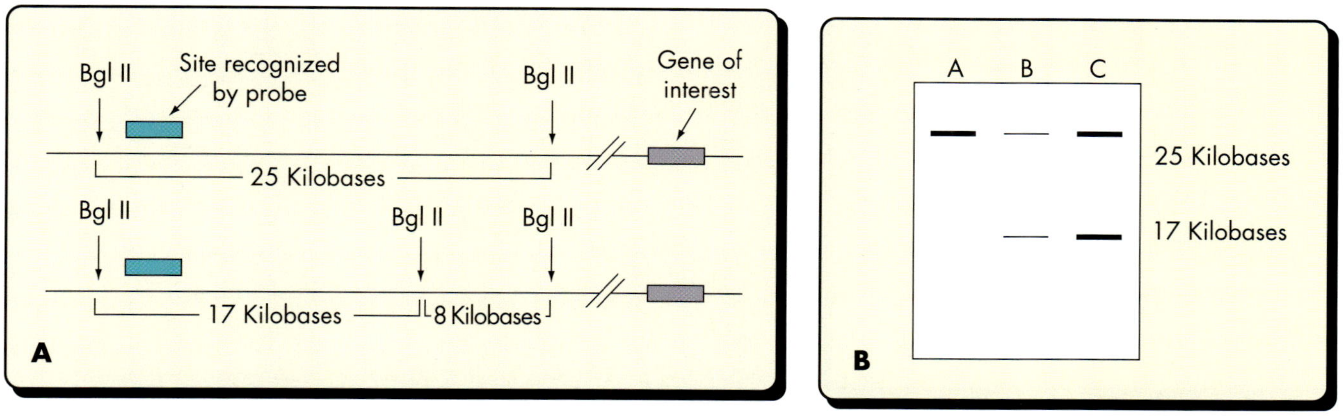

Figure 12-15. Restriction fragment length polymorphisms (RFLPs). RFLP analysis presupposes the existence of a marker sequence close to or in a gene of interest, so that marker and gene will be coinherited. The marker must contain a mutation that modifies a restriction site, so that either the presence or absence of the site is inherited with the mutation in the gene of interest. An RFLP of a hypothetical gene is shown. **A**, The region can contain either two or three restriction sites for the enzyme *Bgl* II, so that restriction digestion (see Fig. 12-14) with *Bgl* II followed by hybridization with a DNA probe (see Fig. 12-28) specific for the marker will result in either a 17-kb or a 25-kb labeled fragment. Absence of the center restriction site (called the polymorphic site) is associated with an abnormality in the gene. **B**, After digestion, hybridization, and gel analysis (see Fig. 12-14) three configurations are possible, with the site present (and thus the abnormal gene absent) in neither (lane A), one (lane B), or both (lane C) chromosomes. An example of the use of RFLP analysis in clinical diagnosis shown in Figure 12-16.

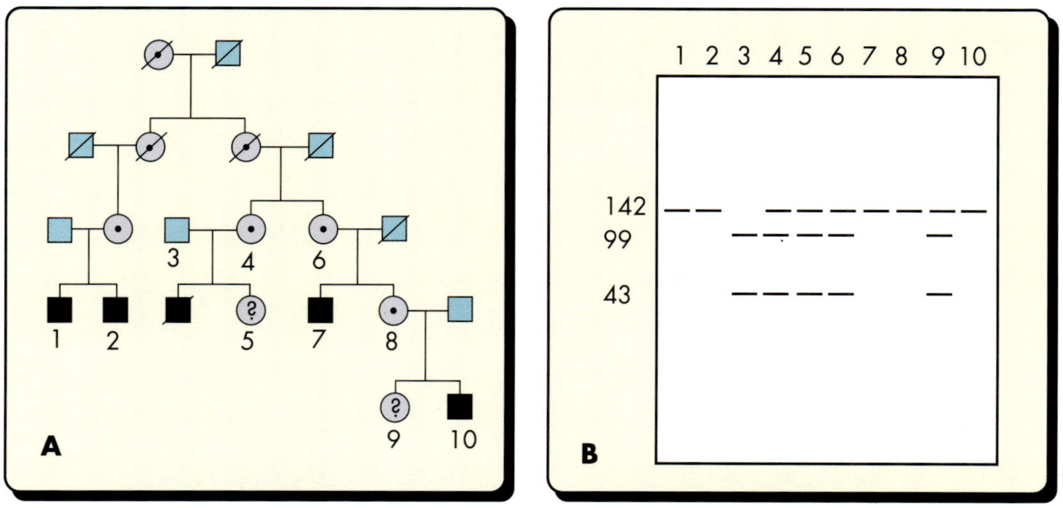

Figure 12-16. Hemophilia detection by restriction fragment length polymorphism (RFLP) analysis. This example employs RFLP analysis (see Fig. 12-15) to identify hemophilia carriers. **A**, Pedigree analysis of a family carrying the hemophilia gene. *Squares* indicate males, *circles* indicate females. *Filled symbols* indicate subjects with hemophilia A, *circles with dots* indicate female carriers, and *diagonal lines* indicate deceased family members. **B** Gel electrophoresis (see Fig. 12-13) of a chromosomal area (amplified by polymerase chain reaction, see Fig. 12-30) carrying a polymorphic site for the restriction enzyme *Bcl* I. The DNA was digested with *Bcl* I prior to gel analysis. Presence of the site is associated with the hemophilia gene. In the absence of the site a 142-bp band results (indicating a normal gene), whereas in its presence a 99-bp plus a 43-bp band indicate a chromosome carrying disease. Lane numbers indicate subjects in the family described in A. Not only homozygous patients but also heterozygous carriers are easily identified. Note the verification of carrier status for subjects 5 and 9, and the homozygous state of subject 8 [9,10]. (*From* Kogan and coworkers [9]).

DNA SEQUENCING

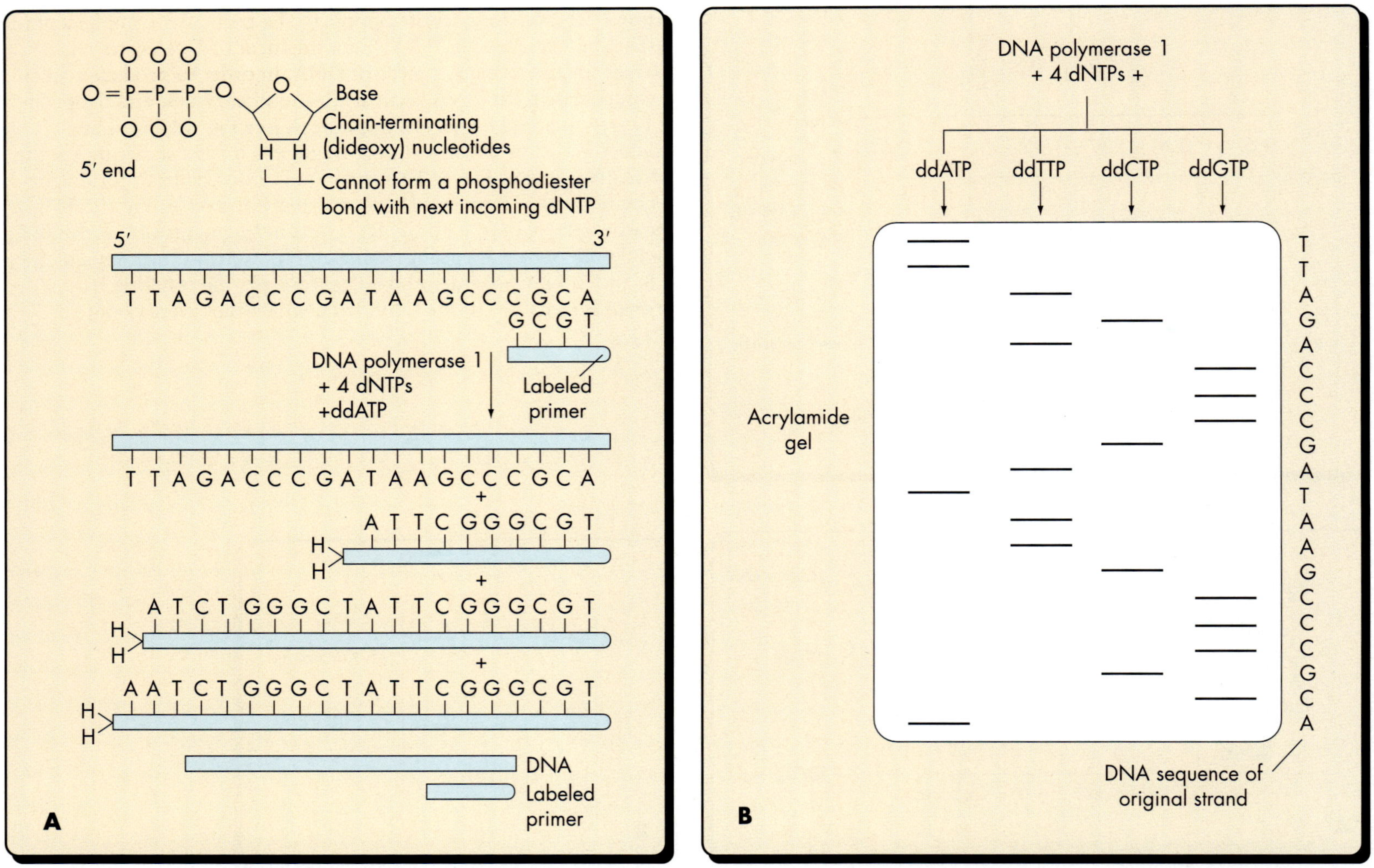

Figure 12-17. DNA sequencing technique. Often, analysis must go beyond restriction maps (see Fig. 12-14), and complete sequencing of a DNA fragment may be necessary, *eg*, during the study of newly cloned genes (see Fig. 12-35), or for the analysis of mutations (see Fig. 12-43). The Sanger dideoxy sequencing technique is still used most commonly. Dideoxynucleotides (**A**) are nucleotides in which the 3′ hydroxyl group has been removed. Although they can be incorporated normally into a growing DNA chain, it is not possible to link another nucleotide to a dideoxynucleotide, because the formation of a phosphodiester bond requires the presence of a 3′ hydroxyl group. Therefore, they are chain elongation terminators. When a DNA strand to be sequenced is incubated with a labeled primer, DNA polymerase, the four normal nucleotides (dNTPs), and a small amount of dideoxy-ATP (ddATP), the result will be a series of labeled DNA fragments that terminate at places where the ddATP was incorporated (*ie*, places corresponding to a T in the original strand). Similar reactions are run with the other three dideoxynucleotides, and the resulting fragments (**B**) are separated by gel electrophoresis (see Fig. 12-13). The sequence of the original strand can be directly read from the autoradiogram of the gel. Novel techniques, employing fluorescent tags, allow this process to be fully automated. Sequences thus obtained can then be analyzed by computer (see Fig. 12-18). An example of a sequencing gel is presented in Figure 12-32. (*From* Watson and coworkers [3].)

```
(Linear) MAP of: ml. seq check: 9236 from: 143 to: 1525

LOCUS        RATACHRMA    2622 bp ds-DNA    ROD    15-JUN-1988
DEFINITION   Rat ml muscarinic acetylcholine receptor gene.
ACCESSION    M16406
KEYWORDS     acetylchonine; muscarinic acetylcholine receptor; neurotransmitter.
SOURCE       Rat DNA and cDNA to mRNA.
  ORGANISM   Rattus norvegicus . . .

                  May 6, 1994 11:54 ..

     ATGAACACCTCAGTGCCCCCTGCTGTCAGTCCCAACATCACTGTCTTGGCACCAGGAAAG
143  ------------+-----------------+----------------+-----------------+---------------+------------------+--  202
     TACTTGTGGAGTCACGGGGGACGACAGTCAGGGTTGTAGTGACAGAACCGTGGTCCTTTC

b    M  N  T  S  V  P  P  A  V  S  P  N  I  T  V  L  A  P  G  K  -

     GGTCCCTGGCAGGTGGCCTTCATCGGGATCACCACAGGCCTCCTGTCTCTAGGCTACAGTG
203  ------------+-----------------+----------------+-----------------+---------------+------------------+--  262
     CCAGGGACCGTCCACCGGAAGTAGCCCTAGTGGTGTCCGGAGGACAGAGATCGATGTCAC

     G  P  W  Q  V  A  F  I  G  I  T  T  G  L  L  S  L  A  T  V

               (Middle part of sequence not shown.
               Last part of sequence shown below.)

     CGCTGGCGCAAGATCCCCAAGCGCCCTGGCTCTGTGCACCGCACCCCCTCCCGCCAATGC
1463 ------------+-----------------+----------------+-----------------+---------------+------------------+--  1522
     GCGACCGCGTTCTAGGGGTTCGCGGGACCGAGCACGTGGCGTCCCCCAGGGCGGTTACG

     R  W  R  K  I  P  K  R  P  G  S  V  H  R  T  P  S  R  Q  C  -

     TAA
1523 ------- 1525
     ATT

A    *  -
```

Figure 12-18. DNA sequencing by computer sequence analysis. Often, analysis of obtained DNA sequence (see Fig. 12-17) is performed using computers. In fact, the sequence obtained can be directly stored in computer-accessible format [11]. Complex programs are available for manipulating computerized DNA sequences. Here, two examples are shown. **A**, The computer has been used to translate the DNA sequence (in this case of the m1 muscarinic acetylcholine receptor) into the appropriate amino acid code (one-letter amino acid abbreviations are used). In addition, the complementary DNA sequence has been determined. Only a portion of the translation is shown. Note the initiation codon, the initiation methionine, and the stop codon at the end of the sequence (see Fig. 12-9).

(Continued on next page)

```
 BESTFIT of: ml. pep  check: 7341  from:  1  to: 461

TRANSLATE of: ml.seq  check: 9236  from: 143  to: 1525
generated symbols 1 to: 461.
LOCUS          RATACHRMA   2622 bp  ds-DNA     ROD        15-JUN-1988
DEFINITION     Rat ml muscarinic acetylcholine receptor gene.
ACCESSION      M16406
KEYWORDS       acetylchonine; muscarinic acetylcholine receptor; neurotransmitter. . . .

 to: at.pep  check: 4456  from: 1 to: 360

TRANSLATE of: at.seq  check: 9446  from: 260  to: 1339
generated symbols 1 to: 360.
LOCUS          RATACHRMA   1450 bp  ss-mRNA    ROD        10-JUN-1992
DEFINITION     Rat angiotensin II receptor mRNA, complete cds.
ACCESSION      M74054
KEYWORDS       angiotensin II receptor . . . .

 Symbol comparison table:
/seqgcg/gcgcore/data/rundata/swgappep.cmp
CompCheck: 1254

       Gap Weight:  3.000        Average Match:  0.540
    Length Weight:  0.100     Average Mismatch: -0.396

          Quality:  143.8               Length:    486
            Ratio:  0.409                 Gaps:     11
Percent Similarity: 49.845    Percent identity: 26.625

   ml.pep x at.pep           May 24, 1994 13:21 ..

  1 MNTSVPPAVSP.NITVLAPGKGPWQVAFIGITTGLLSLATVTGNLLVLIS  49
    :|.|..:::.. .. :|: .: ..:|.. ::::..:  | | ||:|
  3 LNSSAEDGIKRIQDDCPKAGRHSYIFVMIPTLYSIIFVVGIFGNSLVVIV  52

 50 FKVNTELKTVNNYFLLSLACADLIIGTFSMNLYTTYLLMG.HWALFTLAC  98
    : .  .||||.. |||.|| |||.: :. |:..| | : :|::|.  |
 53 IYFYMKLKTVASVFLLNLALADLCF.LLTCPLWAVYTAMEYRWPFGNHLC 101

 99 DLWLALDYVASNASVMNLLLISFDRYFSVTRPLSYRAKRTPRRAALMIGL 148
    .: |  .. |||: | :|:|||:.:.:|:. | :||   | : . :
102 KIASASVTFNLYASVFLLTCLSIDRYLAIVHPMKSRLRRTMLVAKVTCII 151

149 AWLVSFVLWAPAILFWQYLVGERTVLAGQCYIQFLSQ....PI.ITFGTA 193
     ||:. : . ||:: :. .. |.| :|| | ::: |.   || :.:...
152 IWLMAGLASLPAVIHRNVYFIENTNITV.CAFHYESRNSTLPIGLGLTKN 200

194 MAAFYLPVTVMCTLYWRIYRETENRARELAALQGSETPGKGGGSSSSER 243
    : :|.:|. :: | |  |::.
201 ILGFLFPFLIILTSYTLIWKA                              221
```
B

Figure 12-18. (*Continued*) B, Here the program has determined similarities between two translated DNA sequences (the m1 muscarinic receptor and the AT_{1A} angiotensin II receptor). Again, only a portion of the sequence is shown. amino acids connected by *lines*, *dots*, or *double dots* indicate various degrees of similarity between the sequences. In this manner evolutionary relationships between DNA segments can be determined [12].

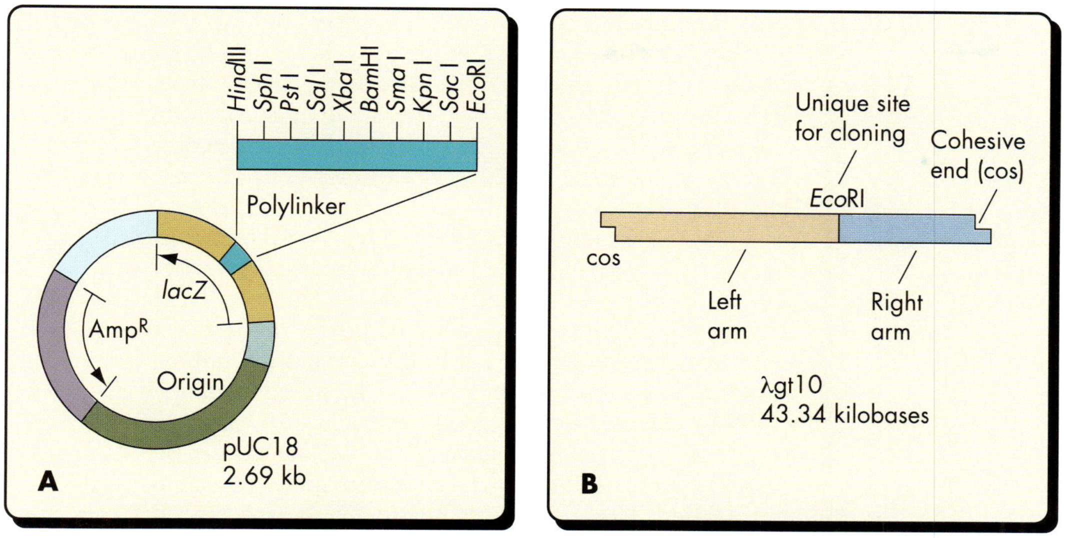

Figure 12-19. Vector types. Loose pieces of DNA, cut out of chromosomes using restriction enzymes (see Fig. 12-11), are difficult to handle. Amplification (increasing the amount of the DNA), sequencing (see Fig. 12-17), and other manipulations cannot be performed on such segments. Although the development of polymerase chain reaction PCR (see Fig. 12-30) has allowed some of these issues to be circumvented, the standard method for manipulating segments of DNA is still to insert them into vectors. Vectors were originally derived from plasmids, naturally occurring circular DNA molecules in bacteria that often confer antimicrobial resistance. Currently used vectors are largely synthetic and contain many useful features. **A** A typical plasmid-derived vector. It contains an origin of replication necessary to permit autonomous replication in bacteria. One or more drug-resistance genes (*Amp*^{R} for ampicillin resistance) allow selection of bacteria carrying the plasmid by growing them in medium containing the selection antibiotic. The polylinker site consists of a series of unique restriction sites (see Fig. 12-11), a convenient one of which can be used to linearize the vector to introduce the foreign DNA. The polylinker is embedded within the *lacZ* gene, which encodes beta-galactosidase. When the vector is propagated in bacteria, this enzyme is expressed and cleaves a colorless compound in the culture medium, X-gal, to a blue product. However, when foreign DNA has been inserted into the polylinker site it will interrupt the *lacZ* gene, and colonies will be white (blue-white selection). This feature is used to select bacteria harboring vectors with foreign DNA (see Fig. 12-20). In vectors designed for expression, two strong promoters (see Fig. 12-5) flank the polylinker site, so that DNA introduced in the vector can be selectively transcribed from either direction (see Fig. 12-24).

B, A different kind of vector: one derived from bacteriophage. This type is particularly used for library screening (see Fig. 12-27). Here, foreign DNA is inserted, using the unique cloning site, between two phage arms, and the phage (packaged in protein *in vitro*) is allowed to infect bacteria, where it will multiply. (*From* Watson and coworkers [3].)

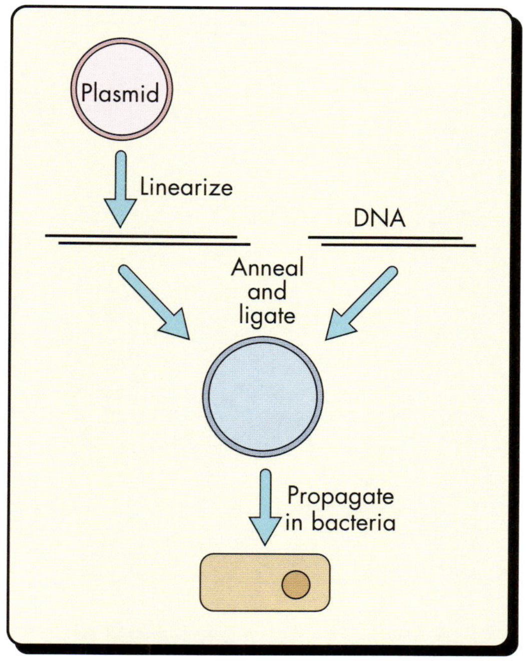

Figure 12-20. Cloning of vectors. The process of inserting a segment of DNA (called the *insert*) into a vector is called *cloning*. Vectors can be linearized with a restriction enzyme (see Fig. 12-11) that has a site in the polylinker, and mixed with a segment of free DNA, first cut with an enzyme that produces identical overhangs. The overhangs from vector and DNA segment will anneal and can be linked with DNA ligase (see Fig. 12-12), resulting in a vector containing the insert. Subsequently, the vector can be introduced into bacteria using a process called transfection; one standard method called electroporation uses electrical current to create temporary holes in the bacterial cell wall. The bacteria are then propagated, and after selection for those who actually carry the vector (using blue-white selection; see Fig. 12-19), the DNA, now amplified, can be extracted (see Fig. 12-21).

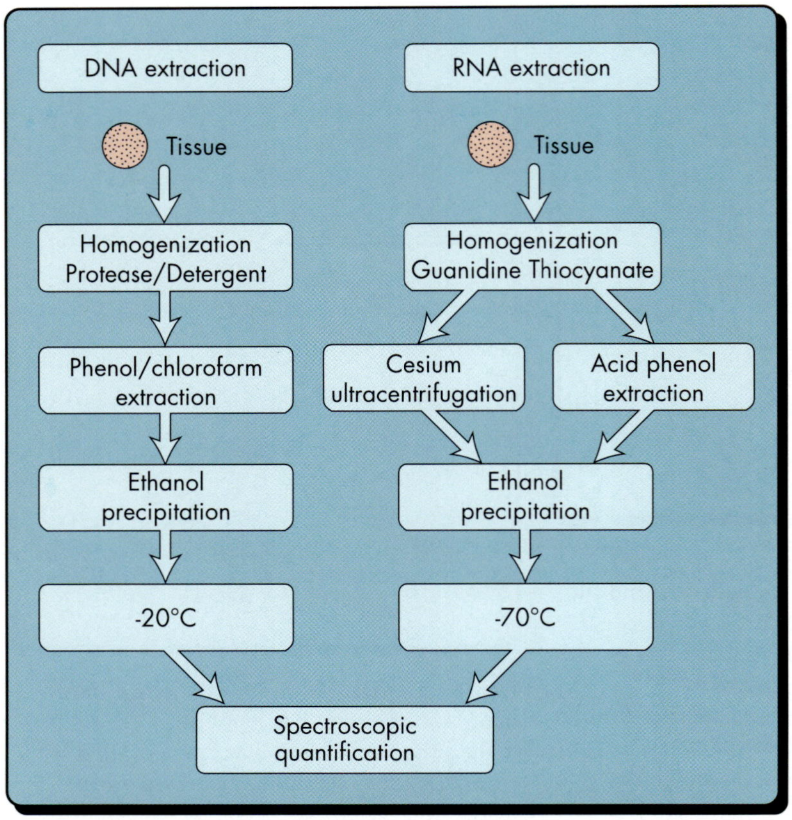

Figure 12-21. Extraction of DNA and RNA. Because each cell in the body contains the full set of genomic material, DNA extraction will in principle always yield the same set of genetic information, independent of the tissue used. RNA extraction, in contrast, will yield various complements of mRNA, dependent on the genes expressed in the particular tissue or cell type studied. Hence, these techniques have totally different purposes. DNA extraction is most often performed to create genomic libraries or as a step in amplifying cloned genetic material (see Figs. 12-20 and 12-26), whereas RNA extraction is used to find out about tissue-specific gene expression (Northern blotting; see Fig. 12-28).

In DNA extraction, the tissue is homogenized to disrupt cells and treated with proteases and detergent to allow access to the nucleus. DNA is separated from protein by phenol-chloroform extraction. The DNA in the aqueous phase is then selectively precipitated in ammonium acetate and ethanol. The precipitate is dried and redissolved in water or an aqueous buffer. DNA can be stored indefinitely at -20°C.

RNA extraction is more taxing than DNA extraction, because the compound is less stable, and a variety of ribonucleases (RNAses) are present in tissue and must be inactivated to prevent significant RNA degradation. To prevent contamination with exogenous RNAses, sterilized glassware, plastic ware, and water is used. Tissue is homogenized in the RNAse inhibitor guanidine thiocyanate as rapidly as possible after removal from the body and then separated from the large amount of DNA present in the cell. A common technique is ultracentrifugation on a layer of cesium chloride, although selective extraction in acidic phenol is also possible. After separation from DNA, the RNA can be purified by ethanol precipitation and stored at -70°C. The resulting RNA is a mixture of mRNA, rRNA, and tRNA. The mRNA fraction can be enriched using poly-A selection (see Fig. 12-22).

Nucleic acids can be conveniently quantified using spectroscopy at a wavelength of 260 nm. Determining the ratio of absorbencies at 260 and 280 nm (proteins absorb at both wavelengths) gives an indication of the degree of protein contamination.

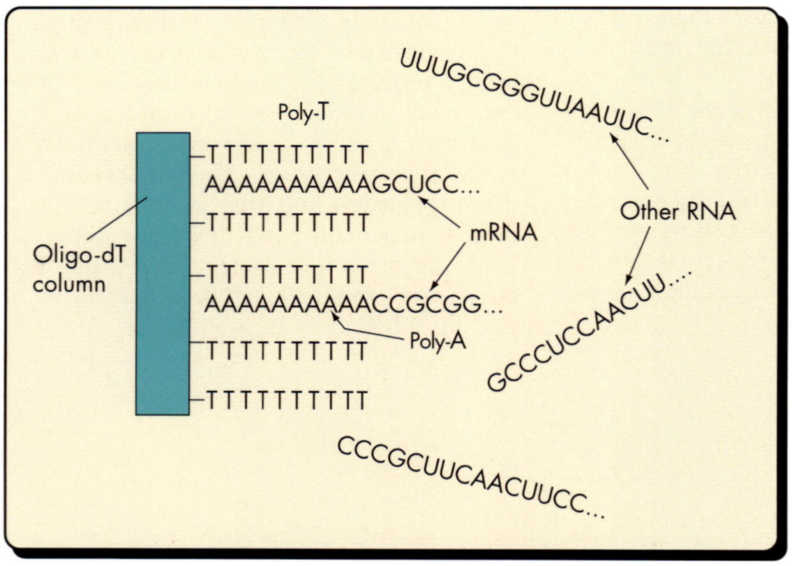

Figure 12-22. Poly-A selection. The RNA fraction of usual interest, mRNA, forms only 1% to 5% of total RNA content. Therefore, a selection step is often necessary to separate mRNA from the other types, rRNA and tRNA (see Fig. 12-8). Poly-A selection performs this function. As shown in Figure 12-6, mature mRNA has a poly-A tail at its 3′ end, and this feature is used to enrich the mRNA fraction by affinity chromatography on a column containing short sequences of oligodeoxythymidine (oligo-dT column). After extraction of total RNA (see Fig. 12-21) the RNA is passed over this column, and poly-A tails will anneal to the oligo-dT, whereas RNA without a poly-A tail will pass through. The enriched fraction can be eluted and recirculated through the column for further selection. This technique tends to reduce the amount of RNA to 1% or 2% of the original, but it retains a much higher fraction of mRNA.

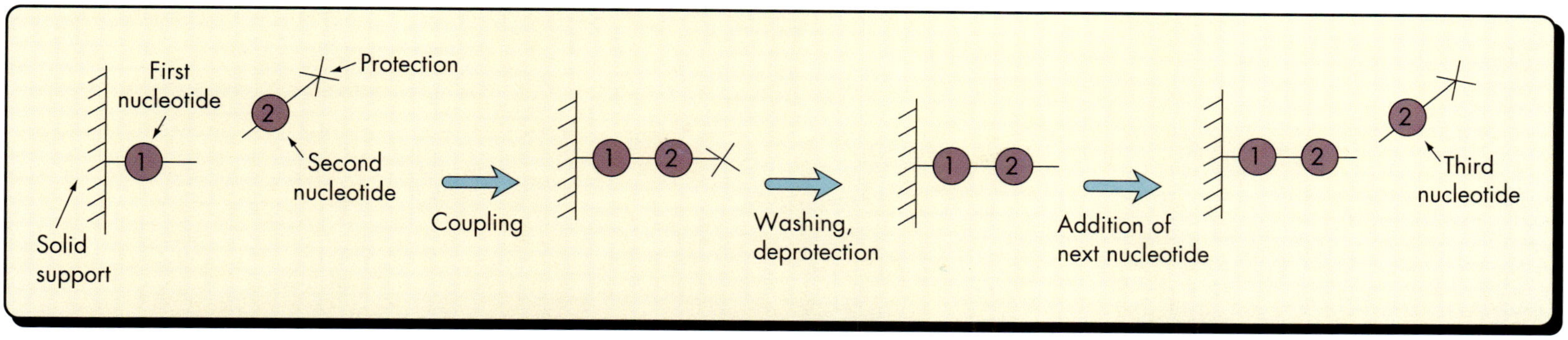

Figure 12-23. Oligonucleotides. Figures 12-21 and 12-22 dealt with nucleic acids extracted from tissue. However, these compounds can also be synthesized in the laboratory, as outlined here and in Figures 12-24 and 12-25. Oligonucleotides, short (10 to 100 nucleotides) synthetic DNA fragments, play essential roles in polymerase chain reaction analysis (see Fig. 12-30) and as molecular probes (see Fig. 12-28). Their synthesis is one of the few occasions in molecular biology where manipulation of nucleic acid is performed by purely chemical means. Several techniques exist, but all use the principle of attaching the first nucleotide to a solid support and, after protection of the appropriate groups, sequentially adding new nucleotides. The support matrix is washed between each step. After the final nucleotide has been added the oligonucleotide is released from the support matrix and purified. Fully automated systems exist to perform these functions.

In a variation on this technique, a mixture of nucleotides, rather than a single type, can be added at any step. This results in a mixture of oligonucleotides with various bases at specific points. Such degenerate oligonucleotides are employed in cloning (see Fig. 12-35).

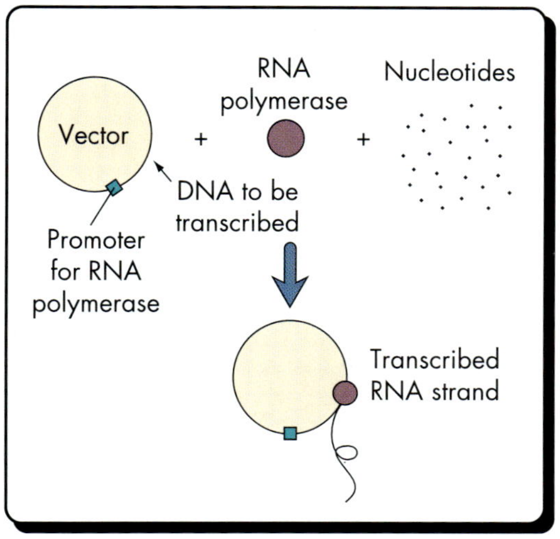

Figure 12-24. *In vitro* transcription. Because of its stability and the ease with which it is incorporated into vectors (see Fig. 12-20), DNA is the preferred material for manipulation and cloning. However, for expression purposes (see Fig. 12-34) and for generation of labeled probes (see Fig. 12-29), RNA is a necessary intermediate. RNA can be transcribed (see Fig. 12-5) *in vitro* employing the RNA polymerase promoters present in many vectors (see Fig. 12-19). If such a vector, carrying a DNA of interest, is incubated with polymerase and the four nucleotides in an appropriate buffer, the polymerase will transcribe RNA from the vector. Radioactively or otherwise labeled nucleotides can be added to the mixture, resulting in radiolabeled RNA strands, useful in several settings (see Fig. 12-29). If expression in eukaryotic systems is planned (see Fig. 12-34), an analogue of the cap structure (see Fig. 12-6) can be added as well.

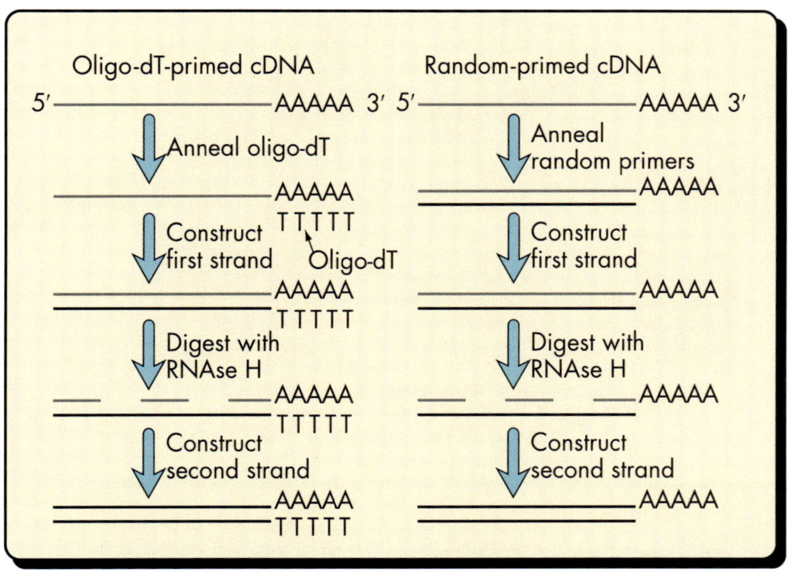

Figure 12-25. Reverse transcription. Reverse transcription is a process basically the reverse of *in vitro* transcription (see Fig. 12-24): it prepares DNA complementary to extracted mRNA. Such complementary DNA (cDNA) can be used for several purposes, including library construction (see Fig. 12-26). Reverse transcription employs a retroviral enzyme, reverse transcriptase, that synthesizes double-stranded DNA on an RNA template. This enzyme needs a double-stranded region to start with, which can be created conveniently by adding oligo-dT (see Fig. 12-22) to the mRNA. This will anneal to poly-A tails (see Fig. 12-6) and function as primer (oligo-dT-primed cDNA). Alternatively, short random nucleotide sequences can be mixed with the RNA, which will anneal at irregular intervals, initiating multiple transcription sites that may yield better transcription (random-primed cDNA). The intermediate product of either procedure is an RNA-DNA hybrid. The RNA is removed using RNAse H, an RNAse (see Fig. 12-21) that digests the RNA strand into a number of short fragments. These become primers for DNA synthesis using DNA polymerase (see Fig. 12-30). Hence, these techniques allow synthesis of either single- or double-stranded cDNA. This cDNA can either be studied directly, *eg*, using polymerase chain reaction (see Fig. 12-30) or incorporated into a vector (see Fig. 12-20) for further manipulation, *eg*, library construction (see Fig. 12-26).

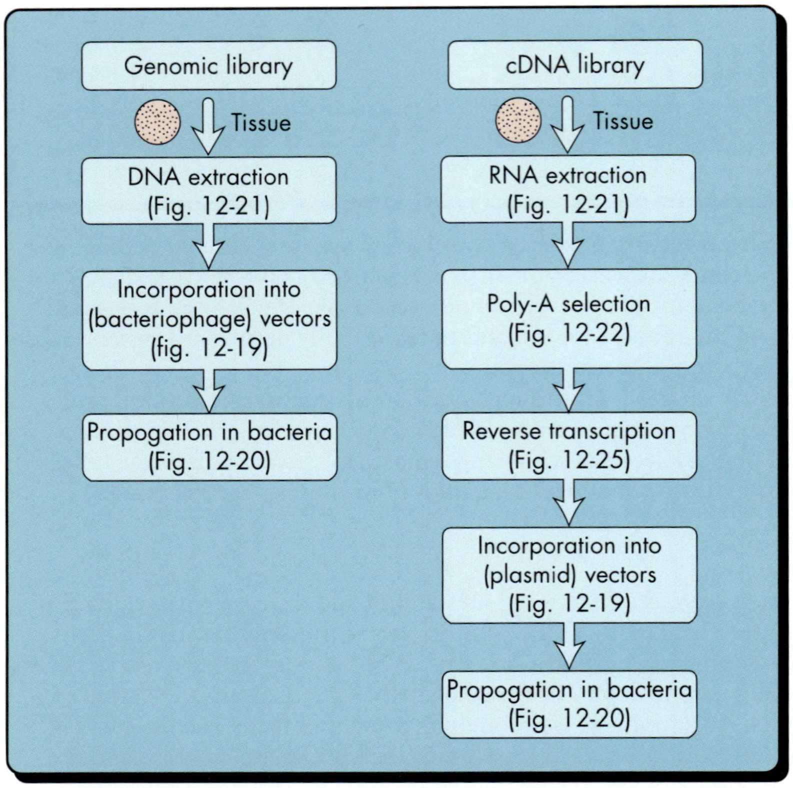

Figure 12-26. Library construction. The construction of libraries, collections of genetic material in vectors, propagated in bacteria, brings together many of the techniques described previously in this chapter. A collection of mRNA incorporated in vectors as cDNA is termed a cDNA library. cDNA libraries derived from different organs will contain different complements of genetic material. Genomic libraries, created by incorporating extracted DNA directly into vectors, will contain the full genomic information of the species they are prepared from. Libraries can be screened to search for specific genetic information.

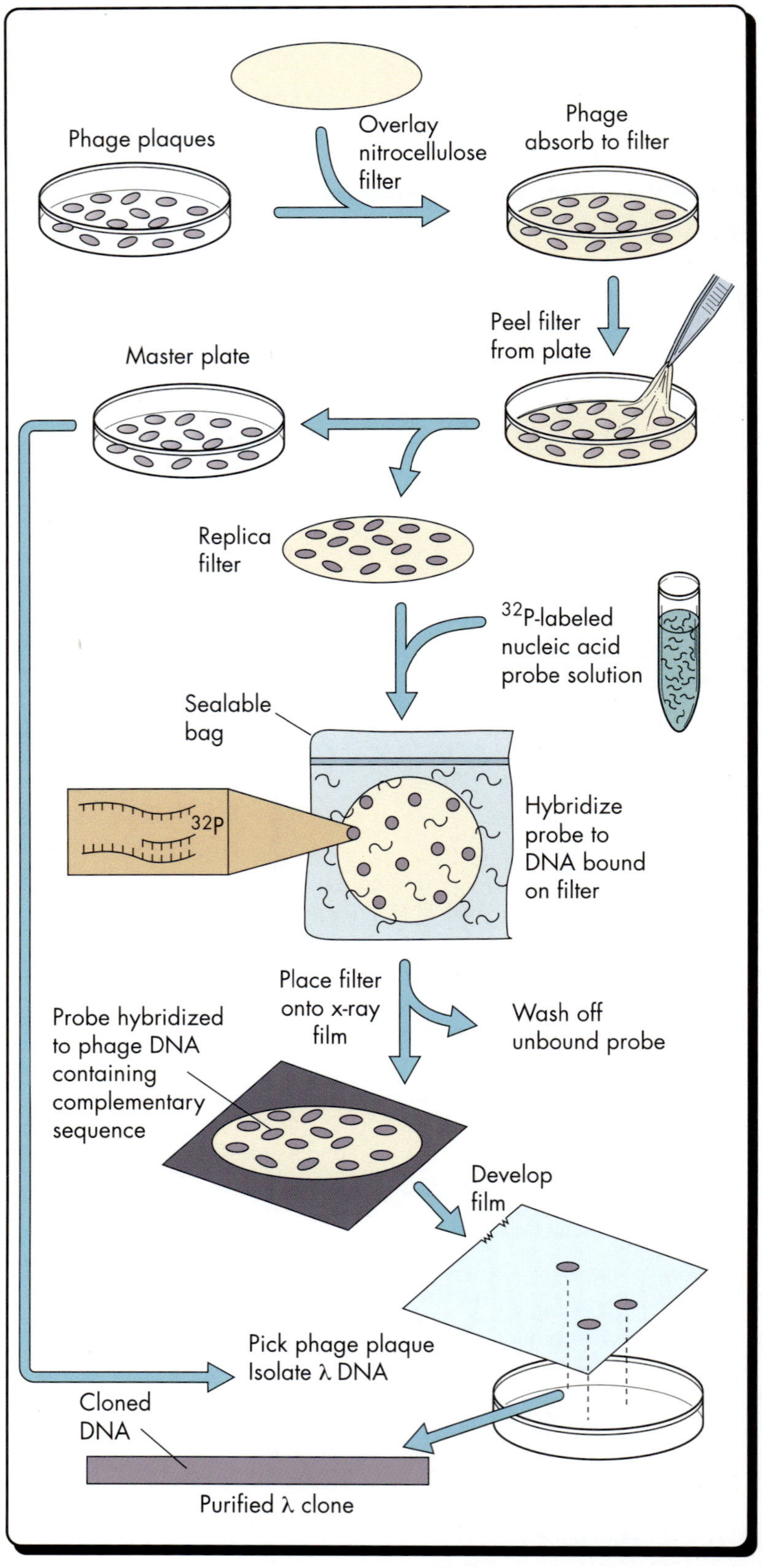

Figure 12-27. Library screening. Library screening, the process of searching for specific information in a DNA library (see Fig. 12-26), as well as a number of blotting procedures (see Figs. 12-28 and 12-29), depend on hybridization: the process of annealing (hybridizing) a labeled nucleic acid fragment (probe) to a collection of RNA or DNA. Unbound probe is washed away, and techniques to visualize the bound, labeled probe will reveal the presence, amount and (depending on the technique) size of the hybridizing species in the DNA and RNA. Although novel nonradioactive techniques are rapidly gaining acceptance, the standard method of labeling nucleic acid probes is still the incorporation of radiolabeled nucleotides during oligonucleotide synthesis (see Fig. 12-23) or *in vitro* RNA (see Fig. 12-24) or DNA (see Fig. 12-25) synthesis.

During library screening a labeled probe is used to determine the presence of a specific DNA species in a library. If the procedure is done in order to clone a novel gene, the nucleotide sequence of the probe can derive either from the amino acid of a protein searched for (see Fig. 12-35), or from the DNA sequence of a known, related gene. The latter approach is based on the fact that under appropriate conditions (termed low stringency) probes will hybridize to DNA sequences that are an incomplete match.

Screening is often performed on phage libraries (see Fig. 12-19). First, the clones in the library are physically separated by plating phage on agar plates covered with bacteria. Plaques develop that are then replicated on paper. The phage DNA is bound to the paper and incubated with the labeled probe. Autoradiography of the paper will show if and where hybridization took place. Lining up the autoradiogram with the original plate will show which phage carries the sequence of interest. This phage can then be isolated, amplified (see Fig. 12-20), and further analyzed by sequencing (see Fig. 12-17) and expression (see Figs. 12-33 and 12-34). Figure 12-36 provides an example. (*From* Watson and coworkers [3].)

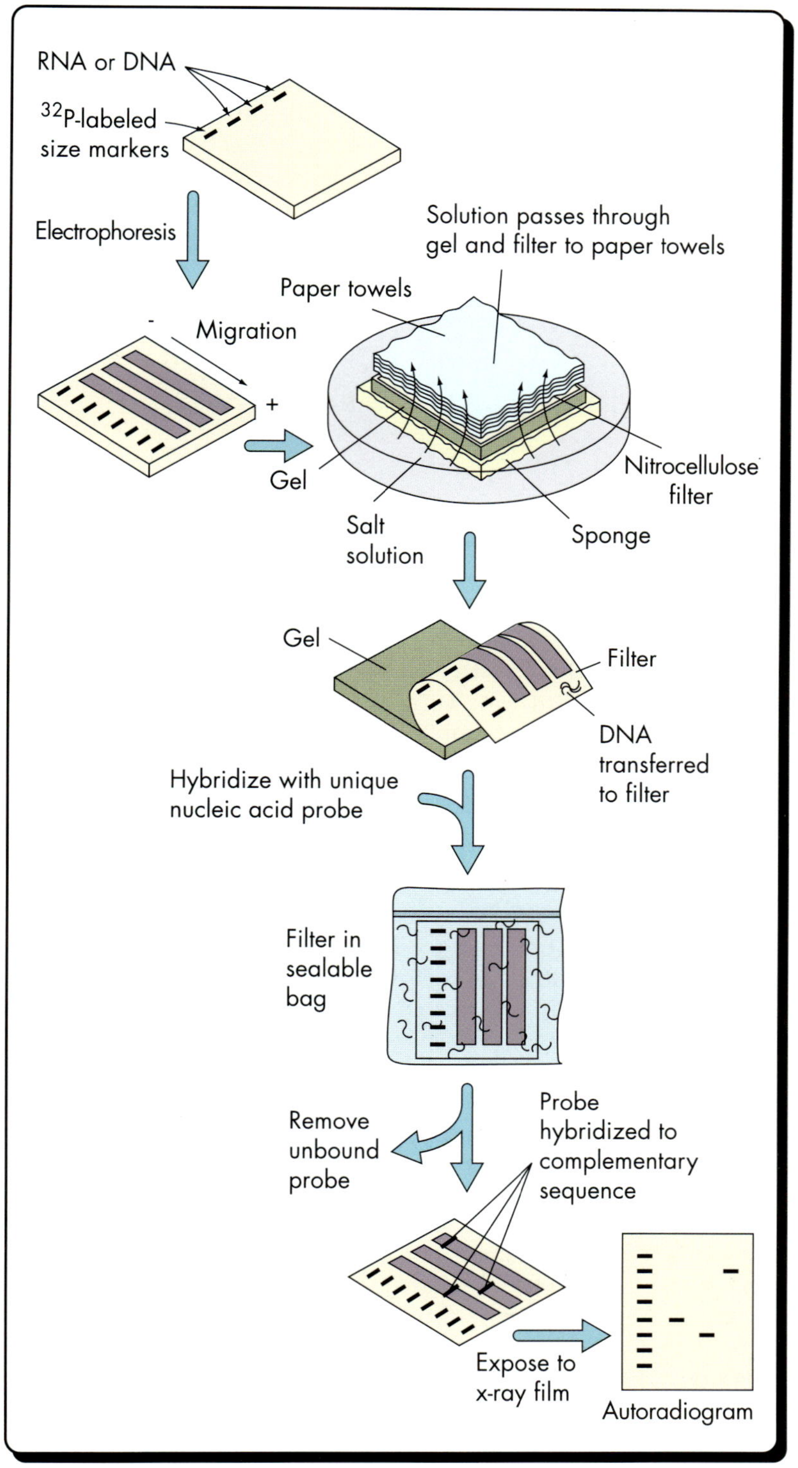

Figure 12-28. Blotting. Whereas library screening (see Fig. 12-27) can reveal whether a specific clone is present in a library constructed from a specific tissue and species, it does not give quantitative information. Blotting techniques allow quantitative assessment of both the amount of nucleic acid and its molecular size. The original technique of Southern blotting (invented by E.M. Southern) is used to determine the presence of a specific sequence in genomic DNA. More commonly used is the technique, by analogy named Northern blotting, whereby the presence of a specific sequence in extracted RNA is determined. (Western blotting is an unrelated technique that uses labeled antibodies to detect the presence of a specific protein in extracted protein separated on a gel.) If knowledge of the size of the nucleic acid is not important, it can simply be mixed with the labeled probe in a technique called slot blotting. An example of this method is shown in Figure 12-31.

Northern blotting is a combination of gel electrophoresis (see Fig. 12-13) and hybridization (see Fig. 12-27). RNA is extracted from the tissue of interest and separated by size on agarose gel. The RNA in the gel is then transferred to paper placed on top of the gel (blotting), bound tightly to the paper, and incubated with labeled probe (see Fig. 12-27). After hybridization, the paper is washed to remove nonhybridized probe and exposed to x-ray film. If mRNA complementary to the probe is present in the RNA on the blot, its presence and size will be revealed by a band on the film. The intensity of the band will be proportional to the amount of mRNA present in the tissue.

Southern blotting basically performs the same procedure with DNA. The material analyzed is genomic DNA (see Fig. 12-21) cut in manageable fragments using a restriction enzyme (see Fig. 12-11). The technique is particularly useful for determining the number of genes in a genome encoding a specific message, as well as for interspecies comparisons (using zoo blots). An example is discussed in Figure 12-36. (*From* Watson and coworkers [3].)

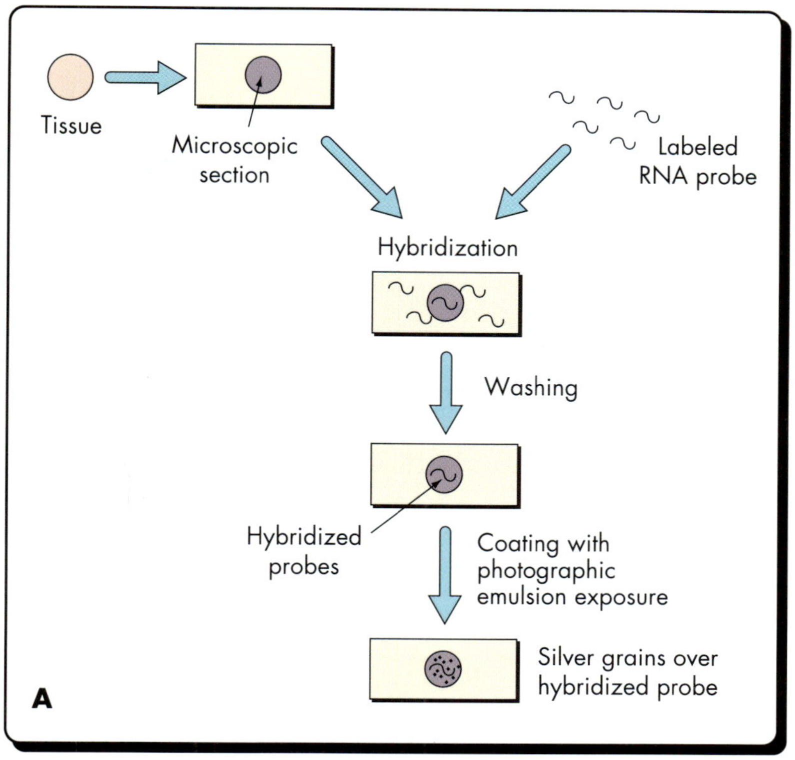

Figure 12-29. Via *in situ* hybridization. **A**, The spatial resolution of Northern gels (see Fig. 12-28) is limited by the size of the organ or organ part from which mRNA can be extracted. To localize mRNA with a higher resolution, the technique of *in situ* hybridization has been developed. Here tissue is removed from an animal and prepared as microscopic sections. These sections are then incubated with labeled probe, which will hybridize with mRNA present in cells. The slides are coated with photographic emulsion, and, after exposure, studied under the microscope. Silver grains will be present over areas where the probe annealed, allowing highly detailed maps of mRNA distribution to be constructed.

(*Continued on next page*)

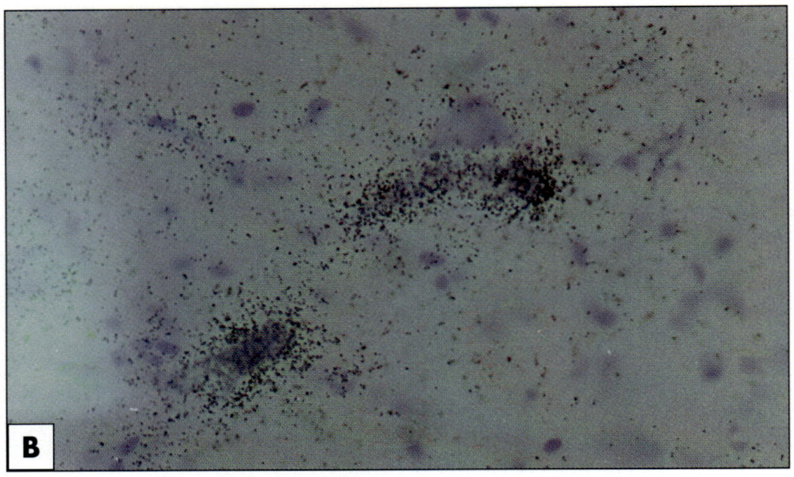

Figure 12-29. (*Continued*) B, The example shows labeling of cells containing mRNA encoding preproenkephalin, a precursor to one of the endogenous opioid receptor agonists, in the gigantocellular field of the ventral medulla.

The usefulness of blotting techniques and *in situ* hybridization is limited by the smallest amount of RNA needed to create a measurable signal. This general problem of manipulating low-abundance messages has been largely overcome by the development of polymerase chain reaction analysis (see Fig. 12-30). (*Part B courtesy of* R. Stornetta, University of Virginia.)

POLYMERASE CHAIN REACTION

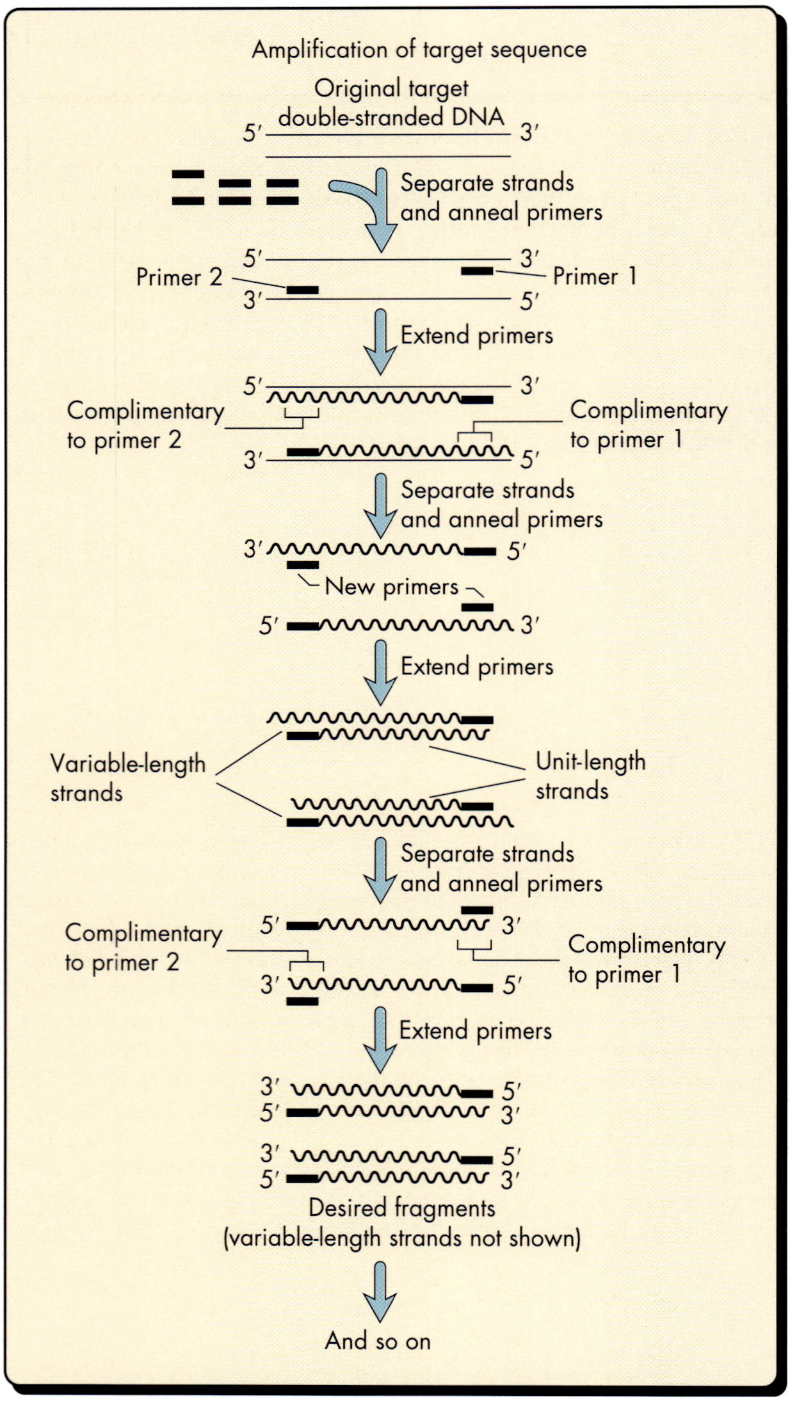

Figure 12-30. Polymerase chain reaction (PCR) technique. The development of PCR has in many ways revolutionized molecular biology. It allows selective amplification of tiny amounts of DNA by more than a millionfold, and it is able to work from unprepared DNA, without the need for vectors. Basically, PCR is a clever modification of DNA replication allowing exponential multiplication of double-stranded DNA [13].

A PCR reaction consists of cycles of three steps: denaturing, annealing, and extension. The starting material is double-stranded DNA, although incorporating a reverse transcription reaction as an initial step allows mRNA to be used as a substrate (RT-PCR). During the denaturing step, the DNA is heated to 94°C, resulting in separation of the strands. Two oligonucleotides (see Fig. 12-23), called primers, each complementary to one of the two strands, a few hundred nucleotides apart, are present in the reaction. During the second phase, annealing, the temperature is decreased (usually to around 55°C, but lower if decreased stringency is desired) and these primers anneal to the now single-stranded DNA. In the third step, extension, the temperature is taken to 72°C, the optimum temperature for the DNA polymerase employed, which extends the primers, assembling a second strand on each single-stranded DNA molecule. Therefore, the total amount of DNA in the area flanked by the primers is now doubled. During the second cycle, this DNA will denature, anneal more primer, and again be doubled. This doubling during each cycle results in a theoretical amplification after 22 cycles of more than 1 millionfold. This number is particularly impressive considering that each cycle takes only about 10 minutes. This extreme sensitivity allows such feats as amplification of DNA from single hairs, blood spots, or even from mummies thousands of years old; at the same time, it makes the technique also extremely prone to artifacts, because even the smallest amount of contaminating DNA will result in a band on a gel.

Use of PCR to amplify material for restriction fragment length polymorphism analysis (see Fig. 12-15) is described in Figure 12-16. Other examples of the use of PCR for diagnosis are shown in Figures 12-31 and 12-32; the first of these uses genomic DNA, the second cDNA as substrate. (*From* Watson and coworkers [3].)

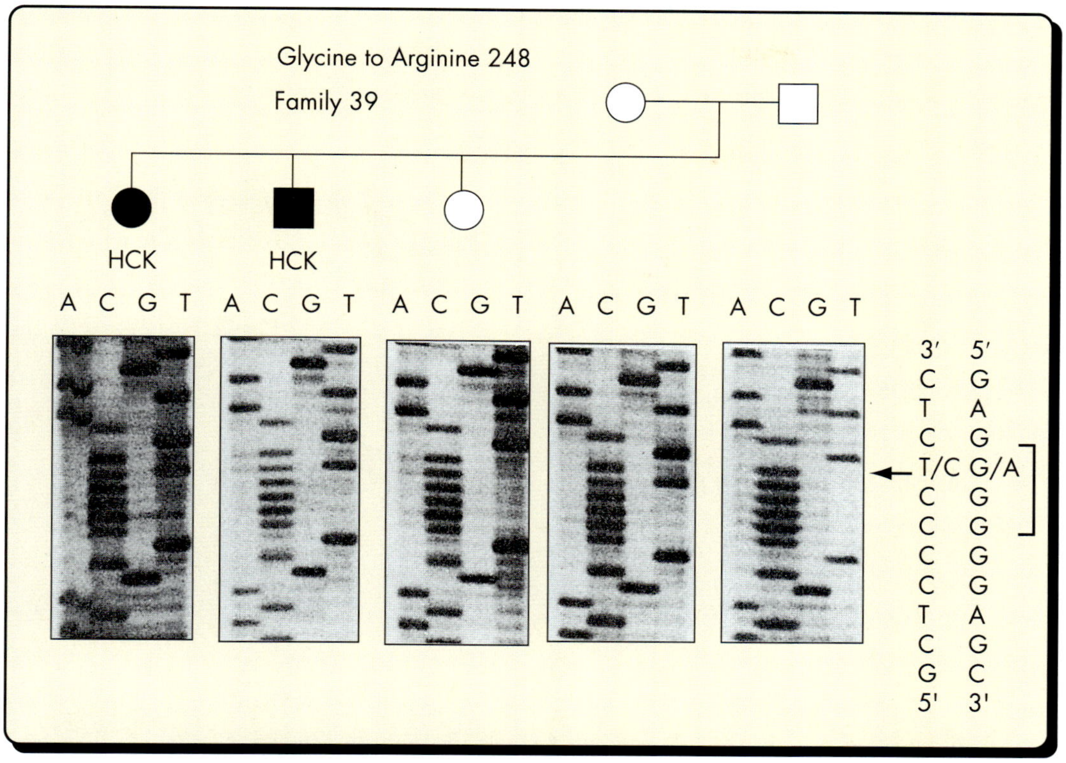

Figure 12-31. Use of polymerase chain reaction (PCR) in detection of malignant hyperthermia (MH). Although the MH syndrome encompasses a spectrum of diseases, it is clear that abnormalities in the skeletal muscle Ca^{2+} release channel (ryanodine receptor) play a major role. The gene for this channel has been cloned, and PCR has been used to search for mutations in the gene linked to MH.

Messenger RNA was obtained from muscle biopsy specimens of three MH-susceptible subjects, and cDNA was obtained using random priming (see Fig. 12-25). The cDNA was amplified using PCR (see Fig. 12-30) and sequenced (see Fig. 12-17), and the sequences obtained were tested for variants. Twenty-one changes from the normal gene sequence were noted in these three patients. Four of these nucleotide substitutions resulted in a change in amino acid sequence, and these substitutions could therefore have a causative role. Thirteen of the changes resulted in loss or gain of a restriction site (see Fig. 12-11) and could therefore be used for restriction fragment length polymorphism (RFLP) analysis (see Fig. 12-15).

Forty-five families with MH-susceptible members were studied to determine the presence or absence of the four amino acid substitutions and linkage of their presence to MH. Because three of these substitutions also created an RFLP, they could easily be analyzed by PCR amplification of genomic DNA, followed by digestion with the appropriate restriction enzyme and gel electrophoresis (compare Fig. 12-16). The remaining substitution was analyzed by PCR amplification followed by sequencing of the PCR product. One of the mutations (Arg for Gly in position 248) indeed segregated with MH susceptibility in one of the 45 families shown [15]. C—positive caffeine test; H—positive halothane test; K—positive halothane and caffeine test. *Squares* denote males and *circles* females. *Filled symbols* indicate MH susceptibility; *open symbols* indicate no diagnosis. (*From* Gillard and coworkers [15].)

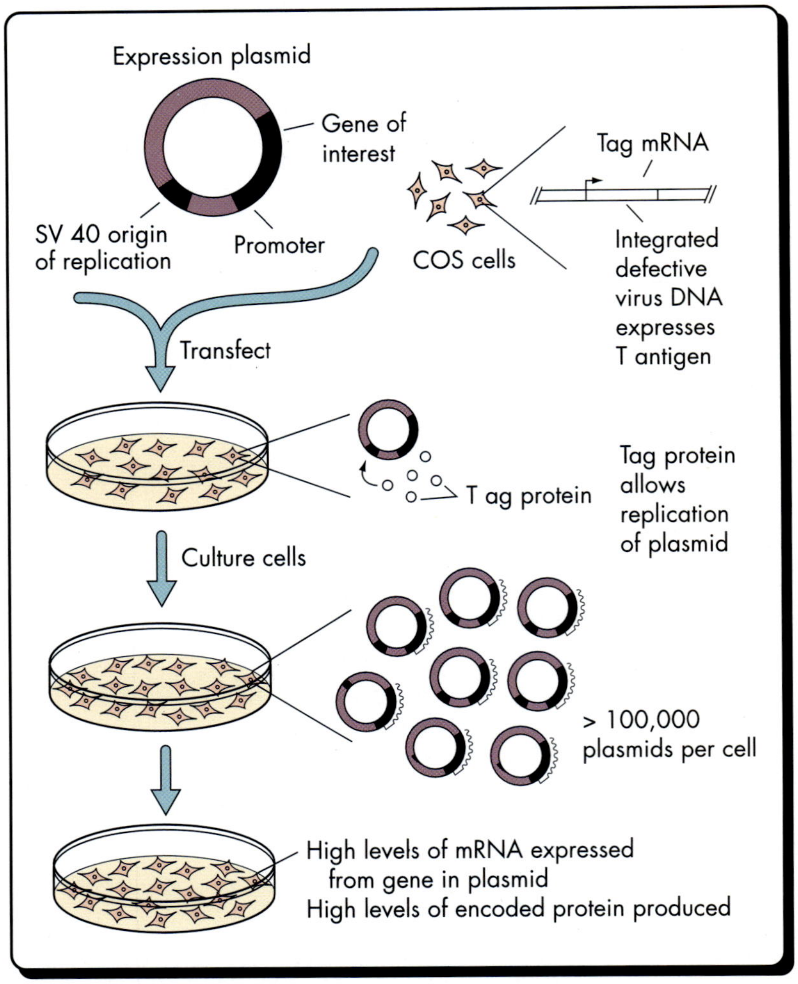

Figure 12-32. COS cells. For study of proteins encoded by mRNA, either extracted or created using genetic engineering, the mRNA must be translated in a well-defined system. This is called expression. Although *in vitro* translation, a technique in which ribosomes translate a message in a cell-free system, is technically a form of expression, the term is usually reserved for translation of recombinant messages in cells. One of the most commonly used systems employs COS cells, monkey kidney cells that carry the SV40 virus T antigen (Tag), involved in virus replication. When vectors carrying the SV40 origin of replication (see Fig. 12-19) are transfected (see Fig. 12-20) into COS cells, the vector is replicated to very high copy number, and as a result a large amount of protein is synthesized. The excess of protein often overwhelms intracellular signaling systems, so that for functional studies, a system such as *Xenopus* oocytes must be used (see Fig. 12-34). Other systems employed to generate large amounts of recombinant protein are yeast, baculovirus, and vaccinia virus. (*From* Watson and coworkers [3].)

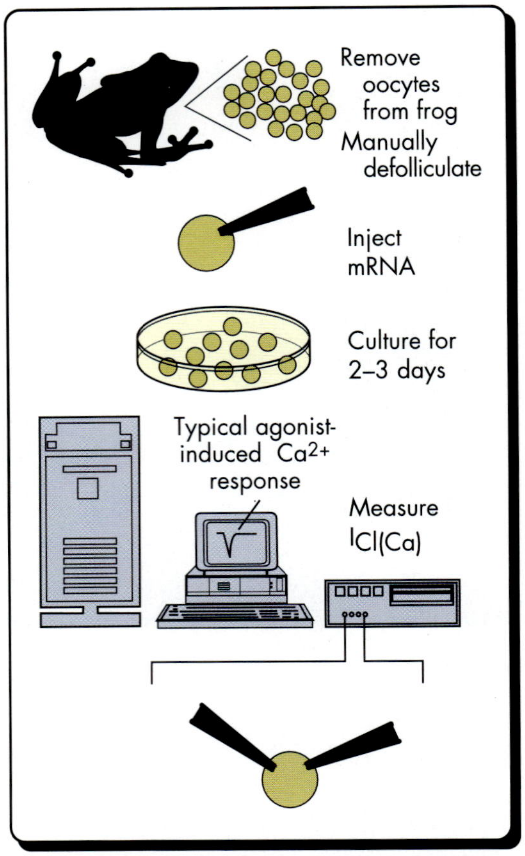

Figure 12-33. *Xenopus* oocytes. Oocytes of the toad *Xenopus laevis* are particularly useful for functional expression systems. These large cells can be easily injected with mRNA, and they have a very active protein-synthesizing machinery. In addition, posttranslational modifications and routing to correct intracellular positions are usually accomplished correctly. Their size makes electrophysiology straightforward, and the system has been used extensively for the study of ion channels. Ca^{2+}-mobilizing receptors can be studied electrophysiologically as well, because the oocyte membrane contains an endogenous Ca^{2+}-activated Cl^- channel.

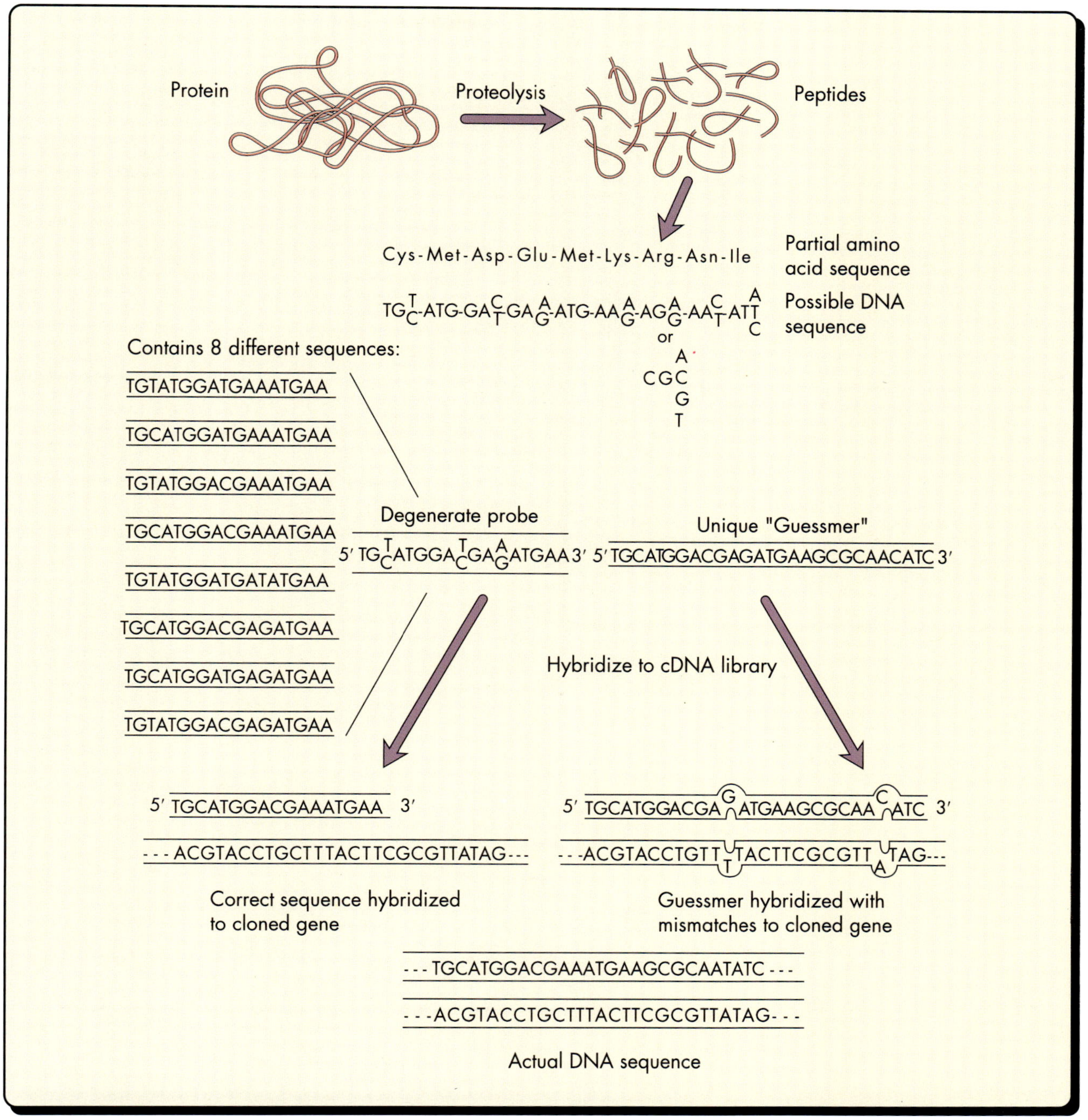

Figure 12-34. Protein sequencing. Although, in contrast to many of the techniques illustrated previously in this chapter, cloning of genes is performed primarily by specialized molecular biology laboratories, the subject receives sufficient media attention to warrant mention in this chapter. Figures 12-35 through 12-40 illustrate some of the most frequently used cloning techniques. In addition, these examples illustrate clearly how a number of the molecular biology approaches mentioned previously can be integrated into a larger project.

Although the method is laborious, often the only way a short segment of DNA encoding a protein can be obtained is by purifying and partially sequencing the protein. The amino acid sequence obtained can then be back-translated to nucleotide sequence, using the genetic code (see Fig. 12-9). An oligonucleotide is then prepared (see Fig. 12-23) and used to screen a library by hybridization (see Fig. 12-27). The degeneracy of the genetic code complicates this technique, because multiple codons may encode a sequenced amino acid. This problem can be resolved either by synthesizing degenerate oligonucleotides, thus specifying every potential DNA sequence, or by constructing a unique guessmer based on the most likely distribution of codon usage. An example of cloning by protein sequencing is shown in Figure 12-36. (*From* Watson and coworkers [3].)

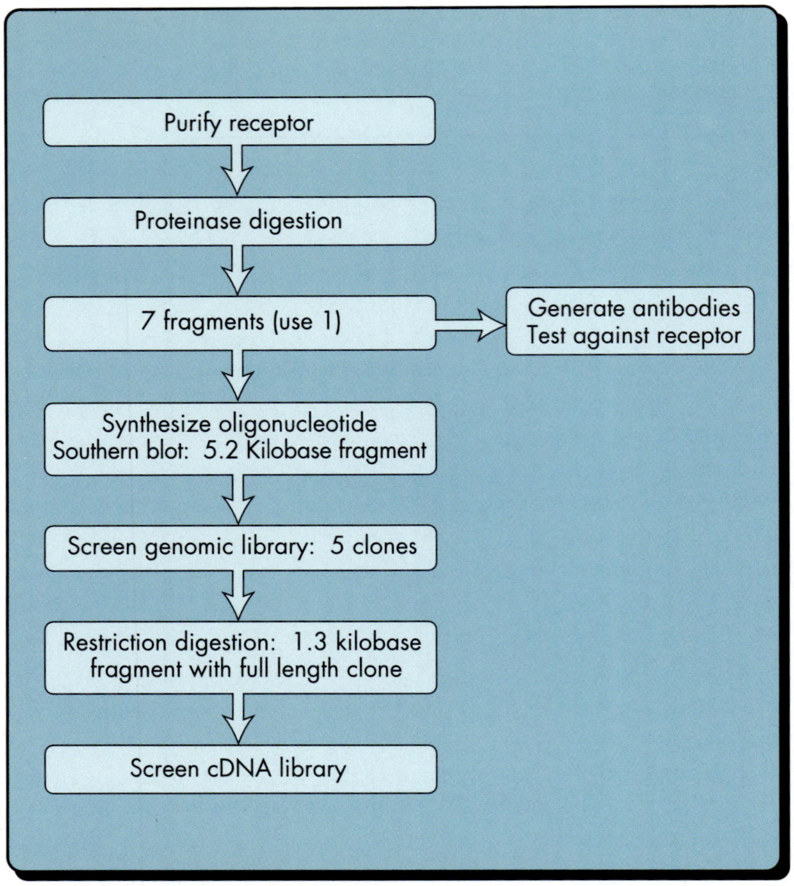

Figure 12-35. β-Adrenergic receptor. In 1986 cloning of the first adrenergic receptor subtype was reported. The technique used was protein sequencing (see Fig. 12-35). The investigators had purified the receptor protein to homogeneity, using affinity chromatography, and then cleaved it in several fragments using protease digestion. The seven most abundant peptides were partially sequenced, and one of those was used in the subsequent experiments. To verify that this fragment was indeed part of the adrenergic receptor, antibodies were raised against it. This was done by synthesizing an oligonucleotide encoding the fragment (see Fig. 12-23), and linking it to the sequence of a carrier protein, thus creating a fusion protein. This protein was injected into rabbits, and the resulting antibodies were shown to bind purified β-adrenergic receptor.

Several oligonucleotides complementary to the deduced DNA sequence of this same peptide fragment were synthesized. These were first used on Southern blots (see Fig. 12-28) with hamster genomic DNA and were shown to result in a single band on the blot, 5.2 kb in size. This indicated that a genomic sequence complementary with the oligonucleotide could be identified, although the 5.3-kb fragment must contain more sequence than that encoding the receptor, as estimated by molecular weight. A hamster genomic library (see Fig. 12-26) was screened using the same oligonucleotide (see Fig. 12-27), and five clones were isolated. Restriction mapping (see Fig. 12-14) of each of these clones showed that treatment with the restriction enzyme *Hind*III (see Fig. 12-11) created a 1.3-kb fragment that still hybridized the oligonucleotide. This fragment was subcloned (see Fig. 12-20) and sequenced (see Fig. 12-17) and was found to contain an area encoding a 435-amino-acid protein. The sequences of all seven peptide fragments mentioned previously were contained within the sequence. The genomic clone had been isolated successfully.

However, the presence of a genomic sequence does not guarantee that the gene is actually expressed. Using the *Hind*III fragment as a probe, a hamster cDNA library (see Fig. 12-26) was screened. Clones obtained from this library confirmed that the message encoded by the genomic clone was indeed expressed as mRNA, and they also demonstrated absence of introns (see Fig. 12-6) [16]. Figure 12-37 illustrates computer analysis of this sequence.

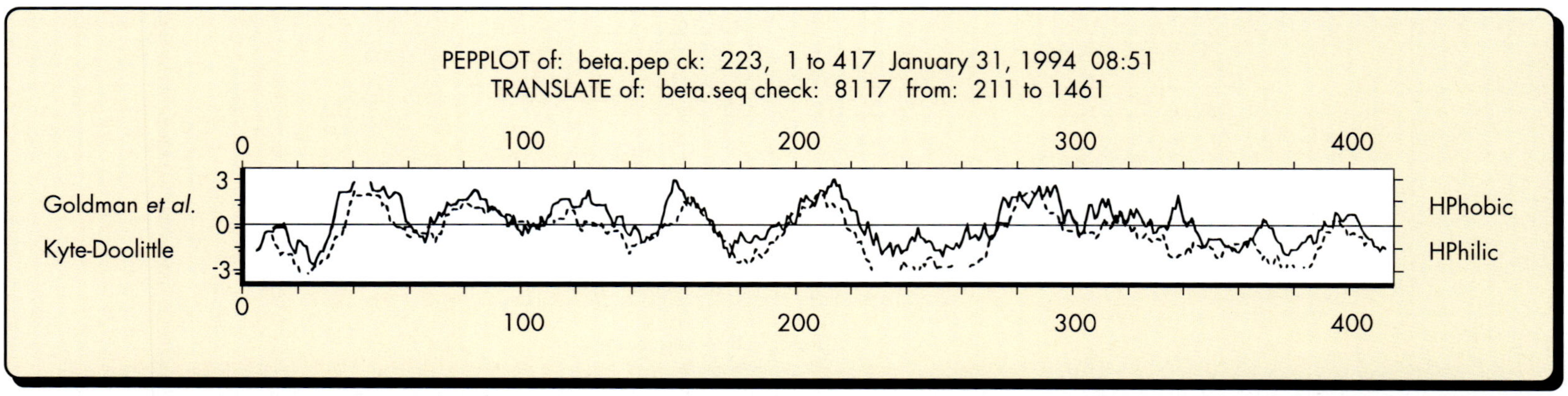

Figure 12-36. Hydropathy plot of the β-adrenergic receptor. To analyze the β-adrenergic receptor sequence (see Fig. 12-36) a hydropathy plot was constructed. This indicates hydrophobic (HPhobic) and hydrophilic (HPhilic) areas within the protein and can localize putative membrane-spanning domains. The plot showed seven such domains, a configuration remarkably similar to the rhodopsins, the light-transducing receptors in the eye. We now know that the rhodopsins, the adrenergic receptors, the odorant receptors, and a multitude of other systems transducing through G proteins all exhibit this heptahelical configuration [12,17].

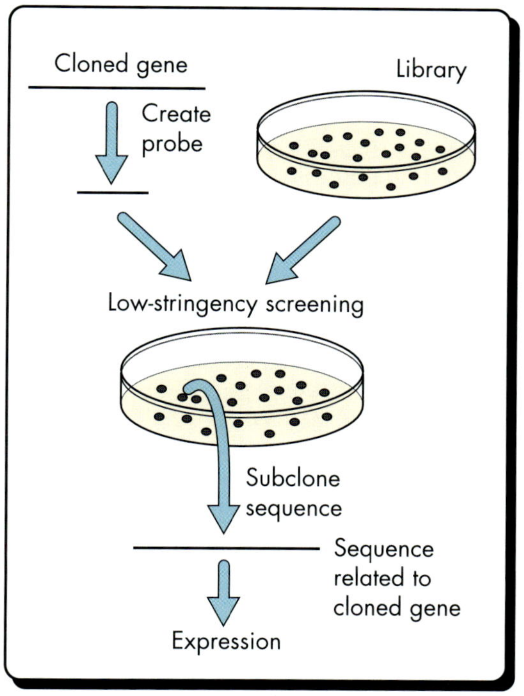

Figure 12-37. Homology screening. Because many genes cluster in related gene families, cloning of a single gene within a family makes it possible to clone other members based on their homology. This is done by screening a library at low stringency (see Fig. 12-27) using a probe derived from the known member. This approach is much easier than cloning by protein sequencing and has been quite successful in cloning subtypes of many proteins.

Demonstration that a cloned gene indeed encodes a functional member of the family is essential, because many cDNAs have been cloned that, based on sequence similarity, are members of a family, yet are either not expressed (pseudogenes) or have no known function (orphans).

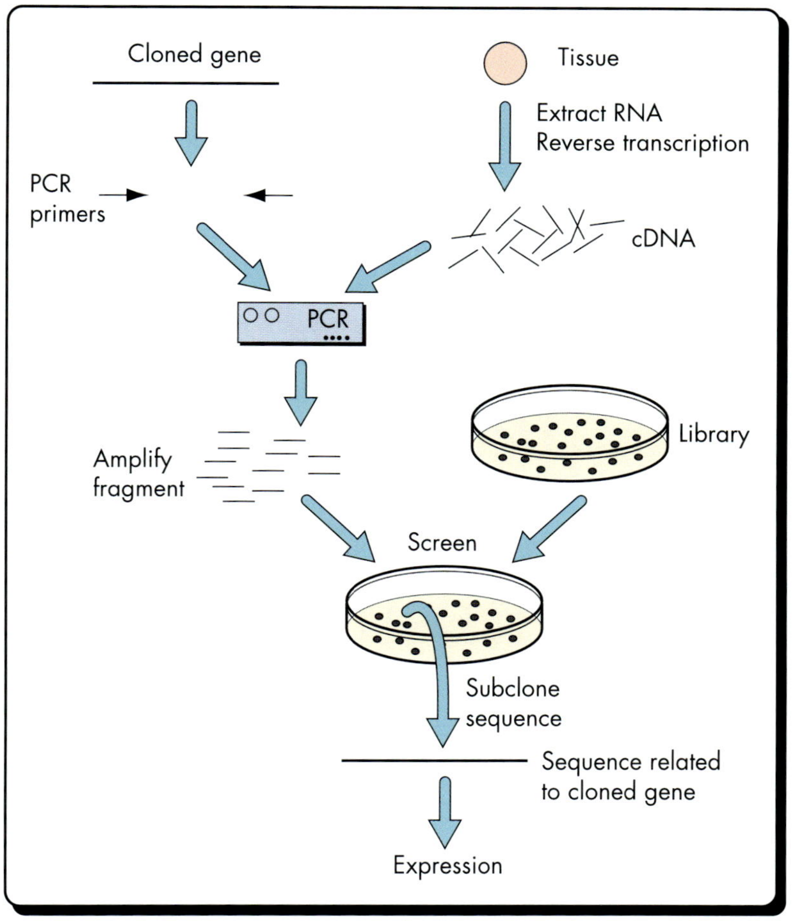

Figure 12-38. Use of polymerase chain reaction (PCR) analysis in homology cloning. Homology cloning (see Fig. 12-38) is even more straightforward with the use of PCR (see Fig. 12-30). PCR primers are designed based on a known subtype of a gene family, or a consensus sequence is determined based on computer alignment of multiple known subtypes (see Fig. 12-18). These primers are then used in a PCR reaction at low stringency employing as a substrate cDNA prepared from tissue expected to express other subtypes of the gene. The resulting PCR product is then used to screen a library (see Fig. 12-27) to obtain the full-length clone. As in homology screening, it is essential that function of the product is confirmed in an expression system such as *Xenopus* oocytes (see Fig. 12-34).

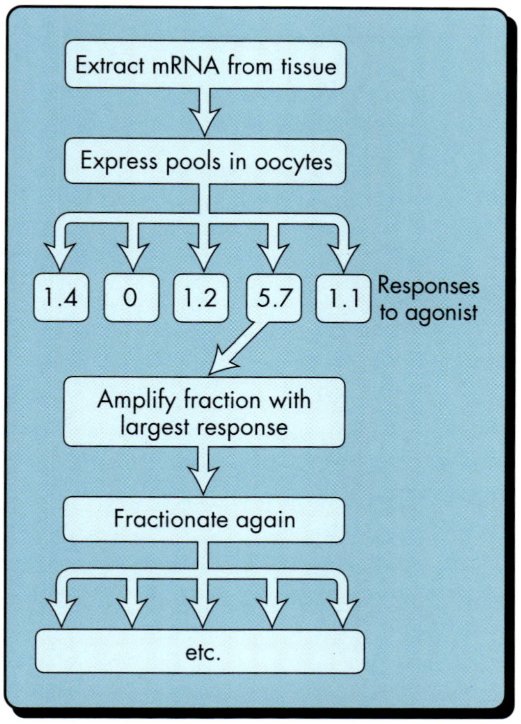

Figure 12-39. Cloning by expression. This method has the major advantage that it does not require any knowledge of the structure of the gene sought. mRNA is extracted (see Fig. 12-26) from tissue and a cDNA library is prepared (see Fig. 12-26). This cDNA is then expressed in an appropriate system, *eg*, by *in vitro* transcription (see Fig. 12-24) and injection of the RNA in *Xenopus* oocytes (see Fig. 12-34) or by expression in COS cells (see Fig. 12-33). The clone is isolated from the library through a process called sib selection, whereby the cDNA is divided into pools that are tested individually for signs of expression of the clone of interest (binding, response to a ligand, or ion conductance). The pool giving the largest response is presumed to hold the highest amount of message for the clone of interest. It is amplified by propagation in bacteria (see Fig. 12-20), and again divided in pools, which are tested individually. This process is repeated until a single cDNA is obtained. One limitation of this technique is that it is virtually impossible to clone multisubunit proteins in this manner.

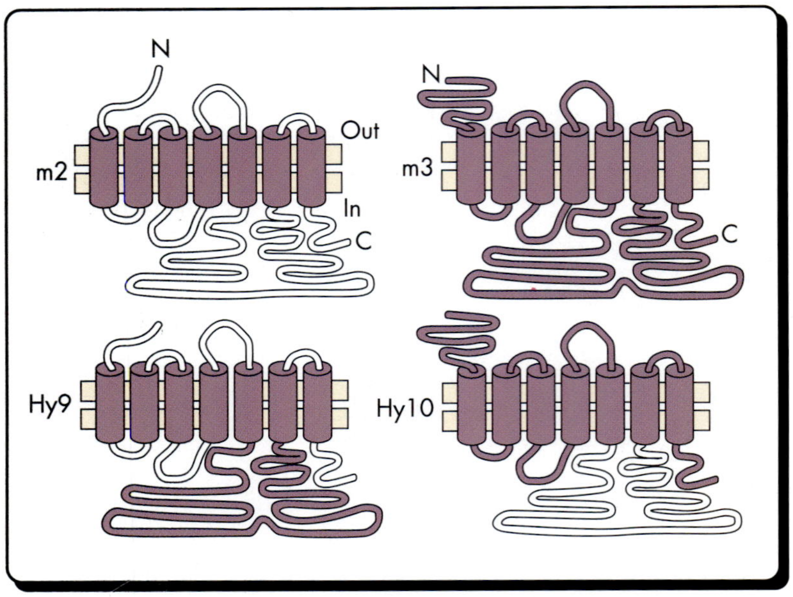

Figure 12-40. Chimeras. One of the remarkable inventions of molecular biology is the ability to modify proteins by engineering the DNA that directs their synthesis. In addition, selective expression of these proteins in living organisms can be accomplished. These techniques form the basis for experimental attempts to correct genetic defects: genetic engineering.

Chimeras are proteins constructed out of fragments of different molecules. Usually functional domains are exchanged. For example, if the third intracellular loops of the m2 (*white line*) and m3 (*solid line*) muscarinic acetylcholine receptor subtypes are exchanged, the resulting chimeras (Hy9 and Hy10) now couple to different G proteins and intracellular signaling systems, indicating that this loop is involved in G protein coupling and selectivity [19]. The techniques for constructing chimeras are quite involved but are basically built up out of complex sequences of restriction digestion (see Fig. 12-11) and linking (see Fig. 12-12). Recently, polymerase chain reaction (see Fig. 12-30) has been used to amplify a selected area of a gene, which can then be cloned into another gene to create a chimera. (*From* Lechleiter and coworkers [18].)

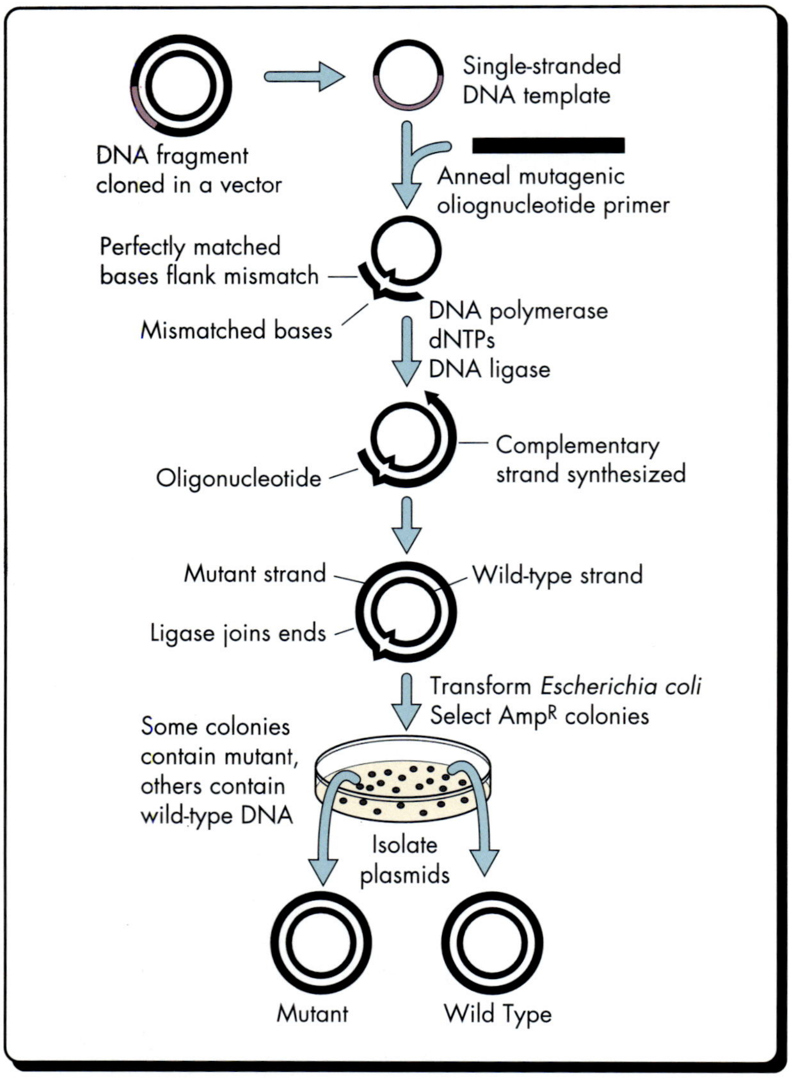

Figure 12-41. Site-directed mutagenesis. Some of the most powerful techniques in molecular biology are those allowing the generation of specific changes in protein structure, by modifying the underlying nucleotide sequence. The technique of site-directed mutagenesis is based on the use of a mismatched primer during DNA synthesis (see Fig. 12-3). The DNA fragment to be modified is cloned into a vector (see Fig. 12-17) and a single-stranded copy is prepared. An oligonucleotide (see Fig. 12-30) is designed, containing the desired mutation flanked by a number of correct nucleotides that will anneal to the DNA. *In vitro* DNA synthesis will result in a double-stranded DNA containing both a normal (wild-type) strand and a mutated strand. When these constructs are propagated in bacteria, DNA repair mechanisms quickly convert these hybrids to either double-stranded wild-type or double-stranded mutant. These can be isolated and screened by sequencing (see Fig. 12-20). Mutated DNA segments can also be obtained with polymerase chain reaction (see Fig. 12-33), using mutated primers. (*From* Watson and coworkers [3].)

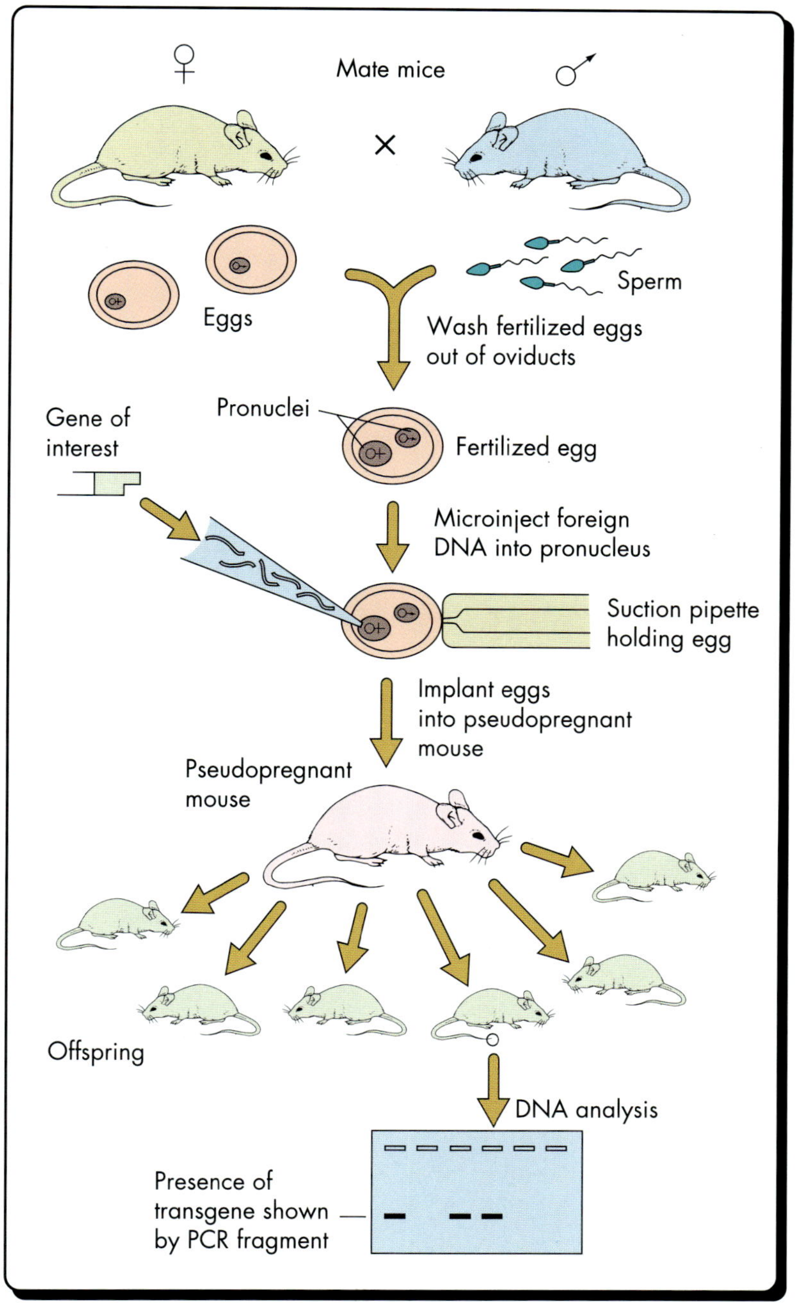

Figure 12-42. Transgenics. Transgenic techniques allow directed expression of a gene, either a wild-type or mutated (see Fig. 12-43), in animals. Mice are most commonly used for this purpose. Fertilized eggs are removed from females and the cDNA of interest is microinjected into one of the two pronuclei. The eggs are then transferred to pseudopregnant foster mothers. In some eggs, the cDNA will become integrated into the genome and passed on during cell division. After birth the offspring is checked for the presence of the transgene by polymerase chain reaction analysis (PCR) (see Fig. 12-30) or Southern blotting (see Fig. 12-28), using as substrate a small amount of genomic DNA obtained from a tail biopsy specimen. Advanced techniques allow for targeting gene expression to specific tissues, by linking the gene to tissue-specific regulatory sequences. Related methods can selectively knock out specific genes. Although results from these studies are not always easy to interpret (because compensatory changes in expression of other genes may occur; see Fig. 12-10), transgenics has provided very powerful methods for studing gene function and the effect of specific mutations [10]. (*From* Watson and coworkers [3].)

REFERENCES

1. Young BD: Molecular biology in medicine. *Postgrad Med J* 1992, 68:251–262.
2. Blau HM, Springer ML: Gene therapy: a novel form of drug delivery. *N Engl J Med* 1995, 333:1204–1207.
3. Watson JD, Gilman M, Witkowski J, Zoller M: *Recombinant DNA*, edn 2. New York: WH Freeman; 1992.
4. Alberts B, Bray D, Lewis J, *et al.*: *Molecular Biology of the Cell*, edn 2. New York: Garland Publishing; 1989.
5. Rosenthal N: DNA and the genetic code. *N Engl J Med* 1994, 331:39–41.
6. Rosenthal N: Tools of the trade: recombinant DNA. *N Engl J Med* 1994, 331:315–317.
7. Rosenthal N: Stalking the gene: DNA libraries. *N Engl J Med* 1994, 331:599–600.
8. Rosenthal N: Regulation of gene expression. *N Engl J Med* 1994, 331:931–933.
9. Kogan SC, Doherty M, Gitschier J: An improved method for prenatal diagnosis of genetic diseases by analysis of amplified DNA sequences: application to hemophilia A. *N Engl J Med* 1987, 317: 985–990.
10. Chehab FF: Molecular diagnostics: past, present, and future. *Hum Mutat* 1993, 2:331–337.
11. Fuchs R, Rice P, Cameron GN: Molecular biological databases: present and future. *Trends Biotechnol* 1992, 10:61–66.
12. Genetics Computer Group: *Program Manual for the GCG Package*, version 7. Madison, WI: Genetics Computer Group; 1991.
13. Lenstra JA: The applications of the polymerase chain reaction in the life sciences. *Cell Mol Biol* 1995, 41:603–614.
14. Lemna WK, Feldman GL, Kerem B, *et al.*: Mutation analysis for heterozygote detection and the prenatal diagnosis of cystic fibrosis. *N Engl J Med* 1990, 322: 291–296.
15. Gillard EF, Otsu K, Fujii J, *et al.*: Polymorphisms and deduced amino acid substitutions in the coding sequence of the ryanodine receptor (*RYR1*) gene in individuals with malignant hyperthermia. *Genomics* 1992, 13:1247–1254.
16. Dixon RAF, Kobilka BK, Strader DJ, *et al.*: Cloning of the gene and cDNA for mammalian beta-adrenergic receptor and homology with rhodopsin. *Nature* 1986, 342:75–79.
17. Kyte J, Doolittle RF: A simple method for displaying the hydropathic character of a protein. *J Mol Biol* 1982, 157:105–132.
18. Lechleiter J, Hellmiss R, Duerson K, *et al.*: Distinct sequence elements control the specificity of G protein activation by muscarinic acetylcholine receptor subtypes. *EMBO J* 1990, 9:4381–4390.

13

Mechanisms of Anesthetic Action

Leonard Firestone, Joseph Quinlan, and Ferenc Gyulai

General anesthesia gained worldwide acceptance almost immediately after its clinical introduction 150 years ago. Yet our understanding of the truly relevant cellular sites and pharmacologic mechanisms of general anesthetics remains well-informed speculation. This stands in marked contrast to certain other agents essential to the practice of anesthesia, namely local anesthetics and opiates, whose important sites and mechanisms have been substantially identified in the last two decades. Fortunately, the recent intensity of research into general anesthetic mechanisms [1] suggests that analogous advances are likely to be forthcoming.

At the start of the present century, the chemical industry had finally matured to the point that large-scale synthesis of pure chemicals became feasible. This, in turn, enabled meaningful biological assays to be performed, and the first durable observations of anesthetic properties and their detailed effects on animals were recorded shortly thereafter. The flammability, pungency, and other toxicities of the clinical inhalation agents led to an ardent search for safer drugs, and an ever-expanding cadre of chemicals with anesthetic properties emerged from the laboratory.

By mid-century, the tools of physical biochemistry were applied to the membranes of cells, and their fluid-mosaic, bilayer nature was revealed. Perturbation of these macromolecular structures by the plethora of anesthetics was now readily observable, and tests of both lipid-based [2] and protein-based [3] theories of general anesthesia were devised. Specific tests of these theories have lately exploited advances in chemical synthesis (resulting in highly resolved anesthetic optical isomers and other novel compounds) and molecular biology (enabling assays of anesthetic effects on pure proteins and receptors expressed *in vitro*).

As we enter the 21st century, technologic breakthoughs such as genetic engineering of mammals and *in vivo* human brain imaging promise to finally yield the essential insights. Animals with preplanned mutations or deletions in the most likely target proteins may demonstrate altered anesthesia responses (or even no responses at all!), while imaging the human brain in the course of anesthesia may prove to be the most direct experimental approach of all. But even these leading-edge approaches ultimately depend on the subtle accumulation of inferences, derived from more than a hundred years of painstaking observation as discussed in this chapter.

PHYSICAL-CHEMICAL OBSERVATIONS

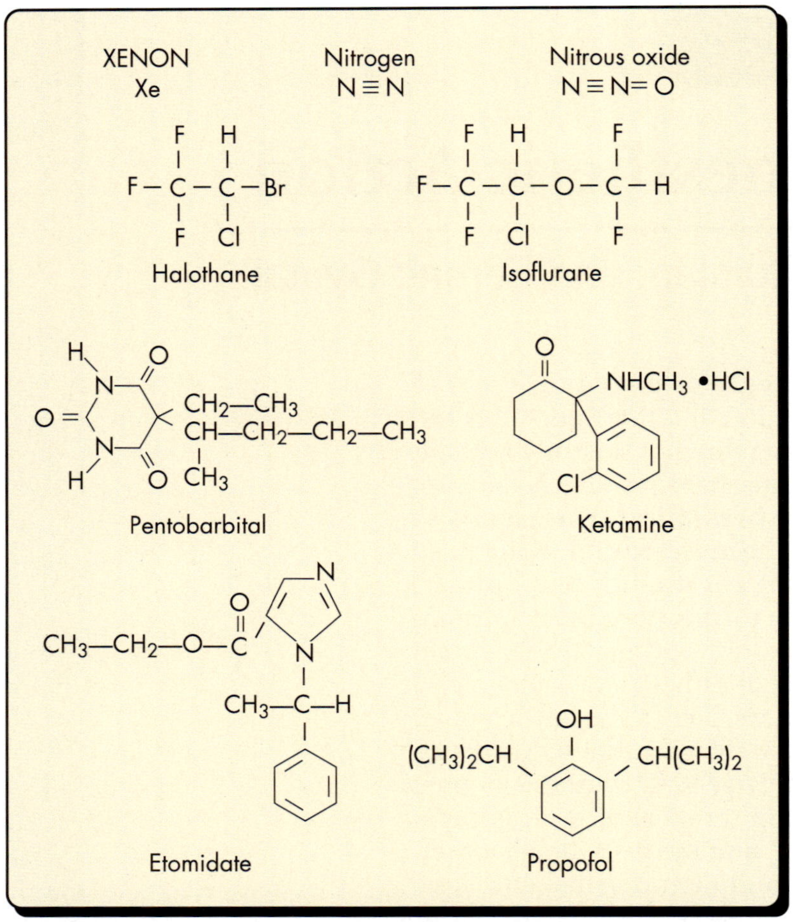

Figure 13-1. Chemical structures of selected anesthetics. Note the remarkable structural heterogeneity among this group. At standard temperature and pressure, the physical state of these agents is heterogeneous as well, with gases, liquids, and solids represented. Anesthetics range from simple atoms, to complex ring structures, and thus their molecular size may vary by more than 10-fold. Even the major constituent of earth's atmosphere, nitrogen, can produce anesthesia, albeit at hyperbaric (50 atm) pressure. The clinical volatile agents in common use (*eg*, halothane and isoflurane) are halogenated, but the unhalogenated parent compounds and close congeners are anesthetics as well (although they are far less potent and more flammable). The lack of an association between a particular functional group and the anesthetic characteristic, so evident in this figure, seemed to argue against a specific site-based mechanism for anesthetic action.

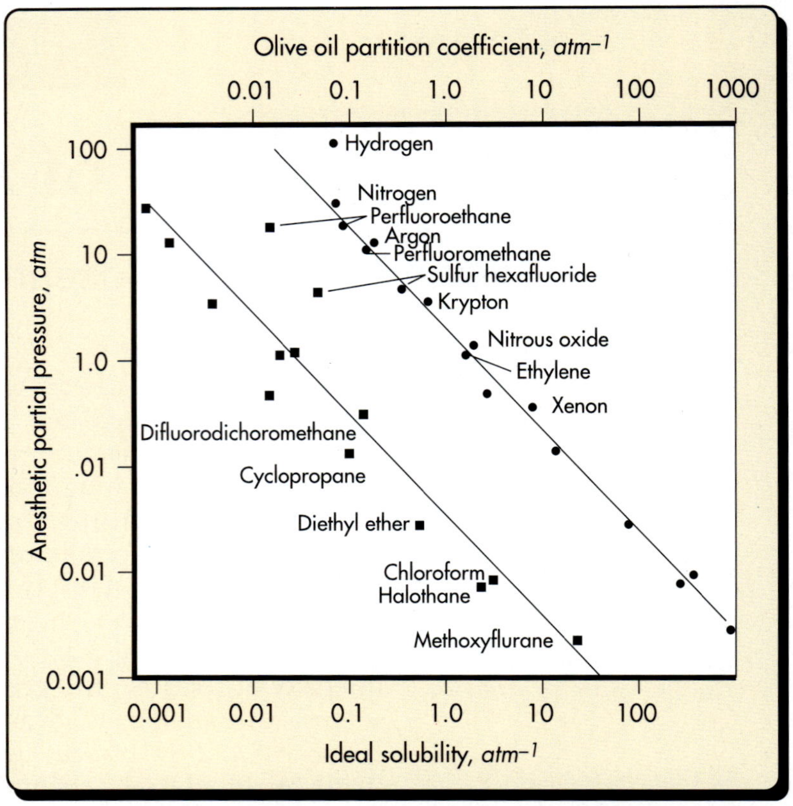

Figure 13-2. Illustration of the Meyer-Overton rule (right upper plot), and Ferguson's rule (left lower plot). The excellent correlation between anesthetic potency (ordinates) and solubility in olive oil (upper abcissa) is known as the Meyer-Overton correlation [4]. With few exceptions, it has proven to be remarkably accurate in predicting anesthetic potency. Ferguson's rule is an attempt to further refine the anesthetic potency–oil solubility relation, by correlating potency with thermodynamic activity, equivalent to ideal solubility (lower abscissa). Thus it predicts that for all anesthetics, obtundation will be achieved at a constant thermodynamic activity. Note that perfluorinated agents such as perfluoroethane and sulphur hexafluoride defy Ferguson's rule but obey the Meyer-Overton rule. (*From* Miller [5]; with permission.)

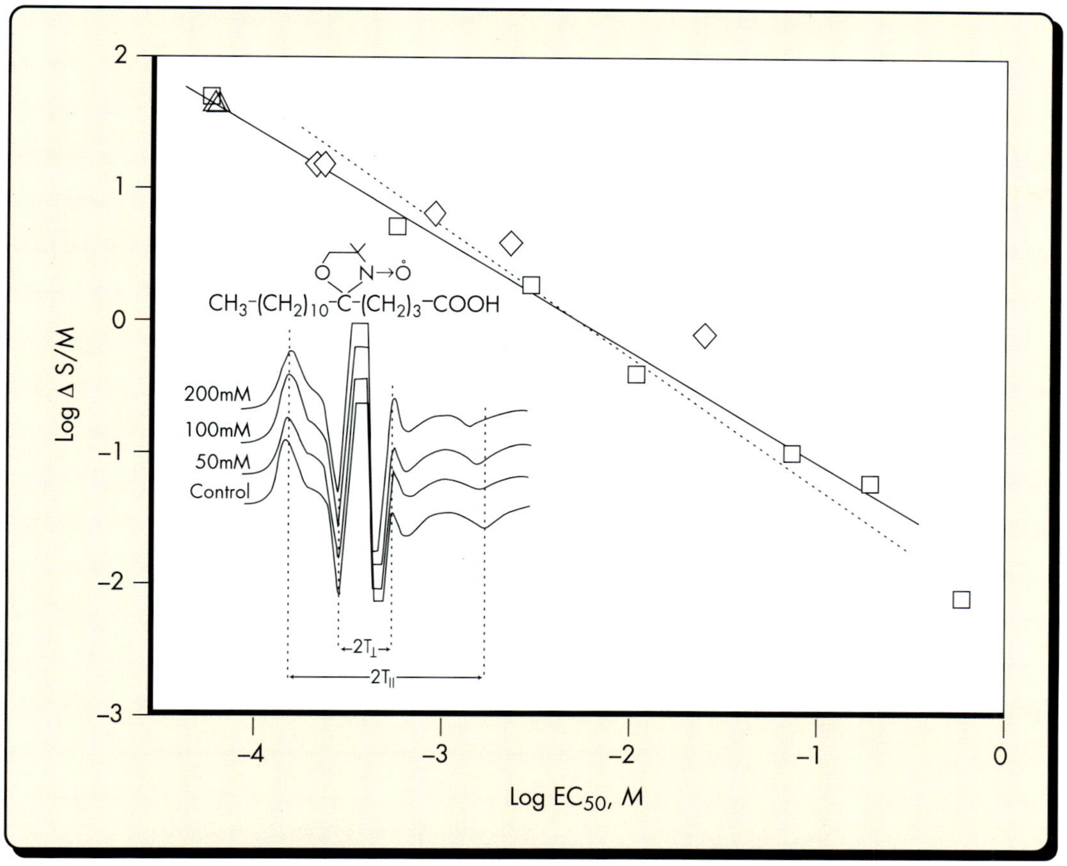

Figure 13-3. Effect of general anesthetics on membrane lipid order. Despite the success of the Meyer-Overton correlation, it reveals little about the mechanism by which an anesthetic acts once dissolved in the membrane. The advent of physical methods to probe the interior of membranes, however, made it possible to obtain direct physical evidence about how dissolved anesthetics affect lipid membranes. Electron paramagnetic resonance (EPR) spectroscopy is one such method that uses free radical reporter-labeled native molecules (*inset*). The particular "spin probe" illustrated partitions into the lipids and orients perpendicular to the plane of the membrane, and senses molecular motions of its neighbors. The series of EPR spectra in the *inset* indicate that diethylether increases molecular motion in the membrane's interior (disorders) as a function of concentration. The plots in the figure correlate the potencies with which a heterogenous array of anesthetics increase disordering (represented on the ordinate by the order parameter, "S") vs. median effective anesthetic concentration (EC_{50}) in animals. The *solid line* is a free fit of these data; the *dashed line* shows the position of a perfect correlation. (Inset *from* Firestone and coworkers [6]; with permission.)

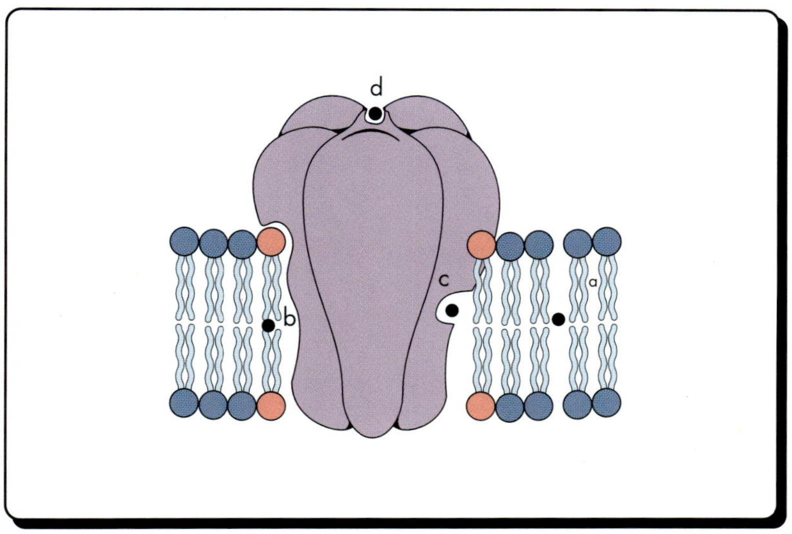

Figure 13-4. Possible membrane sites of general anesthetic action. In the biomembrane, there is a lipid bilayer and a large, irregularly shaped, transmembrane protein (*ie*, a ligand-gated or voltage-gated ion channel). Each lipid molecule consists of a polar head-group oriented toward the aqueous phase, and two highly mobile fatty acyl chains oriented toward the hydrophobic core of the biomembrane. These lipids form a bimolecular leaflet 4 nm in thickness, whose hydrophobic interior can dissolve general anesthetic molecules (*small black circles*). Thus general anesthetics may nonspecifically dissolve in the bulk lipid bilayer (site *a*) as a function of their membrane/buffer partition coefficient or in the "boundary" lipids relatively adherent to the protein (site *b*) and distinguished in this illustration by the *orange* polar head-groups. With either type of lipid, general anesthetics may increase their molecular motions, "disordering" the neat packing array (see Fig. 13-3 legend). General anesthetic molecules may also bind specifically to a pocket within the membrane protein, either in a transmembrane domain (site *c*), or in an aqueous domain (site *d*). It is important to note that sites *a*, *b*, *c*, and *d* are all hydrophobic, and thus anesthetic interaction with any or all of them would be compatible with the Meyer-Overton rule. (*Adapted from* Franks and Lieb [7].)

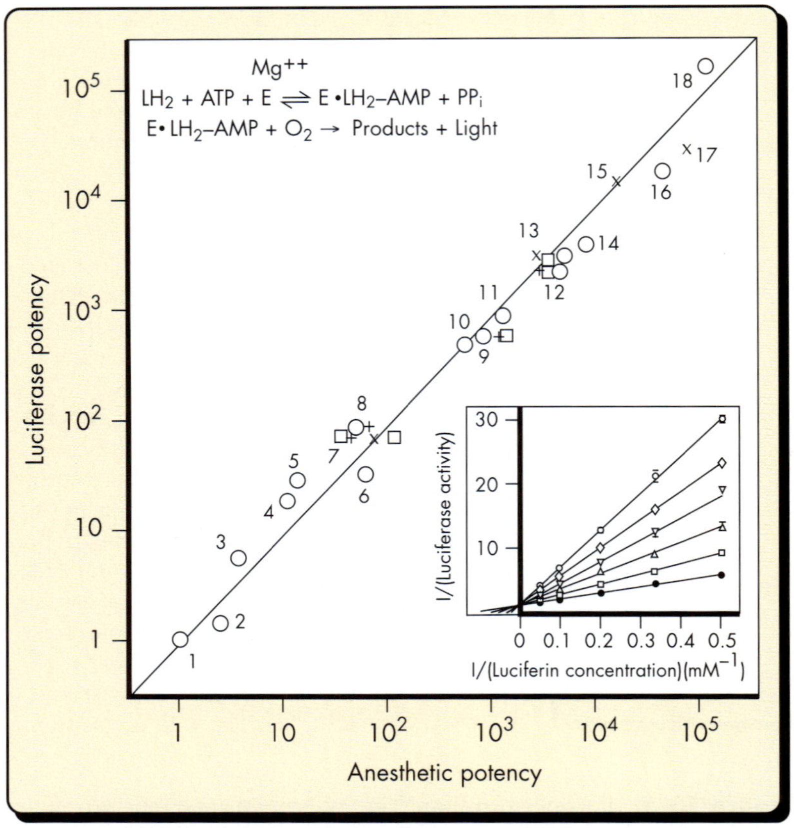

Figure 13-5. Correlation between anesthetic potency and potency for inhibiting luciferase. Luciferase, the light-forming enzyme purified from the North American firefly *Photinus pyralis*, is lipid-free. Thus the excellent correlation observed between an anesthetic's ability to inhibit luciferase activity and its ability to produce obtundation in animals is not dependent upon the presence of lipid. This supports a specific, protein-based mechanism of halothane action at this model site. *Top left*: Light-forming reaction of luciferase, where LH_2 represents the substrate luciferin and E represents the enzyme, luciferase. *Bottom inset*: Lineweaver-Burke plot of reciprocal enzyme activity (ordinate) as a function of reciprocal substrate concentration (abcissa), in the presence of varying concentrations of halothane (0.15 mM [*squares* on graph] - 0.75 mM [*open circles* on graph]. Halothane acts competitively with luciferin for the active site on luciferase, strengthening the case for a direct protein-based mechanism of anesthetic inhibition. For specific anesthetic agents tested, see Franks and Lieb [8]. AMP—adenosine monophosphate; ATP—adenosine triphosphate; PPi—inorganic phosphate. (*Adapted from* Franks and Lieb [8]; with permission.)

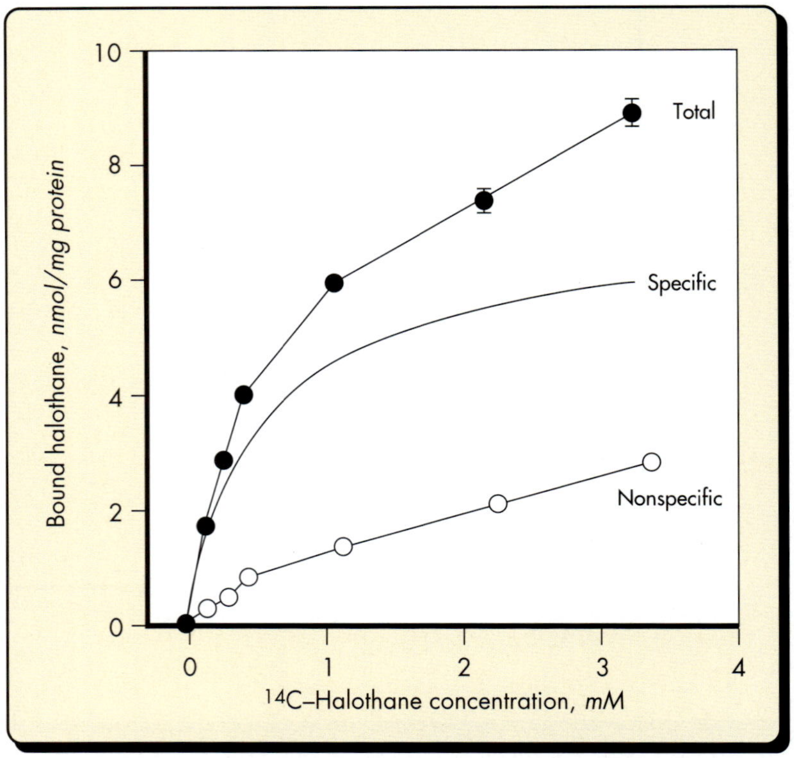

Figure 13-6. Binding isotherm for ^{14}C-labeled halothane to bovine serum albumin (BSA). These data indicate saturable binding to BSA by halothane, lending further support for the possibility that general anesthetics bind directly to a key, excitable protein in the nervous system. A direct, photoaffinity labeling technique was used to study the binding of halothane to BSA, an abundant, well-characterized model protein. Exposure of BSA-containing solutions to ultraviolet light for 10 sec results in a large increase in label incorporation, as a function of halothane concentration. When nonspecific binding (determined in the presence of excess unlabeled halothane) was subtracted from the total binding isotherm, a specific binding isotherm with a plateau (indicating saturation) was obtained. The apparent equilibrium dissociation constant for label incorporation was 260 μM, close to the value for 1 MAC (minimum alveolar concentration) halothane in humans at 37°C. (*From* Eckenhoff and Shuman [9]; with permission.)

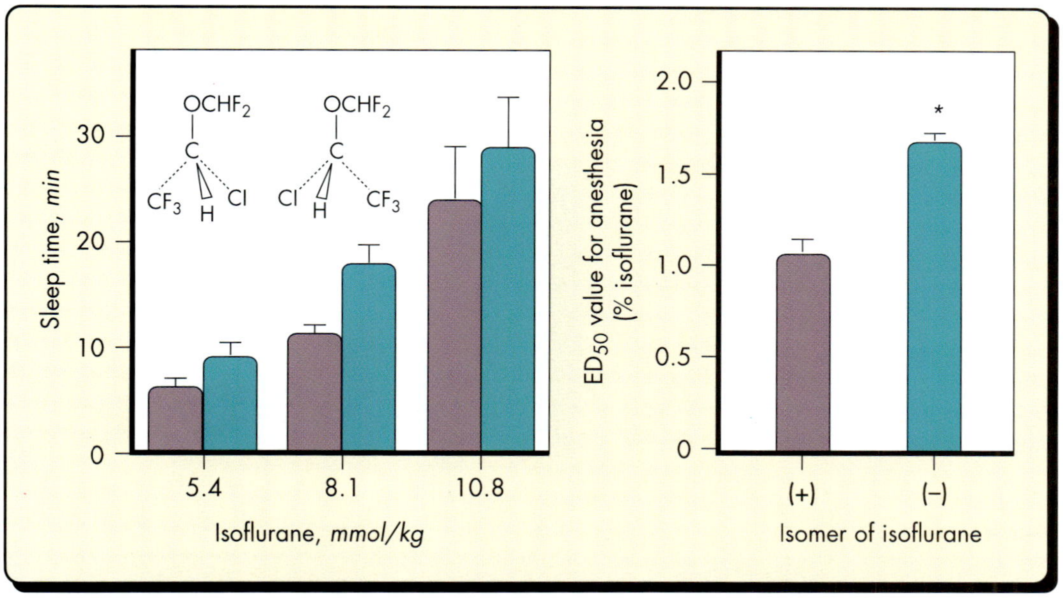

Figure 13-7. Comparative potencies of isoflurane's enantiomers *in vivo*. Differential potency of isoflurane's enantiomers (optical isomers; illustrated in the *inset*) supports a protein site of action in living animals. *Left panel*: Sleep time was measured in mice following a single intraperitoneal injection of either (+)- or (-)-isoflurane (*purple* or *aqua bars*, respectively). Both stereoisomers produced a dose-dependent increase in sleep time, with statistically significant differences ($p < 0.005$) observed at all doses [(+)>(-)]. To rule out pharmacokinetic confounders inherent to the sleep time assay, isomer potencies (*right panel*) were also compared using a more conventional equilibrium inhalation method in rats, with response to a painful stimulus as the endpoint. Once again, a significant difference in ED_{50} was observed, with (+)-isoflurane 60% more potent than the (-) isomer ($p < 0.05$). (*From* Moody and coworkers [10]; Harris and coworkers [11]; and Lysko and coworkers [12].)

SPECIFIC RECEPTOR/CHANNEL SITES

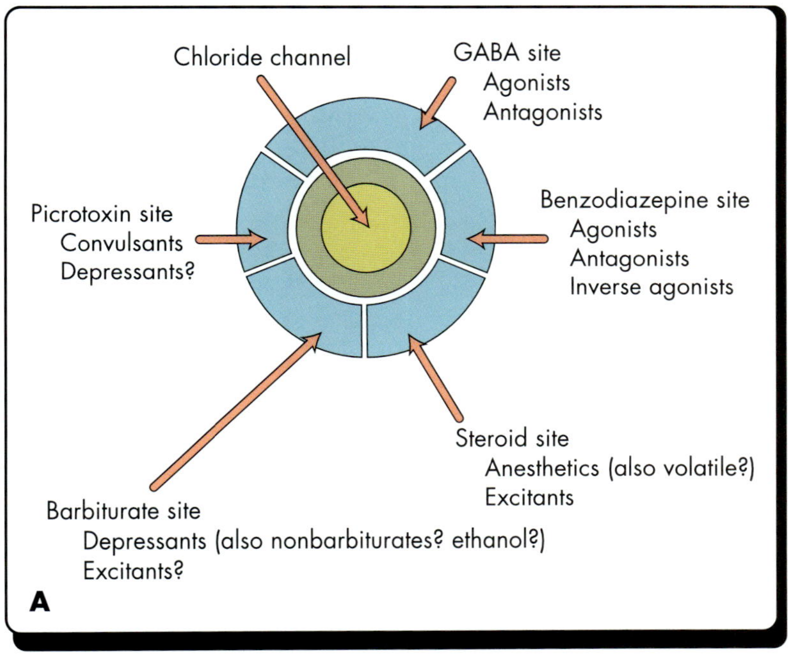

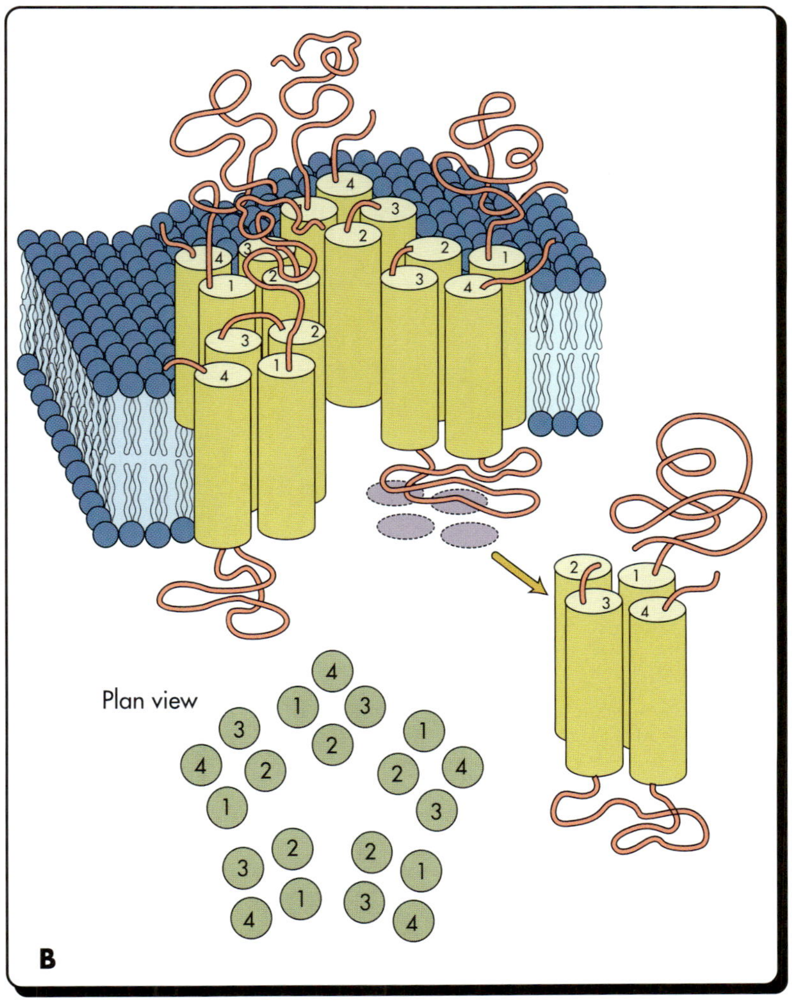

Figure 13-8. Representations of the central nervous system $GABA_A$ (gamma-amino butyric acid type A) receptor. If general anesthetics can interact specifically with a protein, what excitable proteins are the likely candidates? Based on prodigious *in vitro* electrophysiologic and ligand binding data [13], demonstrating potent general anesthetic effects and interaction sites with other hypnotics such as benzodiazepines and barbiturates, the $GABA_A$ receptor is a reasonable candidate for a general anesthetic target. A, Schematic of the multimeric $GABA_A$ receptor, containing an integral chloride channel and interaction ("binding") sites for multiple endogenous and drug modulators of the chloride conductance. The GABA site interacts with agonists to gate the channel and is inhibited competitively by antagonists. The benzodiazepine site allosterically interacts with the agonist site, but fails to gate the channel; in contrast, the barbiturate and steroid (anesthetic? ethanol?) sites appear to gate the channel with varying efficacies.

B, Model of the GABA-A receptor–chloride ion channel protein complex, composed of a heterooligomer of 5 subunits, including alpha, beta, and gamma, delta or rho polypeptides. Each subunit has 4 putative membrane-spanning domains (numbered *1*, *2*, *3*, *4* and represented by cylinders), one or more of which contribute to the wall of the ion channel. The *plan view inset* illustrates how the subunits are arranged around the hypdrophilic ionophore like staves of a barrel. (Part A *adapted from* Olsen and coworkers [14]; part B *adapted from* Olsen and Tobin [14a]; with permission.)

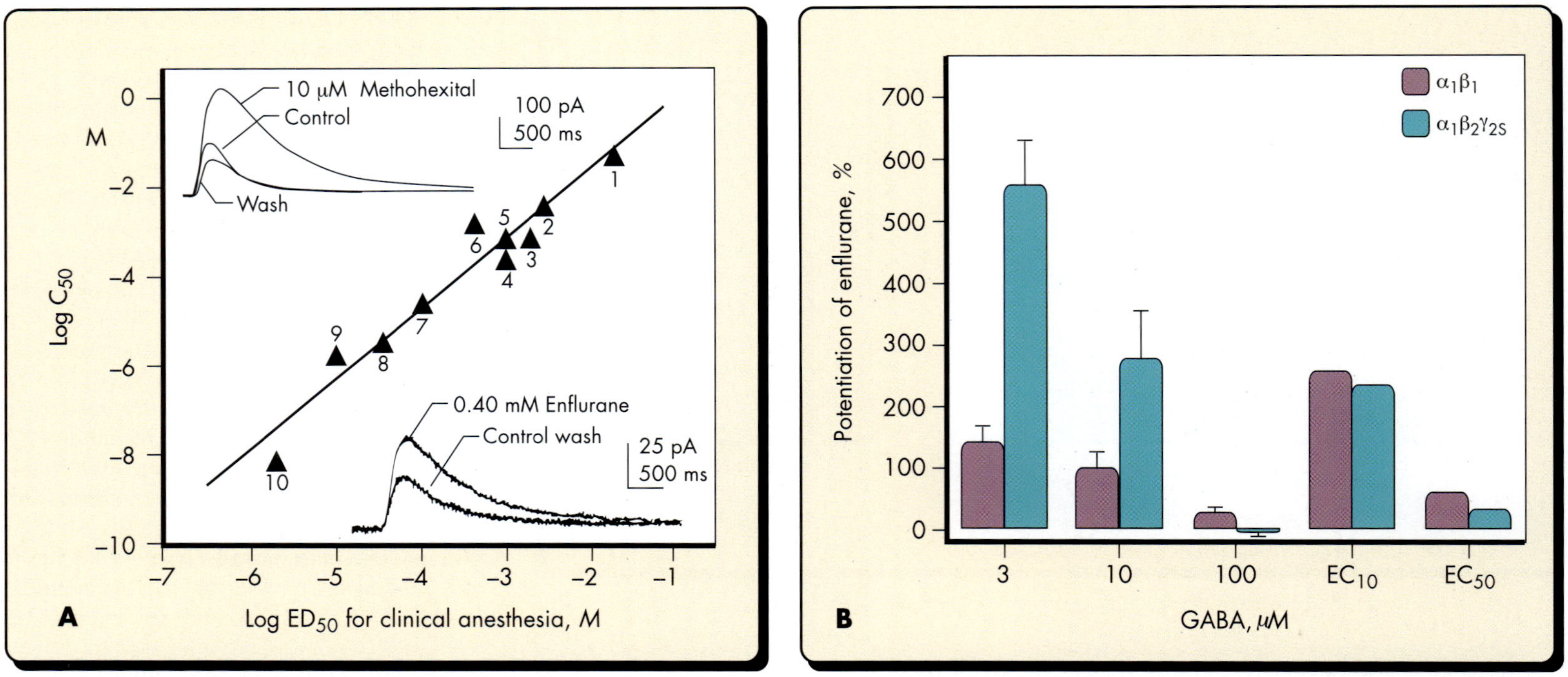

Figure 13-9. $GABA_A$ receptor and anesthetic potency. **A**, Anesthetic potency for modulation of $GABA_A$ receptors is highly correlated with *in vivo* anesthetic potency. These data support the case that potentiation of $GABA_A$ receptor-gated currents is an important anesthetic action. C_{50}, the concentration required to produce a 50% increase in the duration of GABA-activated currents (see *upper left* for methohexital and *lower right* for enflurane), is plotted against the median effective dose ED_{50} for surgical anesthesia. The correlation coefficient, r, = 0.97. The agents represented are: urethane (*1*), chloroform (*2*), trichloroethanol (*3*), isoflurane (*4*), enflurane (*5*), halothane (*6*), pentobarbital (*7*), methohexital (*8*), propofol (*9*), alphaxalone (*10*). **B**, Potentiation of GABA action by enflurane depends on subunit composition of the receptor as well as the concentration of GABA. Percent potentiation is shown as a function of GABA concentration both as absolute concentration (in micromolar) and as the effective concentration (EC) for receptors with either subunit composition. Such data indicate that the specific residue composition of the $GABA_A$ receptor influences the magnitude of general anesthetic effects, as predicted by a protein-based anesthetic mechanism. (Panel A *from* Zimmerman and coworkers [15]; with permission; panel B *from* Harris and coworkers [16].)

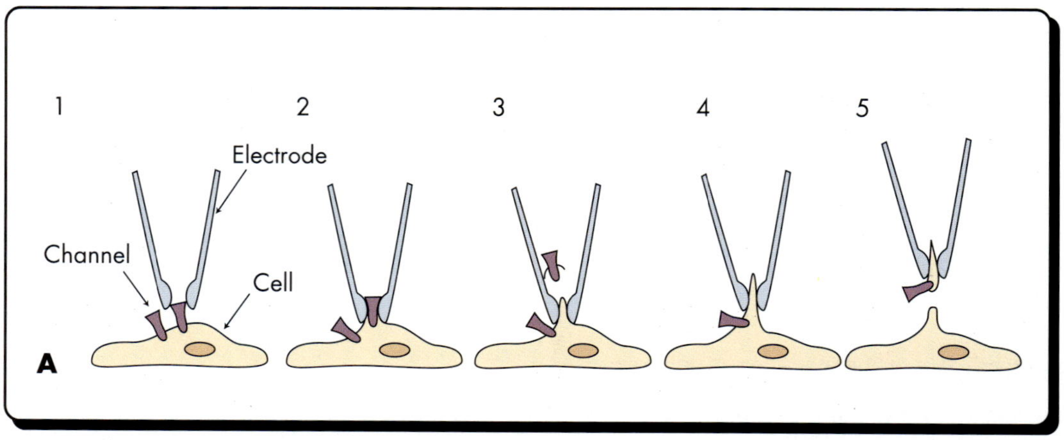

Figure 13-10. Effects of general anesthetics on nicotinic acetylcholine receptor (nAChR) channels. High-resolution patch clamp techniques used for measuring the tiny current that flows through single open nAChR channels reveal that this excitatory channel is acutely sensitive to blockade by general anesthetics, and are useful in elucidating the mechanisms involved. **A**, Serial formation of an outside-out patch containing an nAChR on the tip of a glass electrode. After electrode positioning (*1*), a seal is formed such that the glass pipette tip isolates a section of membrane (*2*) containing one or a few channels. Next, the cell-attached patch is disrupted (*3*), the electrode is withdrawn (*4*), and the outside-out patch, containing a channel with proper orientation toward the extracellular face, is excised (*5*).

(*Continued on next page*)

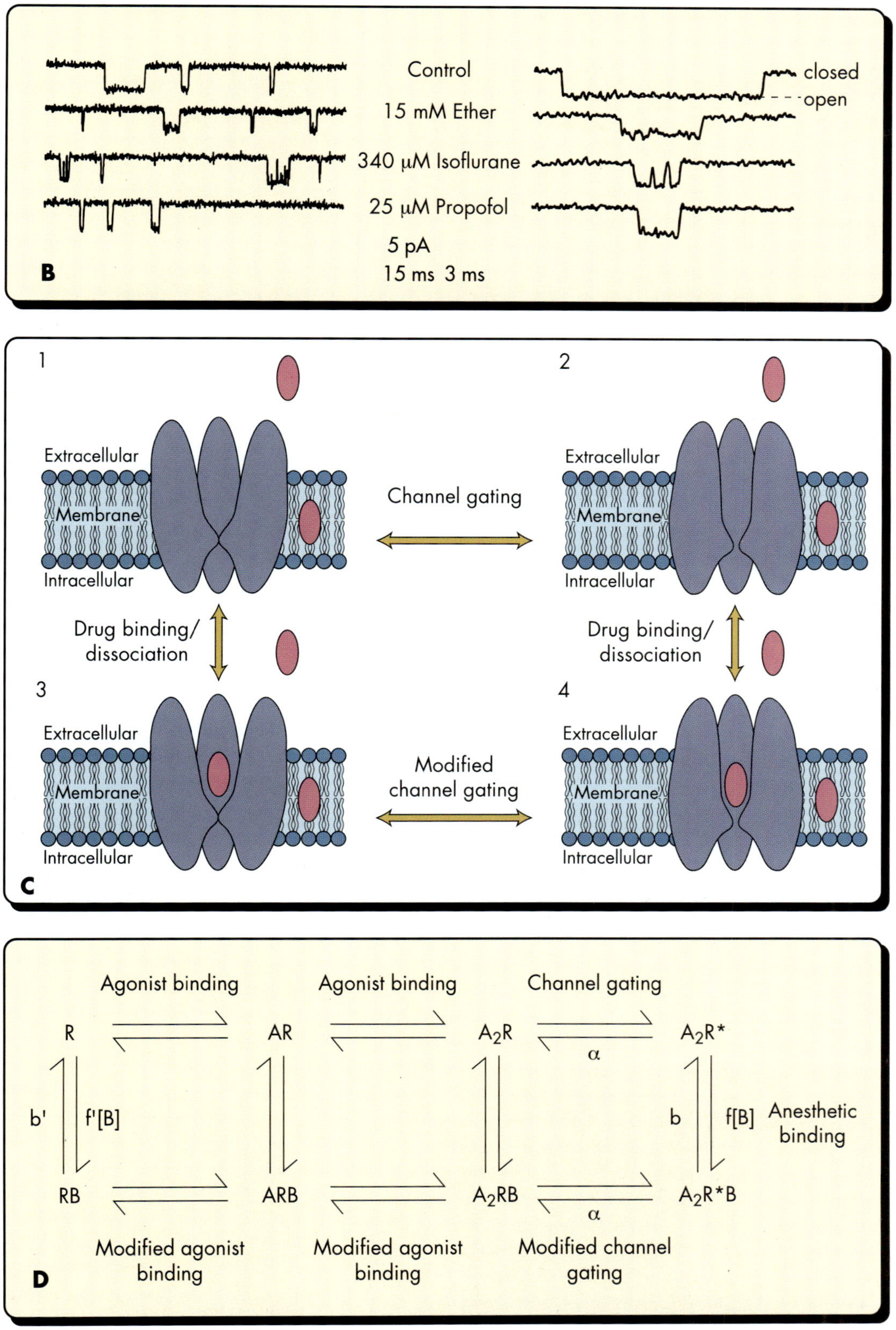

Figure 13-10. (*Continued*) B, Single AChR channels activated by 200 nM ACh and perfused with no drug (control), 15 mM ether, 340 μM (0.7%) isoflurane, or 25 μM propofol. Channel openings are shown as downward transitions. Traces on the right illustrate the "bursts" on an expanded time scale. Typically, ether causes amplitude to be smaller and noisier than normal; isoflurane induces a flickery pattern of brief openings; propofol causes the channels to appear as isolated brief openings. C, In principle, nAChRs exist in both closed (*1*) and open (*2*) states, and general anesthetic molecules may bind to either one (becoming states *3* and *4*, respectively). This gives rise to the kinetic scheme depicted in **D**, where the anesthetic (*B*) may bind to the open, liganded state (*top row*), or one of several closed states (*bottom row*). Using this scheme, the rate constants for anesthetic binding and dissociation can be estimated, leading to a unified mechanism for anesthetic action at nAChRs, where all anesthetics bind directly to the channel protein and block ion flow. The difference in current pattern is determined by the duration of anesthetic blockade. A—agonist; AR—liganded receptor; ARB—anesthetic bound to liganded receptor; A_2R—doubly liganded receptor (two agonist molecules); b—reverse rate constant for anesthetic dissociation from the unliganded receptor; F—forward rate constant for anesthetic binding; Fv′—forward rate constant for anesthetic binding to the lignded receptor. R—receptor; *—open (permeable) state of receptor. (Panels A and C *from* Dilger and coworkers [17]; part B *from* Dilger [18]; with permission.)

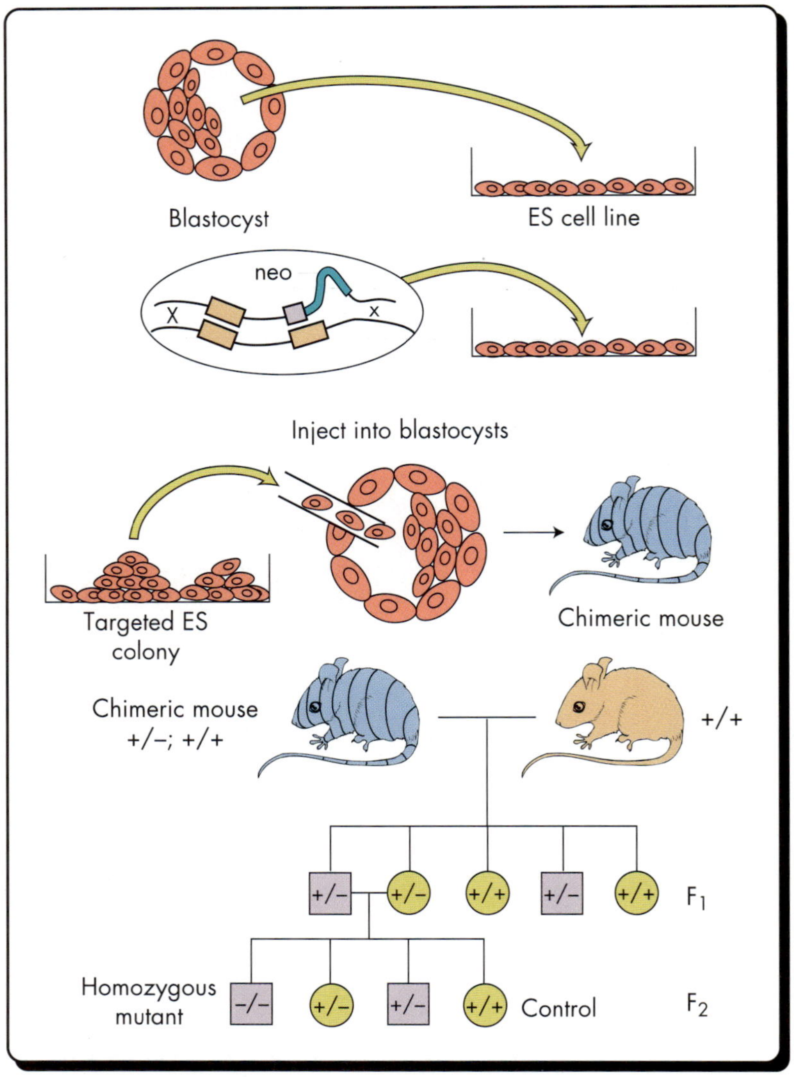

Figure 13-11. Schematic of gene targeting by homologous recombination in embryonic stem (ES) cells. This technology is used to create mice with preplanned mutation or complete deletion of a specific gene, encoding a specific gene product of interest (*ie*, a subtype of the $GABA_A$ receptor, nACh receptor, or α2-adrenergic receptor). Abnormal responses to general anesthetics in such a "knock-out" mouse would be strong evidence for the involvement of the targeted gene's product in the anesthesia process. The process begins with generation of an ES cell line, cultured from an early embryo (blastocyst). The next step is to disrupt the gene of interest in ES cells by homologous recombination with a targeting construct, which is a genomic clone of a significant segment of the gene to be knocked-out, ligated to mutant DNA designed to disable the normal transcription or translation process. In the example illustrated, a neomycin-resistance gene (*neo*) is substituted for a segment of the native gene, which disrupts translation and provides a means to select for cells that underwent homologous recombination and incorporated the targeting construct. After using neomycin to select for successfully "targeted" ES cells, such cells are injected into a host blastocyst (of different coat color), and the blastocyst is reimplanted into a pseudopregnant host to generate chimeric mice containing targeted ES cells (indicated grossly by the presence of the original coat color). Subsequent inbreeding yields a homozygous mutant ("knockout mouse") by the F_2 generation. (*From* Silva and Giese [19]; with permission.)

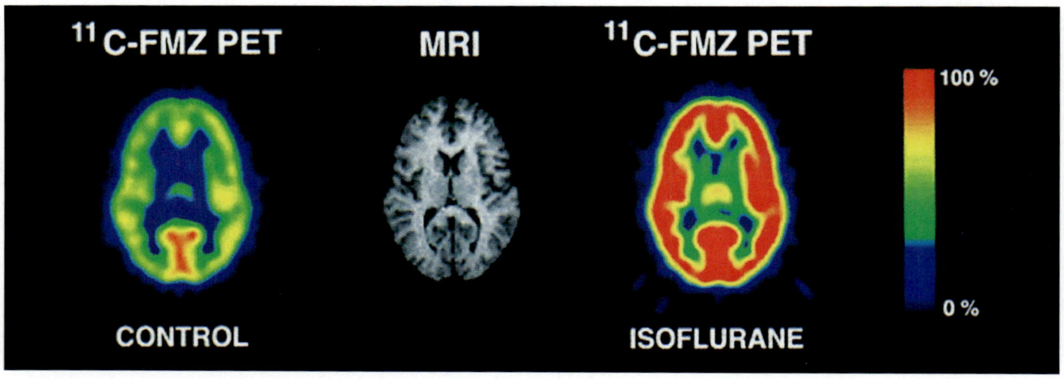

Figure 13-12. Positron emission tomographic (PET) images of ^{11}C-flumazenil (FMZ) distribution in the brain of a single subject before (control) or during (isoflurane) general anesthesia. The color scale (*far right*) indicates relative radioactivity with 0% denoting minimum and 100% maximum intensity. Thus, at a constant ligand dose, the images indicate enhanced $GABA_A$ receptor-specific ligand uptake during isoflurane anesthesia in man, both in cortical and subcortical areas. Preliminary data indicate that this effect of isoflurane is both specific to $GABA_A$ receptors, and dose-dependent, as predicted by a $GABA_A$ receptor-based mechanism of anesthesia. A single transverse slice is illustrated at the level of the occipital lobe, for both the PET and MRI images. The MRI image is used for PET-to-MRI anatomic registration. (*From* Gyulai and coworkers [20].)

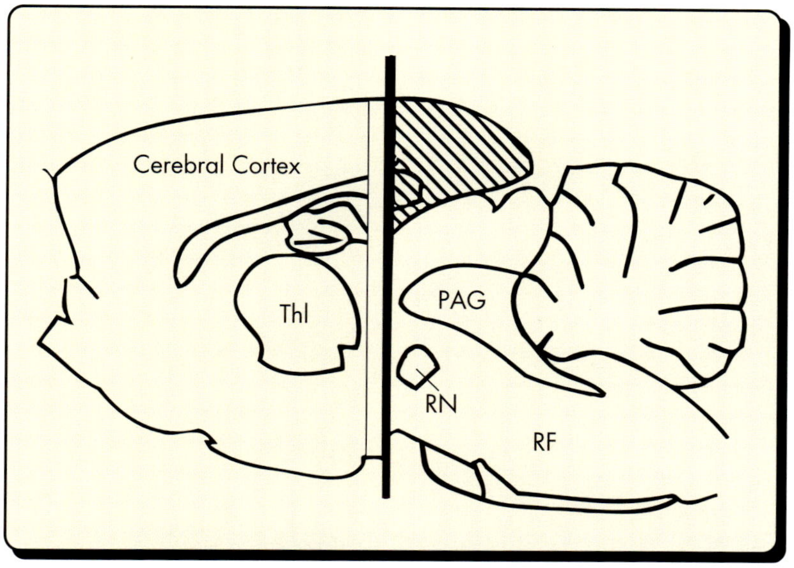

Figure 13-13. Decerebration does not alter minimum alveolar concentration. Decerebrate lesions of rostral cerebral cortex (color area) fails to change the anesthetic requirement in rats. Cortical regions that remain following decerebration were physiologically and anatomically isolated from the midbrain and brainstem. The apparent importance of spinal sites in the production of anesthesia's inhibiting responses to noxious stimuli is reinforced in several separate but related studies. For example, in rats, the threshold concentration of anesthetic necessary to block movements elicited by pain is unchanged by decerebration [21], and concentrations of isoflurane that block pain-evoked movements remain constant after acute spinal cord transection [22]. PAG—periaqueductal grey; Thl—thalamus; RN—red nucleus; RF—reticular formation. (*From* Rampil and coworkers [22].)

ACKNOWLEDGMENTS

This work was supported by grants from the National Institute of General Medical Sciences (GM35900 and GM52035 to LF, and GM15904 for the Harvard Anesthesia Center); the Foundation for Anesthesia Education and Research (Starter Awards to JQ and FG; Young Investigator Award to FG); International Anesthesia Research Society (Clinical Research Scholar Award to LF); University Anesthesiology and Critical Care Medicine Foundation; and, Drs. Susan Firestone and Peter Winter.

REFERENCES

1. Rubin E, Miller KW, Roth SH, eds: Molecular and cellular mechanisms of alcohol and anesthetics. *Ann N Y Acad Sci* 1991, 625:417–475.
2. Janoff AS, Miller KW: A Crititical Assessment of the Lipid Theories of General Anaesthetic Action. In *Biological Membranes*, vol 4. Edited by Chapman D. London: Academic Press; 1982.
3. Franks NP, Lieb WR: Molecular and cellular mechanisms of general anesthesia. *Nature* 1994, 367:607–613.
4. Meyer KH: Contributions to the theory of narcosis. *Trans Faraday Soc* 1937, 33:1062–1068.
5. Miller KW: The nature of the site of general anesthesia. *Int Rev Neurobiol* 1985, 27:1–61.
6. Firestone LL, Alifimoff JK, Miller KW: Does general anesthetic-induced desensitization of the Torpedo acetylcholine receptor correlate with lipid disordering? *Molec Pharmacol* 1994, 46:508–515.
7. Franks NP, Lieb WR: What is the molecular nature of general anesthetic target sites? *Trends Pharmacol Sci* 1987, 8:169–174.
8. Franks NP, Lieb WR: Do general anaesthetics act by competitive binding to specific receptors? *Nature* 1984, 310:599–601.
9. Eckenhoff RG, Shuman H: Halothane binding to soluble proteins determined by photoaffinity labeling. *Anesthesiology* 1993, 79:96–106.
10. Moody EJ, Harris BD, Skolnick P: The potential for safer anesthesia using stereoselective anesthetics. *Trends Pharmacol Sci* 1994, 15:387–390.
11. Harris B, Moody E, Skolnick P: Isoflurane anesthesia is stereoselective. *Eur J Pharmacol* 1992, 217:215–216.
12. Lysko GS, Robinson JL, Casto R, Ferrone RA: The stereospecific effects of isoflurane isomers *in vivo*. *Eur J Pharmacol* 1994, 263:25–29.
13. Tanelian D, Kosek P, Mody I, MacIver MB: The role of the GABA-A receptor/chloride channel complex in anesthesia. *Anesthesiology* 1993, 78:757–776.
14. Olsen RW, Sapp DM, Bureau MH, *et al.*: Allosteric actions of CNS depressants including anesthetics on subtypes of the inhibitory $GABA_A$ receptor-chloride channel complex. *Ann NY Acad Sci* 1991B, 625:145–154.
14a. Olsen RW, Tobin AJ: Molecular biology of $GABA_A$ receptors. *FASEB J* 1990, 4:1469–1480.
15. Zimmerman SA, Jones MV, Harrison NL: Potentiation of GABA-A receptor chloride current correlates with *in vivo* anesthetic potency. *J Pharmacol Exper Therap* 1994, 270:987–991.
16. Harris RA, Mihic SJ, Dildy-Mayfield JE, Machu TK: Actions of anesthetics on ligand-gated ion channels: role of receptor subunit composition. *FASEB J* 1995, 9:1454–1462.
17. Dilger JP, Liu Y, Vidal AM: Interactions of general anesthetics with single acetylcholine receptor channels. *Eur J Anaesthesiol* 1995, 12:31–39.
18. Dilger JP, Vidal AM, Mody HI, Liu Y: Evidence for direct actions of general anesthetics on an ion channel protein. *Anesthesiology* 1994, 81:431–442.
19. Silva A, Giese KP: The "Whys," "Whats," and "Hows" of Gene Targeting in Neuroscience. In *Ins and Outs of Genes: Knockouts and Transfers*. Society for Neuroscience, 1993 Short Course 1 Syllabus, 3–22.
20. Gyulai F, Firestone L, Mintun M, *et al.*: Isoflurane enhances *in vivo* $GABA_A$ receptor binding in humans: quantitative imaging by PET. *Anesthesiology* 1996, 85:A703.
21. Todd MM, Weeks JB, Warner DS: A focal cryogenic brain lesion does not reduce the minimum alveolar concentration for halothane in rats. *Anesthesiology* 1993, 79:139–143.
22. Rampil IJ, Mason P, Singh H: Anesthetic protency (MAC) is independent of forebrain structures in the rat. *Anesthesiology* 1993, 78:707–712.

14

Pharmacology and Physiology of Inhaled Anesthetic Agents

Peter C. Houck, Philip S. Gibbs, and Robert K. Stoelting

The development of new anesthetic agents usually stems from one of two motivations, either the need to eliminate the undesirable properties of an existing compound or in response to changing demands of the marketplace. An example of the former might be the intensive research on nondepolarizing muscle relaxants that has occurred over the past decade. Concerns about cardiovascular side effects, slow onset time, and residual post-operative muscle weakness concerns that were valid for pancuronium can now be avoided by proper selection and use of new relaxant agents with more favorable properties. Is the same true for the newly developed volatile anesthetics? In part yes, but probably not to as great an extent. For instance, it seldom would be necessary to select desflurane or sevoflurane specifically to avoid an undesirable property of isoflurane in adult anesthesia. Rather, changing market forces, driven by the trend toward outpatient surgery and early home discharge, have created a demand for anesthetic agents with shorter durations of action. Thus, the popular interest in desflurane and sevoflurane has arisen because their low blood solubility confers a pharmacokinetic advantage for rapid emergence from anesthesia [1,2]. Indeed, these agents constitute a new class of poorly soluble volatile agents with pharmacokinetic profiles approaching that of nitrous oxide [3].

In addition to solubility, both desflurane and sevoflurane possess unique characteristics that serve to differentiate them from previously available volatile agents and from each other. This chapter provides an overview of these differentiating physiologic and pharmacologic properties in the context of recent research and debate. Recent comprehensive reviews of desflurane and sevoflurane are available to the reader for reference [4–7].

Sevoflurane may possess the most favorable cardiovascular profile of all the volatile agents. Like isoflurane [8] and desflurane [9], sevoflurane [10] causes a dose-dependent decrease in mean arterial blood pressure and maintains cardiac output by decreasing systemic vascular resistance. Unlike with desflurane and isoflurane, heart rate is not significantly increased up to 2 minimum alveolar concentration (MAC) of sevoflurane. Further, the transient sympathetic stimulation caused by large increases in desflurane [11] concentration, and to a lesser degree with isoflurane [11], is absent with sevoflurane [12]. Finally, in a chronically instrumented dog model of coronary steal, sevoflurane caused a reverse steal phenomenon, actually redistributing blood flow toward ischemic myocardium [13].

Metabolism of desflurane is so minimal that the potential for hepatic toxicity is practically nonexistent [14]. The same is true for sevoflurane but for different reasons. Unlike other volatile anesthetics, sevoflurane is not metabolized to a reactive intermediate capable of binding to liver protein, creating neoantigen [15]. Rather, it is metabolized to a unique compound (hexafluoroisopropanol) that is rapidly glucuronidated and excreted in the urine [16]. The potential for desflurane or sevoflurane to cause immune-mediated hepatic injury is remote [15].

Biotransformation of sevoflurane [17], unlike desflurane, is sufficient to increase plasma inorganic fluoride concentrations above 50 μM, the threshold for nephrotoxicity in patients anesthetized with methoxyflurane [18]. Further, sevoflurane degrades in the presence of carbon dioxide absorbent to compound A, a byproduct that is nephrotoxic in rats [19–22]. Multiple clinical studies have failed to demonstrate any clinically significant change in renal function in healthy patients anesthetized with sevoflurane [17,23–28]. Further, sevoflurane has been administered to over 14 million patients worldwide without a single documented case of clinically significant hepatorenal injury related directly to sevoflurane toxicity. Nevertheless, evidence of subclinical renal injury [17] and inadequate studies in patients with preexisting renal insufficiency suggest that sevoflurane should not be administered to this subset of patients until further studies are done [29].

Sevoflurane [30,31], unlike desflurane [32], is nonpungent and is therefore suitable for inhalation induction. Other respiratory effects of sevoflurane and desflurane do not clinically distinguish these agents from isoflurane. Both are respiratory depressants, decreasing ventilation in a dose-dependent fashion. Both increase the resting $PaCO_2$ and depress the carbon dioxide response curve [33,34].

The central nervous system (CNS) effects of desflurane and sevoflurane are qualitatively similar to those of isoflurane. Both are cerebral vasodilators [35,36], capable of increasing intracranial pressure [36,37], and carbon dioxide responsiveness remains intact [38,39]. They have similar effects on electroencephalographic activity, producing burst suppression at approximately 1.25 MAC with increasing periods of electrical silence thereafter [36,40]. Neither causes convulsant activity.

Desflurane and sevoflurane are interesting new volatile anesthetic agents with unique properties that differentiate them from previous inhaled agents and from each other. The remainder of this chapter expands on areas of greatest contrast between these agents, including physiochemical properties and cardiovascular, hepatic, and renal effects.

GENERAL PROPERTIES

CHRONOLOGY OF INHALED ANESTHETIC DEVELOPMENT

Date of Introduction	Compound	Comments
1840s	Nitrous oxide Diethyl ether Chloroform	Most early anesthetics either flammable or organotoxic
1951	Fluroxene	First halogenated ether Flammable at higher concentrations Concerns of organ toxicity
1956	Halothane	Alkanes sensitize myocardium to epinephrine
1960	Methyoxyflurane	Nonflammable Extensive hepatic metabolism Nephrotoxicity
1973	Enflurane	Nonflammable, reduced metabolism, favorable pharmacokinetics
1981	Isoflurane	Nonflammable, reduced metabolism, favorable pharmacokinetics
1992	Desflurane	Pharmacokinetics comparable to nitrous oxide
1995	Sevoflurane	Pharmacokinetics comparable to nitrous oxide

Figure 14-1. Chronology of inhaled anesthetic development. The anesthetic properties of nitrous oxide, diethyl ether, and chloroform were discovered in the 1840s. Eighty years elapsed before the introduction of other agents such as ethylene, cyclopropane, and divinyl ether (not shown). In 1950, all available volatile anesthetics were either flammable or potentially toxic to the liver. Recognition that fluorination reduced flammability led to the introduction of the first halogenated hydrocarbon anesthetic, fluroxene. However, this anesthetic retained flammability at higher concentrations, and concerns about organ toxicity persisted. Halothane, a halogenated alkane, solved the flammability problem but sensitized the myocardium to epinephrine. The tendency for alkanes to enhance the arrhythmogenic effects of epinephrine led to the search for new inhaled anesthetics derived from ethers. Several halogenated methyl ethyl ethers were developed that neither were flammable nor sensitized the myocardium to epinephrine. The first of these, methoxyflurane, was highly soluble, resulting in prolonged induction and prolonged emergence times. Of greater concern was nephrotoxicity secondary to hepatic metabolism and release of inorganic fluoride. Increased fluorination and decreased chlorination produced enflurane, the first modern inhaled anesthetic that combined the favorable properties of moderate solubility, resistance to metabolism, and not sensitizing the myocardium to epinephrine. Isoflurane, the chemical isomer of enflurane, was a further improvement. The most recently introduced agents, desflurane and sevoflurane, hold a pharmacokinetic advantage owing to a blood solubility similar to that of nitrous oxide [3]. Exchanging the sole chlorine on isoflurane for fluorine creates desflurane. The increased stability of the fluorine carbon compared with the chlorine carbon bond nearly eliminates the hepatic metabolism of desflurane [14]. Like desflurane, sevoflurane is halogenated exclusively with fluorine and is thus very insoluble in blood. Unlike desflurane, sevoflurane undergoes significant hepatic metabolism [16] and degradation by soda lime [41].

PHYSICAL AND CHEMICAL PROPERTIES OF INHALED ANESTHETICS

	Nitrous oxide	Halothane	Enflurane	Isoflurane	Desflurane	Sevoflurane
Boiling point, °C		50.2	56.5	48.5	**23.5**	58.5
Vapor pressure, *mm Hg @ 20°C*	Gas	244	172	240	**664**	160
Odor	Sweet	Organic	Ethereal	Ethereal	Ethereal	Ethereal
Pungency	None	None	Moderate	Moderate	**Strong**	**None**
Preservative necessary	No	Yes	No	No	No	No
Stability in moist soda lime						
40°C		Stable		Stable	Stable	**Unstable**
60°C		SI.Unstable		Stable	Stable	**Unstable**
80°C		Unstable		Unstable	SI.Unstable	**Unstable**

Figure 14-2. Physical and chemical properties of inhaled anesthetics. Replacing the sole chlorine in isoflurane with fluorine to produce desflurane markedly increases the vapor pressure, such that desflurane boils at just above room temperature. This property of desflurane renders conventional flow-over vaporizer technology inadequate for controlled vaporization. The TEC 6 vaporizer (Ohmeda, West Yorkshire, England, UK) incorporates a new design that first heats a desflurane reservoir, creating a controlled supply of saturated vapor that is then blended with fresh gas to the desired concentration [42]. Sevoflurane's vapor pressure is compatible with conventional vaporizer technology. Sevoflurane, like halothane, is nonpungent [30] and is suitable for inhalation induction [31]. Desflurane, conversely, is the most pungent of all inhaled agents and is not recommended for inhalation induction, especially in children [32]. Sevoflurane breaks down in the presence of soda lime to compound A, a toxic byproduct, whereas desflurane is the most stable of all the inhaled agents [41,43]. (*Adapted from* Eger [44] and Stoelting [45].)

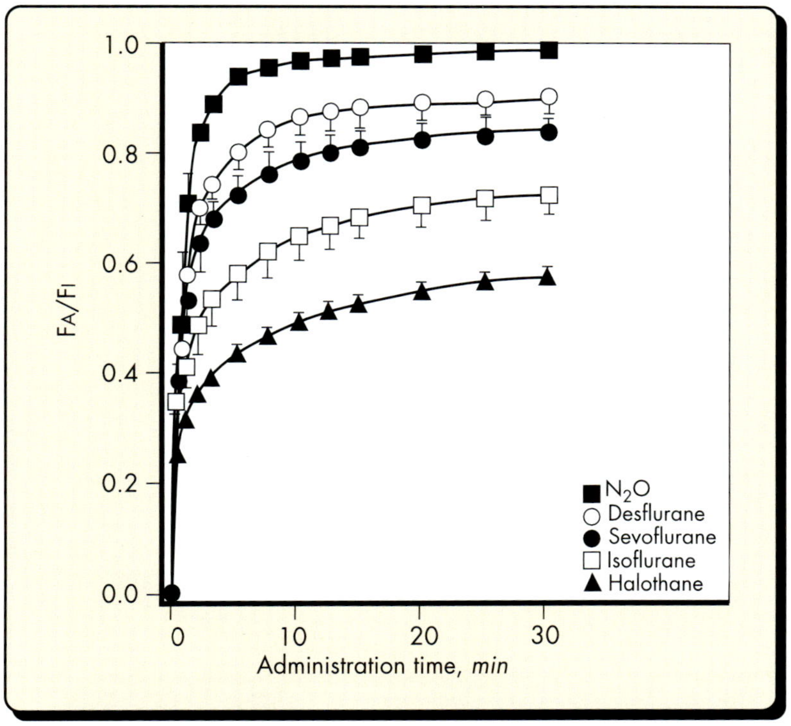

Figure 14-3. Anesthetic wash-in curves. The dynamic interaction between anesthetic uptake and delivery at the lung is described by plotting the rate of rise of the alveolar anesthetic concentration (F_A) toward a constant inspired concentration (F_I), against time. The resultant F_A/F_I curve is useful for comparing the pharmacokinetic behavior of various anesthetics. During the first moments of anesthetic induction alveolar ventilation rapidly increases the F_A. As induction proceeds the partial pressure of anesthetic in the lung increases, allowing for uptake of anesthetic by the blood and tissues. Anesthetic uptake retards the rate of rise of F_A toward F_I, producing the characteristic shape of the F_A/F_I curve. Less soluble anesthetics achieve partial pressure equilibrium between compartments more quickly; hence the rapid rise of F_A toward F_I and rapid induction. Clinically, overpressure can be utilized to compensate for the increased uptake of more soluble anesthetics to achieve rapid induction. Values are mean ± SD. (*Adapted from* Yashuda and coworkers [3].)

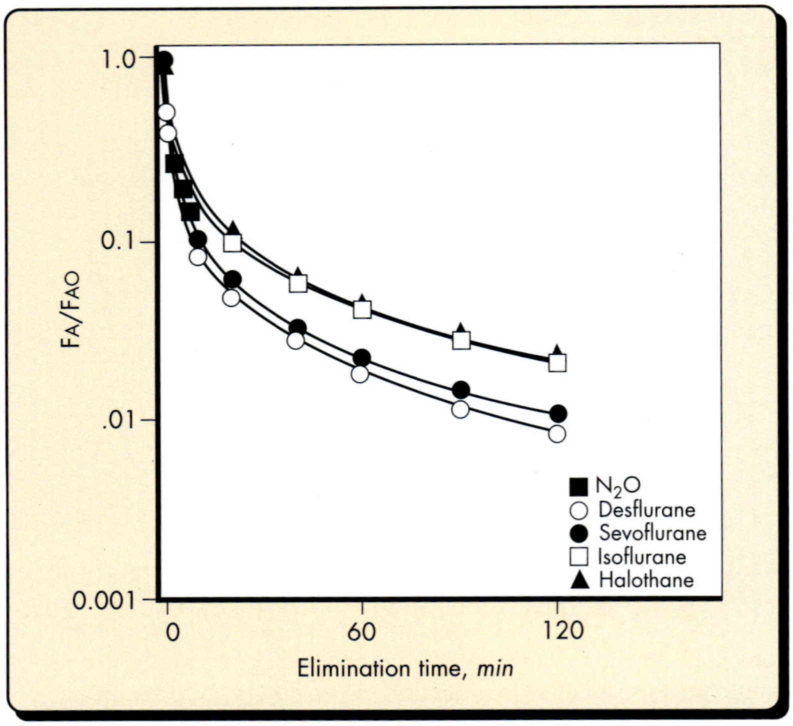

Figure 14-4. Anesthetic wash-out curves. The kinetics of anesthetic elimination are described by the F_A/F_{A0} curve, where F_A is the alveolar anesthetic concentration and F_{A0} is the alveolar anesthetic concentration of the last exhaled breath before the anesthetic is discontinued. These curves illustrate the rapid wash-out of desflurane and sevoflurane (owing to low blood solubility) and predict rapid emergence from anesthesia. Clinical studies suggest that patients awaken approximately twice as fast from equal MAC concentrations of desflurane [1] or sevoflurane [2] compared with isoflurane. Values are mean ± SD. (*Adapted from* Yashuda and coworkers [3].)

CARDIOVASCULAR EFFECTS

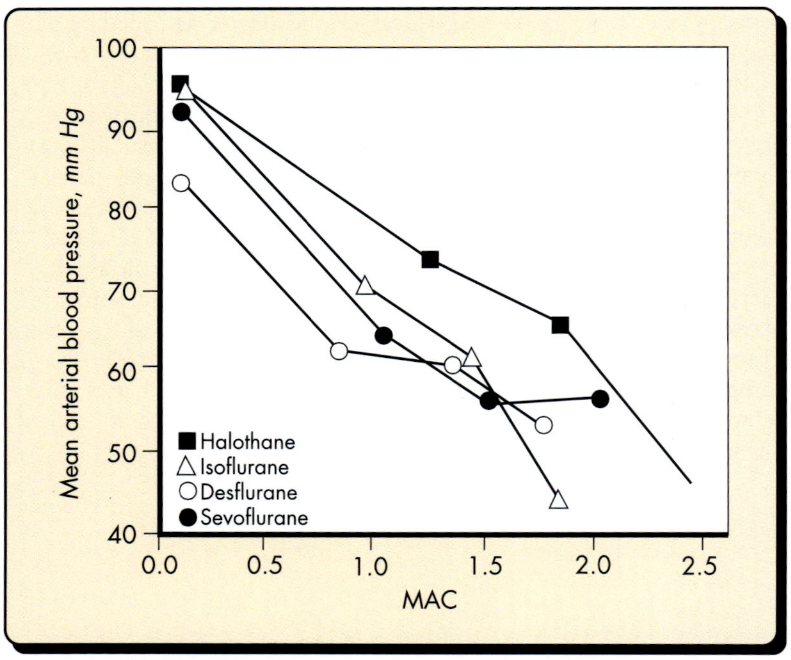

Figure 14-5. Relationship of mean arterial blood pressure to MAC for halothane, isoflurane, desflurane, and sevoflurane. The data in Figures 14-5 through 14-10 present the cardiovascular actions of inhaled anesthetics in young, healthy, human volunteer subjects. All volatile anesthetics decrease mean arterial blood pressure in a dose-dependent fashion, with halothane decreasing blood pressure the least at equal MAC concentrations [8–10,46]. (*Adapted from* Eger [44] and Malan and coworkers [10].)

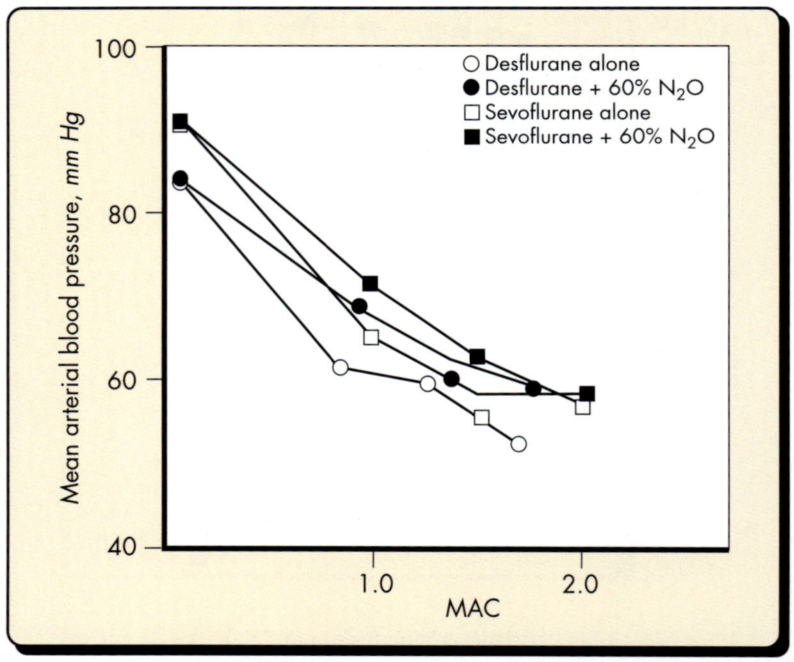

Figure 14-6. Relationship of mean arterial blood pressure to MAC for desflurane alone, deflurane + 60% nitrous oxide (N_2O), sevoflurane alone, and sevoflurane + 60% N_2O. Substituting a portion of the volatile anesthetic with an equal MAC proportion of N_2O attenuates the decrease in blood pressure caused by the volatile anesthetic alone [10,47]. This effect is most likely secondary to the mild sympathomimetic stimulation produced by N_2O, which tends to offset the cardiovascular depressant effect of the volatile agent alone [48]. Although N_2O administered alone or in combination with a volatile agent tends to support the circulation, administration of N_2O in the presence of opioids unmasks the direct cardiac depressant effect of N_2O and can produce profound circulatory depression [49]. (*Adapted from* Cahalan and coworkers [47], Weiskopf and coworkers [9], and Malan and coworkers [10].)

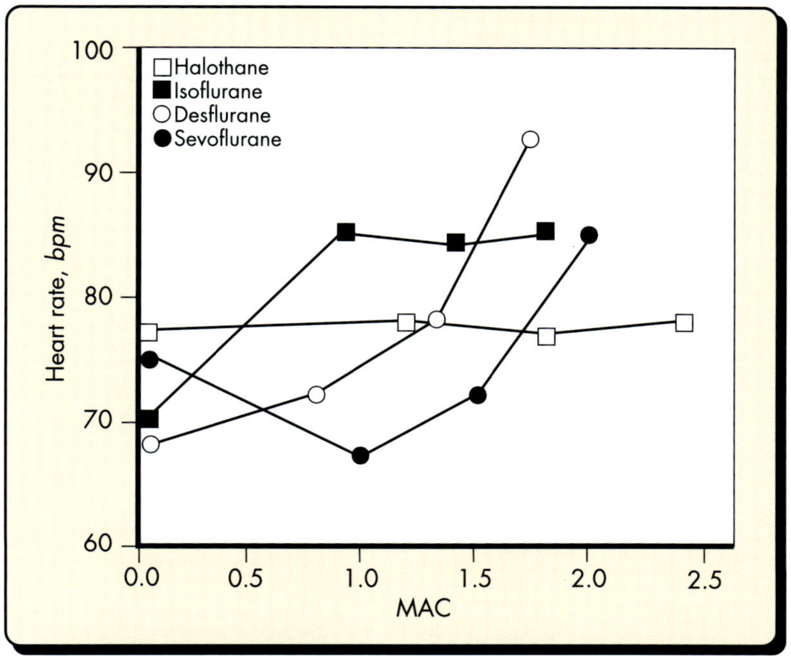

Figure 14-7. Relationship of heart rate to MAC for halothane, isoflurane, desflurane, and seroflurane. Desflurane and isoflurane both increase heart rate [8,9]. Desflurane increases heart rate only at higher concentrations, and then in a dose-dependent fashion. In contrast, isoflurane increases heart rate even at low concentrations, and this effect is not dose related. Sevoflurane [10], like halothane [46], does not increase heart rate (the increase at 2 MAC did not achieve statistical significance). (*Adapted from* Eger [44] and Malan and coworkers [10].)

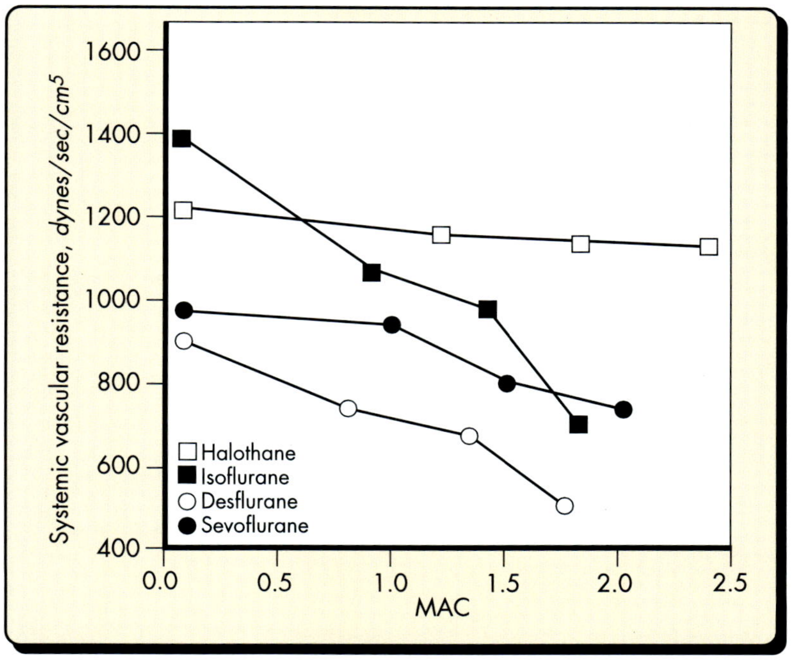

Figure 14-8. Relationship of systemic vascular resistance to MAC for halothane, isoflurane, desflurane, and sevoflurane. Isoflurane, desflurane, and sevoflurane each reduce systemic vascular resistance in a dose-dependent fashion [8–10]. Further, this is the primary mechanism for the decrease in mean arterial blood with these agents, as cardiac output is maintained. In contrast, systemic vascular resistance is unchanged by halothane, indicating that the decrease in blood pressure with this agent occurs in response to the decrease in cardiac output [46]. (*Adapted from* Eger [44] and Malan and coworkers [10].)

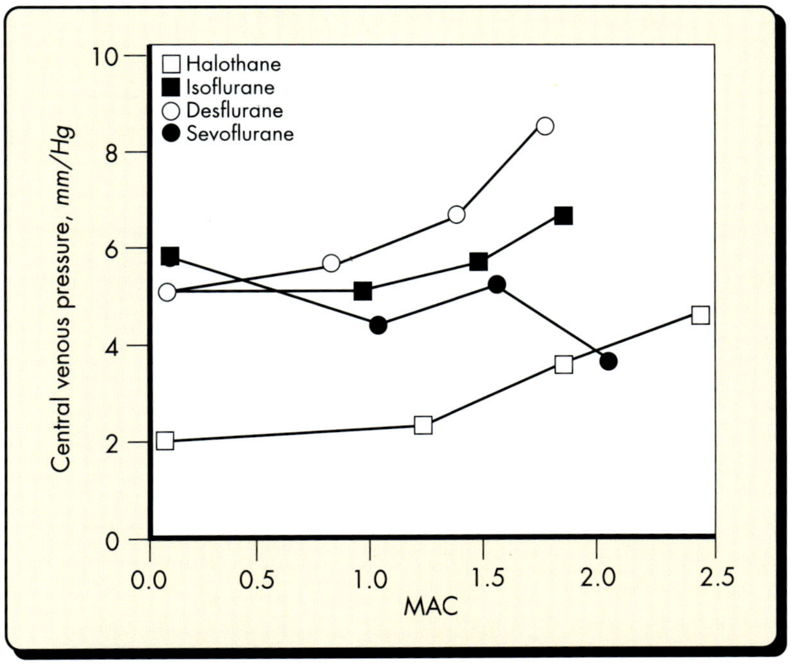

Figure 14-9. Relationship of central venous pressure to MAC for halothane, isoflurane, desflurane, and sevoflurane. Isoflurane, desflurane, and halothane [8,9,46] cause a dose-dependent increase in central venous pressure, whereas sevoflurane [10] does not. One possible explanation for this difference may be related to study protocol. In patients receiving sevoflurane, intravenous fluids were adjusted to maintain end-diastolic area constant, determined by transesophageal echocardiography. When fluids were administered to isoflurane patients in an identical fashion, central venous pressure was likewise unchanged [10]. (*Adapted from* Eger [44] and Malan and coworkers [10].)

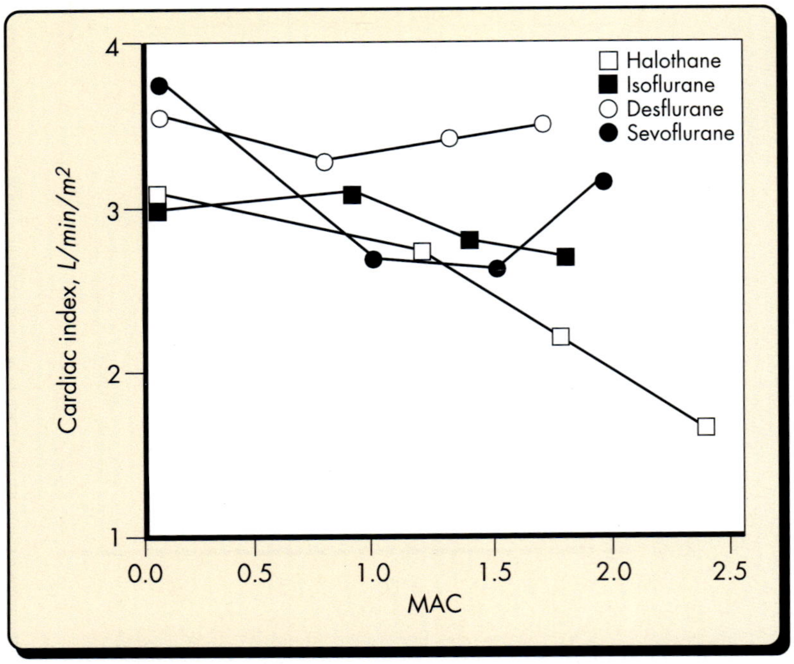

Figure 14-10. Relationship of cardiac index to MAC for halothane, isoflurane, desflurane, and sevoflurane. Desflurane and isoflurane [8,9] maintain cardiac output by a concomitant decrease in systemic vascular resistance. In contrast, halothane [46] causes a decrease in cardiac output whereas systemic vascular resistance is unchanged. At lower concentrations sevoflurane [10], like halothane, causes a modest decrease in cardiac output. At higher concentrations cardiac output returns to control values in response to a decrease in systemic vascular resistance, as occurs with isoflurane and desflurane. The combined hemodynamic effects of unchanged cardiac output associated with decreased systemic vascular resistance and increased or unchanged filling pressures indicate that desflurane and sevoflurane, like other volatile anesthetics, are myocardial depressants. (*Adapted from* Eger [44] and Malan and coworkers [10].)

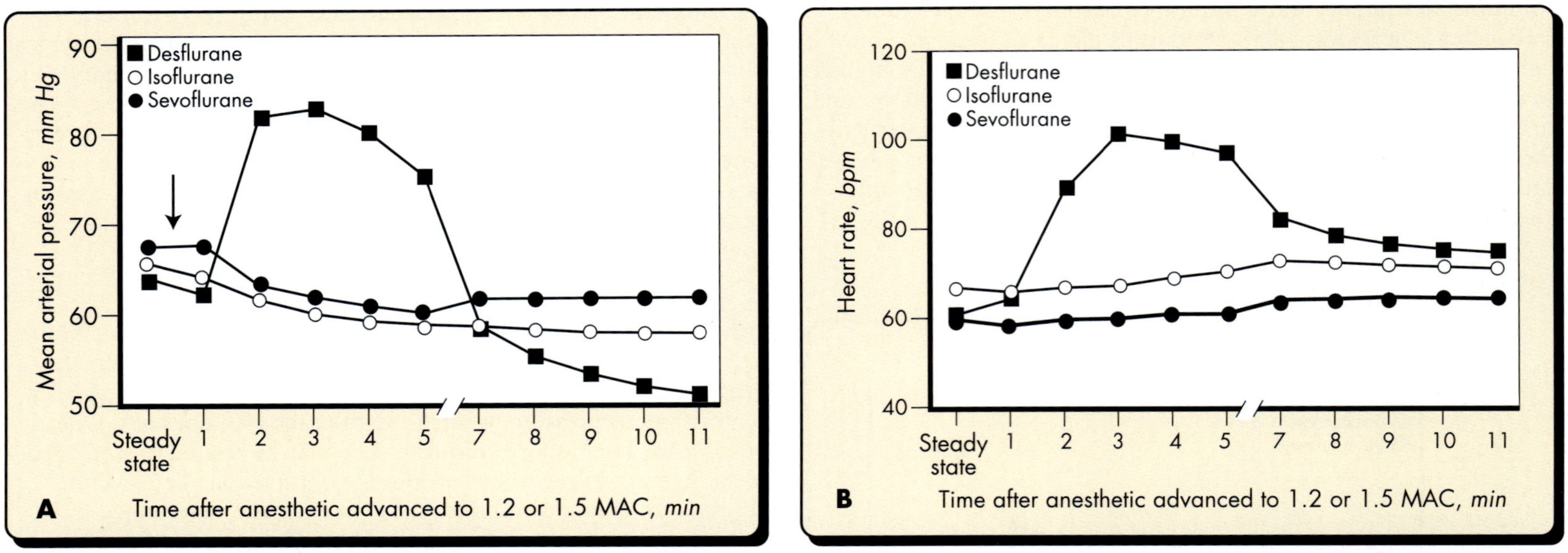

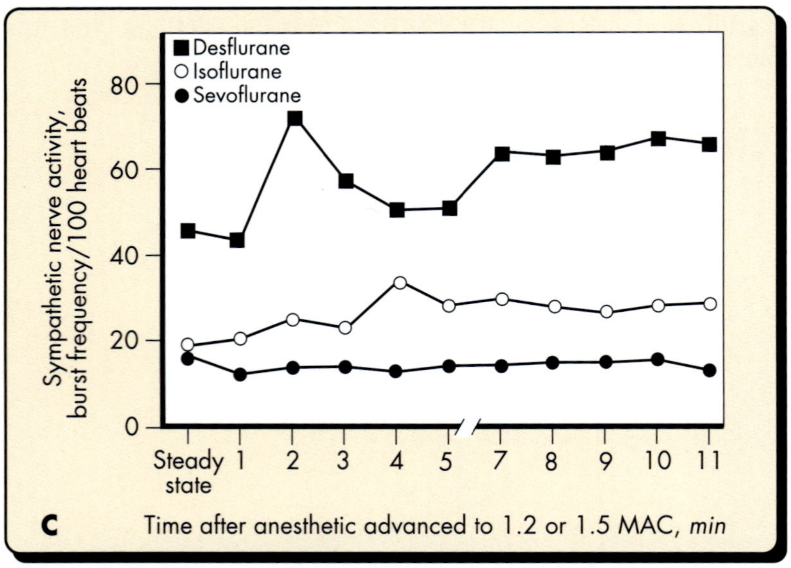

Figure 14-11. The sympathoexcitatory effect of desflurane. Ebert and Muzi [50] demonstrated in human volunteers that rapidly advancing the desflurane vaporizer from 1.0 to1.5 MAC (indicated in figure by *down arrow*) transiently activated the sympathetic nervous system, causing changes characterized by large increases in blood pressure (**A**), heart rate (**B**), and sympathetic nerve activity (**C**). Sympathetic activation was absent in the sevoflurane [12] and isoflurane [50] groups. Further characterization of this effect by others includes these findings: (1) the threshold concentration is 1 MAC [51]; (2) repeated increases in desflurane concentration attenuate the response [52]; (3) smaller increases (1% inspired concentration) are associated with a smaller response [51]; (4) a similar response occurs with isoflurane but to a much lesser degree [11]; and (5) sympathetic activation occurs in response to a direct effect of desflurane in a highly perfused tissue and to a lesser degree in response to stimulation of tracheopulmonary irritant receptors [53]. (*Adapted from* Ebert and coworkers [54].)

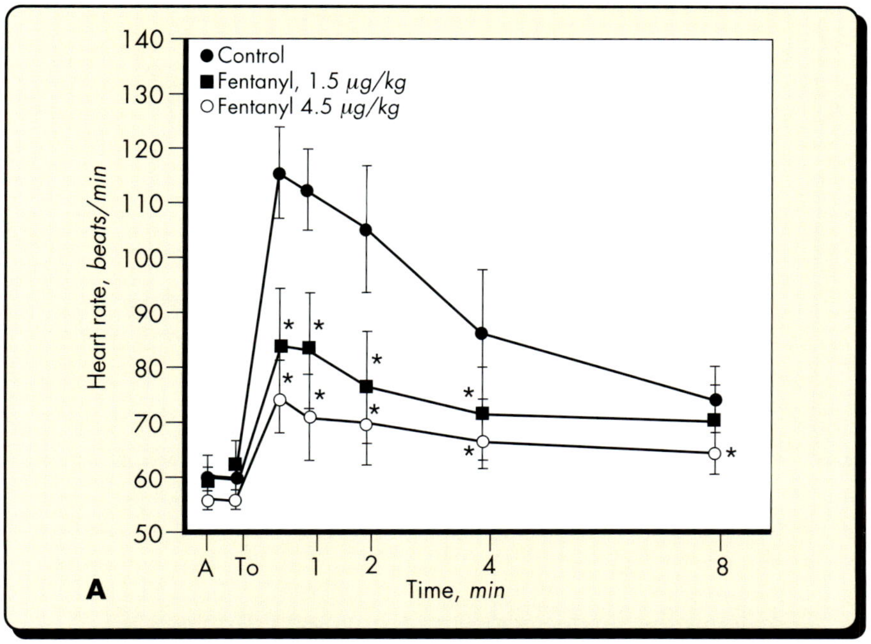

Figure 14-12. Sympathoexcitatory properties of desflurane attenuated by narcotics. Rapidly increasing the inspired concentration of desflurane from 0.55 to 1.1 MAC in human volunteers approximately doubled subjects' heart rate (**A**) and mean arterial blood pressure (**B**). Prior administration of fentanyl (1.5 or 4.5 μg/kg) attenuated the heart rate increases by 61% and 70%, respectively, and the blood pressure increases by 31% and 46%, respectively [55]. The sympathoexcitatory property of desflurane may be clinically significant in patients at risk for myocardial ischemia. Helman *et al.* [56] found that cardiac surgical patients in whom anesthesia was induced with thiopental and desflurane had an increased incidence of hemodynamic lability and myocardial ischemia compared with patients in whom thiopental and opioid were used [56]. Knowledge of the characteristics of desflurane sympathoexcitation and the use of anesthetic adjuvants when appropriate permit the safe administration of desflurane to include patients at risk for myocardial ischemia [57,58]. Values represent mean ± SE. *—$p<0.0.5$ between fentanyl and control value. (*Adapted from* Weiskopf and coworkers [55].)

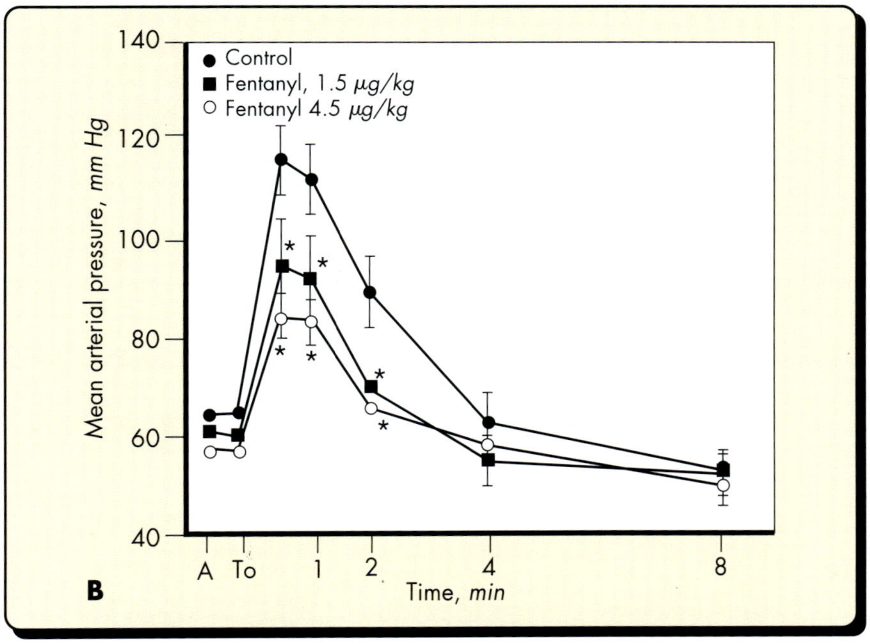

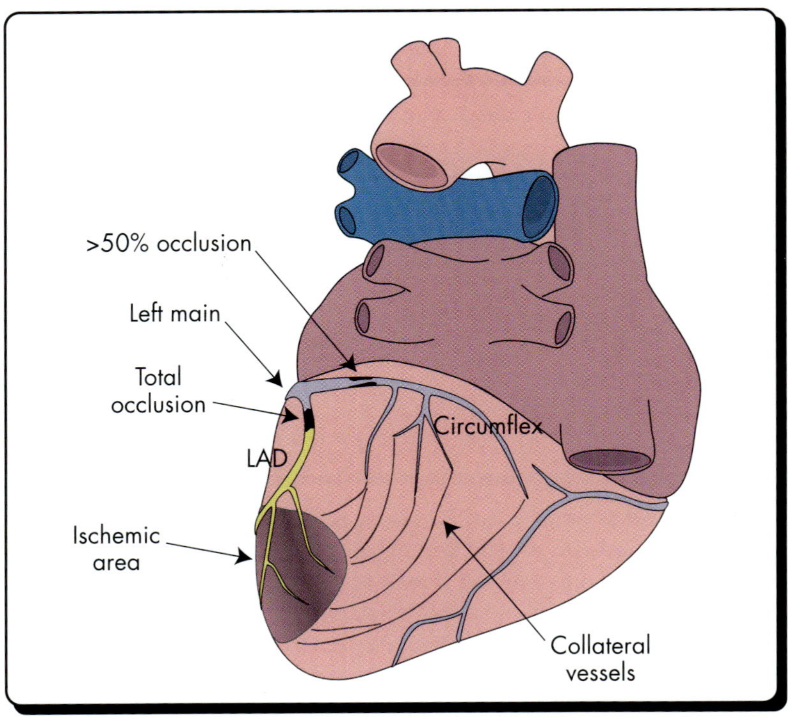

Figure 14-13. Coronary steal–prone anatomy. Coronary steal is defined as the redistribution of myocardial blood flow to nonischemic myocardium at the expense of decreasing collateral flow to ischemic myocardium. The anatomic conditions that predispose ischemic myocardium to intercoronary steal include total occlusion of a major coronary vessel with collateral flow into the ischemic bed distal to the occlusion [59]. Administration of a potent coronary arteriolar vasodilator, *eg*, dipyridamole, although augmenting flow to the nonischemic myocardium, reduces collateral perfusion pressure sufficiently to diminish flow in the already maximally dilated ischemic bed. Conditions for coronary steal are enhanced by a stenosis in the vessel supplying the collaterals [59]. Steal prone anatomy, as illustrated here, is present in approximately 23% of patients presenting for coronary artery bypass surgery [60]. LAD—left anterior descending coronary artery.

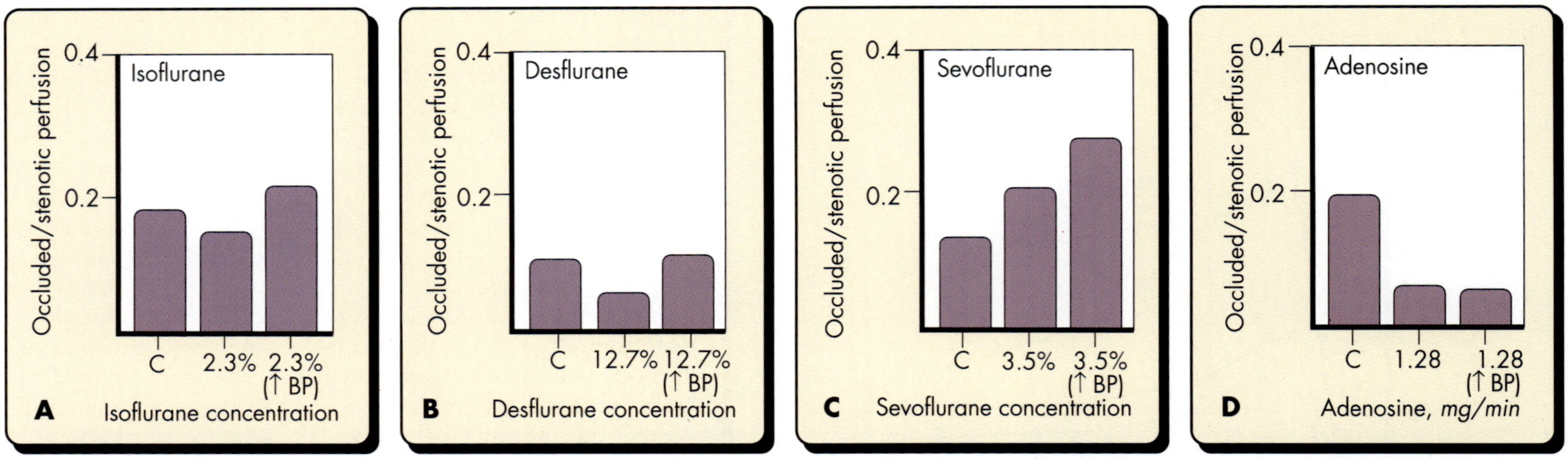

Figure 14-14. Studies addressing use of isoflurane and induction of coronary steal. Isoflurane has been suggested, but not proven, in both clinical [61] and experimental [62] studies to induce coronary steal. Desflurane and sevoflurane, in addition to isoflurane, are coronary vasodilators and therefore may have the potential to induce coronary steal. This question was addressed in separate studies from the same institution in a validated chronically instrumented dog model that reproduced the steal prone anatomy shown in Figure 14-13 [13,63,64]. **A**, **B**, and **C**, Ratio of transmural blood flow in the occluded ischemic zone (left anterior descending coronary artery or LAD region) to the nonischemic stenotic zone (circumflex region supplying collaterals) when the dogs were conscious (1st bar), anesthetized with inhaled agent (2nd bar), and anesthetized, but blood pressure (BP) returned to conscious control levels (3rd bar). Isoflurane and desflurane, but not sevoflurane, tended to redistributed blood flow away from the ischemic zone (LAD) when blood pressure was allowed to fall. Restoration of blood pressure normalized flow distribution, indicating that flow redistribution was secondary to hemodynamic changes rather than to coronary steal. Adenosine, a potent coronary dilator administered to awake control animals (**D**), redistributed blood flow away from the ischemic zone even when blood pressure was restored (coronary steal). These data suggest that isoflurane, desflurane, and sevoflurane are not potent enough coronary vasodilators to induce coronary steal in this validated model. C—conscious. (*Data from* Hartman and coworkers [63,64] and Kersten and coworkers [13].)

HEPATIC EFFECTS

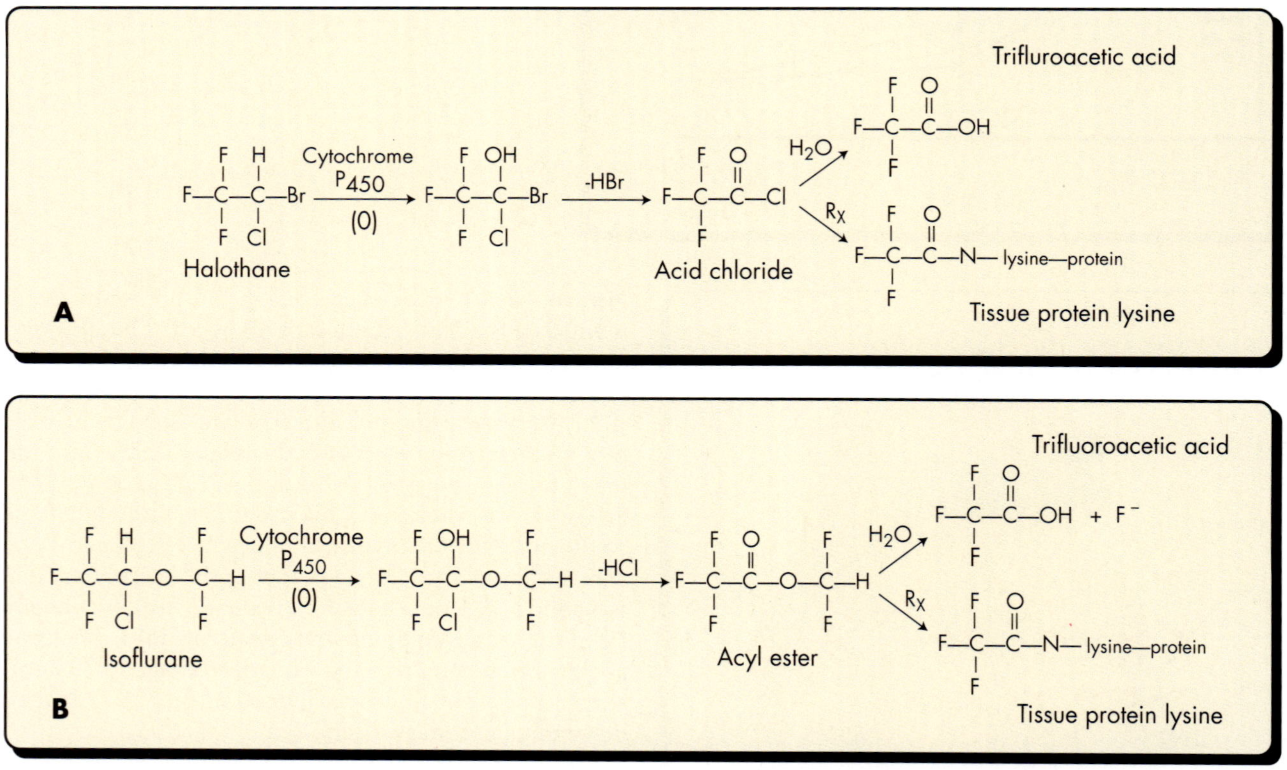

Figure 14-15. Biotransformation of halothane (**A**), isoflurane (**B**), and desflurane (**C**), producing metabolites capable of liver protein binding. Halothane, enflurane, isoflurane, and desflurane are each metabolized to reactive acyl halide intermediates by cytochrome P_{450}, localized to hepatocellular endoplasmic reticulum. The majority reacts with water and is excreted as urinary trifluoroacetic acid. A portion, however, can bind to hepatocellular protein and function as hapten, converting tissue protein from immunologic self to non-self (neoantigen) [65]. All patients exposed to halothane create neoantigen, but only a few are immunologically sensitized to generate IgG antibody [66].

(*Continued on next page*)

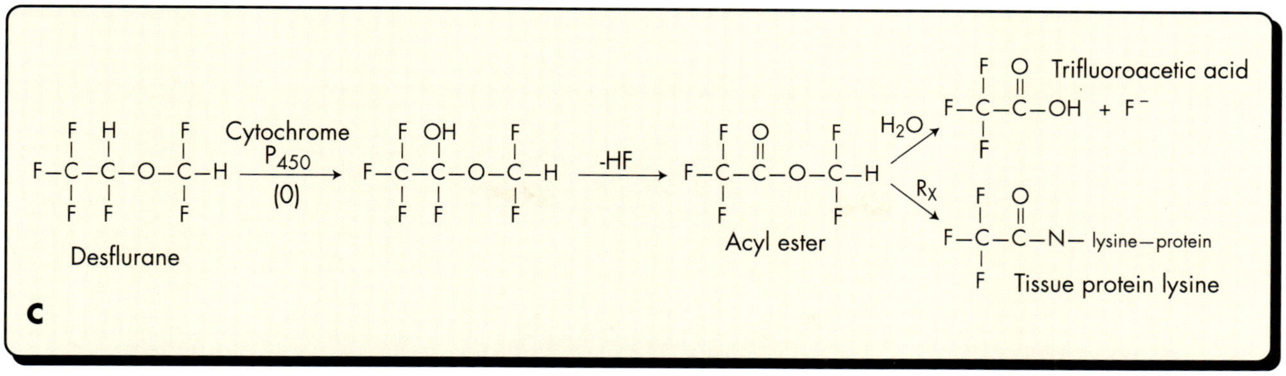

Figure 14-15. (*Continued*) Those patients (approximately 1 in 30,000), are at risk for immunologically mediated massive hepatic necrosis or halothane hepatitis upon subsequent exposure to halothane [66]. The common metabolic pathway for isoflurane, enflurane, and desflurane suggests a similar mechanism for the extremely rare unexplained hepatic failure following use of these anesthetics, although this has not been adequately resolved [67]. (*Adapted from* Frink [68].)

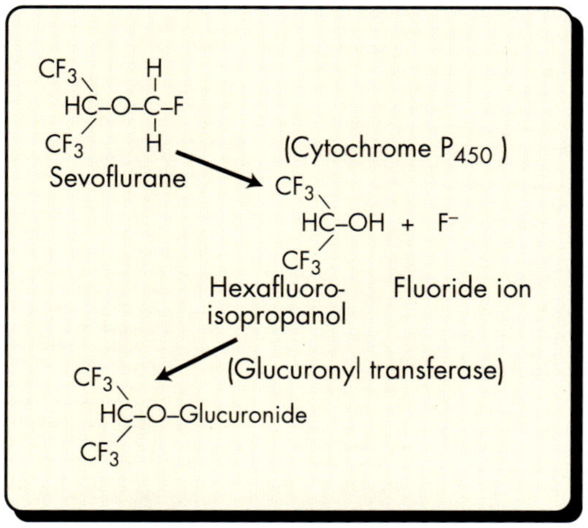

Figure 14-16. Characteristics of sevoflurane biotransformation. These characteristics suggest the potential for hepatic toxicity to be low. Reactive acyl halide intermediates are not formed by sevoflurane metabolism, rather it is biotransformed via cytochrome P_{450} to a unique compound, hexafluoroisopropanol (HFIP), which has low binding affinity for liver protein [15]. Sevoflurane is metabolized rapidly as HFIP appears in the blood only 5 minutes after the start of anesthesia. HFIP is rapidly glucuronidated (only 15% circulates unconjugated) and excreted as urinary metabolite [16]. Studies in human volunteers and patients have demonstrated no abnormalities in hepatic function associated with sevoflurane [26–28]. (*Adapted from* Frink [68].)

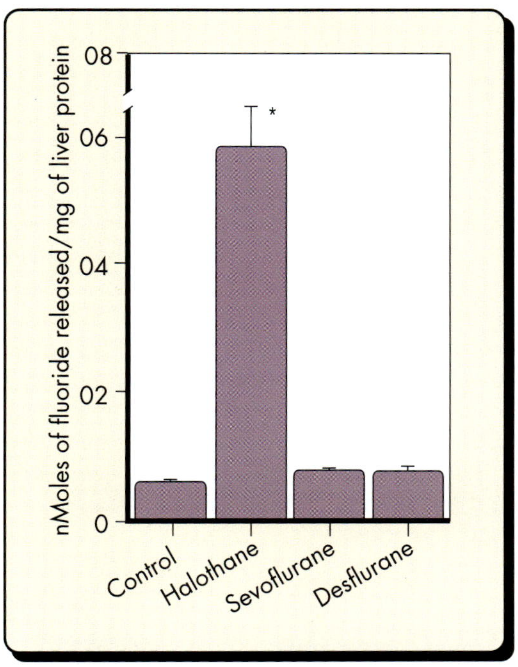

Figure 14-17. Amount of fluorine bound to hepatic protein after exposure to 1.5 MAC of sevoflurane, halothane, or desflurane in rats. Immune-mediated hepatic injury first requires the covalent binding of anesthetic reactive intermediates to hepatic protein to form neoantigen. Green *et al.* [15] measured the hepatic protein binding of organic fluoride metabolites in rats exposed to these three agents. Only the halothane group exhibited significant binding. The minimal extent of desflurane biotransformation and low affinity of hexafluoroisopropanol (sevoflurane metabolite) for liver protein suggest that the potential for immune-mediated hepatic injury is remote for these two anesthetics. (*Adapted from* Frink [68].)

DOSE-DEPENDENT INORGANIC FLUORIDE NEPHROTOXICITY

Peak Serum F⁻, *μM/L*	Laboratory Abnormalities	Clinical Symptoms
< 40	None	None
50–80	Mild urine concentrating deficit	None
90–120	Moderate urine concentrating deficit Low urine osmolality Hypernatremia Serum hyperosmolarity	Mild polyuria
> 120	Severe above abnormalities plus Increased BUN Increased creatinine	High-output renal failure

Figure 14-18. Dose-dependent inorganic fluroide nephrotoxicity. The classic study by Cousins and Mazze [18] described the dose-dependent effects of inorganic fluoride nephrotoxicity in patients anesthetized with methoxyflurane, where the threshold concentration for either laboratory or clinical evidence of fluoride nephropathy was 50 μM. Plasma fluoride concentrations can approach or exceed this threshold following short- to moderate-duration sevoflurane anesthesia (see Fig. 14-21), but without evidence of renal injury [23–28]. Several factors may account for the apparent greater nephrotoxic potential of methoxyflurane, including higher rate of metabolism (see Fig.14-19), greater total extent of metabolism (see Fig. 14-20), and greater intrarenal metabolism (see Fig. 14-23). Further, patients anesthetized with methoxyflurane did not develop clinically significant changes in renal function until fluoride concentrations exceeded 80 μM, which is infrequent with sevoflurane, even after prolonged duration of anesthesia [17,69]. BUN—blood urea nitrogen level. (*Data from* Cousins and Mazze [18].)

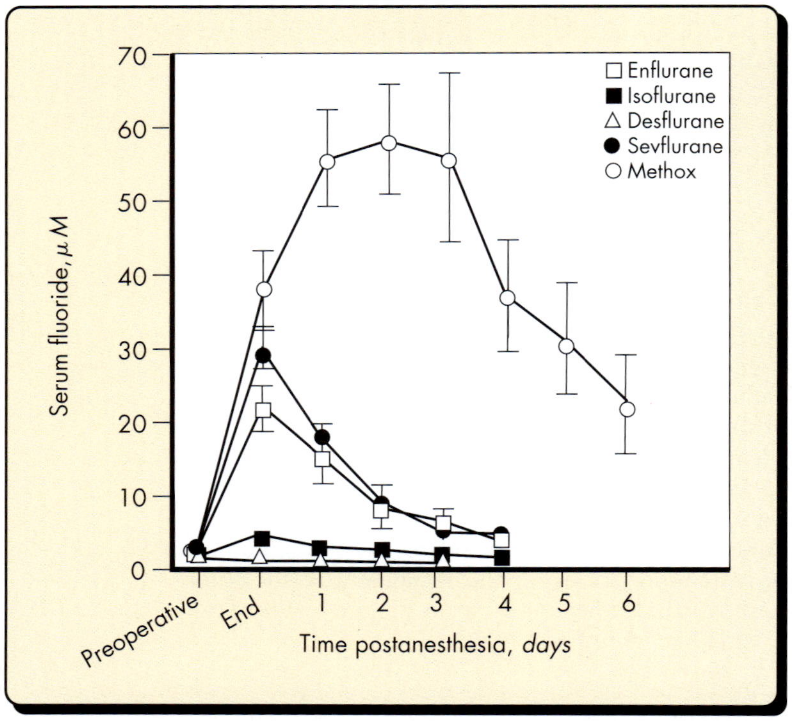

Figure 14-19. Plasma inorganic fluoride concentrations before and after 3 hours of anesthesia (mean ± SE). Extensive biotransformation of methoxyflurane is associated with inorganic fluoride levels that far exceed those of other anesthetics and remain elevated for several days owing to high tissue solubility and continued metabolism. Peak plasma fluoride concentrations with sevoflurane are approximately 1.5 to 2 times greater than those after enflurane administration, but they diminish rapidly, consistent with the rapid pulmonary elimination of sevoflurane [23,24]. The minimal biotransformation of isoflurane and desflurane eliminates concerns about nephrotoxicity for these anesthetics [14,70]. (*Adapted from* Kharasch [71].)

EXTENT OF ANESTHETIC METABOLISM

Agent	% Metabolized
Methoxyflurane	75
Halothane	46
Enflurane	8.5
Sevoflurane	4.9
Isoflurane	0.2
Desflurane	0.02

Figure 14-20. Extent of anesthetic metabolism. Plasma inorganic fluoride concentration is influenced by both the rate and total extent of anesthetic metabolism. For example, the rate of sevoflurane metabolism is approximately twice that of enflurane [23,24], reflected by a peak plasma fluoride concentration that is 1.5 to 2 times greater for sevoflurane (see Fig. 14-19). In contrast, the total extent of sevoflurane metabolism is only half that of enflurane owing to lower blood solubility and rapid pulmonary elimination. This difference may account in part for the apparent safety of sevoflurane despite peak plasma fluoride concentrations that sometimes exceed 50 μM. (*Data from* Sutton and coworkers [14], Kharasch and coworkers [16], Holaday and coworkers [70], and Carpenter and coworkers [72].)

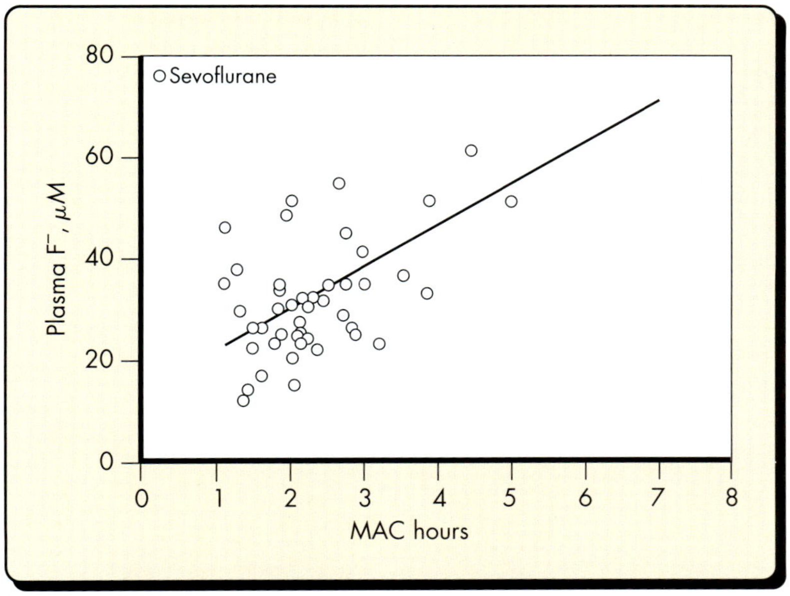

Figure 14-21. Data from Frink *et al.* [27] illustrating the positive correlation between peak plasma inorganic fluoride concentration and MAC-hours of anesthesia in patients anesthetized with sevoflurane. The mean peak fluoride concentration was 29 μM; however, there is considerable variability between patients. In general, these data suggest that after 1.5 to 4 MAC-hours of anesthesia, plasma fluoride is in the 20- to 40-μM range and rarely exceeds 50 μM. In all patients, postoperative renal function was normal by routine serum and urine laboratory tests. $r = 0.65$; $p < 0.01$.(*Adapted from* Frink and coworkers [27].)

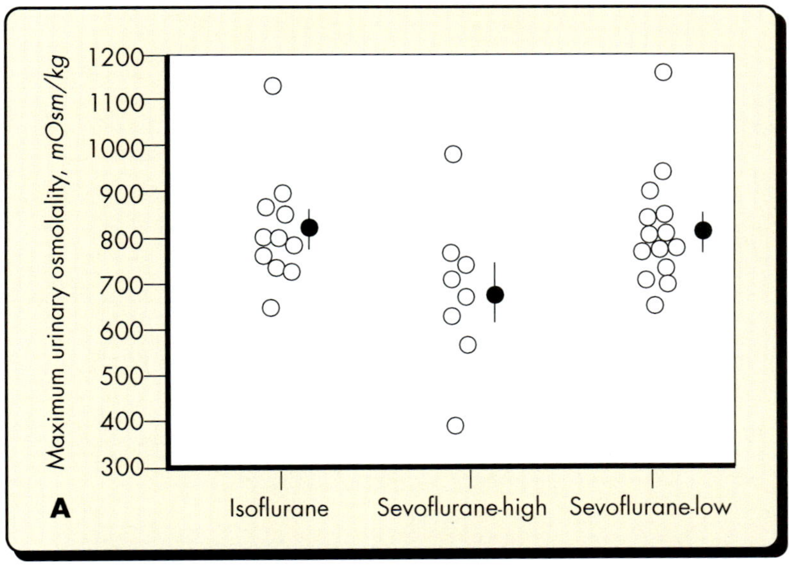

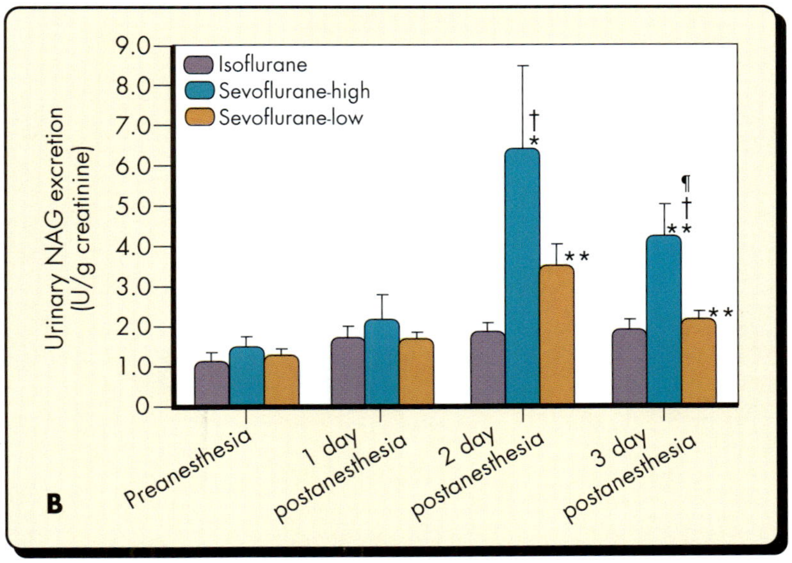

Figure 14-22. Effect of sevoflurane versus isoflurane on renal function. Higuchi *et al.* [17] utilized vasopressin testing (**A**) and urinary N-acetyl-beta-glucosamidase (NAG) excretion (**B**), a sensitive index of renal tubular damage, to detect subclinical renal damage in patients undergoing prolonged isoflurane or sevoflurane anesthesia. For data analysis the sevoflurane group was segregated into patients with peak fluoride concentrations greater than 50 μM (sevoflurane-high; mean MAC hours, 14.0) or less than (sevoflurane-low; mean MAC, hours 9.9) 50 μM. Urinary NAG excretion was increased above isoflurane controls only in the sevoflurane-high group. Maximum urinary osmolality tended to be lower in the sevoflurane-high group but the difference was not statistically significant ($P < 0.068$). These results suggest that prolonged sevoflurane anesthesia with peak plasma fluoride concentrations greater than 50 μM may cause mild subclinical renal damage. Based on these results in healthy patients, studies are warranted in patients with preexisting renal disease, who may be more susceptible to fluoride nephrotoxicity [29]. Values represent mean ± SE. * —P < 0.05; **—p < 0.01 compared with preoperatiave value; daggar—p < 0.05 compared with isoflurane group; paragraph symbol—p < 0.05 compared with sevoflurane-low group. (Adapted from Higuchi and coworkers [17].)

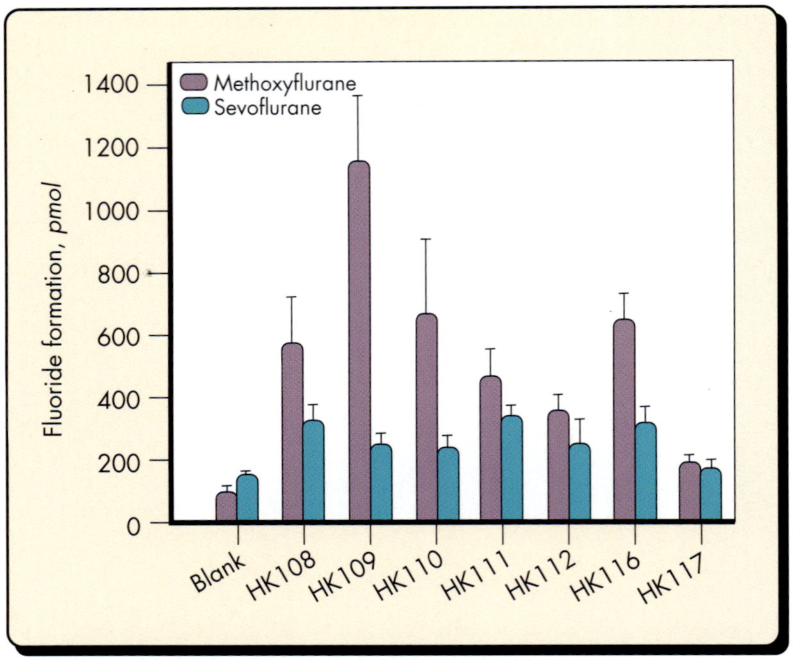

Figure 14-23. Comparative renal microsomal methoxyflurane (*open*) and sevoflurane (*solid*) defluorination (mean ± SD). Because cytochrome P_{450} is present in the kidney, Kharash *et al.* [73] reasoned that greater intrarenal biotransformation of methoxyflurane, compared with other volatile agents, may account in part for the greater apparent nephrotoxic potential of methoxyflurane. Indeed, human kidney microsomes incubated with methoxyflurane generate 3 to 10 times the amount of inorganic fluoride as sevoflurane (Renal microsomes obtained from human cadaveric, HK 110, 111, or donor HK 108, 108, 112, 116, 117 kidneys) [73]. Consistent with these results, cytochrome P_{450} 2E1, the isoform predominantly responsible for sevoflurane metabolism, is minimally present in the kidney [74]. (*Adapted from* Kharasch and coworkers [73].)

COMPARISON OF SEVOFLURANE AND METHOXYFLURANE METABOLISM

	Sevoflurane	Methoxyflurane
Peak inorganic fluoride, *μM*	> 50	> 50
Duration of fluoride increase	< 12 h	2–3 d
Extent of metabolism, %	2–5	75
Systemic elimination	Rapid pulmonary elimination; decreases amount available for metabolism	High tissue solubility; increases amount available for metabolism
Metabolizing enzymes	P_{450}2E1, ?P_{450} 2A6	P_{450} 2E1, P_{450} 2A6, P_{450} 2B6, P_{450} 3A4
Site of metabolism	Liver; kidney (minimal)	Liver (2–3 times greater than sevoflurane); kidney (4 times greater than sevoflurane)

Figure 14-24. Comparison of sevoflurane and methoxyflurane metabolism. Biotransformation of methoxyflurane, and to a lesser degree sevoflurane, can increase inorganic fluoride concentrations above 50 μM. Rapid pulmonary elimination of sevoflurane at the end of anesthesia decreases the residual amount of anesthetic available for metabolism, reflected by the rapid decline in fluoride concentration. In contrast, the area under the fluoride time-concentration curve is much greater for methoxyflurane due to greater tissue solubility and extent of metabolism (see Figs. 14-19 and 14-20). Cytochrome P_{450} 2E1, the predominant isoform metabolizing sevoflurane, is minimally present in the kidney, limiting the amount of intrarenally generated fluoride compared with that generated with methoxyflurane [73,74]. These factors may account in part for the apparent safety of sevoflurane despite fluoride concentrations considered potentially nephrotoxic. (*Adapted from* Kharasch [71].)

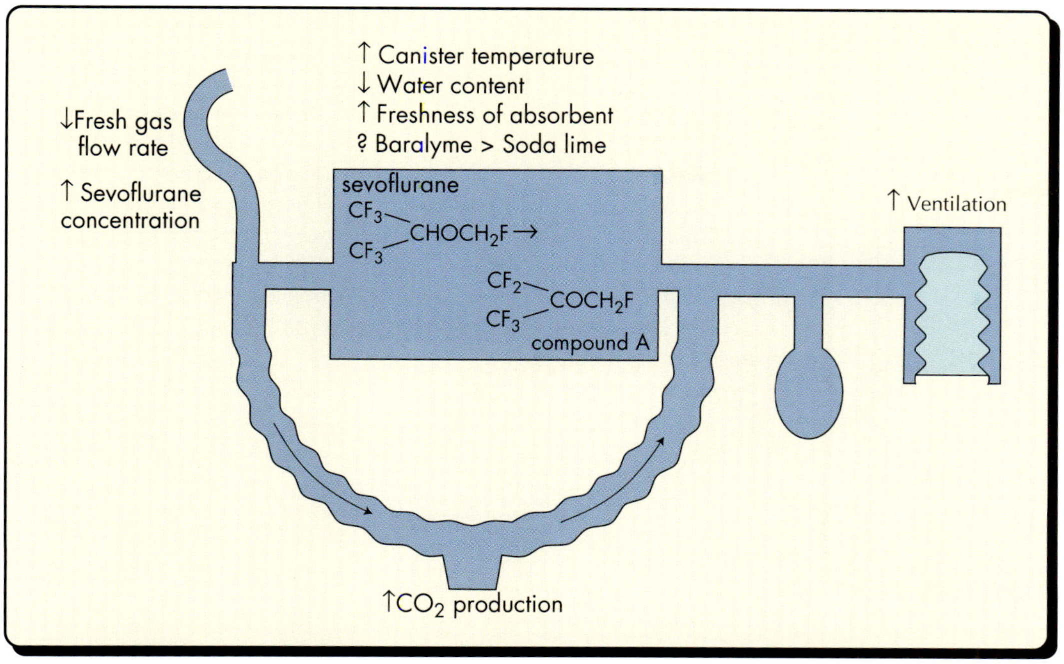

Figure 14-25. Factors increasing sevoflurane degradation in anesthesia circuit. Sevoflurane degrades in the presence of base to compound A, a toxic byproduct [41]. Temperature is a major determinant of compound A production [41,69,75–77]. The conversion of CO_2 to carbonate is exothermic; thus, conditions that increase CO_2 absorption accelerate compound A production. Those factors include increased CO_2 production by the patient [77], increased ventilation [77], fresh absorbent [76], and low fresh gas flow rates, which, in addition, allow compound A to accumulate within the circuit [75,77]. Compound A formation is decreased by moist absorbent, therefore, accumulation of water and partial exhaustion of absorbent over time may serve to limit compound A production as anesthesia progresses [76]. Baralyme (Allied Healthcare Products, Inc., St. Louis, MO) may generate more compound A than soda lime [75,76]. Finally, there is a positive correlation between sevoflurane concentration in the circuit and compound A formation [69].

COMPOUND A TOXICITY IN RATS

Exposure, *h*	Toxic threshold, *ppm*	LC_{50}, *ppm*
1	150–200	1090
3	50	331
6	50	203
12	25	127

Figure 14-26. Compound A toxicity in rats. Toxicity of compound A in rats is associated with renal corticomedullary necrosis [19–22]. Toxic threshold was defined as damage to at least 1% of corticomedullary nephrons on pathologic examination. As compound A approached the LC_{50} (concentration of anesthetic lethal in 50% of animals), injury extended into the cortex and medulla. The concentrations of compound A achieved in long-duration, low-flow, or closed-circuit anesthesia in humans can approach or exceed the toxic threshold in rats, but without significant changes in renal function [69]. The clinical implications of these data are unclear because the relative sensitivity to compound A between the rat and human kidney is unknown. Further, indices of renal function were not measured or correlated with histopathologic changes. (*Data from* Morio and coworkers [19], Kandel and coworkers [20], and Gonsowski and coworkers [21,22].)

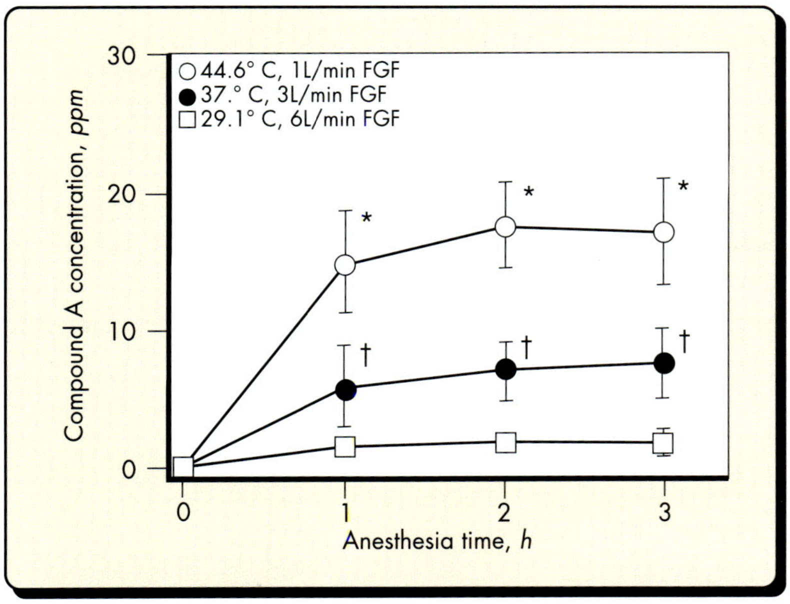

Figure 14-27. The inverse relationship between fresh gas flow (FGF) rate and compound A concentration in patients anesthetized with approximately 1 MAC of sevoflurane [78]. Mean peak compound A concentrations were 19.7 (14 to 27) ppm, 8.1 (4.6 to 12) ppm, and 2.1 (1.1 to 3.9) ppm for 1, 3, and 6 L/min fresh gas flow rates, respectively. Corresponding mean peak CO_2 absorbent temperatures were 44.6°C, 37.0°C, and 29.1°C, respectively. Increasing the fresh gas flow rate reduces compound A concentration by reducing CO_2 absorption and heat generated by exothermic conversion of CO_2 to carbonate and venting of excess gases preventing the accumulation of byproducts. (*Adapted from* Bito and Ikeda [78].)

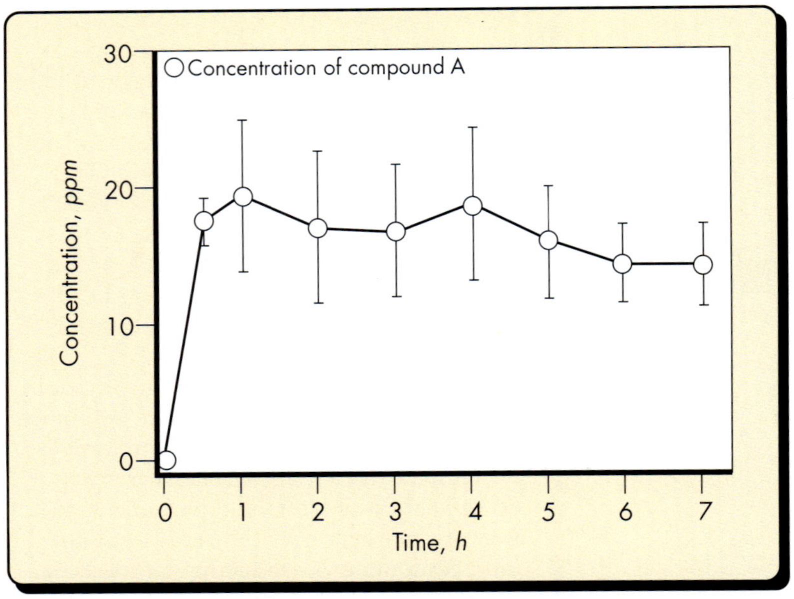

Figure 14-28. Concentration of breakdown products in the anesthesia circuit. Closed-circuit anesthesia should maximize the conditions for compound A formation and accumulation. In patients anesthetized with 1 MAC of sevoflurane utilizing a closed circuit and soda lime, compound A concentrations (mean ± SD) peaked at 1 to 2 hours (mean, 20 ppm; range, 14 to 30 ppm), remained constant until 5 hours, and fell slightly thereafter. These concentrations are approximately half the toxic threshold and 1/10 the LC_{50} (anesthetic concentration lethal in 50% of exposed animals) in rats for a similar 6-hour exposure (see Fig. 14-26). Nevertheless, no patient showed clinical or laboratory evidence of hepatorenal toxicity [28]. (*Adapted from* Bito and Ikeda [28].)

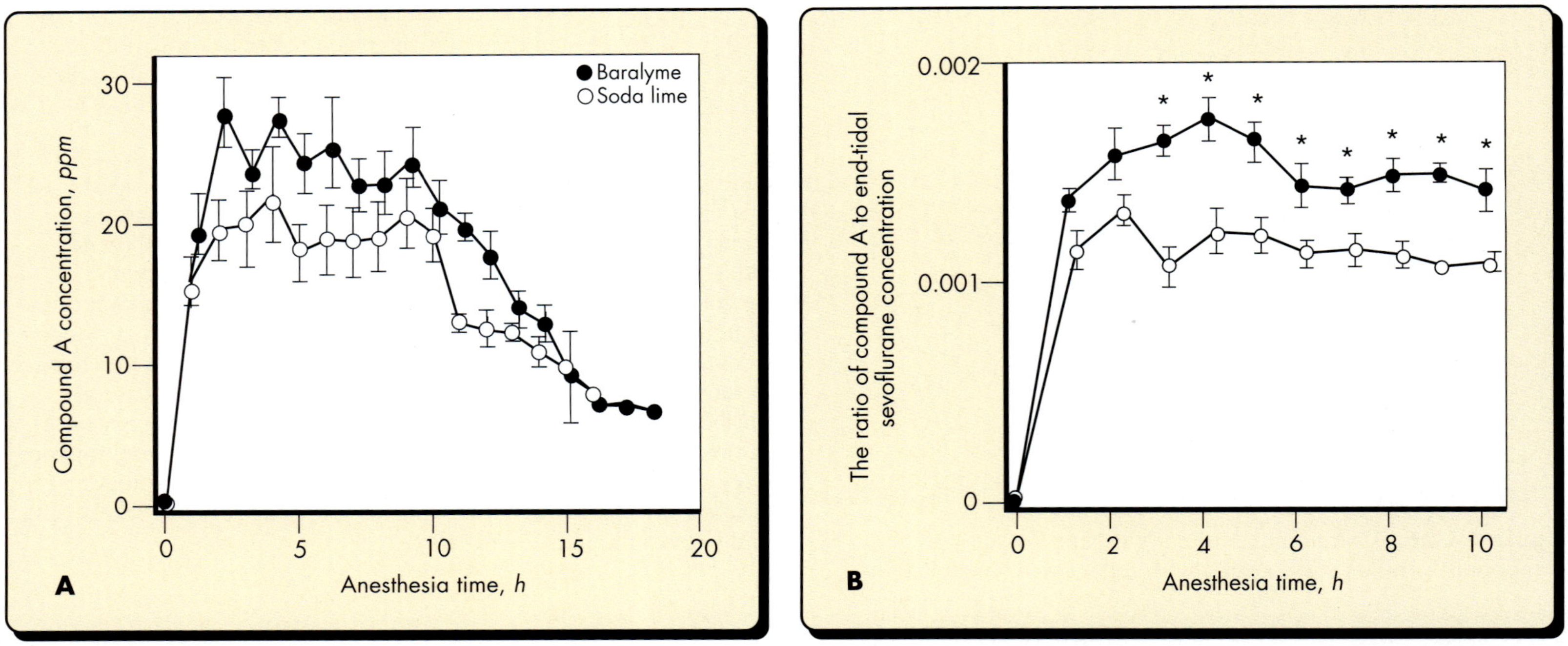

Figure 14-29. Compound A concentrations during long-duration, low-flow, sevoflurane anesthesia with either Baralyme (Allied Healthcare Products, Inc., St. Louis, MO) or soda lime absorbent. The mean peak compound A concentration between Baralyme and soda lime was not statistically different (**A**). However, the ratio of compound A to end-tidal sevoflurane concentration (**B**) was 1.5 to 2 times greater in the Baralyme group ($P < 0.05$), suggesting a moderate increase in sevoflurane degradation by Baralyme over soda lime [79]. Values are mean ± SE. *$P < 0.05$. (Adapted from Bito and Ikeda [79].)

REFERENCES

1. Smiley R, Ornstein E, Mateo R, *et al.*: Desflurane and isoflurane in surgical patients: Comparison of emergence time. *Anesthesiology* 1991, 74:425–428.
2. Frink EJ Jr, Malan TP Jr, Atlas M, *et al.*: Clinical comparison of sevoflurane and isoflurane in healthy patients. *Anesth Analg* 1992, 74:241–245.
3. Yashuda N, Lockhart SH, Eger EI II, *et al.*: Comparison of kinetics of sevoflurane and isoflurane in humans. *Anesth Analg* 1991, 72:316–324.
4. Brown B, Jr.: Sevoflurane: introduction and overview. *Anesth Analg* 1995, 81(suppl):S1–S3.
5. Tinker JH: Desflurane: first new volatile anesthetic in almost 20 years. *Anesth Analg* 1992, 75(suppl):S1–S2.
6. Eger EI II: New inhaled anesthetics. *Anesthesiology* 1994, 80:906–922.
7. Lerman J, Sikich N, Kleinman S, Yentis S: The pharmacology of sevoflurane in infants and children. *Anesthesiology* 1994, 80:814–824.
8. Stevens WC, Cromwell TH, Halsey MJ, *et al.*: The cardiovascular effects of a new inhalation anesthetic, Forane, in human volunteers at constant arterial carbon dioxide tension. *Anesthesiology* 1971, 35:8–16.
9. Weiskopf RB, Cahalan MK, Eger EI II, *et al.*: Cardiovascular actions of desflurane in normocarbic volunteers. *Anesth Analg* 1991, 73:143–156.
10. Malan TP Jr, DiNardo JA, Isner RJ, *et al.*: Cardiovascular effects of sevoflurane compared with those of isoflurane in volunteers. *Anesthesiology* 1995, 83:918–928.
11. Weiskopf RB, Moore MA, Eger EI II, *et al.*: Rapid increase in desflurane concentration is associated with greater transient cardiovascular stimulation than with rapid increase in isoflurane concentration in humans. *Anesthesiology* 1994, 80:1035–1045.

12. Ebert TJ, Muzi M, Lopatka CW: Neurocirculatory responses to sevoflurane in humans: a comparison to desflurane. *Anesthesiology* 1995, 83:88–95.
13. Kersten JR, Brayer AP, Pagel PS, *et al.*: Perfusion of ischemic myocardium during anesthesia with sevoflurane. *Anesthesiology* 1994, 81:995–1004.
14. Sutton TS, Koblin DD, Gruenke LD, *et al.*: Fluoride metabolites after prolonged exposure of volunteers and patients to desflurane. *Anesth Analg* 1991, 73:180–185.
15. Green WB Jr, Eckerson ML, Depa R, Brown BR Jr: Covalent binding of oxidative metabolites to hepatic protein not detectable after exposure to sevoflurane or desflurane [abstract]. *Anesthesiology* 1994, 81:A437.
16. Kharasch ED, Karol MD, Lanni C, Sawchuk R: Clinical sevoflurane metabolism and disposition: I. Sevoflurane and metabolite pharmacokinetics. *Anesthesiology* 1995, 82:1369–1378.
17. Higuchi H, Sumikura H, Sumita S, *et al.*: Renal function in patients with high serum fluoride concentrations after prolonged sevoflurane anesthesia. *Anesthesiology* 1995, 83:449–458.
18. Cousins MJ, Mazze RI: Methoxyflurane nephrotoxicity: A study of dose response in man. *JAMA* 1973, 225:1611–1616.
19. Morio M, Fujii K, Satoh N, *et al.*: Reaction of sevoflurane and its degradation products with soda lime. *Anesthesiology* 1992, 77:1155–1164.
20. Kandel L, Laster MJ, Eger EI II, *et al.*: Nephrotoxicity in rats undergoing a one-hour exposure to compound A. *Anesth Analg* 1995, 81:559–563.
21. Gonsowski CT, Laster MJ, Eger EI II, *et al.*: Toxicity of compound A in rats: Effect of a 3-hour administration. *Anesthesiology* 1994, 80:556–565.
22. Gonsowski CT, Laster MJ, Eger EI II, *et al.*: Toxicity of compound A in rats: Effect of increasing duration of administration. *Anesthesiology* 1994, 80:566–573.
23. Cozen PF, Nuscheler M, Melotte A, *et al.*: Renal function and serum fluoride concentrations in patients with stable renal insufficiency after anesthesia with sevoflurane or enflurane. *Anesth Analg* 1995, 81:569–575.
24. Frink EJ Jr, Malan TP Jr, Isner RJ, *et al.*: Renal concentrating function with prolonged sevoflurane or enflurane anesthesia in volunteers. *Anesthesiology* 1994, 80:1019–1025.
25. Higuchi H, Sumikura H, Satoh T, Kanno M: Urine concentrating ability after prolonged sevoflurane anesthesia. *Br J Anaesth* 1994, 73:239–240.
26. Bito H, Ikeda K: Renal and hepatic function in surgical patients after low-flow sevoflurane or isoflurane anesthesia. *Anesth Analg* 1996, 82:173–176.
27. Frink EJ Jr, Ghantous H, Malan TP Jr, *et al.*: Plasma inorganic fluoride with sevoflurane anesthesia: Correlation with indices of hepatic and renal function. *Anesth Analg* 1992, 74:231–235.
28. Bito H, Ikeda K: Closed-circuit anesthesia with sevoflurane in humans: effects on renal and hepatic function and concentrations of breakdown products with soda lime in the circuit. *Anesthesiology* 1994, 80:71–76.
29. Mazze RI, Jamison R: Renal effects of sevoflurane. *Anesthesiology* 1995, 83:443–445.
30. Doi M, Ikeda K: Airway irritation produced by volatile anaesthetics during brief inhalation: Comparison of halothane, enflurane, isoflurane, and sevoflurane. *Can J Anaesth* 1993, 40:122–126.
31. Naito Y, Tamai S, Shingu K, *et al.*: Comparison between sevoflurane and halothane for paediatric ambulatory anaesthesia. *Br J Anaesth* 1991, 67:387–389.
32. Zwass MS, Fisher DM, Welborn LG, *et al.*: Induction and maintenance characteristics of anesthesia with desflurane and nitrous oxide in infants and children. *Anesthesiology* 1992, 76:373–378.
33. Lockhart S, Rampil I, Yashuda N, *et al.*: Depression of ventilation by desflurane in humans. *Anesthesiology* 1991, 74:484–488.
34. Doi M, Ikeda K: Respiratory effects of sevoflurane. *Anesth Analg* 1987, 66:241–244.
35. Lutz L, Milde J, Milde L: The cerebral functional, metabolic, and hemodynamic effects of desflurane in dogs. *Anesthesiology* 1990, 73:125–131.
36. Scheller MS, Tateishi A, Drummond JC, Zornow MH: The effects of sevoflurane on cerebral blood flow, cerebral metabolic rate for oxygen, intracranial pressure, and the electroencephalogram are similar to those of isoflurane in the rabbit. *Anesthesiology* 1988, 68:548–551.
37. Muzzi DA, Losasso TJ, Dietz NM, *et al.*: The effect of desflurane and isoflurane on cerebrospinal fluid pressure in humans with supratentorial mass lesions. *Anesthesiology* 1992, 76:720–724.
38. Ornstein E, Young WL, Fleischer LH, Ostapkovich N: Desflurane and isoflurane have similar effects on cerebral blood flow in patients with intracranial mass lesions. *Anesthesiology* 1993, 79:498–502.
39. Kitaguchi K, Ohsumi H, Kuro M, *et al.*: Effects of sevoflurane on cerebral circulation and metabolism in patients with ischemic cerebrovascular disease. *Anesthesiology* 1993, 79:704–709.
40. Rampil I, Lockhart S, Eger EI II, *et al.*: The electroencephalographic effects of desflurane in humans. *Anesthesiology* 1991, 74:434–439.
41. Strum DP, Johnson BH, Eger EI II: Stability of sevoflurane in soda lime. *Anesthesiology* 1987, 67:779–781.
42. Andrews JJ, Johnston RV: The new Tec 6 vaporizer. *Anesth Analg* 1993, 76:1338–1341.
43. Eger EI II: Stability of I-653 in soda lime. *Anesth Analg* 1987, 66:983–985.
44. Eger EI II: *Desflurane (Suprane): A Compendium and Reference.* Rutherford, NJ: Healthpress; 1993.
45. Stoelting RK: *Pharmacology and Physiology in Anesthetic Practice*, edn 2. Philadelphia: JB Lippincott; 1991.
46. Eger EI II, Smith NT, Stoelting RK, *et al.*: Cardiovascular effects of halothane in man. *Anesthesiology* 1970, 32:396–409.
47. Cahalan MK, Weiskopf RB, Eger EI II, *et al.*: Hemodynamic effects of desflurane/nitrous oxide anesthesia in volunteers. *Anesth Analg* 1991, 73:157–164.
48. Hornbein TF, Eger EI II, Winter PM, *et al.*: The minimum alveolar concentration of nitrous oxide in man. *Anesth Analg* 1982, 61:553–556.
49. Stoelting RK, Gibbs PS: Hemodynamic effects of morphine and morphine-nitrous oxide in valvular heart disease and coronary artery disease. *Anesthesiology* 1973, 38:45–52.
50. Ebert TJ, Muzi M: Sympathetic hyperactivity during desflurane anesthesia in healthy volunteers: a comparison with isoflurane. *Anesthesiology* 1993, 79:444–453.
51. Moore MA, Weiskopf RB, Eger EI II, *et al.*: Rapid 1% increases of end-tidal desflurane concentration to greater than 5% transiently increase blood pressure and heart rate in humans. *Anesthesiology* 1994, 81:94–98.
52. Weiskopf RB, Eger EI II, Noorani M, Daniel M: Repetitive rapid increases in desflurane concentration blunt transient cardiovascular stimulation in humans. *Anesthesiology* 1994, 81:843–849.
53. Weiskopf RB, Eger EI II, Daniel M, Noorani M: Cardiovascular stimulation induced by rapid increases in desflurane concentration in humans results from activation of tracheopulmonary and systemic receptors. *Anesthesiology* 1995, 83:1173–1178.
54. Ebert TJ, Harkin CP, Muzi M: Cardiovascular responses to sevoflurane: a review. *Anesth Analg* 1995, 81(suppl):S11–S22.
55. Weiskopf RB, Eger EI II, Noorani M, Daniel M: Fentanyl, esmolol, and clonidine blunt the transient cardiovascular stimulation induced by desflurane in humans. *Anesthesiology* 1994, 81:1350–1355.
56. Helman JD, Leung JM, Bellows WH, *et al.*: The risk of myocardial ischemia in patients receiving desflurane versus sufentanyl anesthesia for coronary artery bypass graft surgery. *Anesthesiology* 1992, 77:47–62.
57. Thompson IR, Bowering JB, Hudson RJ, *et al.*: A comparison of desflurane and isoflurane in patients undergoing coronary artery surgery. *Anesthesiology* 1991, 75:776–781.
58. Parsons RS, Jones RM, Wrigley SR, *et al.*: Comparison of desflurane and fentanyl-based anesthetic techniques for coronary artery bypass surgery. *Br J Anaesth* 1994, 72:430–438.
59. Gross GT, Waltier DC: Coronary steal in four models of single or multiple vessel obstruction in dogs. *Am J Cardiol* 1981, 48:84–92.
60. Buffington CW, Davis KB, Gillispie S, Pettinger M: The prevalence of steal-prone coronary anatomy in patients with coronary artery disease: an analysis of the Coronary Artery Surgery Study Registry. *Anesthesiology* 1988, 69:721–727.
61. Reiz S, Balfors E, Sorensen MB, *et al.*: Isoflurane: a powerful coronary vasodilator in patients with coronary artery disease. *Anesthesiology* 1983, 59:91–97.

62. Buffington CW, Romson JL, Levine A, *et al.*: Isoflurane induces coronary steal in a canine model of chronic coronary occlusion. *Anesthesiology* 1987, 66:280–292.
63. Hartman CJ, Kampine JP, Schmeling WT, Waltier DC: Alterations in collateral blood flow produced by isoflurane in a chronically instrumented canine model of multivessel coronary artery disease. *Anesthesiology* 1991, 74:120–133.
64. Hartman CJ, Pagel PS, Kampine JP, *et al.*: Influence of desflurane on regional distribution of coronary blood flow in a chronically instrumented canine model of multivessel coronary artery obstruction. *Anesth Analg* 1991, 72:289–299.
65. Kenna JG, Satoh H, Christ DD, Pohl LR: Metabolic basis for drug hypersensitivity: Antibodies in sera from patients with halothane hepatitis recognize liver neoantigens that contain the trifluoroacetyl group derived from halothane. *J Pharmacol Exp Ther* 1988, 245:1103–1109.
66. Elliott RH, Strunin L: Hepatotoxicity of volatile anesthetics. *Br J Anaesth* 1993, 70:339–348.
67. Kenna GJ, Jones RM: The organ toxicity of inhaled anesthetics. *Anesth Analg* 1995, 81(suppl):S51–S66.
68. Frink EJ Jr: The hepatic effects of sevoflurane. *Anesth Analg* 1995, 81(suppl):S46–S50.
69. Bito H, Ikeda K: Plasma inorganic fluoride and intracircuit degradation product concentrations in long-duration, low-flow sevoflurane anesthesia. *Anesth Analg* 1994, 79:946–951.
70. Holaday DA, Fiserova-Bergerova V, Latto PI, Zumbiel MA: Resistance of isoflurane to biotransformation in man. *Anesthesiology* 1975, 43:325–332.
71. Kharasch ED: Biotransformation of sevoflurane. *Anesth Analg* 1995, 81(suppl):S27–S38.
72. Carpenter RL, Eger EI II, Johnson BH, *et al.*: The extent of metabolism of inhaled anesthetics in humans. *Anesthesiology* 1986, 65:201–205.
73. Kharasch ED, Hankins DC, Thummel KE: Human kidney methoxyflurane and sevoflurane metabolism: intrarenal fluoride production as a possible mechanism of methoxyflurane nephrotoxicity. *Anesthesiology* 1995, 82:689–699.
74. de Waziers I, Cugnenc PH, Yang CS, *et al.*: Cytochrome P-450 isoenzymes, epoxide hydrolase and glutathione transferases in rat and human extrahepatic tissues. *J Pharmacol Exp Ther* 1990, 253:387–394.
75. Liu J, Laster MJ, Eger EI II, Taheri S: Absorption and degradation of sevoflurane and isoflurane in a conventional anesthetic circuit. *Anesth Analg* 1991, 72:785–789.
76. Wong DT, Lerman J: Factors affecting the rate of disappearance of sevoflurane in Baralyme. *Can J Anaesth* 1992, 39:366–369.
77. Fang ZX, Eger EI II: Factors affecting the concentration of compound A resulting from the degradation of sevoflurane by soda lime and Baralyme in a standard anesthetic circuit. *Anesth Analg* 1995, 81:564–568.
78. Bito H, Ikeda K: Effect of total flow rate on the concentration of degradation products generated by reaction between sevoflurane and soda lime. *Br J Anaesth* 1995, 74:667–669.
79. Bito H, Ikeda K: Long-duration, low-flow sevoflurane anesthesia using two carbon dioxide absorbents: quantification of degradation products in the circuit. *Anesthesiology* 1994, 81:340–345.

15

Pharmacology and Physiology of Intravenous Anesthetics

Allison Kinder Ross and Peter S.A. Glass

To date no drug is available that incorporates all the characteristics of the ideal anesthetic agent. We do, however, have numerous intravenous (IV) hypnotics and opioids that are extremely useful in clinical practice. The purpose of understanding and learning about the pharmacology of these IV drugs is to aid the clinician in choosing the most appropriate drug for the desired effect, the pathophysiology of the patient, and the particular surgical intervention. Once the choice of drug has been made, knowledge of the pharmacokinetic parameters of the drug is utilized to determine the dosing regimen so as to optimize the ability to obtain the therapeutic goal. Thus this chapter attempts to provide an overview of the general effects of IV hypnotics and how the differing effects among these drugs affect each organ system.

To determine the appropriate dosing scheme, a clear understanding of pharmacokinetic and pharmacodynamic principles is required. These principles include not only the processes of distribution, redistribution, and metabolism but also new concepts such as the effect site and context-sensitive half-times. An understanding of the effect site and drug onset will affect both drug choice and dosing. Context-sensitive decrement time explains why all hypnotics are fairly short-lasting for induction but longer-lasting after infusions. The use of the context-sensitive decrement time should also facilitate decisions about when to terminate infusions. In addition, because we do not have a single drug that provides all the requirements for anesthesia, a hypnotic is usually combined with an opioid. Such combinations have pronounced effects on the doses required for both induction and maintenance of anesthesia. Recent work in this area is also described in this chapter. Important advances are being made in IV drug delivery systems. It is thus important that this chapter be read in conjunction with the chapters on pharmacokinetic and pharmacodynamic principles as well as the chapter on IV drug delivery systems.

STRUCTURES AND PROPERTIES

PROPERTIES OF AN "IDEAL" IV HYPNOTIC

Physicochemical
- Water soluble
- Long shelf life (> 1 d)
- Stable on exposure to light (> 1 d)
- Small volume (± 10 mL) required for anesthetic induction

Pharmacokinetic/pharmacodynamic
- Small interindividual variation
- Safe therapeutic ratio
- Onset in one arm-brain circulation time
- Inactivated by rapid metabolism to nontoxic metabolites providing short duration of effect with rapid recovery

Hypersensitivity
- No anaphylaxis
- No histamine release

Side effects
- No local toxicity (absence of pain or thrombophlebitis on injection)
- No alterations in body organ function, except primary CNS effects
  - Does not induce nausea and vomiting
  - Preserves oxygen supply and demand for heart, CNS, and other vital organs

Economic
- Inexpensive

Figure 15-1. Properties of an "ideal" intravenous hypnotic. CNS—central nervous system. (*Modified from* Barash and coworkers [1]; with permission.)

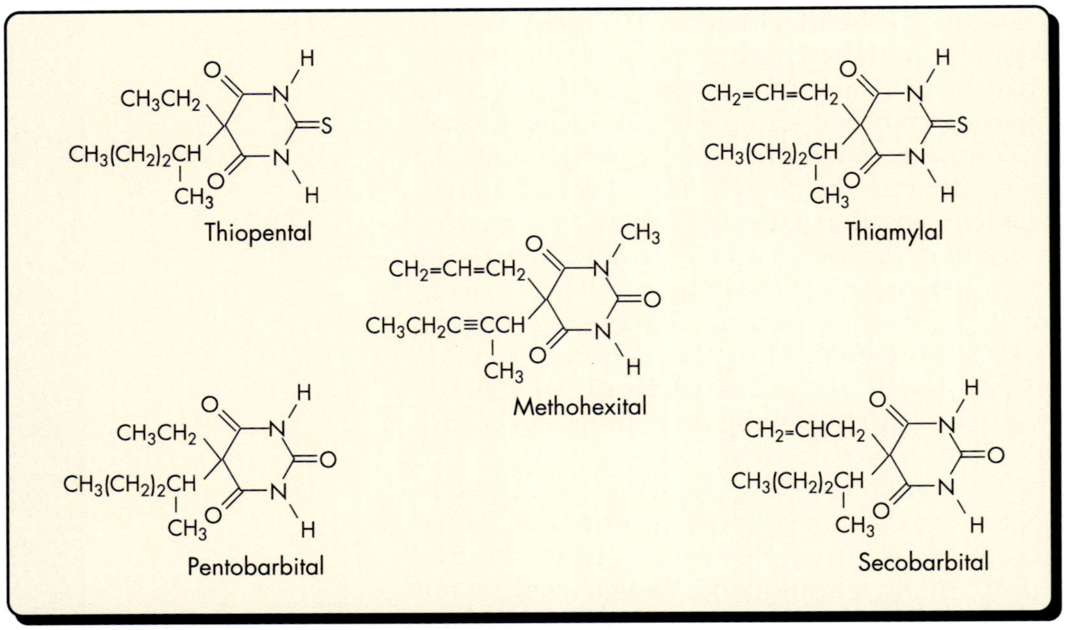

Figure 15-2. Chemical structures of barbiturates. Barbituric acid has no hypnotic activity. However, substitution at position 2 with oxygen or sulfur results in a water-soluble barbiturate salt, and the length of side chains in the 5 position determines potency, *ie*, the longer the chain and extent of branching, the more potent the barbiturate.

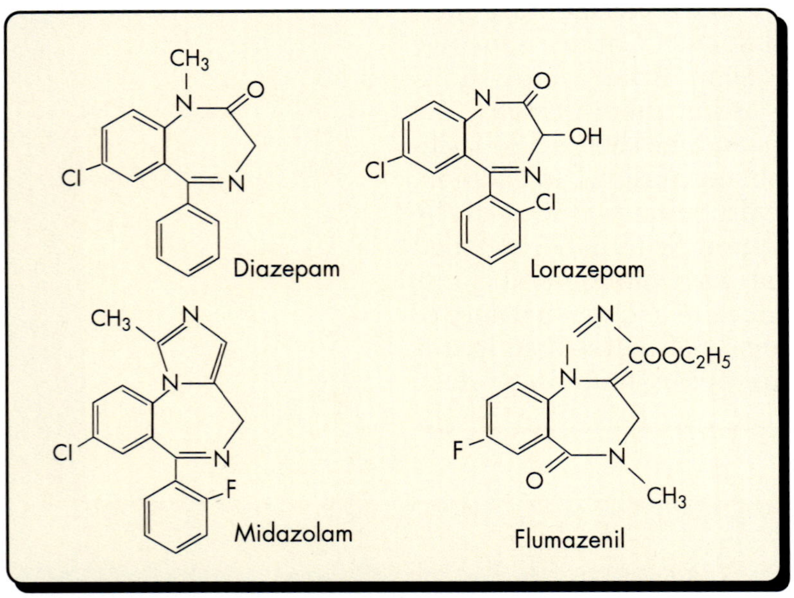

Figure 15-3. Structure of benzodiazepines. Midazolam has an imidazole ring that contributes to its rapid metabolism and water solubility.

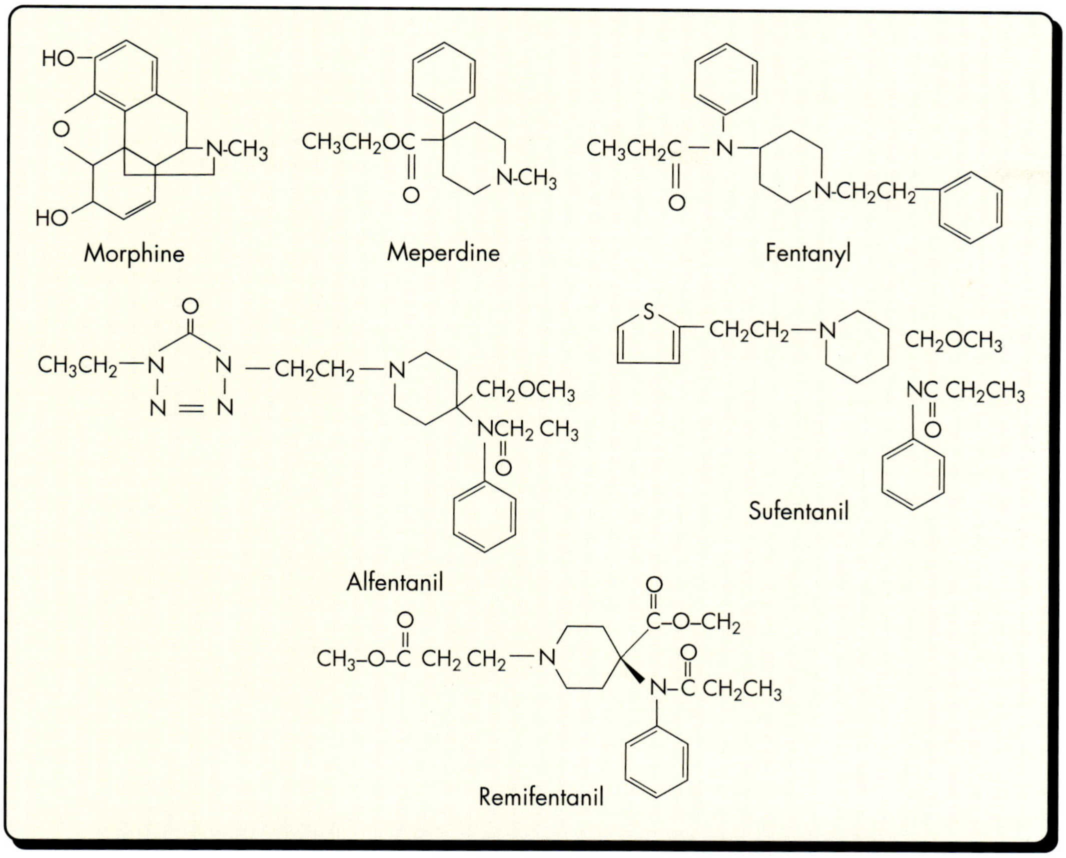

Figure 15-4. Chemical structures of narcotic anesthetics. Morphine is the principal phenanthrene alkaloid present in opium. Synthetic opioids are manufactured but contain the phenanthrene nucleus of morphine.

PHYSICOCHEMICAL PROPERTIES OF IV ANESTHETICS AND OPIOIDS

	pK_a	pH	Solution	Water soluble?	Other
Thiopental	7.45	10.5 – 11	Sodium salt is mixed with anhydrous $NaHCO_3$	Yes	Needs refrigeration and must be mixed within 24 h
Methohexital	7.9	10 – 11	Same as thiopental	Yes	As for thiopental
Etomidate	4.24	4 – 7	Propylene glycol solution	No	
Propofol	11.1	6.0 – 8.5	Oil at room temperature mixed in soybean oil, glycerol and egg phosphatide (intralipid)	No	Not recommended for patients with egg allergy; strict aseptic technique.
Ketamine	7.5	7.0	White crystalline salt in slightly acidic solution	Yes (partially)	
Midazolam	6.2	3.5	Mixed in NaCl	Yes	
Diazepam	3.4	6.2 – 6.9	Mixed in propylene glycol or intralipid	No	
Fentanyl	8.4	4.0 – 7.5	Citrate salt	Yes	
Sufentanil	8.0	3.5 – 6	Citrate salt	Yes	
Alfentanil	6.5	4 – 6	Mixed in NaCl	Yes	
Remifentanil	7.07	2.5 – 3.5	Lyophilized powder containing glycine	Yes	Must be freshly prepared as undergoes slow spontaneous degradation

Figure 15-5. Physicochemical properties of IV anesthetics and opioids. There are many differences among the agents with respect to their physicochemical properties. Etomidate, propofol, and diazepam differ from the other agents in their outlying pK_as and insolubility in water.

PHARMACOKINETICS OF IV HYPNOTICS AND OPIOIDS						
	$T_{1/2}\ k_{e0}$, *min*	Time to Peak Effect, *min*	V_c, *L/kg*	Vd_{ss}, *L/kg*	Clearance, *mL/min/kg*	Elimination Half-Life, *h*
Thiopental	1.5	1.7	0.3 – 0.6	2 – 4	3 – 4	6 – 12
Methohexital			0.2 – 0.4	1.5 – 3	9 – 12	2 – 4
Etomidate	1.5	2	0.11 – 0.2	2.5 – 4.5	18 – 25	3 – 6
Propofol	2.4	2.2	0.31 – 0.4	2 – 10	20 – 30	4 – 8
Ketamine			1 – 2	3 – 4	12 – 17	2 – 4
Midazolam	4.0	2.8	0.15 – 0.2	1.1 – 1.7	6 – 11	1.7 – 2.6
Diazepam			0.2 – 0.4	0.7 – 1.7	0.1 – 0.5	20 – 50
Fentanyl	4.7	3.6	0.5 – 1.0	3 – 5	10 – 20	3 – 5
Alfentanil	1.0	1.4	0.1 – 0.3	0.4 – 1	3 – 8	1 – 2
Sufentanil	3	5.6	2.5 – 3	3 – 6	10 – 15	7 – 10
Remifentanil	1.2	1.5	0.3 – 0.4	40 – 60	0.1 – 0.3	0.1 – 0.2

Figure 15-6. Pharmacokinetics of intravenous hypnotics and opioids. The slower elimination times of thiopental and diazepam are a reflection of their lower hepatic extraction. Conversely, drugs with higher hepatic metabolism, *ie*, etomidate, propofol, and ketamine, have a more rapid clearance. Note the very high clearance of remifentanil due to esterase metabolism when compared with other opioids. $T_{1/2}\ k_{e0}$ is the time required for the biophase (effect compartment in the central nervous system) to have equilibrated by 50% with the plasma. Time to peak effect is the time of maximal drug effect following a bolus dose and is dependent on both the drug's k_{e0} and its distribution pharmacokinetics. The time to peak effect determines the dosing interval when administering the drug by intermittent boluses. V_c—central volume of distribution; Vd_{ss}—volume of distribution at steady state.

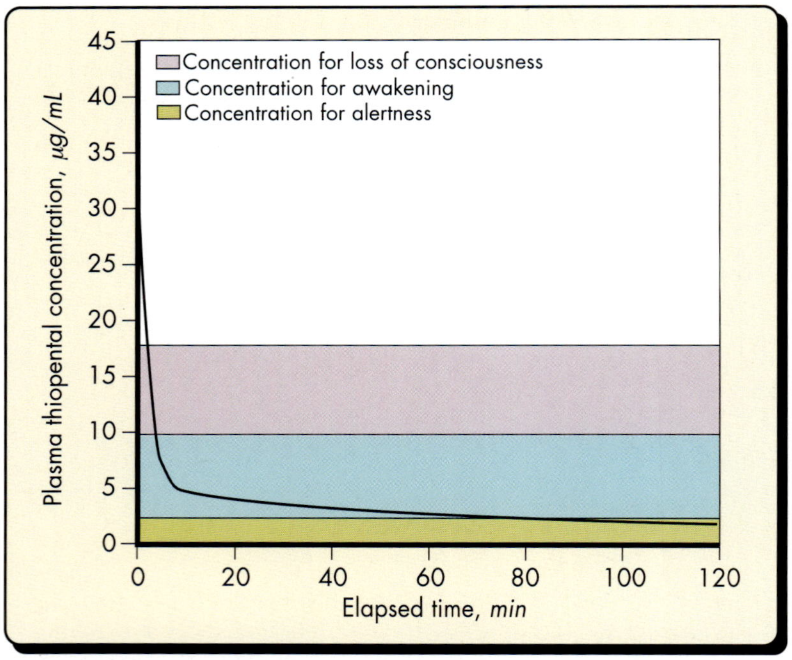

Figure 15-7. The disposition of thiopentone following a bolus of 4 mg/kg. The pharmacokinetic parameters used were those of Maitre and coworkers [2].

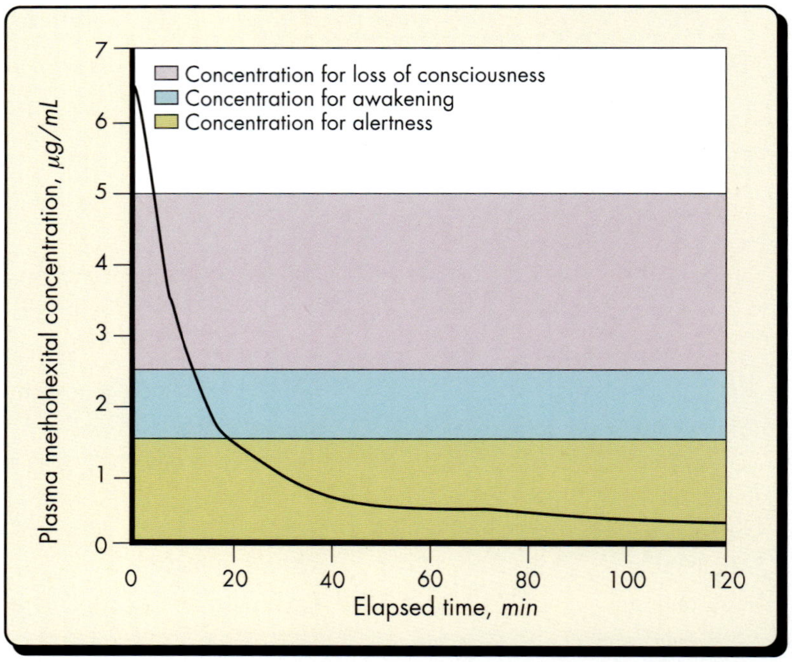

Figure 15-8. The disposition of methohexital following a bolus dose of 2 mg/kg. The pharmacokinetic parameters used were those of Breimer [3].

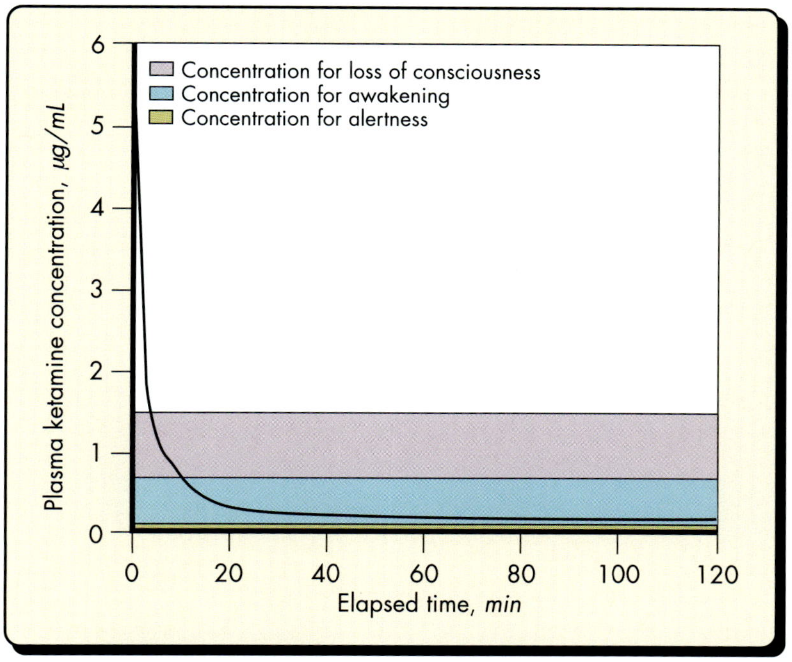

Figure 15-9. The disposition of ketamine following a bolus dose of 2 mg/kg. The pharmacokinetic parameters used were those of Domino and coworkers [4].

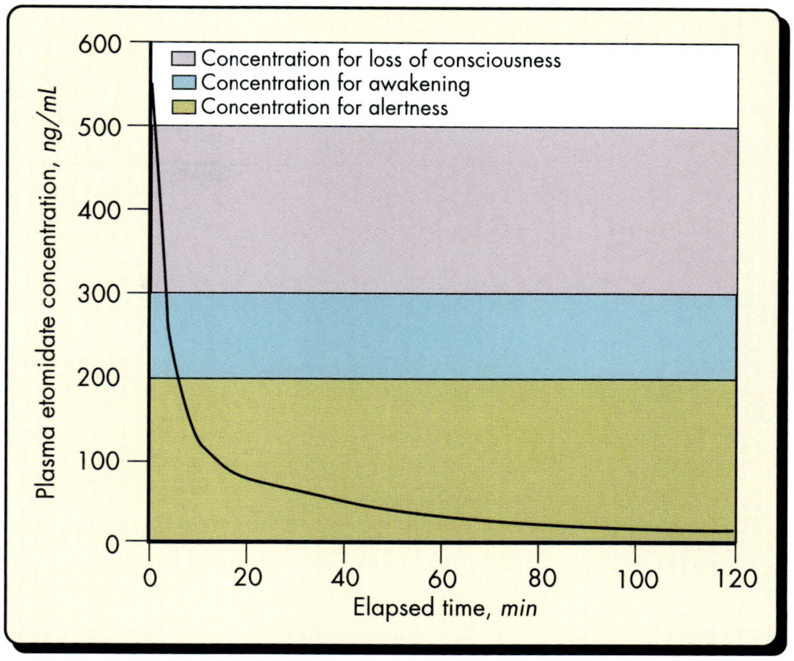

Figure 15-10. The disposition of etomidate following a bolus dose of 0.2 mg/kg. The pharmacokinetic parameters used were those of Arden and coworkers [5].

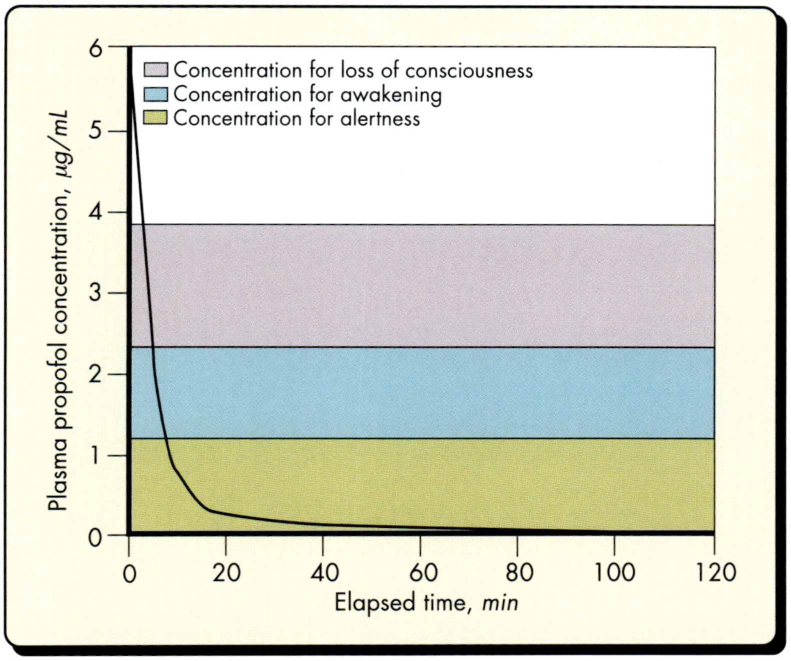

Figure 15-11. The disposition of propofol following a bolus dose of 2 mg/kg. The pharmacokinetic parameters used were those of Gepts and coworkers [6].

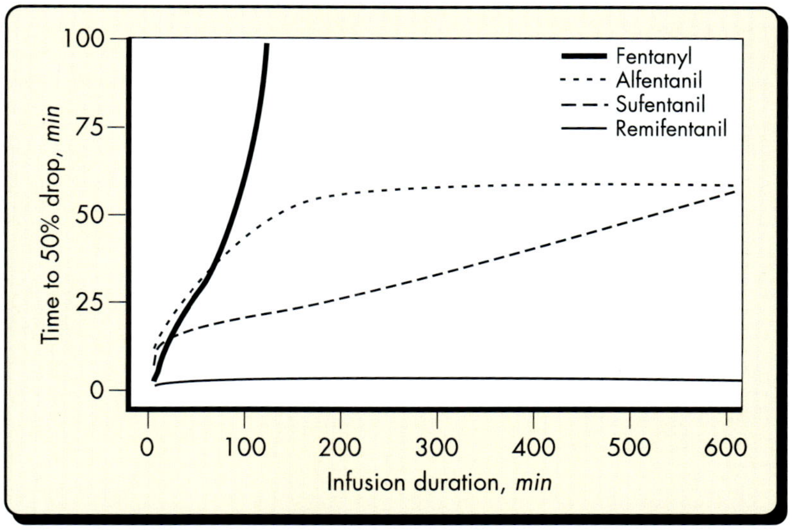

Figure 15-12. Context-sensitive half-time of opioids. The difference between context-sensitive half-time and elimination is clearly illustrated by sufentanil and fentanyl, which have similar elimination half-lives but very different context-sensitive half-times. Also note the extremely short context-sensitive half-time of remifentanil (3 to 5 minutes), which appears to be time independent because of its very rapid esterase metabolism.

METABOLISM AND ELIMINATION OF IV ANESTHETICS

	Metabolism	Primary Metabolite	Elimination
Thiopental	Liver by oxidation	Thiopental-carboxylic acid	Renal
Methohexital	Liver by hydroxylation	None	Fecal
Etomidate	Liver by ester hydrolysis	Carboxylic acid	77.8% renal, 12.9% fecal
Ketamine	Liver demethylation and hydroxylation	Norketamine	91% renal, 3% fecal
Propofol	Liver by conjugation	Propofol glucuronide	Renal
Midazolam	Liver by conjugation	4-Hydroxy- and 1-hydroxymethyl-midazolam	Renal
Diazepam	Liver by oxidation	Desmethyldiazepam, hydroxydiazepam	70% renal, 10% fecal
Fentanyl	*N*-dealkylation and hydroxylation	Norfentanyl	Primarily renal
Alfentanil	Same as for fentanyl	Noralfentanil	Renal
Sufentanil	Same as for fentanyl	Norsufentanil	Renal, fecal
Remifentanil	Ester hydrolysis	G190291	Renal

Figure 15-13. Metabolism and elimination of IV anesthetics. Metabolism occurs in the liver for the induction agents. With the exception of ketamine (norketamine is 30% to 50% as potent) and diazepam (desmethyldiazepam is 90% as potent), the metabolites are inactive. Excretion of the IV agents is primarily renal, with very little active drug being excreted. MethohexitalOs elimination is fecal. (*Adapted from* Attia and coworkers [7].)

PHYSIOLOGIC EFFECTS

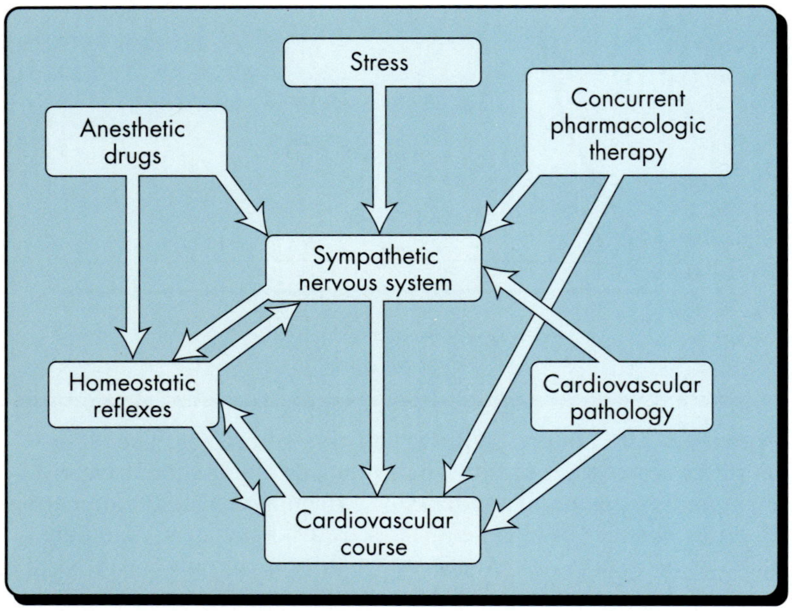

Figure 15-14. The effects of IV anesthetics on the cardiovascular system. Effects are rarely dependent on the drug alone. The net change observed is, rather, a result of multifactorial input.

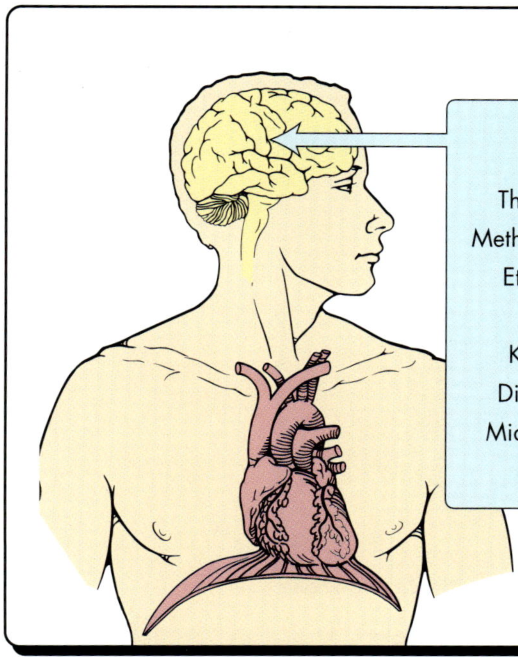

CNS effects of IV anesthetics

	CBF	CPP	$CMRO_2$	ICP	IOP
Thiopental	↓↓	↓↓	↓↓	↓↓	↓
Methohexital	↓↓	↓↓	↓↓	↓↓	↓
Etomidate	↓↓	0	↓↓	↓↓	↓
Propofol	↓↓	↓↓	↓↓	↓↓	↓↓
Ketamine	↑↑	↑	↑	↑	↑
Diazepam	↓	↓	↓	↓	↓
Midazolam	↓	↓	↓	↓	↓
Opioids	↓↑	0	↓	↓↑	0

Figure 15-15. Central nervous system effects of IV anesthetics. The barbiturates provide a dose-dependent (up to a point in which the electroencephalogram flattens) depression of cerebral blood flow (CBF), cerebral metabolism of oxygen ($CMRO_2$), and intracranial pressure (ICP). Because of this decrease in ICP, cerebral perfusion pressure (CPP) tends to be preserved. Intraocular pressure (IOP) decreases by about 40% with a barbiturate induction. Benzodiazepines have a slightly less (dose-dependent) depressive effect on CNS parameters. Midazolam has been shown to have a protective effect in mice with cerebral hypoxia that was less than that of pentobarbital but better than that of diazepam. Propofol will decrease IOP to a greater extent than will thiopental. Ketamine is unique in its stimulatory effects on the limbic system as well as in causing an overall CNS excitatory effect. The anesthetized state induced by ketamine is a Odissociative anesthesiaO displayed by open eyes and preservation of protective reflexes not seen with other induction agents. Etomidate preserves CPP while lowering CBF and $CMRO_2$.

The opioids have been reported to both increase and decrease CBF and ICP. The resultant change appears very dependent on the presence of other drugs and preexisting pathology. The changes that do occur, however, are generally small. Opioids tend to have less of an effect on CNS parameters than do hypnotics. (*Modified from* Barash and coworkers [1]).

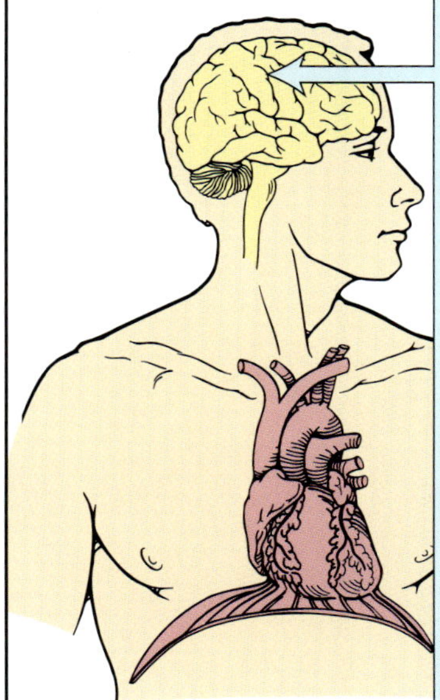

Brainwave effects of IV anesthetics

	Seizures	EEG
Thiopental	↓↓	Depression progresses from alpha to delta and theta, then burst suppression progresses to flat line.
Methohexital	↑↓	Same as for thiopental but may be used to stimulate seizure activity for cortical mapping.
Etomidate	↑↓	Initial increase in alpha amplitute, sharp beta bursts, then delta activity.
Propofol	↑↓	Initial increase in alpha, then shift to delta and theta frequency. May be used to treat siezures but has also been effective in stimulating siezures for cortical mapping
Ketamine	↑	Produces generalized theta wave activity and petit-mal-seizure–like activity in hippocampus
Diazepam	↓	Similar to Midazolam
Midazolam	↓	Rhythmic beta activity appears rapidly after administration followed by delta and theta activity and then general EEG suppression
Opioids	↑ (Rare)	Depression progressing to high voltage delta waves but with ceiling effect

Figure 15-16. Brainwave activity of IV anesthetics. Thiopental produces dose-dependent depression in the electroencephalogram (EEG) leading to a barbiturate coma. Thiopental is also useful as an anticonvulsant because of its augmentation of gamma aminobutyric acid. Methohexital, conversely, has been found to produce epileptiform seizures when used in high doses or administered by infusion. Etomidate differs from the barbiturates in its lack of beta waves on induction. It has been found to produce increased epileptic EEG activity in seizure patients and been associated with grand mal seizures. The myoclonic movements seen with etomidate are not associated with EEG seizurelike activity. Propofol blood levels correlate with percent delta activity and correlate inversely with percent beta activity. PropofolOs effect on seizures is controversial, and the drug has both been used to treat seizures and has been associated with seizures. Ketamine has excitatory central nervous system effects. Midazolam is the popular choice as an immediate anticonvulsant due to its fast onset and long duration. Increasing opioid concentration does not progress to burst suppression and a flat EEG.

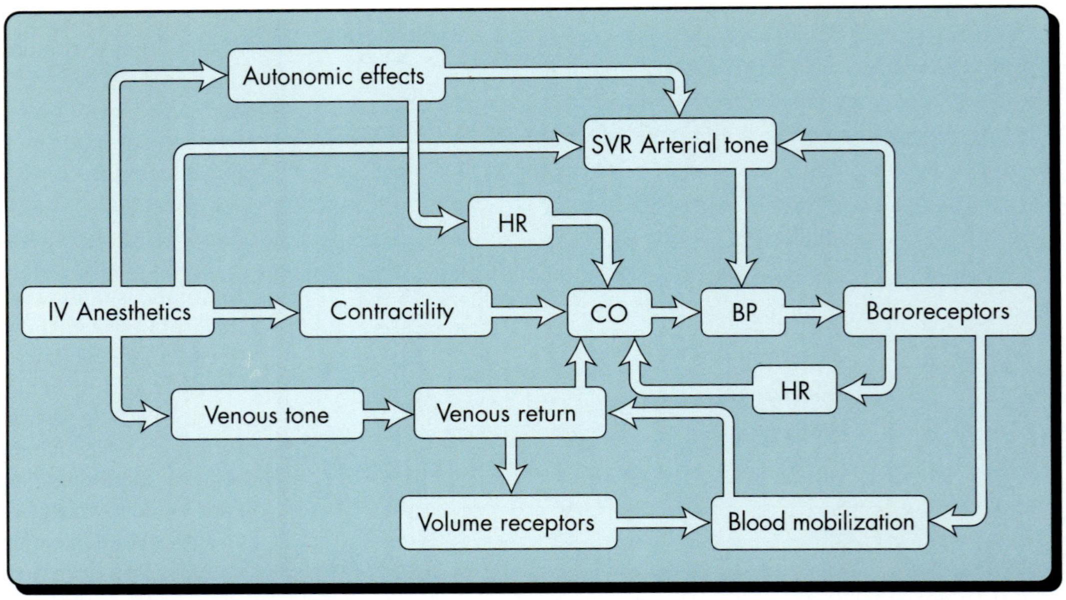

Figure 15-17. The general mechanisms by which IV hypnotics affect the cardiovascular system. Specific drugs have slightly differing actions on contractility, venous tone, and autonomic tone, thus inducing different compensatory mechanisms and providing different net effects on the observed hemodynamic parameters. BP—blood pressure; CO—cardiac output; HR—heart rate; SVR—systemic vascular resistance.

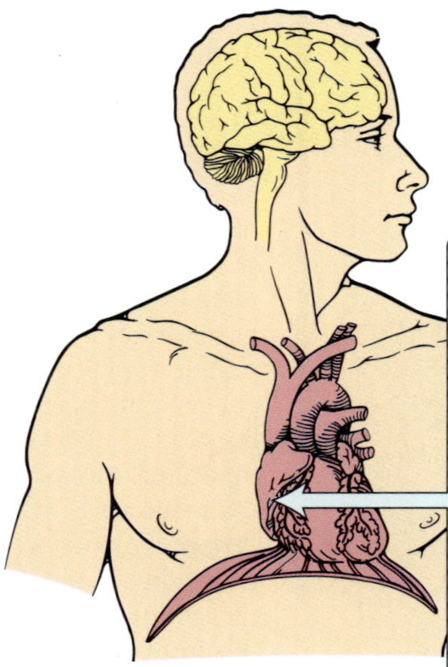

Cardiovascular effects of IV anesthetics

	HR	MAP	CO	SVR	Venodilation	dP/dT
Thiopental	↑	↓	↓	0 to ↑	↑	↓
Methohexital	↑↑	↓	↓	NR	↑	↓
Etomidate	0	0	0	0	0	0
Propofol	↓↑	↓	0	↓	↑	NR
Ketamine	↑↑	↑↑	↑	↑	0	0
Midazolam	↓ to ↑	0 to ↓	0 to ↓	0 to ↓	↑	0
Diazepam	↓ to ↑	0 to ↓	0	↓ to ↑	↑	0
Opioids	↓	0 to ↓	0	0	0 to ↓	0

Figure 15-18. Cardiovascular effects of IV anesthetics. All of the agents listed here affect the cardiovascular system in some way, either by depression or by stimulation of the various parameters. The newer agents, propofol and etomidate, have little effect on cardiac output at normal doses in healthy patients; however, even propofol must be used with caution in a patient with any cardiac compromise or hypovolemia. The same is true for the barbiturates. Ketamine is unique in its ability to increase cardiac output through direct sympathetic stimulation with tachycardia. It has the ability to cause direct vasodilatation; however, this effect is negligible due to the sympathetic outflow. Etomidate is the closest exception to the conclusion that IV agents are cardioactive. Etomidate produces only slight changes in the measured parameters, which makes it useful in the patient with cardiovascular disease. Midazolam and diazepam have little effect at premedication doses. Besides mild bradycardia, opioids produce minimal effects on hemodynamics. Alfentanil and remifentanil may result in a decrease in mean arterial pressure of up to 30%. HR—heart rate; CO—cardiac output; SVR—systemic vascular resistance; dP/dT—contractility; NR—not reported. (*Adapted from* Barash and coworkers [1]).

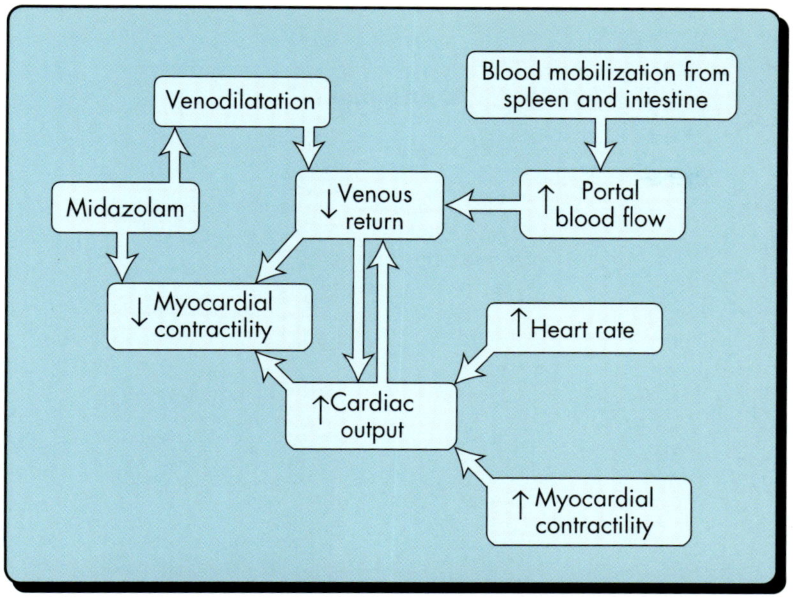

Figure 15-19. Cardiovascular effects following an induction dose of midazolam. (*From* Gelman and coworkers [8]; with permission.)

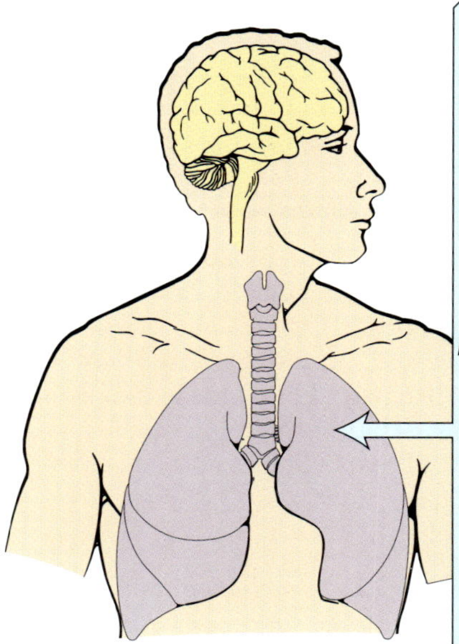

Respiratory effects of IV anesthetics

	Respiratory depression	CO_2 during spontaneous ventilation	Response to increasing CO_2	Mechanics	Bronchial tone	Cilia/Secretions
Thiopental	↑	Acute rise in $PaCO_2$	↓	↓	0 to perhaps increased bronchospasm at lower doses	Increased secretions at lower doses and decreased mucociliary clearance
Methohexital	↑	Acute rise in $PaCO_2$	↓	Initial↑ TV and RR	0	
Etomidate	↑	Slight rise in $PaCO_2$	↓		0	
Propofol	↑	Acute rise in $PaCO_2$	↓	↓TV	Mild bronchodilation	
Ketamine	0	No change	↑	↓RR	Releives bronchospasm	Excessive secretions
Midazolam	↑	Rise in $PaCO_2$	↓	↓TV and ↑RR (normal MV)	0	
Diazepam	↑	Rise in $PaCO_2$	↓		0	
Opioids	↑↑	Dose Dependent ↑ $PaCO_2$	↓↓↓	↓RR	0	Slightly antitussive

Figure 15-20. Respiratory effects of IV anesthetics. With the exception of ketamine, IV agents cause respiratory depression and may result in apnea at normal to high doses. Even ketamine can result in respiratory depression when injected rapidly or given to the spontaneously breathing elderly patient. Thiopental was once thought to increase airway sensitivity; however, this effect may occur only at lower doses and is more likely due to inadequate induction prior to airway manipulation. Propofol provides a more profound respiratory depression of airway reflexes than thiopental and may thus be the better agent for laryngeal mask airway insertion. Ketamine remains the only respiratory stimulant and bronchodilator, although its ability to increase airway secretions mandates use of a concomitant antisialagogue. The benzodiazepines produce respiratory depression; however, the ventilatory response curves flatten rather than shift to the right. Opioids provide dose-dependent respiratory depression primarily by decreasing respiratory rate (RR). MV—minute ventilation; TV—tidal volume.

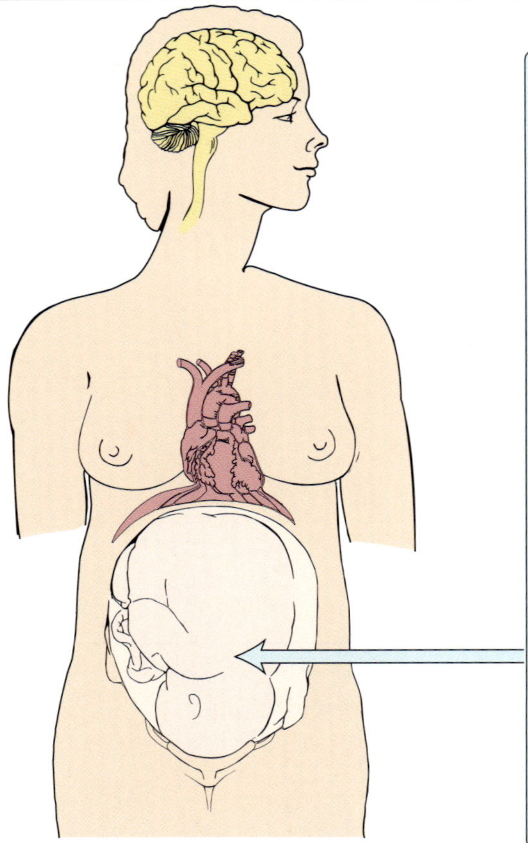

Maternal-Fetal effects of IV anesthetics

	UBF	Ability to cross placenta	Uterine tone	Fetal effects
Thiopental	Decreased 20%	Yes	No change to inhibition of uterine contractility	No effect at doses up to 4mg/kg
Etomidate	No change	Yes	NR	Suppresses cortisol production in neonate
Propofol	No change	Yes	NR	Comparable to thiopental
Ketamine	No change to increased	Yes	Moderate increase	No effect in doses less than 1 mg/kg
Midazolam	NR	Yes	NR	Lower Apgar scores at 5 mg/kg
Diazepam	Decreased at higher doses	Yes	No effect on uterine contractility	Minimal effects other than decreased beat-to-beat variability at small doses (5-10 mg)
Opioids	No change	Yes	No effect (Meperidine may ↑ uterine contractions)	Respiratory depression

Figure 15-21. Pregnancy effects of IV agents. Thiopental is often used as an induction agent during cesarean section and does not depress the fetus at doses up to 6 mg/kg. It reaches peak concentration in umbilical venous blood in 1 minute and in arterial blood at 2 to 3 minutes. Lower neonatal blood concentrations will result from injection at the beginning of a contraction versus during injection at uterine diastole. Fetal effects depend on uptake based on the solubility of the agent in fetal blood, fetal blood flow to the intervillous space, and concentration of the drug in fetal blood flow returning to the placenta. Diazepam can cause hypotonia, lethargy, decreased feeding, and hypothermia at high doses. Opioids may result in profound respiratory depression because metabolism of opioids is impaired in the neonate. Neurobehavioral outcome in the neonate has been altered following administration of certain opioids (*eg*, meperidine). NR—not reported. (*From* Schnider and Levinson [9].)

MISCELLANEOUS EFFECTS OF IV AGENTS

	Action
Thiopental	Histamine release, contraindicated in acute intermittent porphyria, slight increase in blood glucose levels
Methohexital	Hiccoughs, twitching
Etomidate	Pain on injection, myoclonic activity, suppression of adrenal function
Propofol	Opisthotonos, pain on injection
Ketamine	Nystagmus, dilated pupils, emergence reactions, salivation
Midazolam	Anterograde amnesia
Diazepam	Pain on injection

Figure 15-22. Miscellaneous effects of IV agents. Etomidate suppresses adrenal function in induction doses for up to 8 hours. There is a decrease in cortisol, 17-hydroxyprogesterone, aldosterone, and corticosterone production. Although only thiopental is included in the table, the other barbiturates have the same side effects. One of the primary advantages of propofol is its antiemetic action.

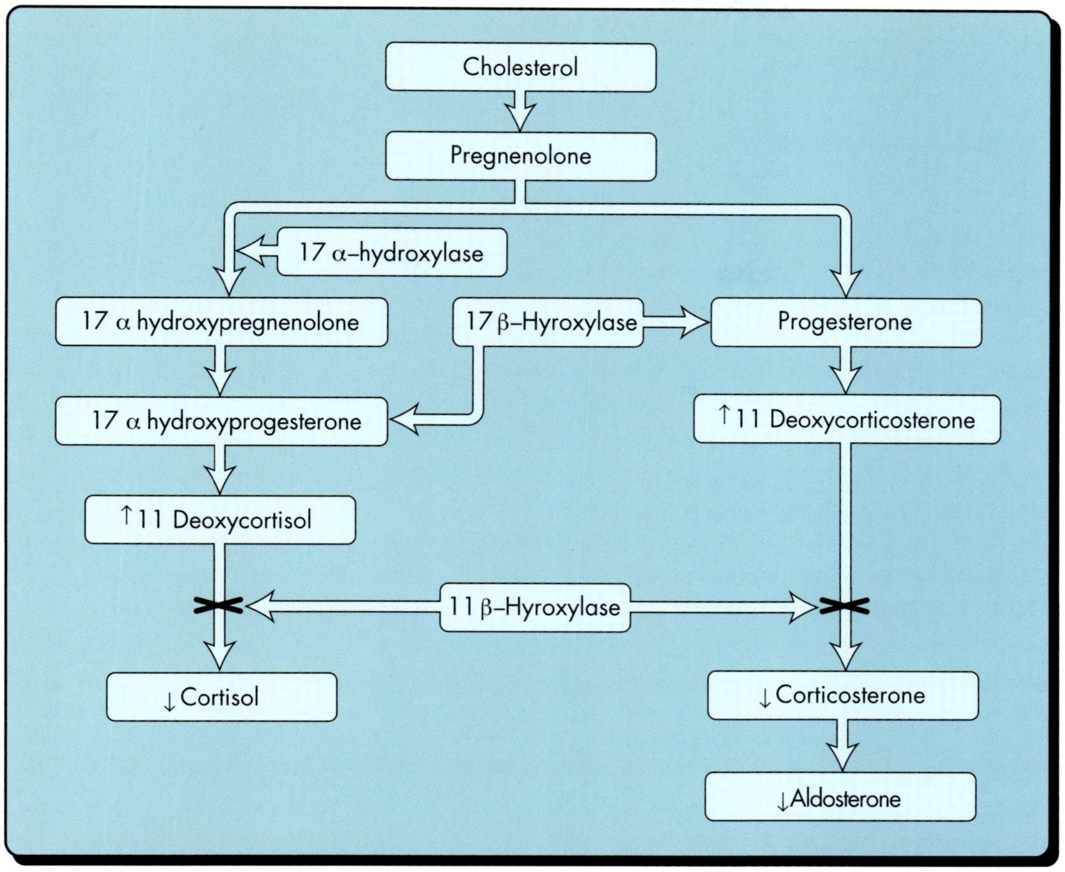

Figure 15-23. Pathway for the biosynthesis of cortisol and aldosterone. The sites at which etomidate affects cortisol/aldosterone synthesis by its action on 11-β-hydroxylase (major site) and 17-α-hydroxylase (minor site) are illustrated. (*From* Miller [10]; with permission.)

INDUCTION CHARACTERISTICS AND DOSES

COMPARISON OF INDUCTION CHARACTERISTICS AMONG ANESTHETIC INDUCTION DRUGS

	Pain	Duration after single dose, *min*	Emergence	Respiratory Effects	Hemodynamic	Phlebitis
Thiopental	No	5	Smooth	Apnea, transient depression	Slight depression	No
Etomidate	Yes	3	Smooth	Transient depression	None	Yes
Ketamine	No	5 – 10	May be stormy	Minimal, reflexes preserved	Increased HR and BP	No
Propofol	No	3 – 5	Smooth (clear headed)	Apnea, transient depression	Slight depression	No
Diazepam	Yes	10	Smooth	Decreased drive	Minimal	Yes
Midazolam	No	5	Smooth	Decreased drive	Slight vasodilation	No

Figure 15-24. Comparison of induction characteristics among anesthetic induction drugs. BP—blood pressure; HR—heart rate.

USES AND DOSES OF IV ANESTHETICS

	Premedication or sedation	Induction	Anesthetic maintentance
Thiopental	25 – 50 mg	2 – 4 mg/kg	NA
Methohexital	20 – 30 mg/kg PR	1 – 2 mg/kg	80 – 150 ´g/kg/min
Etomidate	5 – 8 ´g/kg/min	0.2 – 0.3 mg/kg	10 ´g/kg/min
Propofol	25 – 75 ´g/kg/min	1 – 2.5 mg/kg	80 – 150 ´g/kg/min
Ketamine	0.2 – 0.8 mg/kg IV (2 – 4 mg/kg IM)	1 – 2.0 mg/kg IV (4 – 6 mg/kg IM)	20 – 90 ´g/kg/min
Midazolam	0.5 – 1 mg	0.1 – 0.2 mg/kg	0.25 – 1 ´g/kg/min
Diazepam	2 mg	0.3 – 0.5 mg/kg	0.1 mg/kg PRN

Figure 15-25. Uses and doses of IV anesthetics. The barbiturates are primarily induction agents with the exception of methohexital, which has been used rectally (PR) as a premedicant. Propofol, etomidate, and ketamine maintenance doses are in conjunction with N_2O or an opiate. Prolonged infusions of etomidate should be avoided due to the ability of this agent to inhibit corticosteroid synthesis. Please see chapter on IV drug delivery systems for more detailed infusion schemes. IM—intramuscularly; NA—not applicable; PRN—as needed.

REFERENCES

1. Barash PG, Cullen BF, Stoelting RK: *Clinical Anesthesia*, edn 2. Philadelphia: JB Lippincott; 1989.
2. Maitre PO, Bührer M, Shafer SL, Stanski DR: Estimating the rate of thiopental blood-brain equilibration using pseudo steady-state serum concentrations. *J Pharmocokinet Biopharm* 1990, 18:175–187.
3. Breimer DD: Pharmocokinetics of methohexitone following intravenous infusion in humans. *Br J Anaesth* 1976, 48:643–648.
4. Domino EF, Domino SE, Smith RE, *et al.*: Ketamine kinetics in unmedicated and diazepam premedicated subjects. *Clin Pharmacol Ther* 1984, 36:645–653.
5. Arden JR, Holley FO, Stanski DR: Increased sensitivity to etomidate in the elderly: initial distribution versus altered brain response. Anethesiology 1986, 65:19–27.
6. Gepts E, Jonckheer K, Maes V, *et al.*: Disposition kinetics of propofol during alfentanil anaesthesia. *Anaesthesia* 1988, 43(Suppl):8–13.
7. Attia RR, Grogono AW, Domer FR: *Practical Anesthetic Pharmacology*, edn 2. East Norwalk: Appleton-Century-Crofts; 1987.
8. Gelman S, Reves JG, Harris D: Circulatory responses to midazolam anesthesia: Emphasis on canine splanchnic circulation. *Anesth Analg* 1983, 62:135.
9. Schnider SM, Levinson G: *Anesthesia for Obstetrics*, edn 3. Baltimore: Williams & Wilkins; 1993.
10. Miller RD: *Anesthesia*, edn 3. New York: Churchill Livingstone; 1990.

16

Mechanisms of Local Anesthetic Action

John Butterworth

Local anesthetics are a class of water-soluble but membrane-permeable compounds that reversibly inhibit electrical impulse conduction in nerves and muscle cells. At concentrations below those that completely "block" nerve conduction, systemically administered local anesthetics serve as antiarrhythmic agents, supplement general anesthesia, and provide therapy for central pain syndromes. Local anesthetics dramatically increase the firing threshold of nerves (rendering them less excitable) and, if depolarizations occur frequently, produce "use-dependent" (phasic) block. Local anesthetics also produce spinal, epidural, and intravenous regional anesthesia through mechanisms that are as yet much less well understood than are those that underlie peripheral nerve block.

Local anesthetics reduce the excitability of cardiac cells and neurons by binding to and inhibiting the function of voltage-gated sodium (Na) channels. Na channels are highly selective for Na ions over all other cations prevalent in living organisms. Flow of Na ions from extracellular fluid into the cytoplasm depolarizes (drives the membrane potential toward a positive value) for the period during which ionic flux is occurring. Since the time of Hodgkin and Huxley, biophysicists have generally agreed that Na channels can exist in at least three conformations: "resting," "open," and "inactivated." Conduction through open Na channels ceases spontaneously after only a brief time due to "inactivation" of the channel. Na channels that have bound a local anesthetic do not conduct Na ions. Binding of local anesthetics is favored by depolarizing membrane potentials ("voltage-dependence"), by the open and inactivated conformations of the Na channel ("state-dependence"), and by increased frequency of depolarizations ("use-dependence" or "frequency-dependence"). The greater affinity of local anesthetics for some conformations of the Na channel than for others has been called the *modulated receptor hypothesis*. Local anesthetics show a moderate degree of stereospecificity: Generally, the R^+ isomers have greater potency than do the S^- isomers.

The apparent efficacy of a given local anesthetic concentration at inhibiting nerve conduction depends on the length of nerve exposed to the drug, with greater inhibition occurring when that length is increased. The mechanistic details by which local anesthetics inhibit nerve conduction may depend on the type of nerve involved. Peripheral nerve fibers can be classified into distinct categories based on their size, conduction velocity, presence or absence of myelin, and function. Numerous potential reasons exist for differences in local anesthetic susceptibility among different fiber types, including differences in intrinsic conduction safety, diffusion barriers, the area of nerve membrane exposed to local anesthetic, and location of nerve block. There may also be differences among local anesthetics in their relative tendency to produce block of a specific modality.

Certain physical properties of local anesthetics have been correlated with their rates of onset, potency, and duration. Some authors have linked increased local anesthetic speed of onset (in patients) with decreasing pK_a values. Nevertheless, the small differences in rates of onset of regional anesthesia with different local anesthetics observed in patients are not particularly well-predicted by observations of local anesthetic onset *in vitro*. Alkaline conditions generally increase local anesthetic potency and onset rate *in vivo*; however, pH has a complex influence on local anesthetic action. Both cooling and pregnancy can also increase local anesthetic potency and onset rate. Some authors have linked local anesthetic duration of action with the extent of protein binding in blood. Nevertheless, protein binding (largely to a_2-acid microglobulin) is a reflection of drug hydrophobicity and has no direct relationship with local anesthetic binding to its receptor on the Na channel.

The most important systemic toxic reactions to local anesthetics result from drug actions on the heart and brain or from rare allergic reactions. Local anesthetics, once taken up by the blood stream, rapidly gain entrance to the central nervous system (CNS). In humans, the initial signs of local anesthetic intoxication are those of CNS disinhibition; if the local anesthetic concentration continues to increase, CNS excitation, up to and including seizures, then CNS depression, coma, and respiratory arrest may be seen. Fortunately, cardiovascular toxicity from local anesthetics is rare and usually seen only with blood concentrations three- to fivefold greater than those required to produce CNS side effects. Allergy to local anesthetic solutions is also rare. Reactions may also occur to other constituents of local anesthetic solutions, such as preservatives. Reactions to accidental intravenous injections of plain local anesthetics or local anesthetic-epinephrine solutions may often be misinterpreted as allergy.

In summary, local anesthetics are extremely useful drugs in clinical practice. When applied to peripheral nerves, these anesthetics produce reversible voltage-, frequency-, and state-dependent inhibition of Na channels. These actions can be exploited to produce the many forms of regional anesthesia.

LOCAL ANESTHETIC STRUCTURES

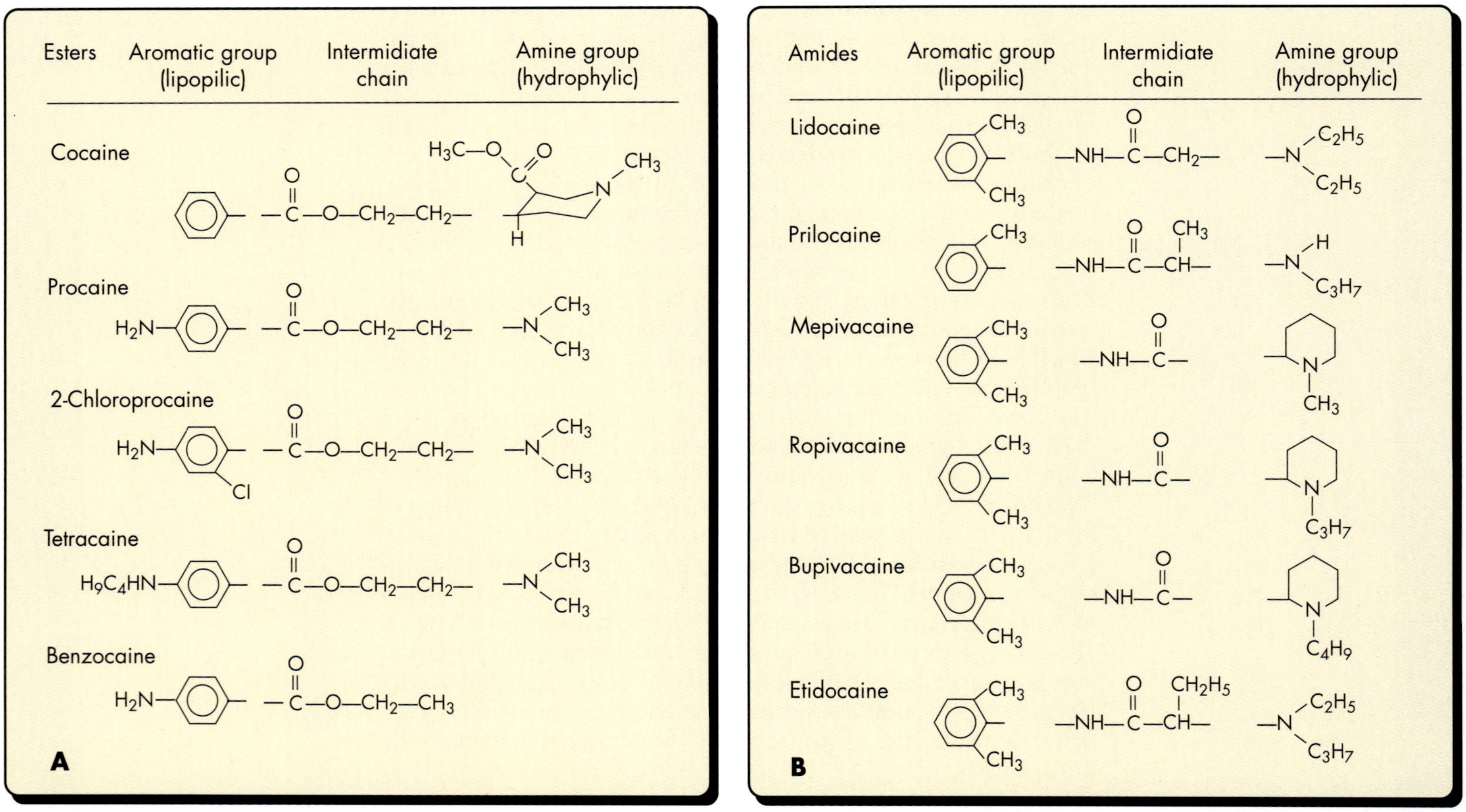

Figure 16-1. Local anesthetic structures. Clinically useful local anesthetics consist of an aromatic (benzene ring) moiety connected through either an ester (**A**) or an amide (**B**) bond to an aliphatic (hydrocarbon) chain and, with one exception, all contain a tertiary amine nitrogen. Benzocaine, an agent used primarily for topical anesthesia, is the only local anesthetic used clinically lacking a tertiary amine group. The aromatic region of the molecule contributes to the high degree of lipid solubility of local anesthetics. The tertiary amine nitrogen can exist (at physiologic pH) as either the free base or, after binding a proton, as a positively charged form. Increasing pH favors free-base local anesthetic forms over positively charged forms. The free-base forms are considerably more membrane-permeable than are the positively charged forms. Local anesthetics connected through an ester bond are metabolized in blood by nonspecific esterases; local anesthetics connected through an amide bond are metabolized in the liver by mixed-function oxidases.

BIOCHEMISTRY OF SODIUM CHANNELS

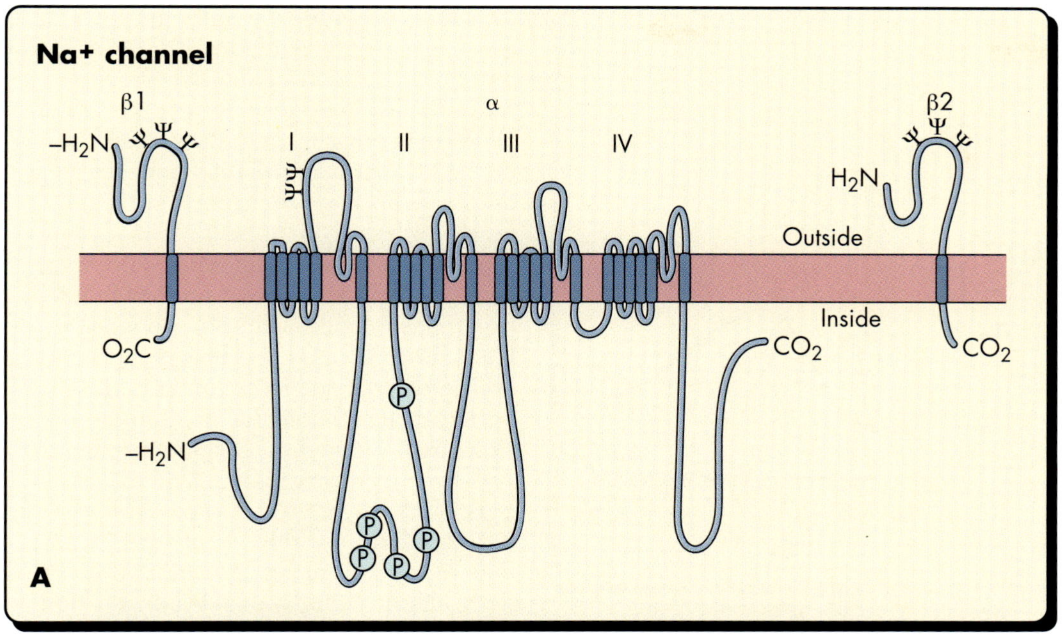

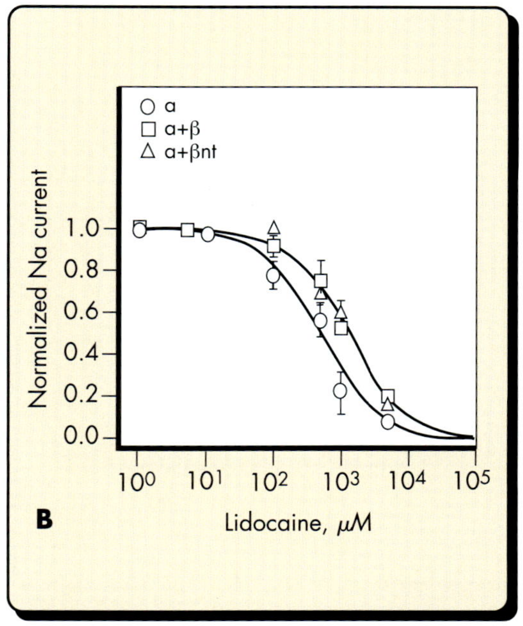

Figure 16-2. A, Structure of the sodium (Na) channel. Na channels are heavily glycosylated integral membrane proteins containing up to three subunits. Na channels from mammalian neurons contain one larger (α) subunit of roughly 260 kD molecular weight with four membrane-spanning domains (*I, II, III,* and *IV*). Mammalian Na channels contain varying numbers of secondary (β) subunits. Channels from rat brain contain one (β1) subunit of approximately 36 kD and another smaller (β2) subunit of approximately 33 kD. β2 subunits are bonded to the α subunit through disulfide links, and β1 subunits are noncovalently associated with the α subunit. All three subunits are heavily glycosylated (as is typical for integral membrane proteins). Na channel α subunits have been cloned for the electric organ from the electric eel, rat brain (where there are three distinct subtypes), skeletal muscle, and heart. These various forms of Na channels demonstrate great homology in segments S1 through S6 (located in all four membrane-spanning domains). The two β subunits in rat brain Na channels have also been cloned. Both the β1 and β2 subunits have relatively small cytoplasmic domains, a single membrane-spanning segment, and large extracellular domains [1].

In this figure, the sites of potential glycosylation are indicated by ψ and those of phosphorylation by *P*. Cylinders denote regions assumed to be in α-helical formation, although the actual three-dimensional structure of the Na channel, particularly that of the ion-conducting pore, remains controversial. In addition, the pore itself may not be lined by α-helices and β-strands, as is commonly assumed [2].

B, Ionic conduction and selectivity and drug binding appear to be primarily functions of the α subunits. The β subunits influence peak current, activation, and inactivation; however, the relative importance of the subunits for physiology and pharmacology depends on the tissue of origin. Isolated alpha subunits from mammalian brain and skeletal muscle have slower decay of Na currents than do native (complete) Na channels. Cardiac Na channel α subunits produce Na currents resembling those from native (complete) channels. On the contrary, β1 subunits, even when missing the cytoplasmic "tail" of the subunit (βnt), inhibit lidocaine block of Na current with cardiac α subunits, as shown in this figure [3]. (*Part A from* Catterall [1]; *Part B from* Makielski [3].)

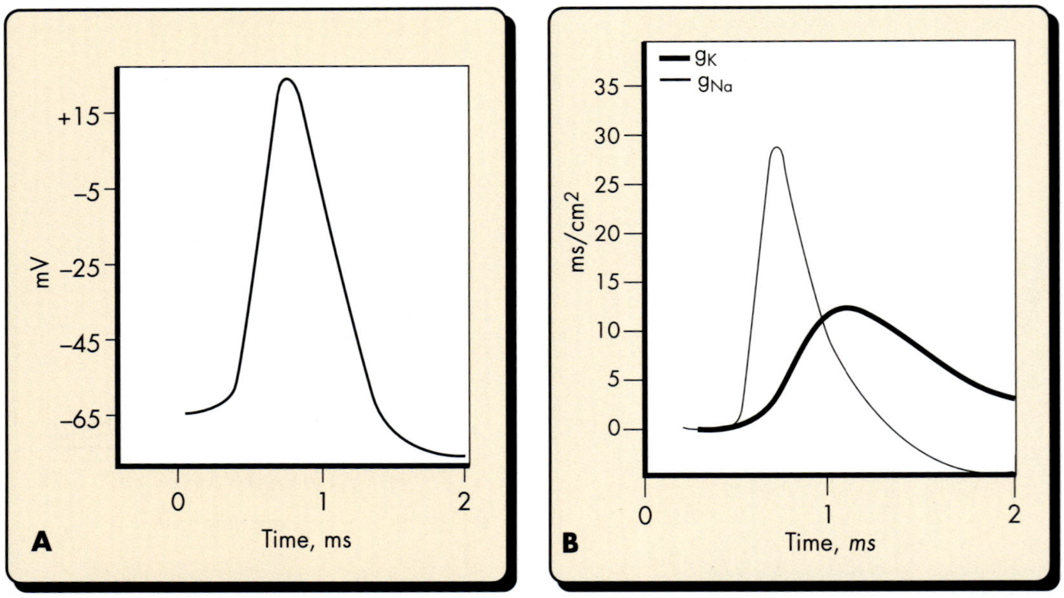

Figure 16-3. Healthy cells exist in a state of ionic disequilibrium, having excesses of sodium (Na) and chlorine (Cl) ions externally and potassium (K) and magnesium (Mg) ions in the cytoplasm. The ionic disequilibrium between Na and K arises from Na–K adenosine triphosphatase, an energy-consuming integral membrane protein that moves three Na ions out of the cell for every two K ions moved into the cell, and a small "leak" current of K ions exiting the cytoplasm driven by the concentration gradient. In neurons, action potentials result when a stimulus or an invading wave of depolarization causes Na channels to "open" briefly, allowing Na ions to enter the cytoplasm driven by their concentration gradient. In myelinated nerve, Na channels are found nearly exclusively in nodes of Ranvier and, rarely, in internodal membrane, permitting waves of depolarization to proceed in jumps from node to node (saltatory conduction). Here, the time course of changes in membrane potential and ionic conductances during an action potential in a squid giant axon are illustrated. **A**, Membrane potential rises from its resting value of -65 mV to a peak of 15 mV or greater, then returns to the resting value, all within about 1 ms. **B**, The time course of changes in membrane potential is almost perfectly matched by the time course of changes in Na conductance (g_{Na}). A late increase in K conductance (g_K) contributes to (but is not essential for) repolarization of the membrane. (*From* Butterworth and Strichartz [4].)

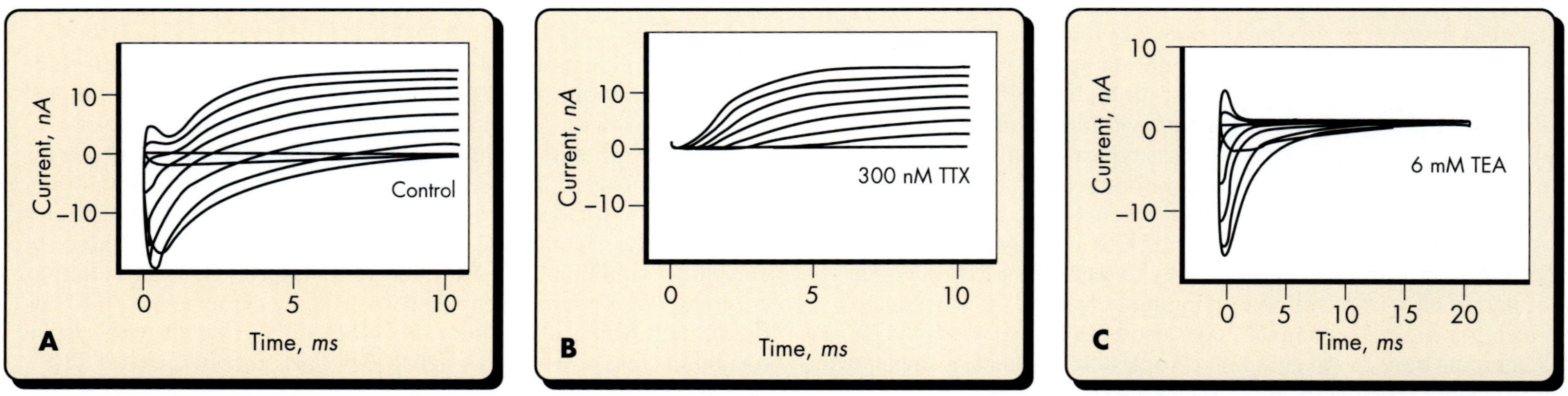

Figure 16-4. Sodium (Na) and potassium (K) channels can be selectively inhibited. Under control conditions (**A**), a node of Ranvier under a voltage clamp exhibits an early inward current and a later outward current from activation of Na and K channels, respectively. **B**, In the presence of the highly selective Na channel inhibitor tetrodotoxin (*TTX*), only the later outward current from K channels remains. **C**, Con-versely, in the presence of tetraethylammonium (*TEA*) ions, the later outward current from K channels is selectively inhibiting, leaving the transient inward current (Na) still present (*From* Hille [5].)

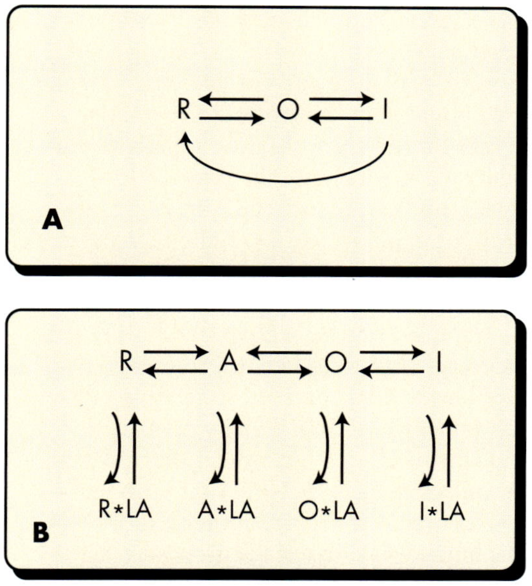

Figure 16-5. Proposed models for sodium (Na) channel behavior in the presence and absence of local anesthetics. Since the time of Hodgkin and Huxley, neuronal Na channels have been recognized to exist in at least three forms: resting (*R*), open (*O*), and inactivated (*I*). In addition, the relative likelihood that a channel will be in any one of these conformations is determined by the current value and recent history of the membrane potential, as shown in the simplified scheme **A**, The resting and inactivated forms are relatively stable, *ie*, at resting membrane potential, most Na channels will remain in the resting conformation. Similarly, with a maintained depolarization, most channels will assume the inactivated conformation. Inactivated Na channels can neither conduct Na ions nor "open" again in response to a depolarization without first returning to the resting information. This latter characteristic distinguishes inactivated channels from other conformations in which Na ionic currents are not conducted. The open (ion-conducting) form of the channel is present only early on during an induced (voltage clamp) depolarization, but will rapidly shift into the inactivated form during depolarization. Other Na conformations may (and likely do) exist.

B, Because the process by which a resting channel is reconfigured into an open channel is called *activation*, many investigators believe that an *activated* (but not yet open and no longer closed) form of a channel must be present to account for the actions of local anesthetics. Here, local anesthetics (*LA*) may bind to any of four native Na channel conformations, yielding four additional nonconducting channel conformations. The modulated receptor hypothesis, proposed by Bertil Hille (described in detail in reference 5), tries to account for voltage- and frequency-dependent actions of local anesthetics. It assumes that different Na channel conformations have differing affinities for local anesthetics. Thus, use-dependent block must result from increased local anesthetic affinity for some conformation of the Na channel, which is more often present during repeated depolarizations than during infrequent ones. Investigators have argued whether the conformation with greatest affinity for local anesthetics during frequent depolarizations is an open or an inactivated one. It appears that the correct answer may depend on whether cardiac or neuronal tissue is being studied. For both neuronal and muscular Na channels the data are conclusive that resting conformations have relatively low affinity for local anesthetics.

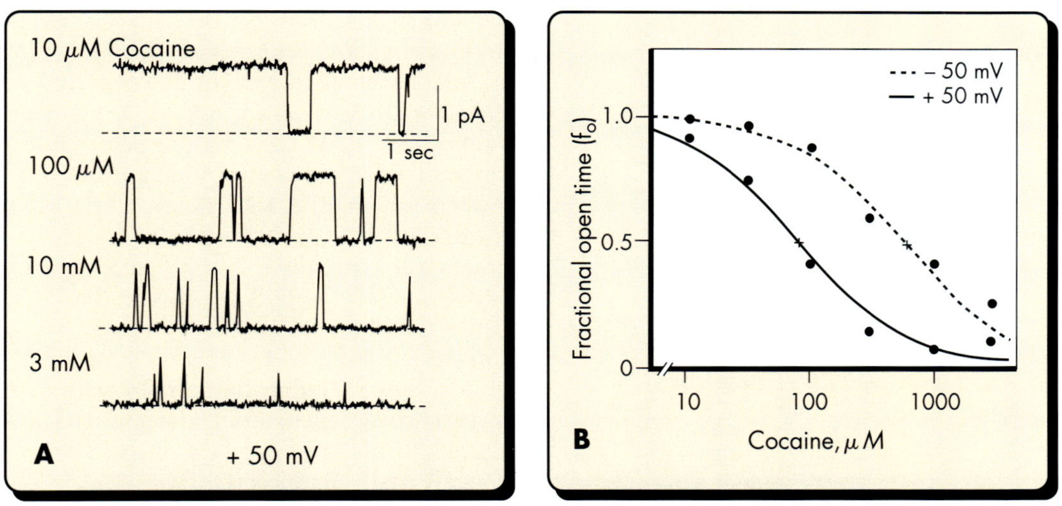

Figure 16-6. Voltage- and concentration-dependence of cocaine binding to individual mammalian sodium (Na) channels. Single Na channels from rabbit skeletal muscle were partially purified using centrifugation and incorporated into planar lipid bilayers (synthetic membrane analogues). Batrachotoxin (which causes Na channels to stay "open" nearly always when membrane potentials are 50 mV or greater) has been applied. Because local anesthetics and batrachotoxin bind to different sites on Na channels, batrachotoxin-activated channels represent a useful system in which to study interactions between local anesthetics and the open state of the Na channel. **A**, Increasing concentrations of cocaine cause progressive reduction in the time during which the ion channels stay open. With 10 μM cocaine, the channel stays open most of the time and only infrequently ceases to conduct current (indicated by the downward square-wave forms). With 3 mM cocaine, the channel is only rarely open and conducting current (here indicated as roughly 1 picoampere (pA) upward deflections from the line indicating zero current). **B**, A more depolarized membrane potential increases binding of cocaine and reduces the amount of time during which the batrachotoxin-activated ion channel is open and conducting Na ions. (*From* Wang [6].)

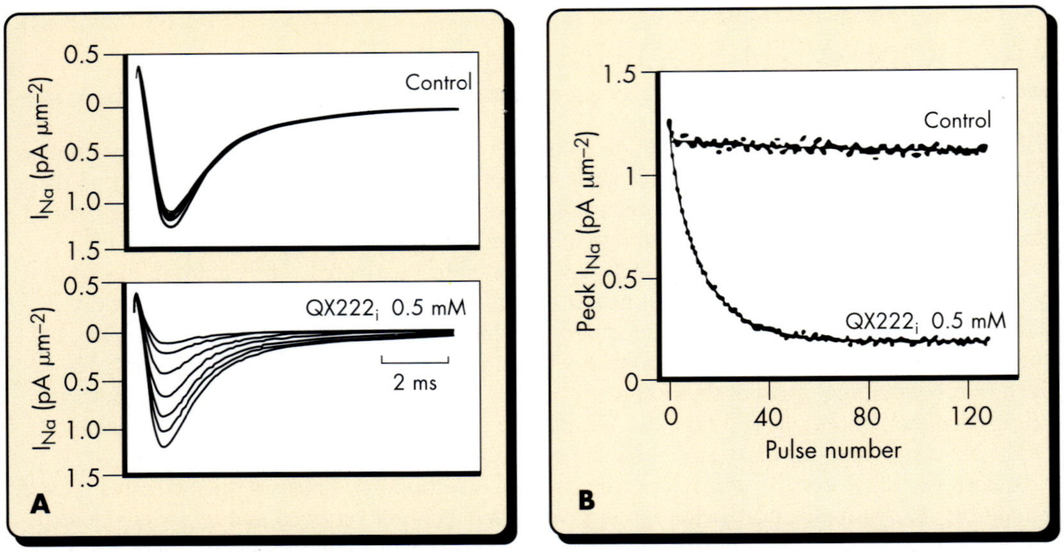

Figure 16-7. Membrane potential, frequency of depolarization, and sodium (Na) channel conformation are closely related. Na channels "open" (briefly) at depolarizing membrane potentials, but almost never open at resting membrane potential. Local anesthetics bind open and "inactivated" channels more quickly than do resting channels. When membranes depolarize frequently, Na channels spend much more time in open and inactivated conformations than they do when the membrane is depolarized less frequently, favoring binding of local anesthetics. **A**, under control conditions, canine cardiac Purkinje fibers were subjected to voltage clamp. Membrane potential was held constant at -150 mV, then depolarized to a constant 0 mV for 10 ms. Under control conditions, the brief depolarizations open Na channels and elicit inward (*downward in the figure*) current, which rapidly inactivates the channels (the current decreases despite continued depolarization). The overlapping traces on the control figure represent currents recorded during depolarizations 1, 2, 4, 8, 16, 32, 64, and 128 in a 130-pulse train of depolarizations. Note that the peak Na current was nearly the same during every depolarization. After intracellular exposure to the lidocaine derivative *QX222*, repetitive depolarizing stimuli elicit progressively smaller inward currents, indicative of use-dependent block. **B**, The peak inward current measured after the indicated number of pulses is plotted. Note that with an increasing number of depolarizations, the decline in Na current progresses to a minimum value, greater than zero current. (*From* Hanck and coworkers [7].)

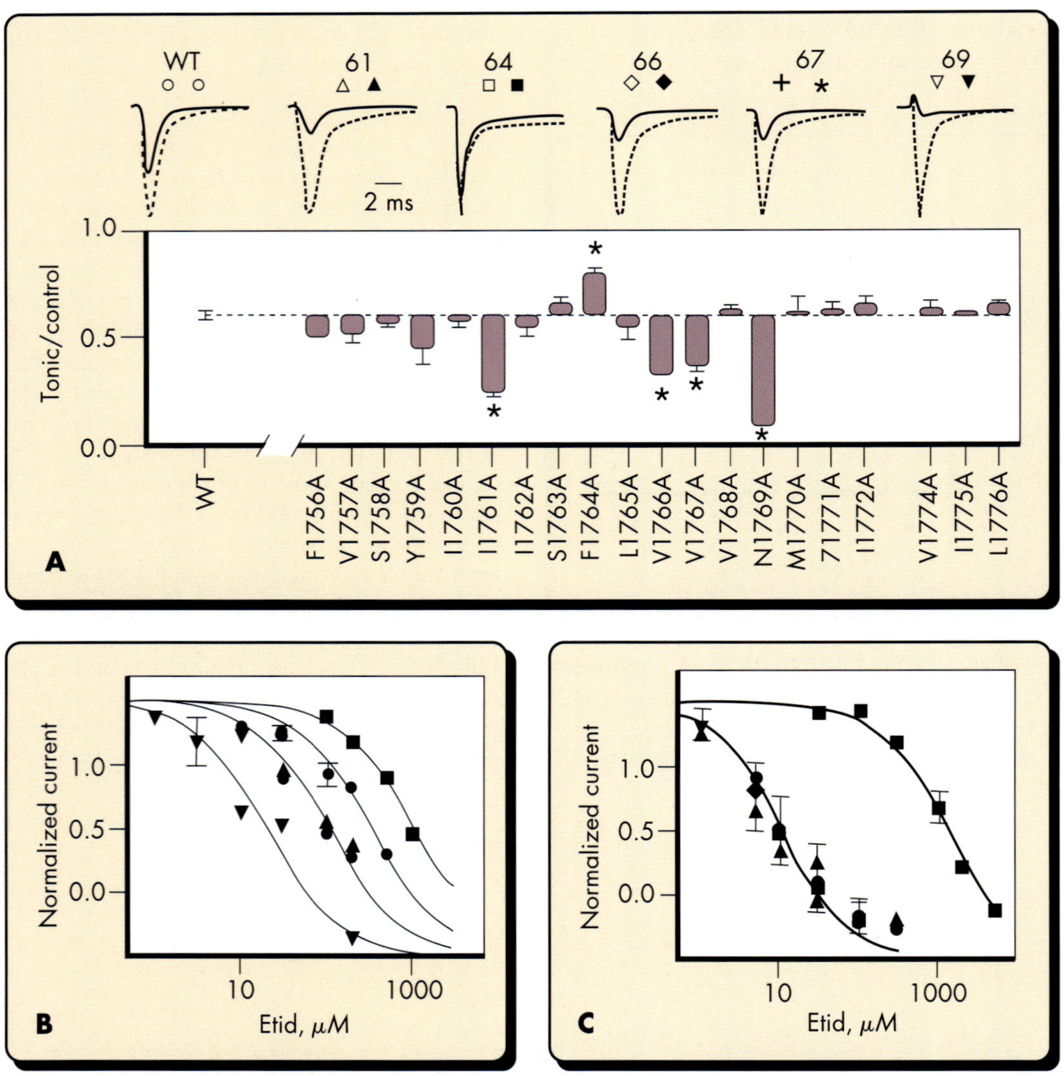

Figure 16-8. Local anesthetic binding to sodium (Na) channel subunits. Ragsdale *et al.* [8] selectively mutated the amino acid sequence of (transmembrane segment S6 of domain IV) rat brain Na channel α subunits to determine the locations at which local anesthetics bind. At each of 21 consecutive sites, alanine was substituted for the native amino acid. **A**, As indicated, some of these mutants were more susceptible to tonic ("open" channel) block by etidocaine (*Etid*), 200 μM (*eg*, N1769A), whereas others were considerably less susceptible to etidocaine (*eg*, F1764A), than was the native wild-type (*WT*) channel whose Na current was reduced roughly 60% by etidocaine, 200 μM. Interestingly, there was also divergence as to whether a given mutation altered the block of open channels (**B**) or of "inactivated" channels (**C**).

(*Continued on next page*)

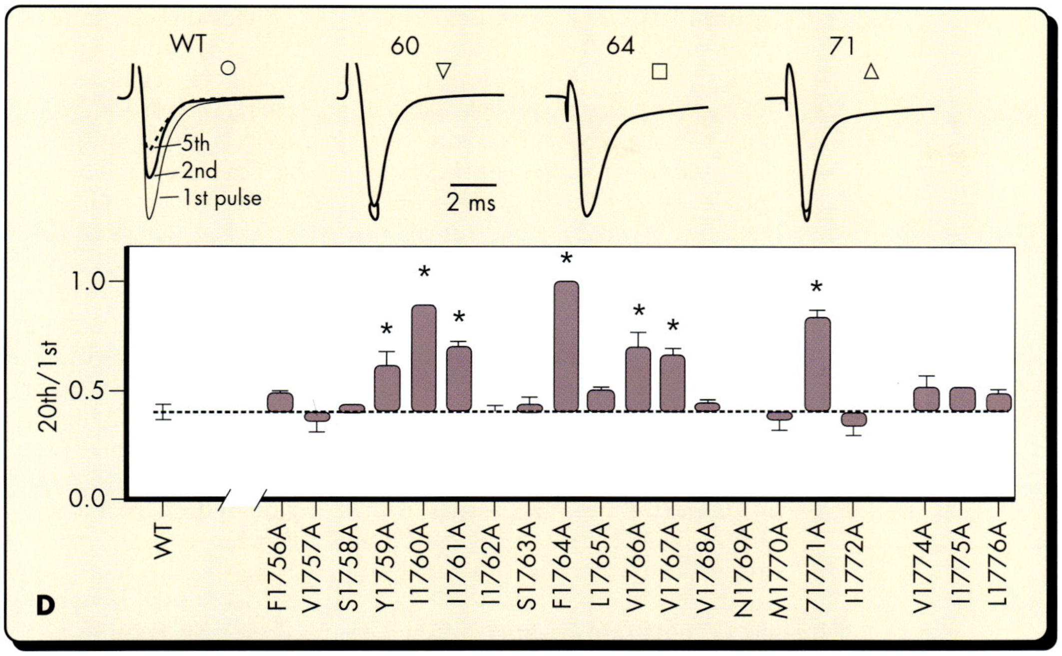

Figure 16-8. (*Continued*) Note that mutant F1764A was particularly resistant to block of inactivated channels. Some of these mutations also reduced use-dependent block (**D**). Note that the WT channels showed typical use-dependent block—the inward Na current (*downward deflection in the figure*) declined as the number of pulses increased from 1 to 20. On the contrary, three of the mutants demonstrated almost no use-dependent block at all. These results led Ragsdale *et al.* to conclude that the local anesthetic binding site was related to amino acids F1764 and Y1771, and that substitution of alanine for these two relatively hydrophobic amino acids destabilizes local anesthetic binding by reducing hydrophobicity. Other mutations that increased tonic block without increasing the affinity for the inactivated state may have altered drug affinity by altering protein conformation in such a way that the inactivated site was mimicked. (*From* Ragsdale and coworkers [8].)

INFLUENCE OF NERVE FIBERS ON NERVE BLOCK

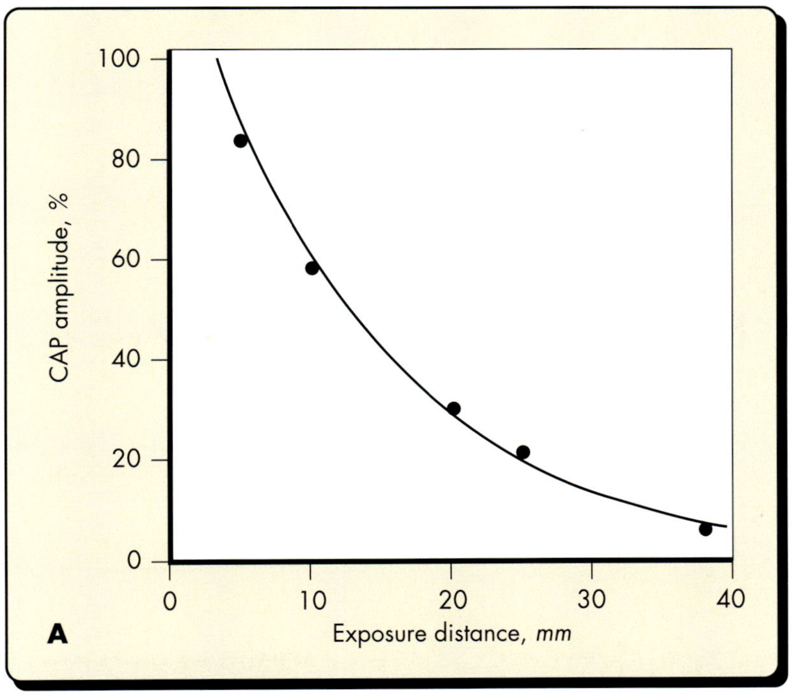

Figure 16-9. The length of nerve exposed to local anesthetics modulates block. Local anesthetics block impulses in nerves by decreasing sodium (Na) currents to levels inadequate to depolarize adjacent plasma membranes. Thus, complete block of Na current is not a necessary condition to block impulse conduction. Raymond [9] quantitatively assessed the relationship between length of drug exposure and drug concentration in producing block of compound action potentials in nerves and of action potentials in single axons. **A**, As the length of a whole bullfrog sciatic nerve exposed to lidocaine 0.8 mM, increased from 6 to 38 mm, inhibition of the action potential amplitude increased from less than 20% to over 90% [9].

(*Continued on next page*)

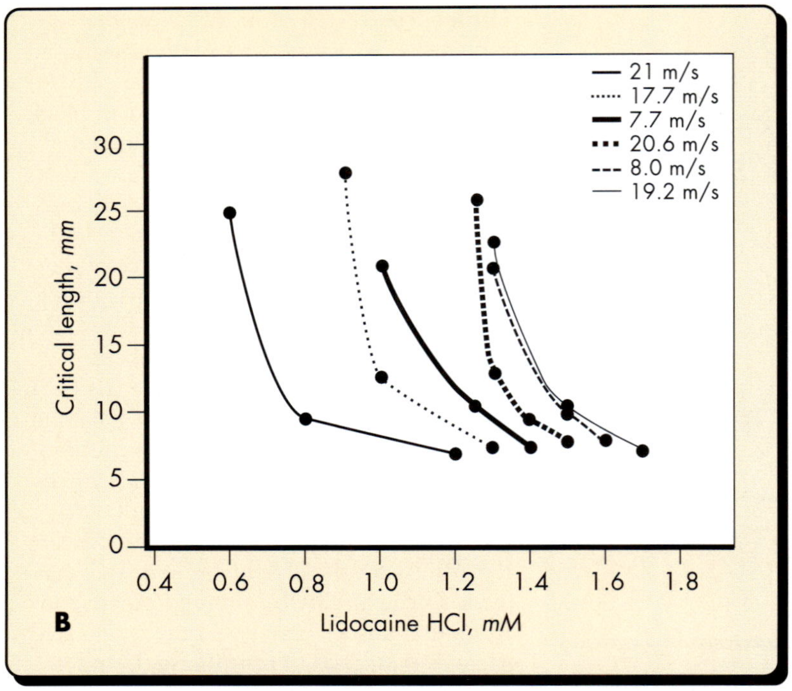

Figure 16-9. (*Continued*) B, Similarly, the drug concentration at which 50% of impulses failed to conduct through an individual axon diminished as the length of nerve exposed to drug increased, and as the length of nerve exposed to drug approached a certain minimal value, the drug concentration required increased dramatically [10]. Note also that no apparent relationship exists between the fiber conduction velocity (given in the figure) and the susceptibility to block by lidocaine. Because fiber size directly correlates with conduction velocity, these data contradict the size principle, which is discussed in a subsequent section on differential nerve block. These results confirm that at any given concentration of lidocaine, there is a direct relationship between the length of nerve exposed to the drug and the likelihood that the nerve fiber will be inhibited. At long exposure lengths the drug concentration appears to approach an asymptotic minimal concentration. These results contradict the common assumption that beyond three nodes of Ranvier the length of drug exposure is not a factor; indeed these data suggest that the region of decremental conduction could exceed 20 nodes of Ranvier. Differences in length of drug exposure (*eg*, with intravenous regional anesthesia, where large expanses of nerve are likely to be exposed to drug vs peripheral nerve block) could explain differences in effective drug concentrations. Moreover, differential nerve block might be produced by restricting the exposure length of a mixed nerve to local anesthetic (if two nerve fiber populations had a differing length-related susceptibility to local anesthtic inhibition. HCl—hydrochloric acid. (*From* Raymond and coworkers [9].)

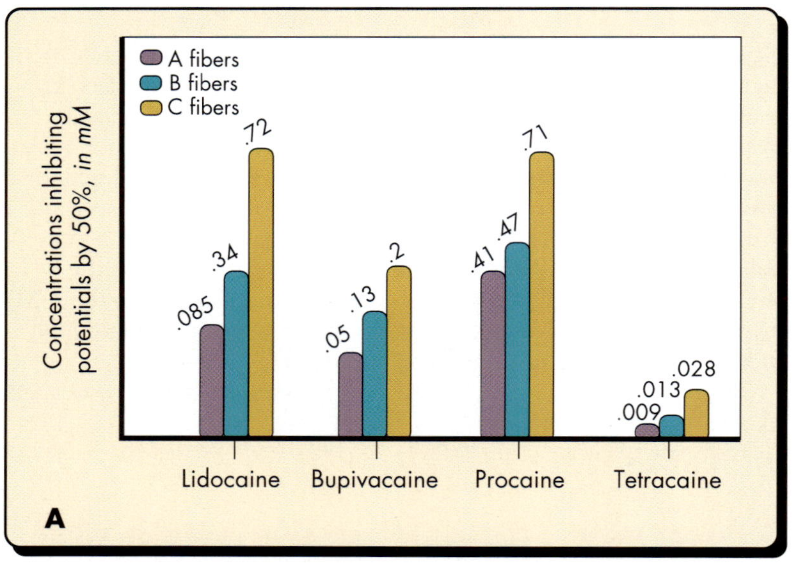

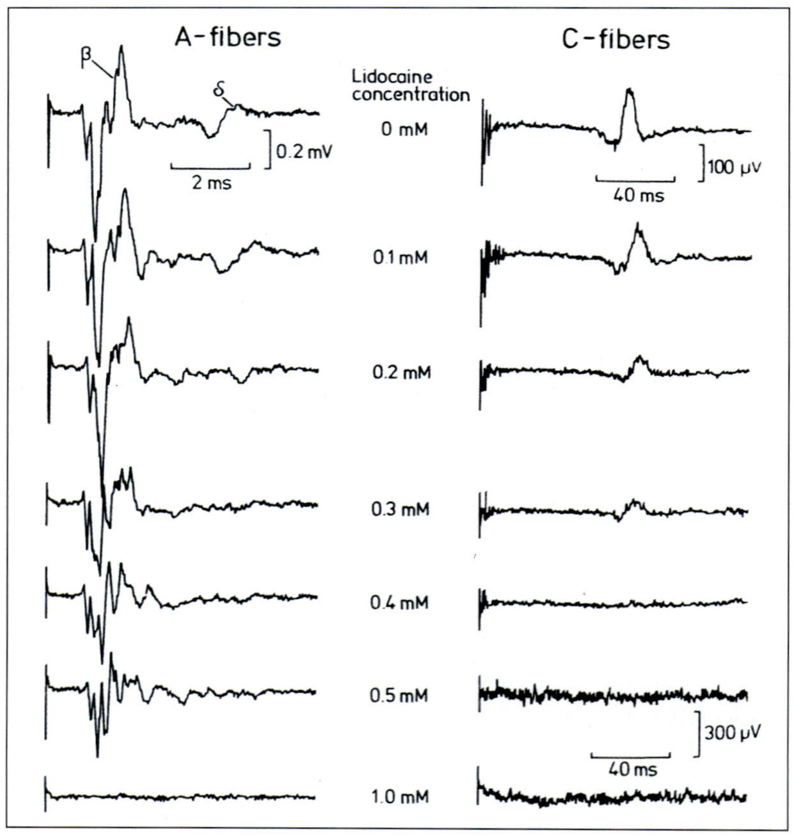

Figure 16-10. Differential inhibition of nerve fiber types. Clinicians have long searched for local anesthetics that would inhibit pain sensation without altering other sensory modalities or motor function. The traditional teaching has been that smaller-diameter nerve fibers of a given class are more susceptible to block than are larger fibers; however, recent studies have not fully supported this principle. Generally speaking, the larger Aα fibers are less susceptible to local anesthetics than are the smaller Aδ or Aγ fibers. The comparative susceptibility of A and C fibers is less easily characterized (*see* Fig. 16-9).

A, Currently available local anesthetics goals only partially produce differential block. In a series of in vitro studies, Gissen et al. [10,11] demonstrated that, in a wide variety of local anesthetics, unmyelinated C fibers were more resistant to block than were B fibers, which in turn were more resistant to block than were A fibers. Thus, unmyelinated fibers are less susceptible to block than are certain larger myelinated fibers. (Note that the bars are not drawn to a consistent scale.)

B, On the contrary, when studied *in vitro*, unmyelinated C fibers (*right*) appear to be more resistant to block by local anesthetic than do smaller Aδ (*left*) myelinated fibers. In recordings from the sural nerve in anesthetized cats, note that signals from small myelinated fibers (Aδ) were lost before any other after application of lidocaine, and that the unmyelinated C fibers were inhibited at lower concentrations than were Aβ fibers [12]. In summary, smaller myelinated (Aδ and Aγ) fibers are more sensitive to local anesthesia than are any other class of nerve fibers. Large Aα fibers appear to be least sensitive, and C fibers and other classes appear to have intermediate susceptibility to block. (*Part B from* Courtney and Strichartz [12].)

FACTORS INFLUENCING LOCAL ANESTHETIC POTENCY

OCTANOL/BUFFER PARTITION COEFFICIENTS				
Drug	25 °C		36 °C	
	P^{+*}	P^{0*}	P^{+*}	P^{0*}
Ester-linked				
Procaine	0.002±0.001	81±6	0.004±0.01	100±10
2-Chloroprocaine	0.026±0.006	720±63	0.042±0.010	810±58
Tetracaine	0.46±0.03	3615±294	0.79±0.05	5822±325
Benzocaine	NA	81	NA	132
Amide-linked				
Procainamide	0.0021±0.0005	7.3±0.1		
Mepivacaine	0.09±0.01	90±11	0.15±0.05	130±15
Ropivacaine	0.46±0.03	775±53	ND	ND
Bupivacaine	1.5±0.03	2565±218	2.0±0.05	3420±263
Lidocaine	0.060±0.005	304±23	0.085±0.01	366±31
Prilocaine	0.30±0.02	129±11	ND	ND
Etidocaine	0.48±0.03	4900±386	0.81±0.05	7317±523

* Partition coefficients expressed as relative concentrations (mol/L) in octanol and buffer.

Figure 16-11. Octanol/buffer partition coefficients (PD) measured at 25°C and 36°C (and pH 7.4) for common local anesthetics. More highly lipid-soluble local anesthetics tend to be more potent at nerve block, to have a longer duration of action, to be more highly protein-bound, to be more potent at producing toxic side effects in the heart and brain, and to have a longer onset time. The lipid solubility of these agents was determined by comparing the relative concentrations of agents distributing between sodium chloride solution (150 mM NaCl, 5 mM 2-(N-morpholino) ethanesulfonic acid, 5 mM morpholino-propane sulfonic acid, 5 mM [3-cyclohexylamino]-propane sulfonic acid), or octanol. The relative concentrations (in mol/L) as distributed between octanol and the buffer for positively charged forms of the local anesthetics are denoted by P^+; the relative concentration of the neutral (uncharged) forms of the local anesthetics is denoted by P^0. Note the relatively high PD for the protonated forms of tetracaine, bupivacaine, and etidocaine; thus, it would be expected that the charged forms of these local anesthetics would be more membrane-permeable than would other charged local anesthetics. The neutral forms of these same three potent local anesthetics have extremely high PDs. The underlying reason that local anesthetic potency increases with increasing lipophilicity is unclear but could result from the increased access to the local anesthetic binding site (increased lipid solubility could favor permeation through diffusion barriers or favor accumulation of drug within the plasma membrane) or increased affinity for that binding site. (From Strichartz and coworkers [13].) NA—not applicable; ND—not determined.

IONIZATION CONSTANTS OF LOCAL ANESTHETICS FROM SPECTROPHOTOMETRIC METHOD*				
	25 °C		36 °C	
Drug	pK	Samples, *n*	pK	Samples, *n*
Ester-linked				
Procaine	9.06±0.10	3	8.89±0.08	3
2-Chloroprocaine	9.30±0.08	3	9.06±0.05	3
Tetracaine	8.59±0.04	3	8.38±0.03	3
Amide-linked				
Mepivacaine	7.92±0.03	3	7.72±0.06	3
Ropivacaine	8.16±0.02	3		ND
Bupivacaine	8.21±0.04	3	8.10±0.02	3
Lidocaine	8.19±0.03	12	7.77±0.04	8
Prilocaine	8.02±0.05	3		ND
Etidocaine	8.11±0.02	3	7.87±0.03	3

* Determined in 150 mEq/L NaCl, 5 mM 2-(N-morpholino)ethanesulfonic acid, 5 mM morpholino-propane sulfonic acid, 5 mM (3-cyclohexlamino)-propane sulfonic acid.

Figure 16-12. Ionization constants of local anesthetics measured by the spectrophotometric method at 25°C and 36°C. Many authors have linked local anesthetics with lower pK_a values with faster speeds of onset of local anesthesia. Nevertheless, it is notable that of the two local anesthetics of fastest onset during clinical anesthesia (etidocaine and 2-chloroprocaine), 2-chloroprocaine has the highest and etidocaine the lowest pK_a value of the agents in common clinical use. Moreover, of the esters, tetracaine has the lowest pK_a value, yet it usually is regarded as having the slowest onset of all local anesthetics connected with an ester bond. Thus, local anesthetic permeation of tissue barriers, nonspecific binding, and concentration may be more predictive of the rate of onset than is the pK_a value. ND—not determined. (*Adapted from* Strichartz and coworkers [13].)

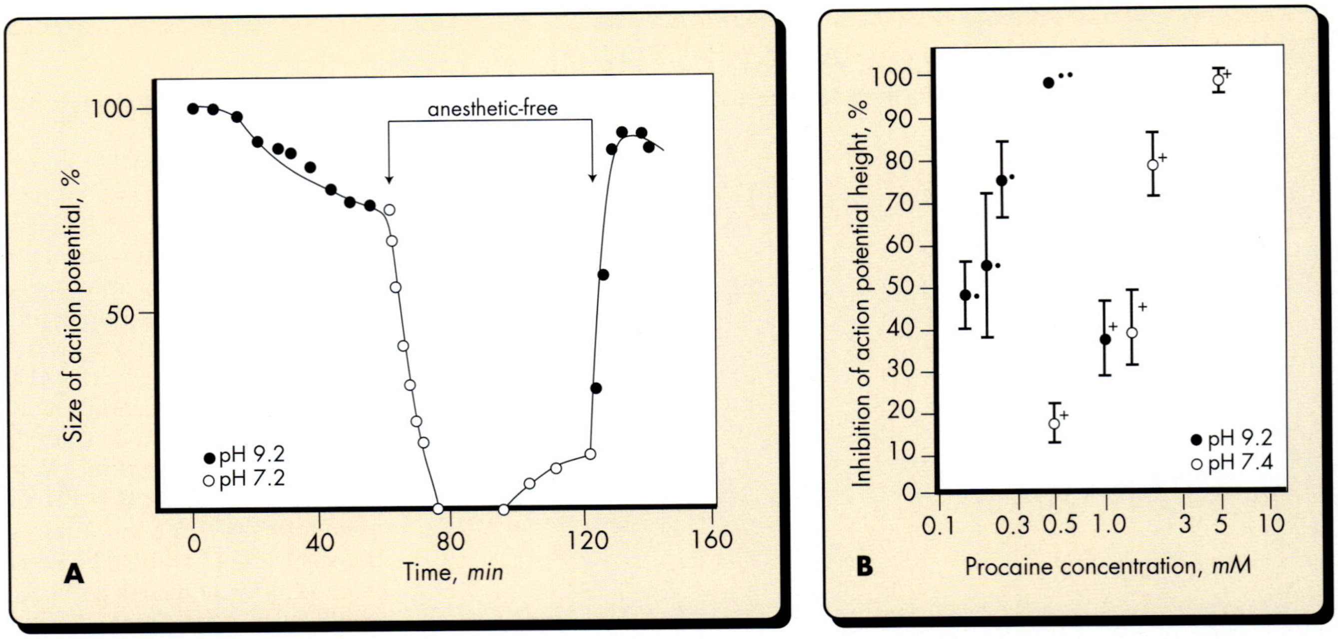

Figure 16-13. The interaction between pH and the tonic block by local anesthetics is complex. Clinicians often add $NaHCO_3$ to local anesthetic solutions in the hope of speeding the onset of anesthesia. Conversely, acidification of the solution bathing an isolated nerve that already has bound local anesthetics will increase the apparent potency of the local anesthetic at producing both tonic and use-dependent blocks. **A**, Action potentials were recorded in C fibers from rabbit vagus nerve after equilibration with dibucaine, 5 μM, at pH 9.2 (*solid circles*). Note the progressive decline in the amplitude of the compound action potential. When the nerve was washed with *anesthetic-free* solution at pH 7.2 (*open circles*) note that the inhibition *intensified*, presumably from hydrogen ions protonating dibucaine molecules already bound (or very near) to Na channels, intensifying their effectiveness. Finally, note that the extent of inhibition *declined* when dibucaine, 5 μM, at pH 9.2 was again applied to the nerve [14]. **B**, In a phenomenon more familiar to clinical anesthetists [15], the apparent potency of procaine at inhibiting action potentials in frog sciatic nerve fibers was increased roughly 10-fold at pH 9.2 over that at pH 7.4, which is consistent with increased membrane loading of the more lipid soluble neutral procaine species at pH 9.2. Such dramatic increases in potency generally cannot be achieved in clinical practice (through addition of $NaHCO_3$ to standard local anesthetic solutions) owing both to limitations of solubility and to the relatively high pH of the plain local anesthetic solutions. Clinical solutions of local anesthetics prepackaged with epinephrine generally are more acidic (to increase the shelf life of the epinephrine) than are the epinephrine-free solutions. Substantially greater increases in pH and commensurate decreases in onset time can be obtained with solutions prepackaged with epinephrine through addition of $NaHCO_3$. (*Part A from* Ritchie and coworkers [14]; *part B from* Butterworth and coworkers [15].)

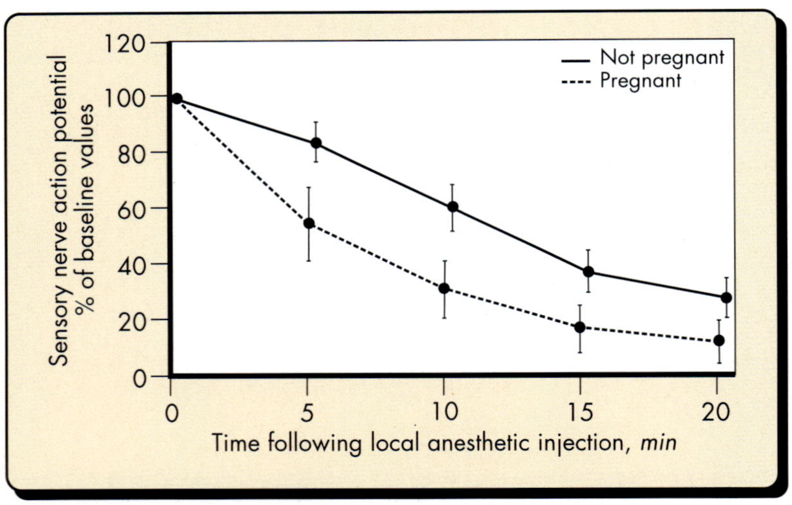

Figure 16-14. Pregnancy increases the susceptibility of nerves to local anesthetic block. For years clinicians have reduced the volume of local anesthetic given to pregnant women undergoing epidural or spinal anesthesia based on the clinical belief that a more extensive block was obtained with a given volume of local anesthetic solution in women who are pregnant than in women who are not pregnant. A series of studies by Datta *et al.* [16] suggested that nerve fibers (from the vagus nerve) of pregnant rabbits were more susceptible to local anesthetics than were similar fibers from rabbits that were not pregnant. In this figure, median nerve block using 1% lidocaine, 5 mL, was compared in pregnant and nonpregnant female volunteers. Inhibition of sensory nerve action potentials was significantly greater in pregnant than in nonpregnant volunteers, confirming that human peripheral nerve is more susceptible to block by local anesthetics during pregnancy (*From* Butterworth and coworkers [17].)

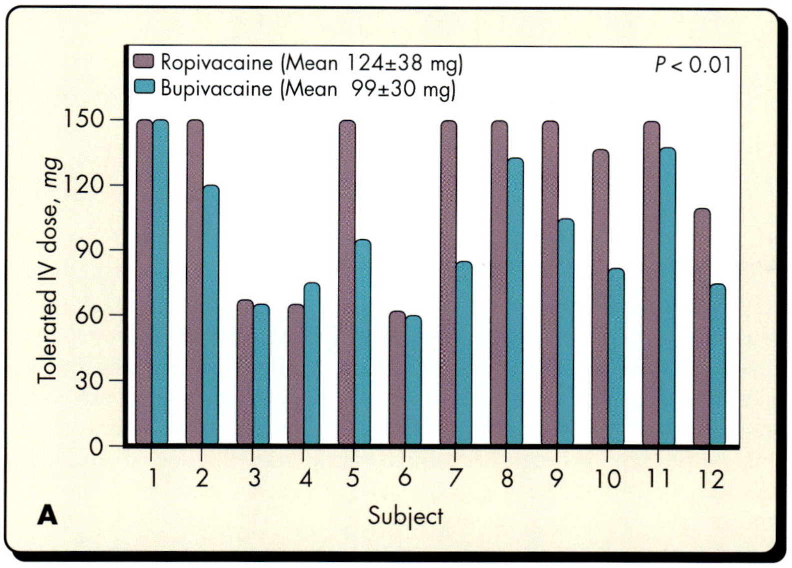

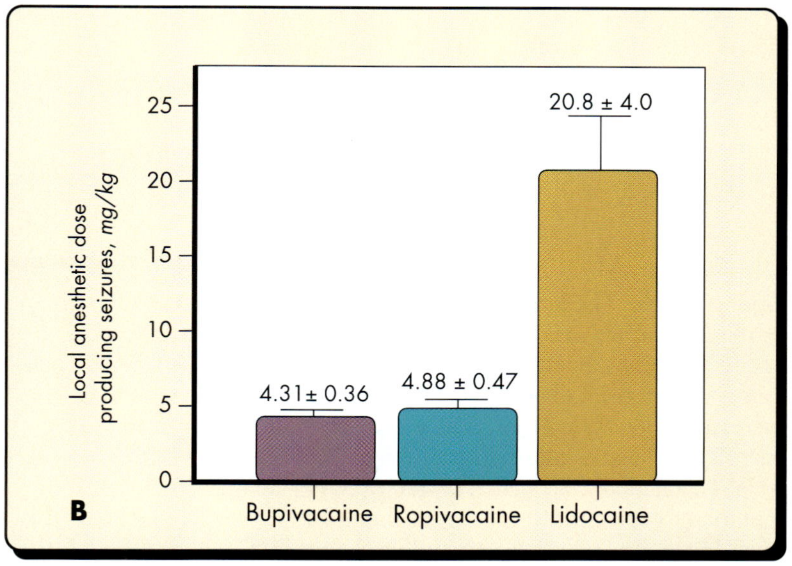

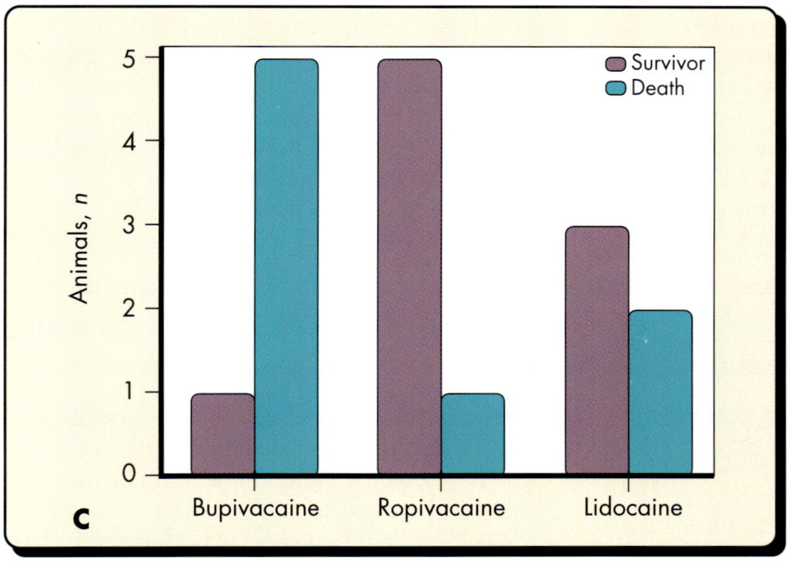

Figure 16-15. The potency of local anesthetics at producing central nervous system (CNS) toxic effects is consistent with their potency at inhibiting conduction in peripheral nerves. **A**, Scott *et al.* [18] infused various local anesthetics in 12 human volunteers until they reported symptoms of local anesthetic intoxication. Note that the more potent local anesthetic (in terms of peripheral nerve block) bupivacaine produced CNS toxic effects at a lower total dose and a lower blood concentration than ropivacaine.

The more potent longer-lasting local anesthetics such as bupivacaine and etidocaine have been associated with cardiovascular depression from which resuscitation can be difficult. The mechanisms underlying differences in cardiac toxicity between bupivacaine and etidocaine and the other local anesthetics are not clear, although a variety of electrophysiologic and biochemical differences have been cataloged. When local anesthetic infusions were administered to awake dogs, it was noted that local anesthetic potency at producing peripheral nerve block predicted the agents that would produce generalized seizures and cardiovascular collapse at the lowest doses.
B, Feldman *et al.* [19] compared the doses producing seizures of three local anesthetics. The most potent agent was bupivacaine. One day later, these same animals were given a bolus injection of twice the convulsive dose of bupivacaine, ropivacaine, or lidocaine, respectively, and received standard resuscitation measures and drugs.
C, Despite resuscitation, nearly every animal receiving twice the convulsive dose of bupivacaine died, whereas nearly every animal receiving twice the convulsive dose of ropivacaine survived. (*Data from* Feldman and coworkers [19].)

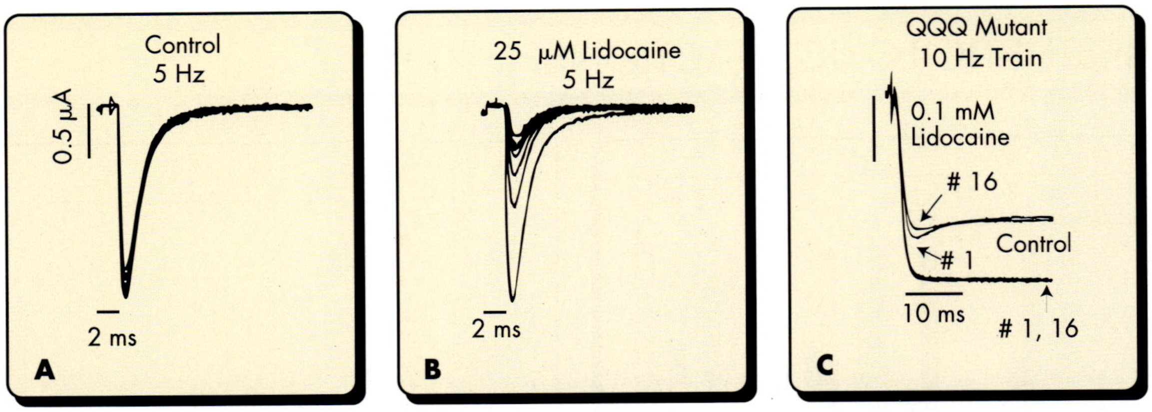

Figure 16-16. The local anesthetic receptor in cardiac sodium (Na) channels. Cardiac action potentials are much longer than are nerve action potentials owing to the slow inward calcium (Ca) current. These longer durations of exposure to depolarizing membrane potentials increase the likelihood that local anesthetics will encounter an "inactivated" Na channel rather than an "open" Na channel, relative to neuronal Na channels. Bennett *et al.* removed Na channel inactivation by mutating three amino acids in the subunit III-IV interdomain [20]. This mutation caused no other measurable change in Na channel function. In this figure, the wild-type Na currents are not affected by repetitive depolarizations in the absence of local anesthetics (**A**) [20]. **B**, Exposure to lidocaine, 25 μM, during repetitive depolarizations produces marked use-dependent block, with very little tonic block (compare the limited inhibition of the first pulse with the marked reduction of current elicited by the 16th pulse). **C**, The mutated Na channels (QQQ) did not inactivate (note the long action potential in the absence of lidocaine). Even though a fourfold more concentrated solution of lidocaine was applied, very little tonic or use-dependent block was obtained. These results are consistent with the observed behavior of lidocaine on the mammalian heart, and they help to explain the observed differences between local anesthetic action on heart and nerve. In nerves, where action potentials are brief, there is little opportunity for drug binding to the inactivated state of the channel because a comparatively small fraction of all channels are inactivated during any one depolarization. Therefore, many studies have emphasized the importance of open channel block with the higher concentrations of local anesthetics that are used to inhibit Na currents in neurons. On the contrary, cardiac channels respond to relatively low concentrations of local anesthetics (*eg*, patients stop having ventricular arrhythmias at lidocaine blood concentrations that generally produce no signs of drug action on neurons). Greater susceptibility of cardiac Na channels is the result of more Na channels becoming inactivated during each depolarization (relative to the situation in neurons), and of the great affinity of local anesthetics for the inactivated form of the cardiac Na channel. (*From* Bennett and coworkers [20].)

LOCAL ANESTHETIC ALLERGY

A. RESULTS OF SKIN TESTING FOR ALLERGY TO LOCAL ANESTHETIC IN 14 OF 90 PATIENTS

Agent Causing Reaction by History	Negative Skin Tests and Challenges, *n*	
	To lidocaine	To mepivacaine
Lidocaine (7)	5	2
Procaine (5)	5	ND*
Prilocaine (1)	1	ND
Unknown (1)	1	ND

*Not done.

Figure 16-17. Allergy to local anesthetics. Most anesthesia texts state that allergy to local anesthetics containing an ester bond (especially those metabolized to p-aminobenzoate, or PABA, such as procaine and benzocaine) is more common than to local anesthetics containing an amide bond; however, limited data exist on which to form that conclusion. Although many patients believe (or are told) that they are allergic to local anesthetics, most are not. deShazo *et al.* were referred 90 patients for local anesthetic allergy [21]. In 14 patients with a medical history compatible with an immediate hypersensitivity reaction (including generalized urticaria, laryngeal edema necessitating intubation, or hypotension and shock), most had negative test results on lidocaine intradermal prick test and challenge with the undiluted drug [21] (**A**).

(*Continued on next page*)

B. COMBINED RESULTS OF SKIN TESTING FOR ALLERGY TO LOCAL ANESTHETIC			
Drug	No. of patients with negative skin tests and challenges*	No. of patients with positive skin tests†	No. of patients with positive skin tests challenged without adverse reaction‡
Lidocaine	80	2	2
Procaine	4	5	1
Mepivacaine	6	2	1
Tetracaine	0	1§	0

*No differences in results were noted between testing with agents containing paraben and those without. Challenges were performed with local anesthetics containing paraben.

†All positive tests occurred with intradermal injection of undiluted drug.

‡These were the only patients challenged, *ie*, no adverse reactions occurred. The six individuals with positive skin tests who were not challenged with the drug provoking the skin test all subsequently were challenged to lidocaine without adverse reaction.

§Two normal controls also had equally large reactions.

Figure 16-17. (*Continued*) This was even true for 5 of the 7 patients with a history of immediate hypersensitivity to lidocaine. Skin testing in 76 patients with poorly documented local anesthetic allergy found 10 apparently false-positive reactions to an undiluted 1% local anesthetic (**B**). Four of these 10 patients were challenged uneventfully with the agent to which they reacted. Indeed, in none of the 90 patients could true hypersensitivity to a local anesthetic be identified. At least one local anesthetic could be identified as safe for each of the 90 patients. In the absence of skin testing, the prudent approach would be to use a structurally unrelated agent when a patient presents with history of local anesthetic allergy. (*Part A from* deShazo and Nelson [21].) ND—not determined.

REFERENCES

1. Catterall WA: Structure and function of voltage-gated ion channels. *Ann Rev Biochem* 1995, 64:493–531.
2. Perez-Garcia MT, Chiamvimonvat N, Marban E, Tomaselli GF: Structure of the sodium channel pore revealed by serial cysteine mutagenesis. *Proc Natl Acad Sci USA* 1996, 93:300–304.
3. Makielski JC, Limberis JT, Chang SY, *et al.*: Coexpression of β 1 with cardiac sodium channel α subunits in oocytes decreases lidocaine block. *Mol Pharmacol* 1996, 49:30–39.
4. Butterworth JF IV, Strichartz GR: Molecular mechanisms of local anesthesia: a review. *Anesthesiology* 1990, 72:711–734.
5. Hille B: The selective inhibition of delayed potassium currents in nerve by tetraethylammonium ion. *J Gen Physiol* 1967, 50:1287–1302.
6. Wang GK: Cocaine-induced closures of single batrachotoxin-activated Na^+ channels in planar lipid bilayers. *J Gen Physiol* 1988, 92:747–765.
7. Hanck DA, Makielski JC, Sheets MF: Kinetic effects of quarternary lidocaine block of cardiac sodium channels: a gating current study. *J Gen Physiol* 1994, 103:19–43.
8. Ragsdale DS, McPhee JC, Scheuer T, Catterall WA: Molecular determinants of state-dependent block of Na^+ channels by local anesthetics. *Science* 1994, 265:1724–1728.
9. Raymond SA, Steffensen SC, Gugino LD, Strichartz GR: The role of length of nerve exposed to local anesthetics in impulse blocking action. *Anesth Analg* 1989, 68:563–570.
10. Gissen AJ, Covino BG, Gregus J: Differential sensitivities of mammalian nerve fibers to local anesthetic agents. *Anesthesiology* 1980, 53:467–474.
11. Wildsmith JA, Gissen AJ, Gregus J, Covino BG: Differential nerve blocking activity of amino-ester local anaesthetics. *Br J Anaesth* 1985, 57:612–620.
12. Courtney KR, Strichartz GR: Structural elements which determine local anesthetic activity. In *Local Anesthetics*. Edited by Strichartz GR. Berlin: Springer-Verlag; 1987:53–94.
13. Strichartz GR, Sanchez V, Arthur GR, *et al.*: Fundamental properties of local anesthetics. II. Measured octanol: buffer partition coefficients and pK_a values of clinically used drugs. *Anesth Analg* 1990, 71:158–170.
14. Ritchie JM, Ritchie B, Greengard P: The active structure of local anesthetics. *J Pharmacol Exp Ther* 1965, 150:152–159.
15. Butterworth JF IV, Lief PA, Strichartz GR: The pH-dependent local anesthetic activity of diethylaminoethanol, a procaine metabolite. *Anesthesiology* 1988, 68:501–506.
16. Datta S, Lambert DH, Gregus J, *et al.*: Differential sensitivities of mammalian nerve fibers during pregnancy. *Anesth Analg* 1983, 62:1070–1072.
17. Butterworth JF IV, Walker FO, Lysak SZ: Pregnancy increases median nerve susceptibility to lidocaine. *Anesthesiology* 1990, 72:962–965.
18. Scott DB, Lee A, Fagan D, *et al.*: Acute toxicity of ropivacaine compared with that of bupivacaine. *Anesth Analg* 1989, 69:563–569.
19. Feldman HS, Arthur GR, Covino BG: Comparative systemic toxicity of convulsant and supraconvulsant doses of intravenous ropivacaine, bupivacaine, and lidocaine in the conscious dog. *Anesth Analg* 1989, 69:794–801.
20. Bennett PB, Valenzuela C, Chen LQ, Kallen RG: On the molecular nature of the lidocaine receptor of cardiac Na^+ channels. Modification of block by alterations in the α-subunit III-IV interdomain. *Circ Res* 1995, 77:584–592.
21. deShazo RD, Nelson HS: An approach to the patient with a history of local anesthetic hypersensitivity: experience with 90 patients. *J Allergy Clin Immunol* 1979, 63:387–394.

INDEX

00